Biomarker: Theory and Concepts

Biomarker: Theory and Concepts

Edited by **Zach Henderson**

hayle
medical

New York

Published by Hayle Medical,
30 West, 37th Street, Suite 612,
New York, NY 10018, USA
www.haylemedical.com

Biomarker: Theory and Concepts
Edited by Zach Henderson

International Standard Book Number: 978-1-63241-055-9 (Hardback)

Printed in the United States of America.

Contents

Preface

Over the recent decade, advancements and applications have progressed exponentially. This has led to the increased interest in this field and projects are being conducted to enhance knowledge. The main objective of this book is to present some of the critical challenges and provide insights into possible solutions. This book will answer the varied questions that arise in the field and also provide an increased scope for furthering studies.

This book is a detailed and comprehensive medium helping students and researchers to understand the theory and concepts of biomarkers. Biomarkers or biological markers are used as an indicator of a person's health state or condition by scientists or medical professionals. If a biomarker can detect basic symptoms of a disease, differentiate between similar diseases, identify the stage of advancement, work on an easy-to-perform and inexpensive system of diagnosis and is easily accessible to the body; then it is considered to be the ideal biomarker.

I hope that this book, with its visionary approach, will be a valuable addition and will promote interest among readers. Each of the authors has provided their extraordinary competence in their specific fields by providing different perspectives as they come from diverse nations and regions. I thank them for their contributions.

Editor

1

Biomarkers in Gastrointestinal Cancer: Focus on Colon, Pancreatic and Gastric Cancer

Vanessa Deschoolmeester*, Filip Lardon,
Patrick Pauwels and Marc Peeters
*Center for Oncological Research (CORE) Antwerp,
Laboratory of Cancer Research and Clinical Oncology,
University of Antwerp,
Belgium*

1. Introduction

Personalized cancer medicine based on genetic profiling of individual tumors is regarded as the treatment strategy of the future. The targeted drugs for the treatment of cancer have rapidly developed. However, our understanding (at the molecular level) of the precise role that potential targets have in tumorigenesis, and the survival dependence of tumors on these components, has not progressed at the same rate (De Roock et al., 2011). Since patient selection for therapy remains problematic, there has been an increasing interest in biomarkers of cancer risk in predicting future patterns of disease. In the broadest sense, a biomarker is any biological, chemical, or biophysical indicator of an underlying biological process. From a medical perspective, a biomarker is a physiological characteristic that is indicative of health and disease. A cancer biomarker has been defined as "a molecular, cellular, tissue, or process-based alteration that provides indication of current, or more importantly, future behavior of cancer" (Hayes et al., 1996). Cancer biomarkers are employed across the entire healthcare spectrum from the cancer biological research laboratory to patient monitoring in the clinic. Clinical applications include disease risk stratification, chemoprevention, disease screening, diagnosis and prognosis/prediction, treatment planning and monitoring, and posttreatment surveillance. Cancer biomarkers have contributed greatly to our current understanding of the heterogeneous nature of specific cancers and have led to improvements in treatment outcomes. However, full adoption of cancer biomarkers in the clinic has been slow to date, and only a limited number of cancer biomarker products are currently in routine use (http://www.insightpharmareports.com/reports_report.aspx?r=559&id=78452). Two primary challenges in developing cancer biomarkers are the discovery of candidate markers and the validation of those candidates for specific uses. The discovery process depends on the technologies available, and their sensitivity and specificity, to investigate the complex biochemistry of health and disease in order to identify differences that can be detected consistently in diverse populations. The validation process is also arduous and costly, often

* Corresponding Author

requiring collection of or access to many patient samples with extensive clinical annotation and long-term follow-up. In addition, a biomarker must be validated for each specific application for which it will be used. There must be convincing evidence that a surrogate endpoint accurately predicts the clinical endpoint of interest or in the case of screening, a test must have sufficient sensitivity, specificity, and positive predictive value to accurately identify a disease in the general population (US National Academy Press, Institute of Medicine (U.S.). Committee on Developing Biomarker-Based Tools for Cancer Screening, Diagnosis, and Treatment, 2007). Rapidly growing insights in the molecular biology of cancer and recent developments in gene sequencing, global gene expression profiling or genome wide analysis have led to high expectations for the identification, validation and assessment of cancer biomarkers alongside the established "standards of care" for cancer diagnosis and treatment.

In this review, the most promising biomarkers in gastrointestinal cancer are discussed, focusing on the epidermal growth factor receptor (EGFR)-pathway in colon cancer, the serum biomarkers, the glucose transporter (GLUT) receptors, and human equilibrative nucleoside transporter 1 in pancreatic cancer and HER2 in gastric tumors.

2. Colon cancer

2.1 Introduction

Colorectal cancer (CRC) is a major public health problem. CRC results from the cumulative effects of sequential genetic alterations, leading to a progressive and irreversible loss of normal control of cell growth and differentiation. Treatment of CRC consists of complete surgical removal of the primary tumor and the regional lymph nodes. Despite improvements in surgical techniques, dosing and scheduling of adjuvant and neo-adjuvant systemic therapy, five year survival for early stage colorectal cancer, i.e. without invasion or lymph node metastases, is about 90%, but this falls of to 65% for tumors with regional spread and to 10% for late stage disease in which the cancer has metastasized to distant sites (Deschoolmeester et al., 2010). Currently, the tumor-node-metastasis (TNM) stage is the only proven prognostic marker to aid in the identification of patients with aggressive disease (Tejpar et al., 2010). However, its predictive value is limited because even the outcome within each stage group is not homogeneous (Deschoolmeester et al., 2010). CRC should be regarded as a heterogeneous disease defined by different activating mutations in receptor tyrosine kinases (RTKs), or activating or loss of function mutations in downstream components of the RTK-activated intracellular pathways, some of which could occur in the same tumor. The efficacy of targeted drugs is therefore linked to the specific molecular alterations in the tumor (De Roock et al., 2011). The availability and application of various treatment modalities in CRC has resulted in the elucidation of prognostic and predictive biomarkers that will improve outcome through patient classification and selection for specific therapies. A prognostic biomarker provides information about the patient's overall outcome, regardless of therapy, whereas a predictive marker gives information about the effect of a particular therapeutic intervention (Tejpar et al., 2010). Consequently, in recent years a huge amount of research has been devoted to the study of new biological prognostic/predictive markers as recently reviewed by our group (Deschoolmeester et al., 2010). Several criteria must be met to ensure a biomarker is clinically useful. In addition, the biomarker needs to be tested and validated in a large cohort of randomized patients.

Although hundreds of these markers have been proposed in the last 2 to 3 decades, the current reality is that no molecular marker, other than the *KRAS* gene in the case of epidermal growth factor receptor (EGFR)-targeted therapy for metastatic disease, has made it into clinical practice (Duffy & Crown, 2008)(De Roock et al., 2009).

EGFR is a receptor tyrosine kinase belonging to the HER-family. When activated, EGFR phosphorylates and activates other intracellular proteins that affect cell signaling pathways, (Harding & Burtness, 2005) cellular proliferation, and control of apoptosis and angiogenesis (Figure 1) (Tedesco et al., 2004)(Harding & Burtness, 2005). EGFR has been implicated in colorectal tumorigenesis, tumor progression, and metastasis, as reviewed in Lockhart and Berlin (Lockhart et al., 2005)(Ng & Zhu, 2008). Overexpression of EGFR has been described in up to 65%-70% of human colon tumors and has been associated with the progression of CRC to a more advanced stage (Ng & Zhu, 2008). Therefore, EGFR not only represents a possible prognostic marker in the adjuvant setting of primary tumors but primarily a rational molecular target for a new class of anticancer agents, especially in the setting of metastatic CRC (mCRC) (Scartozzi et al., 2006a)(Scartozzi et al., 2006b)(Overman & Hoff, 2007).

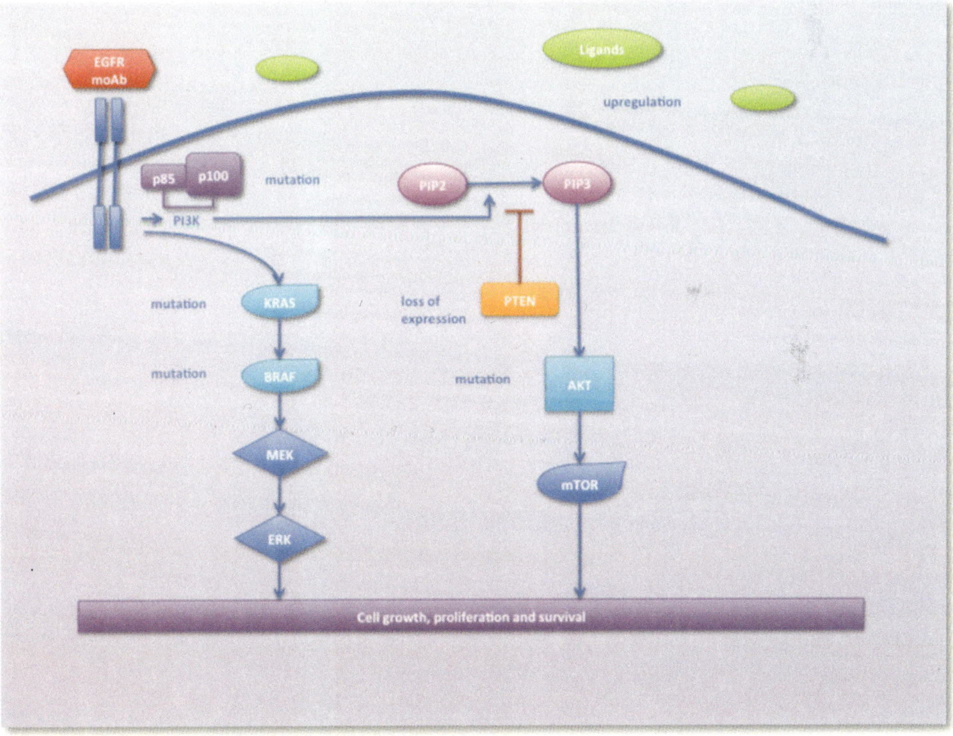

Fig. 1. EGFR signaling pathways and its main transduction pathways.

In preclinical studies, it was found that the inhibition of EGFRs had antitumor activity, and available data suggests synergy with both chemotherapy and radiotherapy (Rivera et al.,

2008). EGFR signaling can be targeted by either monoclonal antibodies (moAb) (cetuximab and panitumumab) or tyrosine kinase inhibitors (TKIs). Cetuximab (a mouse chimeric IgG1) and panitumumab (a fully human IgG2) block ligand induced EGFR tyrosine kinase activation, thereby probably preventing downstream activation of phosphatidylinositol 3-kinase (PI3K)/AKT and RAS/MAPK (mitogen activated protein) signaling pathways, resulting in inhibition of cellular proliferation and induction of apoptosis (Deschoolmeester et al., 2010). Nowadays, anti-EGFR targeted therapy is undergoing extensive clinical evaluation as single agents and in combination with chemotherapy for the treatment of recurrent or first-line mCRC (as reviewed by (Deschoolmeester et al., 2010)). Results of these studies have demonstrated a manageable and acceptable toxicity profile and a promising level of activity. Initially, these therapies were given to unselected populations, but novel insights based on the independent reanalysis of eight randomized trials suggested that these therapies would be effective only in wild type *KRAS* populations (Allegra et al., 2009). Based on these results, the recommended use of these drugs was amended by both the European Medicine Agency (EMEA) and the U.S. Food and Drug Administration (FDA), with important differences, however. The FDA issued a recommendation in 2009 against the use of these drugs in patients with tumors mutated in codon 12 or 13 of *KRAS*, but a label change of the drugs will require additional validation of a single mutation detection assay and reassessment of all randomized trials using this assay. In Europe, the EMEA changed the approval of these drugs for use in wild-type *KRAS* populations only. This has important implications because the exact mutations to be tested are not specified nor is the methodology (see further below) (Bellon et al., 2011).

2.2 KRAS

KRAS belongs to the *RAS* family of genes (*KRAS*, *NRAS* and *HRAS*) that encode guanosine-5′-triphosphate (GTP)-binding proteins. *KRAS* is an important effector of ligand-bound EGFR, mainly, but not exclusively through *BRAF* and *MAPK* axis. KRAS can also activate PI3K through direct interaction with its catalytic subunit (Figure 1) (De Roock et al., 2011). Mutations in the *KRAS* gene are found in 30-40% of CRC and these mutations disable the GTPase activity, causing tumor-associated KRAS to accumulate in the active GTP-bound conformation. About 85-90% of these mutations occur in codons 12 and 13 while the remaining mutations occur in codon 61 (5%) and 146 (5%). The most frequent types of mutations detected are glycine to aspartate on codon 12 (p.G12D, 36.0%), glycine to valine on codon 12 (pG12V, 21.8%), and glycine to aspartate on codon 13 (p.G13D, 18.8%) (Neumann et al., 2009). Several retrospective studies (single-group and randomized clinical trials, summarized by Allegra and colleagues (Allegra et al., 2009)) confirmed the finding by Lievre and colleagues (Lièvre et al., 2006) that mutant *KRAS* is a predictor of resistance to EGFR moAb. This discovery led to the first practical implication of personalized medicine in mCRC. All patients with mCRC are now profiled for seven mutations in *KRAS* codons 12 and 13 before receiving cetuximab or panitumumab (De Roock et al., 2011). However, the picture is not that simple. There is growing evidence for the existence of a whole orchestra of variables and mutations that influence the responsiveness to an anti-EFGR treatment and their role is not fully understood. A European consortium study showed that codon 61 mutations had an adverse effect similar to codon 12 mutations, whereas codon 146 mutations did not affect cetuximab efficacy. Codon 146 mutations co-occurred with other *KRAS* mutations, an additional indication that this might not be an important oncogenic codon (De Roock et al., 2010b). In vitro data also suggest that *KRAS* codon 13 mutations have a weaker transforming activity than codon 12 mutations and some reports also suggest that some of these patients do respond to cetuximab (Koch et al., 2011). Based on these findings, de Roock and colleagues performed a thorough retrospective subgroup analysis in a pooled data set of 579 patients with chemotherapy-refractory CRC. Their data puzzles the picture of the negative predictive value of a *KRAS* mutation, because patients with the p.G13D mutation seem to respond to cetuximab therapy, in contrast to other *KRAS* mutated tumors, albeit with a lower response rate than those with *KRAS* wild type tumors. The prolonged progression-free and overall survival of patients with p.G13D-mutated tumors in comparison with those with other *KRAS*- mutated tumors may not be due to a real reduction in tumor burden but to a delay in progression. A possible explanation of this clinical observation is that p.G13D mutant tumors do not undergo apoptosis (cytotoxic effect) on EGFR inhibition, but proliferation is inhibited (cytostatic effect). However, prospective randomized trials are needed before conclusions about potential beneficial effects of cetuximab in p.G13D-mutated chemotherapy refractory metastatic colorectal cancer should be inferred (De Roock et al., 2010a).

Furthermore, mutations in the *KRAS* gene can be detected by several different molecular methods and no gold standard methodology is currently available. Because the correctness of the *KRAS* test results is of utmost importance for good patient care, a quality control scheme was set up to (a) assess the performance of *KRAS* testing in Europe, (b) provide remedial measures if necessary, and (c) ensure uniform performance over time by repeated testing rounds. In total, 59 laboratories from eight different European countries participated in the regional *KRAS* external quality assessment (EQA) scheme in 2009. Only 70% of laboratories correctly identified the *KRAS* mutational status in all 10 samples. Genotyping mistakes can be the result of several reasons. A very important issue is the starting material and the type of fixative used. Another important issue in *KRAS* genotyping is the method used for testing. The TheraScreen®DxS kit is considered to be the gold standard for *KRAS* testing in Europe for diagnostic use. However, in this EQA scheme, several mistakes were made using this kit. In addition, the kit is designed to detect only one mutation in a sample, and therefore the mutation scoring ignores possible double mutations, interpreting it as crosstalk. Furthermore, there was a very high variability among laboratories in the estimation of the percentage of tumor cells in H&E stained paraffin sections and the general quality of the reports received in the context of this EQA scheme were very poor. Incomplete or inaccurate exams lead to incorrect diagnoses and can have important consequences for a patient. Therefore, further development of the *KRAS* EQA scheme aims to provide a baseline picture of the accuracy and reliability of the analysis of the *KRAS* test, to identify areas of particular difficulty in testing procedures and to provide a mechanism for improvement for the participating laboratories (Bellon et al., 2011).

In addition, up to 50-65% of patients with *KRAS* wild-type tumors are resistant to EGFR moAb therapies. Therefore the quest for predictive markers continues. Genetic alterations in other EGFR effectors, acting downstream of *KRAS* together with alternative *KRAS* mutations (in codon 61 and 146) could drive primary resistance to anti-EGFR therapy and are currently investigated (Sartore-Bianchi et al., 2009a)(Molinari et al., 2009)(Souglakos et al., 2009)(Laurent-Puig et al., 2009)(Meriggi et al., 2009)(Prenen et al., 2009)(Loupakis et al., 2009a)(Loupakis et al., 2009b)(Perrone et al., 2009)(De Roock et al., 2011). Moreover, Sartore-

Bianchi et al., described that when expression of PTEN and mutation of *KRAS, BRAF* and *PIK3CA* are concomitantly ascertained, up to 70% of mCRC patients unlikely to respond to anti-EGFR therapies can be identified (Sartore-Bianchi et al., 2009a).

It is unclear to what extent the effects of mutant *KRAS* are the same for other RTK-targeted therapies. It is possible that *KRAS*-mutant tumors are not dependent on any RTK upstream component, and therefore will not respond to drugs targeting these RTKs. Alternatively, it might be that *KRAS* mutations confer only part of the survival advantage needed for tumor cells, and therefore will still benefit from RTK inhibition. Moreover, to define CRC as *KRAS* mutant versus *KRAS* wild-type probably underestimates additional heterogeneity found within both populations (De Roock et al., 2011).

2.3 BRAF

BRAF, a member of the *RAF* gene family (*ARAF, BRAF* and *CRAF*), encodes a serine-threonine protein kinase, downstream of activated KRAS, and initiates a mitogenic kinase cascade leading to cell proliferation (Figure 1). Activating mutations of *BRAF* have been reported in 5–15% of CRC and >95% of all known mutations involve a thymine to adenine transversion in nucleotide 1799, which leads to a substitution of valine by glutamic acid at amino acid residue 600 (V600E), which results in an upregulation of the ERK signaling pathway independently of *KRAS* mutation (Nash et al., 2010)(Barault et al., 2008)(Oliveira et al., 2004). In addition, the V600E mutation could have additional functions, since *KRAS* and *BRAF* mutations seems to be mutually exclusive in CRC, with very rare exceptions, suggesting they occur in different tumor types and have different outcomes. Moreover, *BRAF* mutations are associated with sporadic microsatellite instability (MSI), CpG island methylator phenotype (CIMP) and right sided tumors, whereas mutant *KRAS* are not (De Roock et al., 2011)(Dasari & Messersmith, 2010).

BRAF mutation status appears to be a valid negative prognostic marker for CRC in the adjuvant and metastatic setting, as demonstrate in the PETACC-3 (Roth et al., 2010), the CRYSTAL (Van Cutsem et al., 2011) and other studies (Yokota et al., 2011)(Park et al., 2011). The presence of CIMP-high appears to eliminate, at least in part, the adverse effect of *BRAF* mutations, whereas the good prognosis associated with MSI-high was abrogated in the presence of a *BRAF* mutation (Ogino et al., 2009a). In contrast, Samowitz et al. (Samowitz et al., 2005) and Roth et al. (Roth et al., 2010) found that *BRAF* mutations were associated with a significantly poorer survival in MSS tumors, but had no effect on the excellent prognosis of MSI-high tumors. Therefore, it has been postulated that it is not the *BRAF* mutation itself which confers a poor prognosis but rather that the mutation has different effects depending on the type of genetic pathway in which it is produced (Barault et al., 2008).

In addition, the currently available data suggest that the *BRAF* V600E mutation confers resistance to EGFR moAb in patients with chemotherapy-refractory *KRAS* wild-type mCRC and might be used as an additional predictive factor in this setting (Siena et al., 2009)(Laurent-Puig et al., 2009)(Sartore-Bianchi et al., 2009a)(Di Nicolantonio et al., 2008)(Tol et al., 2009).

Furthermore, the treatment of *KRAS*-mutated CRC with a selective *BRAF* inhibitor could be an interesting approach since *BRAF* is an important effector downstream of *KRAS* in the ERK signaling pathway. Phase II clinical trials are currently ongoing with the combination of sorafinib (*BRAF* inhibitor) with either FOLFOX, FOLFIRI or cetuximab.

2.4 PIK3CA

The PI3Ks are a family of lipid kinases grouped into three classes with different structure and substrate preferences. Class 1 phosphatidylinositol 3-kinases (PIK3) are heterodimeric proteins composed of a p85 regulatory subunit and one of several p110 catalytic subunits. Among several isoforms of the catalytic subunits, only the α-type, PIK3CA, has been shown to harbor oncogenic mutations or amplifications in its gene in human malignancies (Ogino et al., 2009b)(Jang et al., 2010). Activation of class I PI3K is initiated when a growth factor binds to its cognate RTK, which includes members of the ERBB-family, platelet-derived growth-factor receptor (PDGFR) and the insulin and the insulin-like growth-factor 1 receptors (IGF1R) (De Roock et al., 2011). Activated PIK3CA will phosphorylate phosphatidyl-inositol-4,5-biphospate (PIP2) to produce phosphatidyl-inositol-3,4,5-triphospate (PIP3) which localizes the serine threonine kinase Akt to the cell membrane where it becomes activated (Figure 1). Activated Akt phosphorylates downstream protein effectors and amplifies the signaling cascade, enhancing cell proliferation and survival (Ogino et al., 2009b). Based on the current data, it seems that *PIK3CA* mutation frequency in CRC is probably between 15 and 25% (Dasari & Messersmith, 2010). More than 80% of *PIK3CA* mutations in CRC occur in exon 9 (60-65%) or exon 20 (20-25%). Mutation in *PIK3CA* can co-occur with *KRAS* and *BRAF* mutations. A European consortium recently suggested that only *PIK3CA* exon-20 mutations are associated with a lack of cetuximab activity in *KRAS* wild-type tumors (De Roock et al., 2010b). However, because of the low frequency of this mutation, these data require confirmation in large patient population studies. In contrast, *PIK3CA* exon-9 mutations are associated with *KRAS* mutations and do not have an independent effect on cetuximab efficacy (De Roock et al., 2010b). The apparent difference between exon-9 and exon-20 mutations could explain the conflicting data regarding *PIK3CA* mutations reported by Sartore-Bianchi and colleagues (Sartore-Bianchi et al., 2009b) (lack of response to cetuximab and more exon-20 mutations) and Prenen and colleagues (Prenen et al., 2009) (no correlation). *PIK3CA* mutations as a whole were associated with shorter cancer specific survival in a series of surgically resectable CRC, but exon-9 and exon-20 were not studied separately (Ogino et al., 2009b)(Kato et al., 2007). More studies on large patient populations are needed to establish the prognostic role of *PIK3CA* exon-9 and exon-20 mutations.

2.5 PTEN

PI3K-initiated signaling is inhibited by phosphatase tensin homologue (PTEN). The PTEN protein acts as a phospholipid phosphatase with PIP3 as a substrate. PIP3 is an important lipid second messenger that provides docking sites for multiple downstream components, including AKT, which is activated by phosphorylation and inhibited by PTEN (Figure 1). Since PTEN protein is a negative regulator of the AKT signaling pathway, inactivation of PTEN, which is a common event in human malignancies, facilitates cell proliferation and apoptosis (Sawai et al., 2008)(Goel et al., 2004). PTEN activity may be lost trough various mechanisms, including mutations, deletions, silencing, allelic losses at chromosome 10q23 or hypermethylation of the *PTEN* promoter region (especially in MSI-high CRC). Therefore, ascertainment of PTEN status is usually done on protein level and the recorded frequency of loss of PTEN expression varies from 19% to 36% in CRC. Data on the loss of PTEN are not concordant between primary and metastatic tumors (De Roock et al., 2011)(Dasari & Messersmith, 2010). In addition, PTEN loss in metastatic tumors predicted lack of response to cetuximab and PTEN null metastasis had shorter progression free survival, which was even more significant in *KRAS* wild-type patients. In sharp contrast, the PTEN analysis on the primary tumor did not reveal any predictive or prognostic information. Although the relative low concordance rate between the primary and metastatic tumors for PTEN expression could be secondary to selection of clonal populations during metastasis, it could be the subjective nature of immunohistochemistry testing with significant method and observer variability. This consideration and the possible need to analyze PTEN from metastatic tumors may limit the role of PTEN as biomarker in CRC (Dasari & Messersmith, 2010).

2.6 Conclusion

In summary, both MAPK and PI3K pathways are stimulated by EGFR, with important implication for EGFR targeted therapy and future drug development. Current American Society of Clinical Oncology (ASCO) guidelines recommend testing only for *KRAS* mutations in codon 12 and codon 13, in patients being considered for EGFR moAb therapy (Dasari & Messersmith, 2010). However, evidence shows that other molecular alterations, such as *BRAF*, *PIK3CA* (exon-20) mutations or loss of PTEN expression, could preclude response to EGFR moAb. The subjective nature of PTEN assessment, however, is a significant challenge. In addition, new drugs are being developed against numerous targets in these pathways, and many are in early clinical stages. Finally, a better understanding of the functional interactions within RTK-activated intracellular pathways is essential to target the individual tumor and to deliver more effective medical treatment to patients with mCRC. Furthermore, the ability of the cancer cell to develop drug resistance via new mutations or alternative signaling pathways also needs to be addressed by combination therapy, and, if possible, analysis of tumor tissue upon progression (Dasari & Messersmith, 2010)(De Roock et al., 2011).

3. Pancreatic cancer

3.1 Introduction

Pancreatic cancer has the worst prognosis of all gastrointestinal malignancies with the mortality approaching the incidence (Buxbaum & Eloubeidi, 2010)(Bünger et al., 2011). Late clinical presentation, intrinsic biological aggressiveness, and resistance to conventional chemotherapy and radiotherapy represent the predominant reasons for its poor prognosis (Pizzi et al., 2009). This demonstrates an urgent demand for improved screening tools for early detection (Buxbaum & Eloubeidi, 2010)(Bünger et al., 2011). While surveillance is performed in individuals with genetic syndromes, hereditary pancreatitis, and a strong family history there are no clear guidelines for those with clinical risk factors like diabetes mellitus, tobacco use, and chronic pancreatitis (Buxbaum & Eloubeidi, 2010). Pancreatic ductal adenocarcinoma is the most commonly diagnosed pancreatic neoplasm, and reported to be the forth or fifth leading cause of cancer death in Western countries. Diagnosis of pancreatic cancer at early stages is crucial because successful surgical resection remains the only possibility of cure (Ansari et al., 2011). Only 10-30% of pancreatic tumor patients are operated on with curative intent. The expected 5-year survival rate of R0 resected patients with additional adjuvant chemotherapy is about 4-26%. In contrast, for the remaining patients who present with unresectable UICC stage III and IV carcinomas, no curative therapy is available. These patients have median survival times of 8-12 months (stage III) and 5-8 months (stage IV), respectively (Bünger et al., 2011). In addition, early-stage pancreatic cancer is usually clinically silent, and symptoms only become apparent after the tumor invades surrounding tissues or metastasis to distant organs. Therefore, most persons who present with symptoms attributable to pancreatic cancer have advanced disease (Vincent et al., 2011).

The Holy Grail for pancreatic cancer investigators is to identify early markers, which predict the development of pancreatic cancer, uncover early resectable disease, and guide therapy (Buxbaum & Eloubeidi, 2010).

Potential molecular markers are sought in the pancreatic tissue, juice as well as other body fluids including serum and urine. An important consideration is that pancreatic tumor cells and secreted molecules are found in markedly higher concentrations in the pancreas and pancreatic juice compared to serum. Additionally, molecules and proteins in the serum are overwhelmed by high concentrations of albumin, transferrin, and immunoglobulins (Buxbaum & Eloubeidi, 2010).

Both hypothesis driven and high throughput searches for molecular markers to predict disease, early diagnosis, and treatment response are underway. Challenges include differentiation of cancer from chronic inflammatory disease of the pancreas and achieving reproducible results among diverse patients. Minimally invasive methods including endoscopic ultrasound guided fine needle aspiration (EUS-FNA) to acquire tissue may facilitate these important efforts (Buxbaum & Eloubeidi, 2010). This method enabled not only accurate diagnosis, but also the collection of cancer tissue before surgery or chemotherapy even in inoperable cases. Evaluation of the expression status of multiple molecules within the FNA specimen will lead to the establishment of individualized therapeutic strategies based on the prediction of prognosis or response to chemotherapy (Hamada & Shimosegawa, 2011).

3.2 Serum biomarkers

Improved screening for early diagnosis is essential in order to increase the rate of curatively resectable carcinomas, thereby ameliorating patient's prognosis. In present clinical practice, screening for pancreatic cancer is based on state-of-the-art imaging or even invasive diagnostics. A relatively non-invasive, cost efficient possibility could be provided by the measurement of disease-specific markers in peripheral blood. A wide range of serum markers has been reported to be elevated in pancreatic cancer patients since the eighties. Despite these many markers or their combinations with high diagnostic potential for pancreatic cancer screening, none of them have achieved the levels of sensitivity and specificity necessary to be recommended as a screening tool for asymptomatic patients in the general population (Bünger et al., 2011)(Xu et al., 2011). Only a few markers have shown promising results in recent studies with CA19-9 being the most widely investigated and evaluated single marker (Bünger et al., 2011).

3.2.1 CA19-9

The best-established marker is CA19-9, which is a sialylated Lewis antigen of the MUC1 protein with an overall sensitivity ranging from 41 to 86% and specificity from 33 to 100%

(Bünger et al., 2011)(Buxbaum & Eloubeidi, 2010). As a marker for early pancreatic cancer, there are some important weaknesses. Approximately 10% of the population with the Lewis-negative genotype is not able to produce CA19-9, secondary to a lack of the enzyme involved in its synthesis, even if they have advanced pancreatic cancer. Recently it has been reported that patients with undetectable CA19-9 have a better prognosis than those with elevated levels. Patients with small pancreatic cancers often show false negative CA19-9 values, thus eliminating its value in early diagnosis. In addition, patients with certain blood types are incapable of expressing the antigen recognized by CA19-9. Moreover, CA19-9 elevation is common in patients with obstructive jaundice even without malignancy because of the reduction in clearance by the cholestatic liver. Furthermore, false positive CA19-9 elevation is also frequently observed in patients with cancers of the upper gastrointestinal tract, ovarian cancer, hepatocellular cancer, benign conditions of the hepatobiliary system and chronic pancreatitis (Xu et al., 2011). Nevertheless, continuous evaluation of this marker strongly suggests progressive disease during chemotherapy or recurrence after operation (Hamada & Shimosegawa, 2011). Thus CA19-9 is considered the standard for monitoring response to chemotherapy and recurrence following surgical resection in patients with pancreatic cancer but not for the initial diagnosis of the disease in the asymptomatic population (Xu et al., 2011)(Buxbaum & Eloubeidi, 2010)(Vincent et al., 2011).

In addition to serum it has been shown that pancreatic juice might also be a source of pancreatic cancer tumor markers. Several groups evaluated the diagnostic value of CA19-9 in pancreatic juice. Some groups found that CA19-9 concentrations were significantly higher in patients with cancer than in patients with chronic pancreatitis and other non-neoplastic patients (Malesci et al., 1987) showing a diagnostic value approximately similar to that of serum CA19-9 (Nishida et al., 1988)(Chen et al., 1989). Other studies could not confirm the diagnostic value of CA19-9 in pancreatic juice (Matsumoto et al., 1994). Further investigation into the exact role of CA19-9 in pancreatic juice is required. However, other potentially interesting biomarkers, like *KRAS* mutations, 90K, CEA were identified in this pancreatic juice and need further investigation (Nakaizumi et al., 1999)(Gentiloni et al., 1995).

3.2.2 Micro-RNA

Small non-coding RNAs are now attracting increased attention as robust regulators of various biological processes, including cancer progression. The micro-RNAs (miRs) are a class of conserved small non-coding RNA's of 17-25 nucleotides in length that regulate gene expression by either repressing the translation or causing degradation of multiple target mRNAs. *MiR* genes represent about 1% of the genome in different species and it is estimated that about 30% of the protein-coding genes in the human genome are regulated by miRs (Wang & Sen, 2011). These miRs play a central role in the regulation of cellular functions, such as migration, invasion and stem cell functions (Vincent et al., 2011). Extensive mapping of the known *miR* genes revealed that these are often located in the genomic intervals rearranged in cancers including those displaying amplification, loss of heterozygosity, common breakpoints and fragile sites. Furthermore, functional analyses suggest that miRs play roles in cancer initiation, invasion and progression processes and, therefore, may prove to be informative biomarkers of detection, diagnosis and prognosis besides being potential targets of therapy (Wang & Sen, 2011).

Over 300 miRs have been identified, and widespread alterations in these miRs have been recognized in various types of cancer, including pancreatic cancer, and seem to contribute to their development and progression (see table 1, modified from (Wang & Sen, 2011)). MiR signatures specific for normal pancreas, chronic pancreatitis and cancer tissues have been identified and have been proposed to represent helpful markers for differential diagnosis of pancreatic cancer from chronic inflammatory disease of the pancreas and even other tumors (Hamada & Shimosegawa, 2011)(Vincent et al., 2011)(Wang & Sen, 2011). In addition, these differential-expressing miRs can also be profiled in blood as a minimally invasive biomarker assay for pancreatic cancer. This finding is extremely promising since there is no reliable biomarker assay, much less of minimally invasive nature, currently available for early detection, diagnosis and predicting prognosis of pancreatic cancer patients.

microRNA	Expression profile	References
Let-7f-1	Up	(Lee et al., 2007)
Let-7d	Up	(Lee et al., 2007)
miR-10	Up	(Bloomston et al., 2007)(Zhang et al., 2009b)
miR-15b	Up	(Lee et al., 2007)(Zhang et al., 2009b)
miR-16-1	Up	(Lee et al., 2007)
miR-21	Up	(Lee et al., 2007)(Bloomston et al., 2007)(Zhang et al., 2009b)(Mees et al., 2010)
miR-23	Up	(Bloomston et al., 2007)
miR-24	Up	(Lee et al., 2007)
miR-31	Up	(Szafranska et al., 2007) (Szafranska et al., 2008)
miR-92	Up	(Lee et al., 2007)
miR-95	Up	(Zhang et al., 2009b)
miR-96	Down	(Szafranska et al., 2007) (Szafranska et al., 2008)
miR-99	Up	(Bloomston et al., 2007)
miR-100	Up	(Lee et al., 2007)(Bloomston et al., 2007)
miR-103	Up	(Bloomston et al., 2007)(Zhang et al., 2009b)
miR-107	Up	(Lee et al., 2007)(Bloomston et al., 2007)(Zhang et al., 2009b)
miR-125	Up	(Lee et al., 2007)(Bloomston et al., 2007)
miR-130b	Down	(Szafranska et al., 2007)(Bloomston et al., 2007)(Szafranska et al., 2008)
miR-139	Down	(Lee et al., 2007)
miR-142-P	Down	(Lee et al., 2007)
miR-143	Up	(Szafranska et al., 2007)(Bloomston et al., 2007)(Szafranska et al., 2008) (Zhang et al., 2009b)
miR-145	Up	(Szafranska et al., 2008)(Zhang et al., 2009b)
miR-146	Up	(Szafranska et al., 2007) (Bloomston et al., 2007)
miR-148a	Down	(Szafranska et al., 2007) (Bloomston et al., 2007) (Szafranska et al., 2008)
miR-148b	Down	(Szafranska et al., 2007) (Bloomston et al., 2007)

miR-155	Up	(Lee et al., 2007)(Szafranska et al., 2007)(Szafranska et al., 2008) (Bloomston et al., 2007)(Zhang et al., 2009b)
miR-181a	Up	(Lee et al., 2007)(Bloomston et al., 2007)
miR-181b	Up	(Bloomston et al., 2007)
miR-181c	Up	(Lee et al., 2007)(Bloomston et al., 2007)
miR-181d	Up	(Bloomston et al., 2007)
miR-186	Up	(Zhang et al., 2009b)
miR-190	Up	(Zhang et al., 2009b)
miR-194	Up	{Mees:2010fr}
miR-196a	Up	(Szafranska et al., 2007) (Szafranska et al., 2008)(Zhang et al., 2009b)
miR-196b	Up	(Szafranska et al., 2007)
miR-199a	Up	(Bloomston et al., 2007)
miR-200b	Up	(Zhang et al., 2009b){Mees:2010fr}
miR-200c	Up	{Mees:2010fr}
miR-203	Up	(Ikenaga et al., 2010)
miR-205	Up	(Szafranska et al., 2007) (Bloomston et al., 2007) (Szafranska et al., 2008)
miR-210	Up	(Szafranska et al., 2007) (Bloomston et al., 2007)(Szafranska et al., 2008)(Zhang et al., 2009b)
miR-212	Up	(Lee et al., 2007)
miR-213	Up	(Bloomston et al., 2007)
miR-217	Down	(Szafranska et al., 2007) (Szafranska et al., 2008)
miR-220	Up	(Bloomston et al., 2007)
miR-221	Up	(Lee et al., 2007) (Szafranska et al., 2007)(Bloomston et al., 2007)(Zhang et al., 2009b){Mees:2010fr}
miR-222	Up	(Szafranska et al., 2007) (Bloomston et al., 2007)(Zhang et al., 2009b)
miR-223	Up	(Szafranska et al., 2007)(Bloomston et al., 2007)(Szafranska et al., 2008) (Zhang et al., 2009b)
miR-301	Up	(Lee et al., 2007)
miR-345	Down	(Lee et al., 2007)
miR-375	Down	(Szafranska et al., 2007) (Bloomston et al., 2007) (Szafranska et al., 2008)
miR-376a	Up	(Lee et al., 2007)
miR-424	Up	(Lee et al., 2007)
miR-429	Up	{Mees:2010fr}

Table 1. Deregulated microRNAs in pancreatic ductal adenocarcinoma (modified from (Wang & Sen, 2011)).

In addition, successful therapeutic targeting of miRs (silencing, antisense blocking and miR modification of oncogenic miRs) also holds significant promise towards improved clinical management of patients with cancer, especially those with pancreatic carcinomas, since these patients have very limited treatment options available at this time (Wang & Sen, 2011)(Rachagani et al., 2010).

3.3 Glucose transporter isoforms (GLUT)

Malignant cells have high constitutive glucose uptake and metabolism compared with normal cells (Pizzi et al., 2009). A family of glucose transporter isoforms (GLUT), which is currently composed of 13 members, facilitates the entry of glucose into cells. These are passive carriers and function as an energy-independent system that transports glucose down a concentration gradient. GLUT-1, a member of this family, is considered to be the predominantly upregulated glucose transporter in malignant epithelial tissue and mesothelium, and has been found to correlate with biological behavior in various malignancies (Basturk et al., 2011).

Various studies have shown a close relationship between GLUT-1 expression and tumor aggressiveness and poor prognosis in squamous cell carcinoma of the head and neck and in carcinomas of the lung, stomach, gallbladder, colorectum, kidney, bladder, ovary and cervix. An increased GLUT-1 expression has also proved to be associated with pancreatic cancer invasiveness both *in vitro* and *in vivo* (Basturk et al., 2011). However, literature data regarding the prognostic significance of immunohistochemical GLUT-1 expression in pancreatic ductal adenocarcinoma are limited and non consistent, as a prognostic significance of GLUT-1 expression has been found by some research groups (Sun et al., 2007)(Pizzi et al., 2009) and not by the other (Lyshchik et al., 2007). Differences can be ascribed to heterogeneity of histological types of pancreatic cancer and to the different scoring systems. Overall, GLUT-1 overexpression is regarded as a relative early event in pancreatic carcinogenesis and may be ascribed to local hypoxia. Furthermore, GLUT-1 expression seems to correlate to a higher glucose uptake in undifferentiated and highly proliferative pancreatic cancer cells (Pizzi et al., 2009). Moreover, GLUT-1 promotes cellular invasiveness in pancreatic cancer, which is matrix metalloproteinase 2 (MMP2)-dependent, with MMP-2 being transcriptionally activated by increased GLUT-1 levels (Ito et al., 2004). In addition, an increased expression of GLUT-1 molecules in pancreatic tumors has been suggested to contribute to the higher rate of fluorine 18 fluorodeoxyglucose (^{18}F-FDG) uptake into tumor cells compared with normal pancreatic tissue, as determined by standardized uptake value (SUV). Also, SUV has been found to be a predictor of survival in patients with ductal adenocarcinomas. Therefore, in addition to being of diagnostic value imaging-wise, GLUT-1 may also be a potential therapeutic target to limit glucose uptake and metabolism, thereby limiting the proliferative potential of malignant cells (Basturk et al., 2011). Apigenin, a flavonoid with significant anti-proliferative properties that inhibit pancreatic cancer cell proliferation, has been shown to inhibit glucose uptake as well as both GLUT-1 mRNA and protein expression in human pancreatic cancer cell lines. In addition, the PI3K/Akt pathway may be involved in mediating apigenin's effects on downstream targets such as GLUT-1 (Melstrom et al., 2008). However, literature regarding the biological significance of GLUT-1 expression in pancreatic neoplasia has been limited and controversial (Basturk et al., 2011).

3.4 Human equilibrative nucleoside transporter 1 (hENT1)

Gemcitabine, a pyrimidine nucleoside analogue, has clinically important activity in advanced and metastatic pancreatic adenocarcinoma and for which it is now the standard of care (Maréchal et al., 2009)(Ansari et al., 2011). Gemcitabine is a prodrug that is phosphorylated by deoxycitidine kinase to its mononucleotide in the rate-limiting step of its cellular anabolism. Subsequent nucleotide kinases convert gemcitabine monophosphate to its active metabolites, gemcitabine diphosphate and triphosphate. Permeation of gemcitabine through the plasma membrane requires specialized integral membrane nucleoside transporter proteins. Among these transporters, the major mediators of gemcitabine uptake into human cells appear to be the human equilibrative nucleoside transporter 1 (hENT1) and to a lesser extent the human conservative nucleoside transporter 3 (hCNT3) (Maréchal et al., 2009). Recently, it was reported that tissue mRNA levels of the hENT1, which mediates the cellular entry of gemcitabine, correlated with survival (Ansari et al., 2011). Several subsequent immunohistochemically based studies demonstrated that hENT-1 holds promise as an independent predictive marker to identify those likely to benefit from gemcitabine based monotherapy (Morinaga et al., 2011)(Spratlin et al., 2004)(Farrell et al., 2009) and gemcitabine based chemoradiotherapy (Maréchal et al., 2009)(Murata et al., 2011). In addition, the expression of hENT1 provides independent prognostic information in untreated pancreatic carcinoma patients as well as those treated with adjuvant gemcitabine-based therapy (Kim et al., 2011b)(Maréchal et al., 2009). Whether these assays provide sufficient predictive information to guide treatment decision requires prospective evaluation in randomized clinical trials. However, the consistency and strength of the accumulating preclinical and translational data suggest that nucleoside transporters play an important role in clinical outcomes after gemcitabine adjuvant chemotherapy for pancreatic cancer (Maréchal et al., 2009).

3.5 Conclusion

Although the tumor node metastasis classification provides important prognostic information, it permits only crude stratification of clinical outcome for patients with pancreatic cancer. Although some potential markers were identified, a high degree of inconsistency still exists between reports. Validation through large multicenter prospective studies using standardized protocols is still needed. Considering the complexity of the disease, it seems reasonable to hypothesize that panels of markers, rather than single proteins, might become useful (Ansari et al., 2011).

4. Gastric cancer

4.1 Introduction

Gastric cancer is one of the most common tumors and remains the second leading cause of cancer death worldwide (Gravalos & Jimeno, 2008)(Wagner & Moehler, 2009). Gastric cancer is a heterogeneous disease divided in at least two different tumor entities, the intestinal and the diffuse form, with difference in epidemiology, cause, pathogenesis and disorder. The development of the intestinal form, usually in older patients, is related to *Helicobacter pylori* and usually located in the corpus and the antrum and related to preexisting corpus predominant atrophic gastritis, followed by intestinal metaplasia. In contrast, the diffuse form is usually poorly differentiated, located most frequently in the proximal stomach and its incidence is rising at an alarming rate in overweight young men suffering from gastroesophageal reflux. Diffuse type cancers have usually a worse prognosis (Wagner & Moehler, 2009).

Surgical resection remains the mainstay of treatment and cure in localized, non-metastatic gastric cancer while no globally accepted consensus exists on the best treatment regimen to be used in advanced gastric cancer (De Vita et al., 2010)(Lorenzen & Lordick, 2011). At present, the combination of a fluoropyrimidine and a platinum analogue either alone or in combination with a third drug such as an antracycline or taxanes are the most effective combinations resulting in a median survival of 8-10 months (Lorenzen & Lordick, 2011). These observations suggest the need for new therapeutic approaches, based on the implementation of predictive biomarkers, to further improve the outcome of patients with advanced gastric cancer (De Vita et al., 2010)(Wagner & Moehler, 2009)(Lorenzen & Lordick, 2011). A better understanding of the molecular basis of cancer has contributed to the development of rationally designed molecular targeted therapies, which interfere with the signaling cascades involved in cell differentiation, proliferation and survival (Gravalos & Jimeno, 2008). Recently, the evidence that upregulation of signaling pathways of EGFR-family plays a central role in cell differentiation, proliferation, and survival has supported the development of antitumor strategies against these targets (De Vita et al., 2010). One of the most considerable innovative targets in human cancer is the HER family.

4.2 HER2

The epidermal growth factor receptor (EGFR) family is composed of four members: HER1 also known as EGFR1, HER2, HER3 and HER4, amongst which the EGFR1 and HER2 represents targets for drugs currently under development for gastric cancer (Wagner & Moehler, 2009). The HER2 protein is a 185 kDa transmembrane tyrosine kinase (TK) receptor encoded by a gene located on chromosome 17q21, with an extracellular ligand-binding domain, a short transmembrane domain and an intracellular domain with TK activity. Up to now, no ligands have been identified for its extracellular domain, but it seems to be the preferred heterodimerization partner for other members of the HER family (De Vita et al., 2010). HER2 functions as an oncogene and its amplification or overexpression plays a central role in the initiation, progression and metastasis of some common cancers. Aberrant HER2 expression or function has been implicated in about 10-34% of invasive breast cancers. In addition, HER 2 also appears to be overexpressed in colon, bladder, ovarian, endometrium, lung, uterine cervix, head and neck, and esophageal carcinomas. The first description of HER2 overexpression in gastric cancer, using IHC, was reported in 1986. Since then, a number of studies have confirmed these findings, reporting a HER2 positivity rate in a wide range (6-35%) of gastric carcinomas. Moreover, HER2 expression varies depending on histology and on primary tumor location (Lorenzen & Lordick, 2011)(De Vita et al., 2010). The randomized open-label, multinational phase III ToGA (Trastuzumb for Gastric Cancer) trial, in which by now the largest population of 3807 gastric cancers were centrally screened for *HER2* gene amplification (Fluorescent in situ hybridization (FISH)) and HER2 protein overexpression (IHC 3+), reported a HER2 positivity of 22.1%, with a high degree of concordance between IHC and FISH (87,2%). Furthermore, HER2 positivity rates were found to be higher in esophagogastric junction cancer than in gastric cancer and in intestinal cancer than diffuse or mixed type (Lorenzen & Lordick, 2011)(Croxtall & McKeage, 2010).

Trastuzumab, a recombinant humanized IgG1 monoclonal antibody directed against the extracellular domain of HER2, in combination with chemotherapy agents, has recently received approval in the EU and USA for treatment of metastatic HER2-positive gastric cancer without prior anti-cancer treatment for metastatic disease (Croxtall & McKeage, 2010).

4.3 HER2 as prognostic factor in gastric cancer

The TNM stage is the most important prognostic factor for gastric cancer. Prognosis, however, varies among patients in the same stage. Therefore, additional classification parameters, like HER2 need to be defined in addition to the TNM and the classical pathological characteristics of the tumor in order to better identify the biological subset of this disease (Gravalos & Jimeno, 2008). The role of HER2 as prognostic marker in gastric cancer has been controversial because some of the initial studies failed to find an association with outcome (Zhang et al., 2009a)(De Vita et al., 2010)(Gravalos & Jimeno, 2008)(Lorenzen & Lordick, 2011). Other authors, however, reported a direct correlation between HER2 overexpression and poor outcome (Ananiev et al., 2011)(Kim et al., 2011a)(Im et al., 2005). However, the largest study to date investigating the prognostic significance of HER2 expression in 924 gastric cancer patients showed that HER2 expression is not related to gastric cancer patients outcome (Grabsch et al., 2010). Chua et al. (Chua & Merrett, 2011) performed a systematic examination of the literature to identify translational studies that correlated HER2 with clinicopathologic markers and/or survival. This review included 49 studies totaling 11,337 patients. IHC was most commonly used to assess HER2 expression, identifying a median rate of 18% of gastric cancer demonstrating HER2 overexpression. In patients with and without HER2 overexpression, the median 3-year disease-free survival rate was 58% and 86%, respectively. Of the 35 studies reporting the impact of HER2 overexpression on survival, 20 studies (57%) reported no difference in overall survival, two studies (6%) reported significantly longer overall survival in patients with HER2 overexpression and 13 studies (37%) reported significantly poorer overall survival in patients with HER2 overexpression. HER2 overexpression appears to be associated with poorer survival and with intestinal-type gastric cancer in this group of patients for whom majority undergone curative gastrectomy. Results of the ToGA trial, which are discussed below, seem to refute this suggestion as demonstrated by the longer than expected survival of patients in the control arm, who received chemotherapy alone. However possible confounding factors, such as the wide use of second line treatment and the better prognosis associated with the intestinal histology, should be kept in mind when interpreting these results (Fornaro et al., 2011). In addition, these conflicting results could be due to the lack of a standardized definition of HER2 positivity in gastric cancer (De Vita et al., 2010)(Lorenzen & Lordick, 2011).

Hence, definitive answers about the prognostic role of HER2 in gastric cancer and gastric-esophageal cancer cannot be derived from the available data, which thus emphasizes the need for further research in the field (Fornaro et al., 2011).

4.4 Trastuzumab and the predictive role of HER2 in gastric cancer

Trastuzumab, a recombinant humanized IgG1 monoclonal antibody directed against the extracellular domain of HER2, induces antibody-dependent cellular cytotoxicity, inhibits HER2-mediated signaling and prevents cleavage of the extracellular domain of HER2. In HER2 positive breast cancer, trastuzumab has demonstrated survival benefits for patients with early and metastatic disease and is now the standard of care (Bang et al., 2010)(Croxtall & McKeage, 2010). Several studies indicate antitumor activity of trastuzumab in overexpressing HER2 human gastric cancer cell lines or xenograft models (Matsui et al., 2005)(Tanner et al., 2005)(Fujimoto-Ouchi et al., 2007). Most of these studies used the NCI-N87 and or 4-1ST gastric cell lines, which show HER2 expression in IHC and gene amplification on FISH. These studies showed that trastuzumab suppressed the growth of human gastric cancer with HER2 overexpression *in vitro* and *in vivo* and improved the survival of mice with peritoneal dissemination and ascites of gastric cancer. In addition, trastuzumab administered in combination with chemotherapy agents for gastric cancer showed potent antitumor activity, which was significantly greater than did trastuzumab or the chemotherapy agents as single treatments. A three-drug combination of capacetabine, cisplatin, and trastuzumab achieved remarkable tumor growth inhibition in the N87 model (Fujimoto-Ouchi et al., 2007)(Kim et al., 2008)(Gravalos & Jimeno, 2008). In addition, there are currently no data regarding resistance to trastuzumab in gastric cancer cells and there are no *in vitro* tests available to enable the prediction of resistance (Croxtall & McKeage, 2010).

Based on these results there was a strong rationale to investigate the clinical potential of trastuzumab in gastric cancer patients. Several preliminary single-arm phase II trials paved the way for the registration of the large, randomized controlled, open label, multicenter, international phase III trial which was undertaken in 24 centers in Aisa, Central and South America and Europe. The objective of this "Trastuzumab for Gastric Cancer" (ToGA) study was to assess the clinical efficacy and safety of trastuzumab added to chemotherapy for first-line treatment of advanced gastric or gastro-esophageal junction cancer with overexpression of HER2. Tumors were centrally tested for HER2 status with IHC (Hercep test) and FISH. Because of the inherent difference between breast and gastric tumors, notably tumor heterogeneity and the occurrence of baso(lateral) membrane staining, a new set of IHC scoring criteria were developed that are specific for gastric cancer. Patients were eligible if their tumor samples were scored as 3+ on IHC or if they were FISH positive (Bang et al., 2010) (Bang et al., 2010). As mentioned above, 22,1% of all gastric cancer screened in the ToGA trial were HER2-positive, which is broadly comparable with the incidence in breast cancer. Moreover, there was a high degree of concordance between IHC and FISH. Therefore, IHC is suitable for primary testing of HER2 positivity in gastric cancer with a score of IHC3+ indicating eligibility for treatment with trastuzumab, IHC2+ should be retested by FISH to confirm HER2 positivity and a score of IHC0 or 1+ should be considered as HER2-negative. The incidence of HER2 positivity differed according to tumor location and histological subtype. There was a significantly greater incidence of HER2-positive cancers of the oesophagogastric junction than the stomach and in intestinal than diffuse or mixed cancers. In addition, the incidence of HER2 positive gastric cancers was similar between Europe and Asia, but varied between countries (Croxtall & McKeage, 2010). Patients who satisfied all eligibility criteria (594 patients) were randomized in a 1:1 ratio and

584 patients received treatment with trastuzumab plus chemotherapy (5FU or capecitabine and cisplatin) for six cycles or chemotherapy alone (Lorenzen & Lordick, 2011). The primary objective was to compare overall survival in both treatment arms, and the secondary objectives were to compare progression-free survival, time to progression, overall response rate, control disease, duration of response, and quality of life (Gravalos & Jimeno, 2008). The primary endpoint of the study was met: trastuzumab significantly improved overall survival by nearly 3 months (median 11.1 vs 13.8 months) (Lorenzen & Lordick, 2011). In addition, an exploratory post-hoc analysis showed that trastuzumab plus chemotherapy substantially improved overall survival in patients with high expression of HER2 protein (IHC2+/FISH+ or IHC3+, 16 months) compared with patients with low expression of HER2 protein (IHC0 or 1+ and FISH+) (Bang et al., 2010). The secondary endpoints also showed significant improvements when trastuzumab was added to chemotherapy. The addition of trastuzumab to chemotherapy did not increase toxic effects associated with standard fluoropyrimidine-based and platinum-based chemotherapy and therefore trastuzumab can be combined with standard chemotherapy without affecting the overall safety profile. On the basis of these findings, trastuzumab can be considered as a new standard option for patients with HER2-positive advanced gastric or gastro-oesophageal junction cancer when combined with a chemotherapy regimen consisting of capecitabine plus cisplatin or fluorouracil plus cisplatin (Bang et al., 2010).

On the basis of this evidence, in January 2010 the EMEA and on 20 October 2010, the US FDA granted approval for trastuzumab in combination with cisplatin and fluoropyrimidine (either capecitabine or 5FU), for the treatment of metastatic HER-2 positive gastric or gastro-oesophageal junction adenocarcinoma who have not received prior treatment for metastatic disease (Lorenzen & Lordick, 2011).

Further studies are necessary to investigate the role of trastuzumab in curative gastric cancer treatment, as well its role as monotherapy, maintenance therapy and second line treatment in the palliative setting. Furthermore, additional predictive markers are needed besides a HER2-positive status. In addition, there is an urgent need to improve the knowledge of the mechanisms involved in anti-HER2 sensitivity or resistance, in order to develop other rationally targeted agents in the near future (Fornaro et al., 2011).

4.5 Conclusion

Since there is no internationally accepted standard of care for gastric or gastro-esophageal cancer patients and survival remains poor, new therapeutic strategies are needed. There is mounting evidence of the role of HER2 overexpression in patients with gastric cancer. HER2 overexpression has been correlated to poor outcome and more aggressive disease. Furthermore, the positive results of the randomized phase III ToGA trial have opened up new frontiers. Trastuzumab not only represents a new and effective therapeutic option, but has also stimulated the search for predictive marker in order to refine patient selection (Fornaro et al., 2011). Trastuzumab represents a new reference treatment for patients with HER2-positive metastatic gastric or gastro-esophageal cancer. Routine HER2 testing is suggested for all patients with advanced disease. Other agents directed against members of the HER family (like lapatinib) are currently under investigation (Lorenzen & Lordick, 2011).

5. General conclusion

Ample data shows that only a limited portion of patients may benefit from anti-cancer treatments currently used in the clinic. Personalized cancer medicine, based on genetic profiling of individual tumors and biomarkers, is regarded as the treatment strategy of the future. In this review the most promising biomarkers in colorectal, pancreatic and gastric cancer were discussed (table 2). Currently, the only biomarker that has made it into clinical practice for colorectal cancer is *KRAS* mutation for the selection of patients eligible for cetuximab therapy. Furthermore, evidence shows that other molecular alterations, such as *BRAF*, *PIK3CA* (exon-20) mutations or loss of PTEN expression, could preclude response to EGFR moAb.

Location	Predictive	Prognostic	Stage
Colorectal cancer	KRAS		Clinical stage (since 2008)
	PIK3CA exon 20 mut.		Preclinical stage
		BRAF	Preclinical stage
Pancreatic cancer	CA19-9		Clinical stage
	hENT1	hENT1	Preclinical stage
	miRs	miRs	Preclinical stage
		GLUT	Preclinical stage
Gastric cancer	HER2		Clinical stage (since 2010)
		HER2	Preclinical stage

Table 2. The most promising biomarkers in colorectal, pancreatic and gastric cancer summarized

Improved screening for early diagnosis is essential in order to increase the rate of curatively resectable pancreatic carcinomas, thereby ameliorating patient's prognosis. A relatively non-invasive, cost efficient possibility could be provided by the measurement of disease-specific markers in peripheral blood. However, only a few markers have shown promising results in recent studies with CA19-9 being the most widely investigated and evaluated single marker (Bünger et al., 2011).

In patients with gastric cancer there is mounting evidence of the role of HER2 overexpression since it has been correlated to poor outcome and more aggressive disease. Furthermore, HER 2 overexpression was found to be predictive for treatment of gastric cancer patients with trastuzumab. Routine HER2 testing is now suggested for all patients with advanced disease.

Given the importance of biomarkers in this era of targeted therapies more and especially prospective randomized trials are necessary.

6. References

Allegra, C. J., Jessup, J. M., Somerfield, M. R., Hamilton, S. R., Hammond, E. H., Hayes, D. F., McAllister, P. K., Morton, R. F. & Schilsky, R. L. (2009). American Society of Clinical Oncology provisional clinical opinion: testing for KRAS gene mutations in patients with metastatic colorectal carcinoma to predict response to anti-epidermal growth factor receptor monoclonal antibody therapy. *Journal of clinical oncology : official journal of the American Society of Clinical Oncology* 27(12), 2091–2096.

Ananiev, J., Gulubova, M., Manolova, I. & Tchernev, G. (2011). Prognostic significance of HER2/neu expression in gastric cancer. *Wiener klinische Wochenschrift* 123(13-14), 450–454.

Ansari, D., Rosendahl, A., Elebro, J. & Andersson, R. (2011). Systematic review of immunohistochemical biomarkers to identify prognostic subgroups of patients with pancreatic cancer. *The British journal of surgery* 98(8), 1041–1055.

Bang, Y.-J., Van Cutsem, E., Feyereislova, A., Chung, H. C., Shen, L., Sawaki, A., Lordick, F., Ohtsu, A., Omuro, Y., Satoh, T., Aprile, G., Kulikov, E., Hill, J., Lehle, M., Rüschoff, J., Kang, Y.-K.ToGA Trial Investigators (2010). Trastuzumab in combination with chemotherapy versus chemotherapy alone for treatment of HER2-positive advanced gastric or gastro-oesophageal junction cancer (ToGA): a phase 3, open-label, randomised controlled trial. *Lancet* 376(9742), 687–697.

Barault, L., Veyrie, N., Jooste, V., Lecorre, D., Chapusot, C., Ferraz, J.-M., Lièvre, A., Cortet, M., Bouvier, A.-M., Rat, P., Roignot, P., Faivre, J., Laurent-Puig, P. & Piard, F. (2008). Mutations in the RAS-MAPK, PI(3)K (phosphatidylinositol-3-OH kinase) signaling network correlate with poor survival in a population-based series of colon cancers. *International journal of cancer. Journal international du cancer* 122(10), 2255–2259.

Basturk, O., Singh, R., Kaygusuz, E., Balci, S., Dursun, N., Culhaci, N. & Adsay, N. V. (2011). GLUT-1 expression in pancreatic neoplasia: implications in pathogenesis, diagnosis, and prognosis. *Pancreas* 40(2), 187–192.

Bellon, E., Ligtenberg, M. J. L., Tejpar, S., Cox, K., de Hertogh, G., de Stricker, K., Edsjö, A., Gorgoulis, V., Höfler, G., Jung, A., Kotsinas, A., Laurent-Puig, P., López-Ríos, F., Hansen, T. P., Rouleau, E., Vandenberghe, P., van Krieken, J. J. M. & Dequeker, E. (2011). External quality assessment for KRAS testing is needed: setup of a European program and report of the first joined regional quality assessment rounds. *The oncologist* 16(4), 467–478.

Bloomston, M., Frankel, W. L., Petrocca, F., Volinia, S., Alder, H., Hagan, J. P., Liu, C.-G., Bhatt, D., Taccioli, C. & Croce, C. M. (2007). MicroRNA expression patterns to differentiate pancreatic adenocarcinoma from normal pancreas and chronic pancreatitis. *JAMA : the journal of the American Medical Association* 297(17), 1901–1908.

Buxbaum, J. L. & Eloubeidi, M. A. (2010). Molecular and clinical markers of pancreas cancer. *JOP : Journal of the pancreas* 11(6), 536–544.

Bünger, S., Laubert, T., Roblick, U. J. & Habermann, J. K. (2011). Serum biomarkers for improved diagnostic of pancreatic cancer: a current overview. *Journal of cancer research and clinical oncology* 137(3), 375–389.

Chen, Y. F., Mai, C. R., Tie, Z. J., Feng, Z. T., Zhang, J., Lu, X. H., Lu, G. J., Xue, Y. H. & Pan, G. Z. (1989). The diagnostic significance of carbohydrate antigen CA 19-9 in serum and pancreatic juice in pancreatic carcinoma. *Chinese medical journal* 102(5), 333–337.

Chua, T. C. & Merrett, N. D. (2011). Clinicopathologic factors associated with HER2-Positive gastric cancer and its impact on survival outcomes - a systematic review. *International journal of cancer. Journal international du cancer, DOI: 10.1002/ijc26292.*

Croxtall, J. D. & McKeage, K. (2010). Trastuzumab: in HER2-positive metastatic gastric cancer. *Drugs* 70(17), 2259–2267.

Dasari, A. & Messersmith, W. A. (2010). New strategies in colorectal cancer: biomarkers of response to epidermal growth factor receptor monoclonal antibodies and potential therapeutic targets in phosphoinositide 3-kinase and mitogen-activated protein kinase pathways. *Clinical cancer research : an official journal of the American Association for Cancer Research* 16(15), 3811–3818.

De Roock, W., Biesmans, B., De Schutter, J. & Tejpar, S. (2009). Clinical biomarkers in oncology: focus on colorectal cancer. *Molecular diagnosis & therapy* 13(2), 103–114.

De Roock, W., Jonker, D. J., Di Nicolantonio, F., Sartore-Bianchi, A., Tu, D., Siena, S., Lamba, S., Arena, S., Frattini, M., Piessevaux, H., Van Cutsem, E., O'Callaghan, C. J., Khambata-Ford, S., Zalcberg, J. R., Simes, J., Karapetis, C. S., Bardelli, A. & Tejpar, S. (2010a). Association of KRAS p.G13D mutation with outcome in patients with chemotherapy-refractory metastatic colorectal cancer treated with cetuximab. *JAMA : the journal of the American Medical Association* 304(16), 1812–1820.

De Roock, W., Claes, B., Bernasconi, D., De Schutter, J., Biesmans, B., Fountzilas, G., Kalogeras, K. T., Kotoula, V., Papamichael, D., Laurent-Puig, P., Penault-Llorca, F., Rougier, P., Vincenzi, B., Santini, D., Tonini, G., Cappuzzo, F., Frattini, M., Molinari, F., Saletti, P., De Dosso, S., Martini, M., Bardelli, A., Siena, S., Sartore-Bianchi, A., Tabernero, J., Macarulla, T., Di Fiore, F., Gangloff, A. O., Ciardiello, F., Pfeiffer, P., Qvortrup, C., Hansen, T. P., Van Cutsem, E., Piessevaux, H., Lambrechts, D., Delorenzi, M. & Tejpar, S. (2010b). Effects of KRAS, BRAF, NRAS, and PIK3CA mutations on the efficacy of cetuximab plus chemotherapy in chemotherapy-refractory metastatic colorectal cancer: a retrospective consortium analysis. *The lancet oncology* 11(8), 753–762.

De Roock, W., De Vriendt, V., Normanno, N., Ciardiello, F. & Tejpar, S. (2011). KRAS, BRAF, PIK3CA, and PTEN mutations: implications for targeted therapies in metastatic colorectal cancer. *The lancet oncology* 12(6), 594–603.

De Vita, F., Giuliani, F., Silvestris, N., Catalano, G., Ciardiello, F. & Orditura, M. (2010). Human epidermal growth factor receptor 2 (HER2) in gastric cancer: a new therapeutic target. *Cancer treatment reviews* 36 Suppl 3, S11–5.

Deschoolmeester, V., Baay, M., Specenier, P., Lardon, F. & Vermorken, J. B. (2010). A review of the most promising biomarkers in colorectal cancer: one step closer to targeted therapy. *The oncologist* 15(7), 699–731.

Di Nicolantonio, F., Martini, M., Molinari, F., Sartore-Bianchi, A., Arena, S., Saletti, P., De Dosso, S., Mazzucchelli, L., Frattini, M., Siena, S. & Bardelli, A. (2008). Wild-type BRAF is required for response to panitumumab or cetuximab in metastatic colorectal cancer. *Journal of clinical oncology : official journal of the American Society of Clinical Oncology* 26(35), 5705–5712.

Duffy, M. J. & Crown, J. (2008). A personalized approach to cancer treatment: how biomarkers can help. *Clinical chemistry* 54(11), 1770–1779.

Farrell, J. J., Elsaleh, H., Garcia, M., Lai, R., Ammar, A., Regine, W. F., Abrams, R., Benson, A. B., Macdonald, J., Cass, C. E., Dicker, A. P. & Mackey, J. R. (2009). Human equilibrative nucleoside transporter 1 levels predict response to gemcitabine in patients with pancreatic cancer. *Gastroenterology* 136(1), 187–195.

Fornaro, L., Lucchesi, M., Caparello, C., Vasile, E., Caponi, S., Ginocchi, L., Masi, G. & Falcone, A. (2011). Anti-HER agents in gastric cancer: from bench to bedside. *Nature reviews. Gastroenterology & hepatology* 8(7), 369–383.

Fujimoto-Ouchi, K., Sekiguchi, F., Yasuno, H., Moriya, Y., Mori, K. & Tanaka, Y. (2007). Antitumor activity of trastuzumab in combination with chemotherapy in human gastric cancer xenograft models. *Cancer chemotherapy and pharmacology* 59(6), 795–805.

Gentiloni, N., Caradonna, P., Costamagna, G., D'Ostilio, N., Perri, V., Mutignani, M., Febbraro, S., Tinari, N., Iacobelli, S. & Natoli, C. (1995). Pancreatic juice 90K and serum CA 19-9 combined determination can discriminate between pancreatic cancer and chronic pancreatitis. *The American journal of gastroenterology* 90(7), 1069–1072.

Goel, A., Arnold, C. N., Niedzwiecki, D., Carethers, J. M., Dowell, J. M., Wasserman, L., Compton, C., Mayer, R. J., Bertagnolli, M. M. & Boland, C. R. (2004). Frequent inactivation of PTEN by promoter hypermethylation in microsatellite instability-high sporadic colorectal cancers. *Cancer research* 64(9), 3014–3021.

Grabsch, H., Sivakumar, S., Gray, S., Gabbert, H. E. & Müller, W. (2010). HER2 expression in gastric cancer: Rare, heterogeneous and of no prognostic value - conclusions from 924 cases of two independent series. *Cellular oncology : the official journal of the International Society for Cellular Oncology* 32(1-2), 57–65.

Gravalos, C. & Jimeno, A. (2008). HER2 in gastric cancer: a new prognostic factor and a novel therapeutic target. *Annals of oncology : official journal of the European Society for Medical Oncology / ESMO* 19(9), 1523–1529.

Hamada, S. & Shimosegawa, T. (2011). Biomarkers of pancreatic cancer. *Pancreatology : official journal of the International Association of Pancreatology (IAP) ... [et al.]* 11 Suppl 2, 14–19.

Harding, J. & Burtness, B. (2005). Cetuximab: an epidermal growth factor receptor chemeric human-murine monoclonal antibody. *Drugs of today (Barcelona, Spain : 1998)* 41(2), 107–127.

Hayes, D. F., Bast, R. C., Desch, C. E., Fritsche, H., Kemeny, N. E., Jessup, J. M., Locker, G. Y., Macdonald, J. S., Mennel, R. G., Norton, L., Ravdin, P., Taube, S. & Winn, R. J. (1996). Tumor marker utility grading system: a framework to evaluate clinical utility of tumor markers. *Journal of the National Cancer Institute* 88(20), 1456–1466.

Ikenaga, N., Ohuchida, K., Mizumoto, K., Yu, J., Kayashima, T., Sakai, H., Fujita, H., Nakata, K. & Tanaka, M. (2010). MicroRNA-203 expression as a new prognostic marker of pancreatic adenocarcinoma. *Annals of surgical oncology* 17(12), 3120–3128.

Im, S.-A., Lee, K. E., Nam, E., Kim, D. Y., Lee, J.-H., Han, H.-S., Seoh, J.-Y., Park, H.-Y., Cho, M.-S., Han, W. S. & Lee, S. N. (2005). Potential prognostic significance of p185(HER2) overexpression with loss of PTEN expression in gastric carcinomas. *Tumori* 91(6), 513–521.

Ito, H., Duxbury, M., Zinner, M. J., Ashley, S. W. & Whang, E. E. (2004). Glucose transporter-1 gene expression is associated with pancreatic cancer invasiveness and MMP-2 activity. *Surgery* 136(3), 548–556.

Jang, K.-S., Song, Y. S., Jang, S.-H., Min, K.-W., Na, W., Jang, S. M., Jun, Y. J., Lee, K. H., Choi, D. & Paik, S. S. (2010). Clinicopathological significance of nuclear PTEN expression in colorectal adenocarcinoma. *Histopathology* 56(2), 229–239.

Kato, S., Iida, S., Higuchi, T., Ishikawa, T., Takagi, Y., Yasuno, M., Enomoto, M., Uetake, H. & Sugihara, K. (2007). PIK3CA mutation is predictive of poor survival in patients with colorectal cancer. *International journal of cancer. Journal international du cancer* 121(8), 1771–1778.

Kim, K. C., Koh, Y. W., Chang, H.-M., Kim, T. H., Yook, J. H., Kim, B. S., Jang, S. J. & Park, Y. S. (2011a). Evaluation of HER2 protein expression in gastric carcinomas: comparative analysis of 1,414 cases of whole-tissue sections and 595 cases of tissue microarrays. *Annals of surgical oncology* 18(10), 2833–2840.

Kim, R., Tan, A., Lai, K. K., Jiang, J., Wang, Y., Rybicki, L. A. & Liu, X. (2011b). Prognostic roles of human equilibrative transporter 1 (hENT-1) and ribonucleoside reductase subunit M1 (RRM1) in resected pancreatic cancer. *Cancer* 117(14), 3126–3134.

Kim, S. Y., Kim, H. P., Kim, Y. J., Oh, D.-Y., Im, S.-A., Lee, D., Jong, H.-S., Kim, T.-Y. & Bang, Y.-J. (2008). Trastuzumab inhibits the growth of human gastric cancer cell lines with HER2 amplification synergistically with cisplatin. *International journal of oncology* 32(1), 89–95.

Koch, C., Zeuzem, S. & Trojan, J. (2011). The KRAS p.G13D Mutation in Patients With Metastatic Colorectal Cancer: A Cheat in the Orchestra of Predictive Biomarkers? *Gastroenterology* 141(4), 1527–1528.

Laurent-Puig, P., Cayre, A., Manceau, G., Buc, E., Bachet, J.-B., Lecomte, T., Rougier, P., Lièvre, A., Landi, B., Boige, V., Ducreux, M., Ychou, M., Bibeau, F., Bouché, O., Reid, J., Stone, S. & Penault-Llorca, F. (2009). Analysis of PTEN, BRAF, and EGFR status in determining benefit from cetuximab therapy in wild-type KRAS metastatic colon cancer. *Journal of clinical oncology : official journal of the American Society of Clinical Oncology* 27(35), 5924–5930.

Lee, E. J., Gusev, Y., Jiang, J., Nuovo, G. J., Lerner, M. R., Frankel, W. L., Morgan, D. L., Postier, R. G., Brackett, D. J. & Schmittgen, T. D. (2007). Expression profiling identifies microRNA signature in pancreatic cancer. *International journal of cancer. Journal international du cancer* 120(5), 1046–1054.

Lièvre, A., Bachet, J.-B., Le Corre, D., Boige, V., Landi, B., Emile, J.-F., Côté, J.-F., Tomasic, G., Penna, C., Ducreux, M., Rougier, P., Penault-Llorca, F. & Laurent-Puig, P. (2006). KRAS mutation status is predictive of response to cetuximab therapy in colorectal cancer. *Cancer research* 66(8), 3992–3995.

Lockhart, A. C., Lockhart, C. & Berlin, J. D. (2005). The epidermal growth factor receptor as a target for colorectal cancer therapy. *Seminars in oncology* 32(1), 52–60.

Lorenzen, S. & Lordick, F. (2011). How will human epidermal growth factor receptor 2-neu data impact clinical management of gastric cancer? *Current opinion in oncology* 23(4), 396–402.

Loupakis, F., Ruzzo, A., Cremolini, C., Vincenzi, B., Salvatore, L., Santini, D., Masi, G., Stasi, I., Canestrari, E., Rulli, E., Floriani, I., Bencardino, K., Galluccio, N., Catalano, V., Tonini, G., Magnani, M., Fontanini, G., Basolo, F., Falcone, A. & Graziano, F. (2009a). KRAS codon 61, 146 and BRAF mutations predict resistance to cetuximab plus irinotecan in KRAS codon 12 and 13 wild-type metastatic colorectal cancer. *British journal of cancer* 101(4), 715–721.

Loupakis, F., Pollina, L., Stasi, I., Ruzzo, A., Scartozzi, M., Santini, D., Masi, G., Graziano, F., Cremolini, C., Rulli, E., Canestrari, E., Funel, N., Schiavon, G., Petrini, I., Magnani, M., Tonini, G., Campani, D., Floriani, I., Cascinu, S. & Falcone, A. (2009b). PTEN expression and KRAS mutations on primary tumors and metastases in the prediction of benefit from cetuximab plus irinotecan for patients with metastatic colorectal cancer. *Journal of clinical oncology : official journal of the American Society of Clinical Oncology* 27(16), 2622–2629.

Lyshchik, A., Higashi, T., Hara, T., Nakamoto, Y., Fujimoto, K., Doi, R., Imamura, M., Saga, T. & Togashi, K. (2007). Expression of glucose transporter-1, hexokinase-II, proliferating cell nuclear antigen and survival of patients with pancreatic cancer. *Cancer investigation* 25(3), 154–162.

Malesci, A., Tommasini, M. A., Bonato, C., Bocchia, P., Bersani, M., Zerbi, A., Beretta, E. & Di Carlo, V. (1987). Determination of CA 19-9 antigen in serum and pancreatic juice for differential diagnosis of pancreatic adenocarcinoma from chronic pancreatitis. *Gastroenterology* 92(1), 60–67.

Maréchal, R., Mackey, J. R., Lai, R., Demetter, P., Peeters, M., Polus, M., Cass, C. E., Young, J., Salmon, I., Devière, J. & Van Laethem, J.-L. (2009). Human equilibrative nucleoside transporter 1 and human concentrative nucleoside transporter 3 predict survival after adjuvant gemcitabine therapy in resected pancreatic adenocarcinoma. *Clinical cancer research : an official journal of the American Association for Cancer Research* 15(8), 2913–2919.

Matsui, Y., Inomata, M., Tojigamori, M., Sonoda, K., Shiraishi, N. & Kitano, S. (2005). Suppression of tumor growth in human gastric cancer with HER2 overexpression by an anti-HER2 antibody in a murine model. *International journal of oncology* 27(3), 681–685.

Matsumoto, S., Harada, H., Tanaka, J., Ochi, K., Seno, T., Tsurumi, T. & Kunichika, K. (1994). Evaluation of cytology and tumor markers of pure pancreatic juice for the diagnosis of pancreatic cancer at early stages. *Pancreas* 9(6), 741–747.

Mees, S. T., Mardin, W. A., Wendel, C., Baeumer, N., Willscher, E., Senninger, N., Schleicher, C., Colombo-Benkmann, M. & Haier, J. (2010). EP300--a miRNA-regulated metastasis suppressor gene in ductal adenocarcinomas of the pancreas. *International journal of cancer. Journal international du cancer* 126(1), 114–124.

Melstrom, L. G., Salabat, M. R., Ding, X.-Z., Milam, B. M., Strouch, M., Pelling, J. C. & Bentrem, D. J. (2008). Apigenin inhibits the GLUT-1 glucose transporter and the phosphoinositide 3-kinase/Akt pathway in human pancreatic cancer cells. *Pancreas* 37(4), 426–431.

Meriggi, F., Di Biasi, B., Abeni, C. & Zaniboni, A. (2009). Anti-EGFR therapy in colorectal cancer: how to choose the right patient. *Current drug targets* 10(10), 1033–1040.

Molinari, F., Martin, V., Saletti, P., De Dosso, S., Spitale, A., Camponovo, A., Bordoni, A., Crippa, S., Mazzucchelli, L. & Frattini, M. (2009). Differing deregulation of EGFR and downstream proteins in primary colorectal cancer and related metastatic sites may be clinically relevant. *British journal of cancer* 100(7), 1087–1094.

Morinaga, S., Nakamura, Y., Watanabe, T., Mikayama, H., Tamagawa, H., Yamamoto, N., Shiozawa, M., Akaike, M., Ohkawa, S., Kameda, Y. & Miyagi, Y. (2011). Immunohistochemical Analysis of Human Equilibrative Nucleoside Transporter-1 (hENT1) Predicts Survival in Resected Pancreatic Cancer Patients Treated with Adjuvant Gemcitabine Monotherapy. *Annals of surgical oncology*.

Murata, Y., Hamada, T., Kishiwada, M., Ohsawa, I., Mizuno, S., Usui, M., Sakurai, H., Tabata, M., Ii, N., Inoue, H., Shiraishi, T. & Isaji, S. (2011). Human equilibrative nucleoside transporter 1 expression is a strong independent prognostic factor in UICC T3-T4 pancreatic cancer patients treated with preoperative gemcitabine-based chemoradiotherapy. *Journal of hepato-biliary-pancreatic sciences,* DOI: 10.1007/S00534-011-0440-3

Nakaizumi, A., Uehara, H., Takenaka, A., Uedo, N., Sakai, N., Yano, H., Ohigashi, H., Ishikawa, O., Ishiguro, S., Sugano, K. & Tatsuta, M. (1999). Diagnosis of pancreatic cancer by cytology and measurement of oncogene and tumor markers in pure pancreatic juice aspirated by endoscopy. *Hepato-gastroenterology* 46(25), 31–37.

Nash, G. M., Gimbel, M., Shia, J., Nathanson, D. R., Ndubuisi, M. I., Zeng, Z.-S., Kemeny, N. & Paty, P. B. (2010). KRAS mutation correlates with accelerated metastatic progression in patients with colorectal liver metastases. *Annals of surgical oncology* 17(2), 572–578.

Neumann, J., Zeindl-Eberhart, E., Kirchner, T. & Jung, A. (2009). Frequency and type of KRAS mutations in routine diagnostic analysis of metastatic colorectal cancer. *Pathology, research and practice* 205(12), 858–862.

Ng, K. & Zhu, A. X. (2008). Targeting the epidermal growth factor receptor in metastatic colorectal cancer. *Critical reviews in oncology/hematology* 65(1), 8–20.

Nishida, K., Tasaki, N., Miyagawa, H., Yoshikawa, T. & Kondo, M. (1988). Estimation of carbohydrate antigen (CA) 19-9 levels in pure pancreatic juice of patients with pancreatic cancer. *The American journal of gastroenterology* 83(2), 126–129.

Ogino, S., Nosho, K., Kirkner, G. J., Kawasaki, T., Meyerhardt, J. A., Loda, M., Giovannucci, E. L. & Fuchs, C. S. (2009a). CpG island methylator phenotype, microsatellite instability, BRAF mutation and clinical outcome in colon cancer. *Gut* 58(1), 90–96.

Ogino, S., Nosho, K., Kirkner, G. J., Shima, K., Irahara, N., Kure, S., Chan, A. T., Engelman, J. A., Kraft, P., Cantley, L. C., Giovannucci, E. L. & Fuchs, C. S. (2009b). PIK3CA mutation is associated with poor prognosis among patients with curatively resected colon cancer. *Journal of clinical oncology : official journal of the American Society of Clinical Oncology* 27(9), 1477–1484.

Oliveira, C., Westra, J. L., Arango, D., Ollikainen, M., Domingo, E., Ferreira, A., Velho, S., Niessen, R., Lagerstedt, K., Alhopuro, P., Laiho, P., Veiga, I., Teixeira, M. R., Ligtenberg, M., Kleibeuker, J. H., Sijmons, R. H., Plukker, J. T., Imai, K., Lage, P., Hamelin, R., Albuquerque, C., Schwartz, S., Lindblom, A., Peltomaki, P., Yamamoto, H., Aaltonen, L. A., Seruca, R. & Hofstra, R. M. W. (2004). Distinct patterns of KRAS mutations in colorectal carcinomas according to germline mismatch repair defects and hMLH1 methylation status. *Human molecular genetics* 13(19), 2303–2311.

Overman, M. J. & Hoff, P. M. (2007). EGFR-targeted therapies in colorectal cancer. *Diseases of the colon and rectum* 50(8), 1259–1270.

Park, J. H., Han, S.-W., Oh, D.-Y., Im, S.-A., Jeong, S.-Y., Park, K. J., Kim, T.-Y., Bang, Y.-J. & Park, J.-G. (2011). Analysis of KRAS, BRAF, PTEN, IGF1R, EGFR intron 1 CA status in both primary tumors and paired metastases in determining benefit from cetuximab therapy in colon cancer. *Cancer chemotherapy and pharmacology* 68(4), 1045–1055.

Perrone, F., Lampis, A., Orsenigo, M., Di Bartolomeo, M., Gevorgyan, A., Losa, M., Frattini, M., Riva, C., Andreola, S., Bajetta, E., Bertario, L., Leo, E., Pierotti, M. A. & Pilotti, S. (2009). PI3KCA/PTEN deregulation contributes to impaired responses to cetuximab in metastatic colorectal cancer patients. *Annals of oncology : official journal of the European Society for Medical Oncology / ESMO* 20(1), 84–90.

Pizzi, S., Porzionato, A., Pasquali, C., Guidolin, D., Sperti, C., Fogar, P., Macchi, V., De Caro, R., Pedrazzoli, S. & Parenti, A. (2009). Glucose transporter-1 expression and prognostic significance in pancreatic carcinogenesis. *Histology and histopathology* 24(2), 175–185.

Prenen, H., De Schutter, J., Jacobs, B., De Roock, W., Biesmans, B., Claes, B., Lambrechts, D., Van Cutsem, E. & Tejpar, S. (2009). PIK3CA mutations are not a major determinant of resistance to the epidermal growth factor receptor inhibitor cetuximab in metastatic colorectal cancer. *Clinical cancer research : an official journal of the American Association for Cancer Research* 15(9), 3184–3188.

Rachagani, S., Kumar, S. & Batra, S. K. (2010). MicroRNA in pancreatic cancer: pathological, diagnostic and therapeutic implications. *Cancer letters* 292(1), 8–16.

Rivera, F., Vega-Villegas, M. E. & López-Brea, M. F. (2008). Cetuximab, its clinical use and future perspectives. *Anti-cancer drugs* 19(2), 99–113.

Roth, A. D., Tejpar, S., Delorenzi, M., Yan, P., Fiocca, R., Klingbiel, D., Dietrich, D., Biesmans, B., Bodoky, G., Barone, C., Aranda, E., Nordlinger, B., Cisar, L., Labianca, R., Cunningham, D., Van Cutsem, E. & Bosman, F. (2010). Prognostic role of KRAS and BRAF in stage II and III resected colon cancer: results of the translational study on the PETACC-3, EORTC 40993, SAKK 60-00 trial. *Journal of clinical oncology : official journal of the American Society of Clinical Oncology* 28(3), 466–474.

Samowitz, W. S., Sweeney, C., Herrick, J., Albertsen, H., Levin, T. R., Murtaugh, M. A., Wolff, R. K. & Slattery, M. L. (2005). Poor survival associated with the BRAF V600E mutation in microsatellite-stable colon cancers. *Cancer research* 65(14), 6063–6069.

Sartore-Bianchi, A., Di Nicolantonio, F., Nichelatti, M., Molinari, F., De Dosso, S., Saletti, P., Martini, M., Cipani, T., Marrapese, G., Mazzucchelli, L., Lamba, S., Veronese, S., Frattini, M., Bardelli, A. & Siena, S. (2009a). Multi-determinants analysis of molecular alterations for predicting clinical benefit to EGFR-targeted monoclonal antibodies in colorectal cancer. *PloS one* 4(10), e7287.

Sartore-Bianchi, A., Martini, M., Molinari, F., Veronese, S., Nichelatti, M., Artale, S., Di Nicolantonio, F., Saletti, P., De Dosso, S., Mazzucchelli, L., Frattini, M., Siena, S. & Bardelli, A. (2009b). PIK3CA mutations in colorectal cancer are associated with clinical resistance to EGFR-targeted monoclonal antibodies. *Cancer research* 69(5), 1851–1857.

Sawai, H., Yasuda, A., Ochi, N., Ma, J., Matsuo, Y., Wakasugi, T., Takahashi, H., Funahashi, H., Sato, M. & Takeyama, H. (2008). Loss of PTEN expression is associated with colorectal cancer liver metastasis and poor patient survival. *BMC gastroenterology* 8, 56.

Scartozzi, M., Pierantoni, C., Berardi, R., Squadroni, M. & Cascinu, S. (2006a). Anti-EGFR strategies as an incremental step for the treatment of colorectal cancer patients: moving from scientific evidence to clinical practice. *Expert opinion on therapeutic targets* 10(2), 281–287.

Scartozzi, M., Pierantoni, C., Berardi, R., Antognoli, S., Bearzi, I. & Cascinu, S. (2006b). Epidermal growth factor receptor: a promising therapeutic target for colorectal cancer. *Analytical and quantitative cytology and histology / the International Academy of Cytology [and] American Society of Cytology* 28(2), 61–68.

Siena, S., Sartore-Bianchi, A., Di Nicolantonio, F., Balfour, J. & Bardelli, A. (2009). Biomarkers predicting clinical outcome of epidermal growth factor receptor-targeted therapy in metastatic colorectal cancer. *Journal of the National Cancer Institute* 101(19), 1308–1324.

Souglakos, J., Philips, J., Wang, R., Marwah, S., Silver, M., Tzardi, M., Silver, J., Ogino, S., Hooshmand, S., Kwak, E., Freed, E., Meyerhardt, J. A., Saridaki, Z., Georgoulias, V., Finkelstein, D., Fuchs, C. S., Kulke, M. H. & Shivdasani, R. A. (2009). Prognostic and predictive value of common mutations for treatment response and survival in patients with metastatic colorectal cancer. *British journal of cancer* 101(3), 465–472.

Spratlin, J., Sangha, R., Glubrecht, D., Dabbagh, L., Young, J. D., Dumontet, C., Cass, C., Lai, R. & Mackey, J. R. (2004). The absence of human equilibrative nucleoside transporter 1 is associated with reduced survival in patients with gemcitabine-treated pancreas adenocarcinoma. *Clinical cancer research : an official journal of the American Association for Cancer Research* 10(20), 6956–6961.

Sun, H.-C., Qiu, Z.-J., Liu, J., Sun, J., Jiang, T., Huang, K.-J., Yao, M. & Huang, C. (2007). Expression of hypoxia-inducible factor-1 alpha and associated proteins in pancreatic ductal adenocarcinoma and their impact on prognosis. *International journal of oncology* 30(6), 1359–1367.

Szafranska, A. E., Davison, T. S., John, J., Cannon, T., Sipos, B., Maghnouj, A., Labourier, E. & Hahn, S. A. (2007). MicroRNA expression alterations are linked to tumorigenesis and non-neoplastic processes in pancreatic ductal adenocarcinoma. *Oncogene* 26(30), 4442–4452.

Szafranska, A. E., Davison, T. S., Shingara, J., Doleshal, M., Riggenbach, J. A., Morrison, C. D., Jewell, S. & Labourier, E. (2008). Accurate molecular characterization of formalin-fixed, paraffin-embedded tissues by microRNA expression profiling. *The Journal of molecular diagnostics : JMD* 10(5), 415–423.

Tanner, M., Hollmén, M., Junttila, T. T., Kapanen, A. I., Tommola, S., Soini, Y., Helin, H., Salo, J., Joensuu, H., Sihvo, E., Elenius, K. & Isola, J. (2005). Amplification of HER-2 in gastric carcinoma: association with Topoisomerase IIalpha gene amplification, intestinal type, poor prognosis and sensitivity to trastuzumab. *Annals of oncology : official journal of the European Society for Medical Oncology / ESMO* 16(2), 273–278.

Tedesco, K. L., Lockhart, A. C. & Berlin, J. D. (2004). The epidermal growth factor receptor as a target for gastrointestinal cancer therapy. *Current treatment options in oncology* 5(5), 393–403.

Tejpar, S., Bertagnolli, M., Bosman, F., Lenz, H.-J., Garraway, L., Waldman, F., Warren, R., Bild, A., Collins-Brennan, D., Hahn, H., Harkin, D. P., Kennedy, R., Ilyas, M., Morreau, H., Proutski, V., Swanton, C., Tomlinson, I., Delorenzi, M., Fiocca, R., Van Cutsem, E. & Roth, A. (2010). Prognostic and predictive biomarkers in resected colon cancer: current status and future perspectives for integrating genomics into biomarker discovery. *The oncologist* 15(4), 390–404.

Tol, J., Nagtegaal, I. D. & Punt, C. J. A. (2009). BRAF mutation in metastatic colorectal cancer. *The New England journal of medicine* 361(1), 98–99.

US National Academy Press, Institute of Medicine (U.S.). Committee on Developing Biomarker-Based Tools for Cancer Screening, Diagnosis, and Treatment (2007).

Cancer biomarkers. p 236 Natl Academy Pr. (the promises and challenges of improving detection and treatment).

Van Cutsem, E., Köhne, C.-H., Láng, I., Folprecht, G., Nowacki, M. P., Cascinu, S., Shchepotin, I., Maurel, J., Cunningham, D., Tejpar, S., Schlichting, M., Zubel, A., Celik, I., Rougier, P. & Ciardiello, F. (2011). Cetuximab plus irinotecan, fluorouracil, and leucovorin as first-line treatment for metastatic colorectal cancer: updated analysis of overall survival according to tumor KRAS and BRAF mutation status. *Journal of clinical oncology : official journal of the American Society of Clinical Oncology* 29(15), 2011–2019.

Vincent, A., Herman, J., Schulick, R., Hruban, R. H. & Goggins, M. (2011). Pancreatic cancer. *Lancet* 378(9791), 607–620.

Wagner, A. D. & Moehler, M. (2009). Development of targeted therapies in advanced gastric cancer: promising exploratory steps in a new era. *Current opinion in oncology* 21(4), 381–385.

Wang, J. & Sen, S. (2011). MicroRNA functional network in pancreatic cancer: from biology to biomarkers of disease. *Journal of biosciences* 36(3), 481–491.

Xu, B., Zheng, W.-Y., Jin, D.-Y., Ding, W.-X., Lou, W.-H. & Ramsohok, L. (2011). Predictive value of serum carbohydrate antigen 19-9 in malignant intraductal papillary mucinous neoplasms. *World journal of surgery* 35(5), 1103–1109.

Yokota, T., Ura, T., Shibata, N., Takahari, D., Shitara, K., Nomura, M., Kondo, C., Mizota, A., Utsunomiya, S., Muro, K. & Yatabe, Y. (2011). BRAF mutation is a powerful prognostic factor in advanced and recurrent colorectal cancer. *British journal of cancer* 104(5), 856–862.

Zhang, X. L., Yang, Y. S., Xu, D. P., Qu, J. H., Guo, M. Z., Gong, Y. & Huang, J. (2009a). Comparative study on overexpression of HER2/neu and HER3 in gastric cancer. *World journal of surgery* 33(10), 2112–2118.

Zhang, Y., Li, M., Wang, H., Fisher, W. E., Lin, P. H., Yao, Q. & Chen, C. (2009b). Profiling of 95 microRNAs in pancreatic cancer cell lines and surgical specimens by real-time PCR analysis. *World journal of surgery* 33(4), 698–709.

2

MicroRNAs are Novel Biomarkers for Detection of Colorectal Cancer

Muhammad Imran Aslam[1,2], Maleene Patel[1 2], Baljit Singh[1,2], John Stuart Jameson[2] and James Howard Pringle[1]
[1]*Department of Cancer Studies and Molecular Medicine, University of Leicester, Robert Kilpatrick Clinical Sciences Building, Leicester Royal Infirmary,*
[2]*Department of Colorectal Surgery, University Hospitals of Leicester NHS Trust, Leicester General Hospital, Gwendolen Road, Leicester, United Kingdom*

1. Introduction

Incidence of Colorectal Cancer: Colorectal cancer (CRC) is the third most common neoplasm worldwide. According to the International Agency for Research on Cancer (IARC), approximately 1.24 million new cases of CRC were detected worldwide in 2008 (Ferlay, et al, 2008). It is the third most common cancer in men (10.0% of the total) and the second commonest in women (9.4% of the total) worldwide. IARC data have shown that more than half of all CRC cases occur in the developed regions of the world i.e. Europe, America and Japan (Ferlay, et al, 2008). In the European Union (EU27) alone 334,000 new cases of CRC were detected in 2008 and approximately 38,000 people were diagnosed with CRC in the UK alone (National UK Statistics). The incidence of CRC is on rise in Europe, particularly in southern and Eastern Europe, where rates were originally lower than in Western Europe (Coleman, et al, 1993 & Bray, et al, 2004). Contrary to the current trend in Europe, the incidence rate of CRC in the USA has fallen in the last two decades (NCI-SEER, 2006). Epidemiological studies have identified that a rapid trend of 'Westernization', with change in diet and life style has resulted in increased incidence rates of CRC in developing countries (Marchand, et al, 1999, Flood, et al, 2000, Boyle, et al, 2008, & Ferlay, et al, 2010). The occurrence of CRC is strongly related to age, with nearly 80% of cases arising in people who are 60 years or older, although there has been a recent increase in incidence in people younger than 60. The lifetime risk for developing CRC in men is 1 in 16 whereas in women it is 1 in 20 (National Statistics, UK).

2. The need for improved biomarkers

The survival and prognosis of patients suffering from CRC depends on the stage of the tumour at time of detection. "Five year survival" significantly reduces from 93% for localized early cancerous lesions (Dukes A) to < 15% for advanced metastatic cancers (Dukes D). Unfortunately, approximately one third of patients with CRC have regional or distant spread of their disease at time of diagnosis (Ferlay, et al, 2008). Currently, bowel cancer screening programmes in Europe use either flexible sigmoidoscopy (FS) or guaiac-based faecal occult blood testing (FOBT) as the primary screening tool, with the current gold standard colonic imaging modality of colonoscopy being reserved for patients testing positive. Both primary screening tests have proven to be of benefit in reducing the death rate from CRC in randomised controlled trials but are generally considered to lack the desired convenience or accuracy for use as a general screening test (Hewitson, et al, 2007). A comparative study of diagnostic sensitivities of FOBT, faecal immunochemical stool testing (FIT), flexible sigmoidoscopy (FS), colonoscopy and CT colonography (CTC) has revealed 20%, 32%, 83.3% 100% and 96.7% sensitivity, respectively for the detection of CRC and advanced adenomas (Graser, et al, 2009) . Endoscopic and radiological diagnostic modalities are expensive and are associated with risks such as bleeding, infection, bowel perforation and exposure to radiation. This explains why there is still a need for an improved, reliable, accurate and non-invasive biomarker for colorectal cancer detection.

3. Colorectal cancer development

The development of CRC follows the sequential progression from adenoma to the carcinoma (Vogelstein, et al, 1988). Carcinogenesis pathways for colorectal neoplasia have become much clearer and precise in the past two decades. The common pathway for CRC development is dependent on Adenomatous Polyposis Coli (APC) & Tumour Protein-53 (TP53) gene mutations and is initiated through WNT signalling (Segditsas, et al, 2006). In this pathway colonic carcinoma originates from the colonic epithelium as a consequence of accumulation of genetic alterations in the tumour suppressor gene TP53 and oncogenic APC genes. The initial genetic alterations result in adenoma formation in which cells exhibit autonomous growth. During the further course of carcinogenesis, intestinal epithelial cells acquire the characteristics of invasion and the potential for metastasis. Another carcinogenesis pathway has recently gained acceptance and is commonly named as the serrated-neoplasia pathway. This pathway is for the most part APC and TP53 independent and shows distinct molecular features of somatic mutations such as BRAF mutation and concordance with high CpG islands methylation phenotype (CIMP-H), microsatellite instability (MSI+) and MutT homologue 1 (MLH1) methylation (Casey, et al, 2005 & Spring, et al, 2006,) . Sequential progression of colorectal neoplasia from adenoma to carcinoma highlights that opportunities exist to improve cancer specific survival by altering the natural course of disease development. Such interventions could potentially be chemo preventive for high risk individuals, the early detection of colorectal neoplasia, chemotherapy to down stage the cancer prior to surgical resection and therapy for palliation of symptoms in advanced stage cancer. Recent advances in proteomics and genomics provide a vast amount of information about the role of micro-molecules in several cancer related pathways. These advances have focused on the detection of micro molecules released from tumour cells and their utility as diagnostic biomarkers. The discovery of tumour specific microRNAs (miRNAs) has opened a new era of biomarker research that holds great potential for future cancer detection strategies.

4. What are MicroRNAs

MicroRNAs are single-stranded, evolutionarily conserved, small (17–25 ribonucleotides) noncoding (Lee, et al, 1993) RNA molecules. MiRNAs function as negative regulators of target genes by directing specific messenger RNA cleavage or translational inhibition through the RNA induced silencing complex (RISC) (Bartel, et al, 2004 & 2009). So far around 1400 mature human miRNAs have been described in the Sanger miRBase version 17 (An international registry and database for miRNA nomenclature, targets, functions and their implications in different diseases). In the database, each mature miRNA in human and non-human species is assigned a unique identifier number for universal standardization. For example human microRNA 21 is designated as hsa-miR-21. Table 1 summarizes the different types of RNAs by size, mechanism of action and function in human cells.

Types of Non Coding RNA	Size No of Nucleotides	Mechanism of Action	Function
MicroRNA (miRNA)	17-23	RNA induced silencing complex (RISC)	Translational Inhibition
Messanger RNA (mRNA)	900-1500	Conveys genetic information from DNA to the ribosomes	Protein synthesis
Small interfering RNA (SiRNA)	20-25 Double stranded	RNA interference and RNA interference related pathways	Interference with gene expression
Piwi-interacting RNA (piRNA)	26-31	RNA-protein complex formation with piwi proteins	Transcriptional gene silencing of retrotransposons and other genetic elements in germ line cells
Small Nucleolar RNA (SnoRNA)	70-200	Act as ribonucleoprotein (RNP) complexes to guide the enzymatic modification of target RNAs at sites determined by RNA:RNA antisense interactions	Chemical modifications of other RNAs e,g methylation, pseudouridylation
Transfer RNA (tRNAs)	73 to 93 Clover Leaf	Transfers a specific active amino acid to a growing polypeptide chain at the ribosomal site of Protein	Amino acid carriers and protein synthesis during translation.
Ribosomal RNA (rRNA)	120-5050	Decode mRNA into amino acids	Protein synthesis in ribosomes

Table 1.

5. MicroRNA biogenesis in human cells

MiRNAs are mostly transcribed from intragenic or intergenic regions by RNA polymerase II into primary transcripts (pri-miRNAs) of variable length (1 kb- 3 kb). In the nucleus Pri-miRNA transcript is further processed by the nuclear ribo-nuclease enzyme 'Drosha' thereby resulting in a hairpin intermediate of about 70–100 nucleotides, called pre-miRNA. The pre-miRNA is then transported out of the nucleus by a transporting protein exportin-5.

In the cytoplasm, the pre-miRNA is once again processed by another ribonuclease enzyme 'Dicer' into a mature double-stranded miRNA. The two strands of double stranded miRNA (miRNA/miRNA* complex) are separated by Dicer processing. After strand separation, the mature miRNA strand (miRNA- also called the guide strand) is incorporated into an RNA-induced silencing complex (RISC), whereas the passenger strand, denoted with a star (miRNA*) is commonly degraded (Hammond, et al, 2000, Lee, et al, 2003, Bohnsack, et al, 2004 & Thimmaiah, et al, 2005). This miRNA/RISC complex is responsible for miRNA function. If on miRNA cloning or array the passenger strand is found at low frequency (less than 15% of the guide strand) it is named miR*. However, if both passenger and guide strand are equal in distribution, then these two strands are named 3p and 5p version of miRNA depending on their location to either 5' or 3' of the miRNA molecule. In this case both strands can potentially incorporate in RISC complex and have a biological role. Nevertheless, quite a few miRNA* strands are found to be conserved and play an important role in cell homeostasis. However, only recently studies have focussed on the functional role of the miRNA* strand. Well-conserved miRNA* strands may prove important links in cancer regulation networks (Stark, et al, 2007, Okamura, et al, 2008, Zhou, et al, 2010 & Guo, et al, 2010). Figure 1 illustrates the biogenesis of miRNAs in the cellular nucleous, its transport to cytoplasm, and processing by Drosha and Dicer Enzymes. Figure 1 also illustrates the RISC incorporation of miRNAs for functional activity in different pathways of translational inhibition or activation.

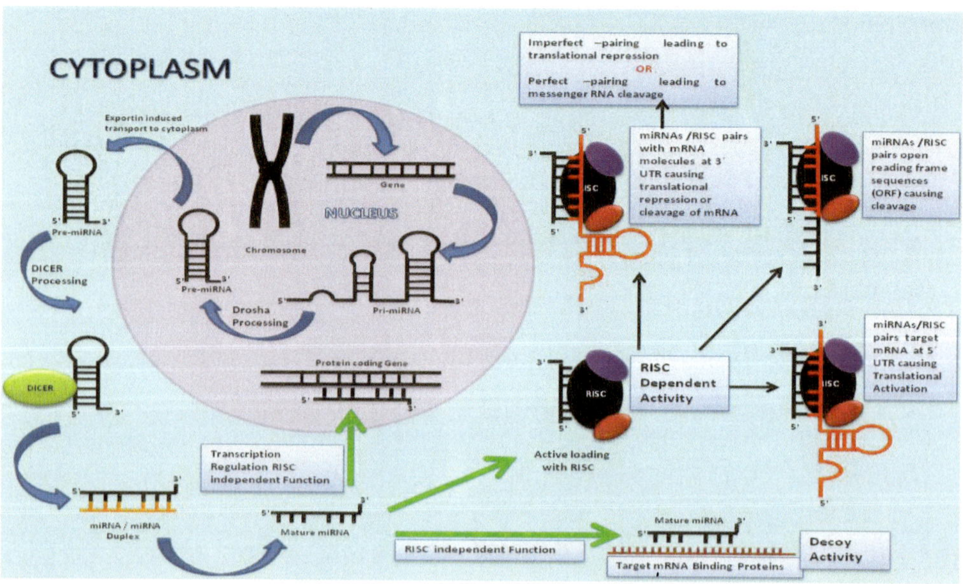

Fig. 1.

6. Mechanism of action & cellular function of MicroRNA

The specificity of miRNA targeting is defined by Watson–Crick complementarities between positions 2 to 8 from the 5 primed end of miRNA sequence with the 3′ untranslated region

(UTR) of their target mRNAs. When miRNA and its target mRNA sequence show perfect complementarities, the RISC induces mRNA degradation. Should an imperfect miRNA–mRNA target pairing occur, translation into a protein is blocked (Bartel, et al, 2004 & 2009). Regardless of which of these two events occur, the net result is a decrease in the amount of the proteins encoded by the mRNA targets. Each miRNA has the potential to target a large number of genes (on average about 500 for each miRNA family). Conversely, an estimated 60% of the mRNAs have one or more evolutionarily conserved sequences that are predicted to interact with miRNAs (Friedman, et al, 2009). MiRNAs have been shown to bind to the open reading frame or to the 5′ UTR of the target genes and, in some cases, they have been shown to activate rather than to inhibit gene expression (Ørom, et al, 2008). It has also reported that miRNAs can bind to ribonucleoproteins in a seed sequence and a RISC-independent manner and then interfere with their RNA binding functions (decoy activity) (Eiring, et al, 2010). MiRNAs can also regulate gene expression at the transcriptional level by binding directly to the DNA (Khraiwesh, et al, 2010) as illustrated in Figure 1.

7. Methods of MicroRNA analysis and quantification

Numerous approaches have been developed to analyze and quantify the expression of miRNAs. A commonly adopted strategy is to perform mass scale expression profiling/signature of miRNAs on a small cohort of patients to identify most significantly dysregulated miRNAs. Expression profiling is usually followed by a validation of selected miRNAs on an independent cohort by using QRT-PCR. Expression profiling has been performed using Hybridization-Microarray, Real Time Polymerase Chain Reaction (QRT-PCR) Array and most recently Deep-Sequencing (Meyer, et al, 2010). Most of these approaches are developed against the gold standard 'Northern Blotting'. Each has its unique advantages and disadvantages, such as throughput, sensitivity, ease of use and cost. QRT-PCR can detect very low concentrations of molecules with much superior sensitivity and expenditure of time and money (Chen, et al, 2005). Microarray-based techniques have the advantage of being relatively cost-effective, quick and simple to utilize (Pradervand, et al, 2010). Ultra high throughput miRNA sequencing allows de-novo detection and relative quantification of miRNAs, but requires a considerable amount of time and cost for data generation and data analysis (Wang, et al, 2007). A key issue of miRNA detection and quantification is the selection of endogenous controls for relative quantification. In QRT-PCR based detection systems, several small nuclear and small nucleolar RNAs (e.g. RNU6B) are recommended for normalising miRNA expression signature/profiles in tissues, cell lines, and human body fluids. However, RNU6B is heat unstable and rapidly degrades resulting in poor reproducibility of experiments. That's why many researchers have used the invariant and most stable miRNAs as endogenous controls (Meyer, et al, 2010). In order to overcome this problem of normalization in QRT-PCR and other detection systems, researchers have used different statistical strategies including: global mean expression; quantile; scaling; and normalizing factor. However, some normalization methods have been challenged whereas others were adapted to the specific nature of miRNA profiling experiments. At present, there is no generally agreed normalization strategy for any of the known detection approaches. Table 2 shows the comparison of different detection systems by practical application, throughput, cost and time expenditure.

Detection Systems	MicroRNA QRT-PCR Expression Profiling	MicroRNA-Array	MicroRNA-Sequencing
Method	PCR	Hybridization	Deep Sequencing
Initial RNA Concentration	10ng	100 ng	250ng
Time Required	< 24 hours	24-48 hours	>1 week
Cost	Low-medium for Pool Profiling. Even lower for custom designed individual assays.	Low-medium for Pool Profiling	High
Throughput	Medium-high	High	Ultra-high
Utility	Relative and absolute quantification of miRNAs	Relative and absolute quantification of miRNAs	Relative quantification of known miRNAs. Identification of novel miRNA sequences.

Table 2.

8. Role of MicroRNA in colorectal cancer development

MiRNAs have been shown to play an important role in colorectal cancer oncogenesis, progression, angiogenesis, invasion and metastasis (Lee, et al, 2007, Huang, et al, 2008 & Liu, et al, 2011). Esquela-Kerscher & Slack in their review have suggested that the dysregulation of miRNA genes that target mRNAs for tumour suppressor or oncogenes can influence tumourigensis (Esquela-Kerscher, et al, 2006). The miRNA expression profiling studies on colonic tumour and adjacent normal tissue have identified several differentially expressed miRNAs in cancerous tissue. Table 1 summarizes the relatively over-expressed and under-expressed miRNAs studied in CRC tissue from different studies. Studies focussing on the functional and mechanistic involvement of miRNAs in colon cancers have reported that selected groups of distinct miRNAs are commonly and concurrently upregulated or downregulated in colon cancer tissues and are often associated with distinct cytogenetic abnormalities (Xi, et al, 2006, Schepeler, et al, 2008 & Schetter, et al, 2008). Table 3 shows the summary of dysregulated miRNAs in colorectal tumour tissue compared to adjacent normal colonic mucosa. Over expressed or under expressed miRNAs identified by two or more studies are underlined and the miRNAs with conflicting expression levels in different studies are identified in Bold.

Studies	Downredulated miRNAs in CRC tissue	Upregulated miRNAs in CRC tissue
Michael, et al, 2003	<u>let-7</u>, **miR-16**, miR-24, <u>miR-26a</u>, miR-102, <u>miR-143</u>, <u>miR-145</u>, <u>miR-200b</u>	

Studies	Downredulated miRNAs in CRC tissue	Upregulated miRNAs in CRC tissue
Volinia, et al, 2006	let-7a-1, miR-9-3, miR-23b, miR-138, miR-218	**miR-16**, miR-17-5p, miR-20a, miR-21, miR-29b ,miR-141, **miR-195**, miR-199a
Xi, et al, 2006	let-7b, **let-7 g** , miR-26a , miR-30a-3p, **miR-132**, miR-181a, **miR-181b**, miR-296, miR-320, miR-372	miR-10a, miR-15b ,miR-23a, miR-25, miR-27a, miR-27b, **miR-30c**, miR-107, **miR-125a**, miR-191, miR-200c, miR-339
Bandrés. et al, 2006	miR-133b, miR-145	**miR-31**, miR-96, miR-135b, miR-183
Akao, et al, 2006	miR-143, miR-145, let -7	
Nakajima, et al, 2006		**let-7 g**, miR-181b, miR-200c
Lanza, et al, 2007		miR-17-5p, miR-20, miR-25, miR-92, miR-93-1, miR-106a
Rossi, et al, 2007	miR-200b, miR-210 , miR-224	miR-19a, miR-20, miR-21, miR-23a, miR-25, miR-27a, miR-27b, miR-29a, miR-30e, miR-124b, **miR-132**, **miR-133a**, miR-135b, miR-141, miR-147, miR-151, miR-152, miR-182, miR-185
Slaby, et al, 2007	**miR-31**, miR-143, miR-145	miR-21
Monzo, et al, 2008	miR-145	miR-17-5p ,miR-21, **miR-30c**, miR-106a, miR-107, miR-191, miR-221
Schepeler, et al, 2008	miR-101, miR-145, miR-455, miR-484	miR-20a, miR-92, miR-510, miR-513
Schetter, et al, 2008		miR-20a, miR-21, **miR-106a**, **miR-181b**, miR-203
Arndt, et al, 2009	miR-1, miR-10b, miR-30a-3p, miR-30a-5p, **miR-30c**, **miR-125a**, **miR-133a**, miR-139, miR-143, miR-145, **miR-195**, miR-378*, miR-422a, miR-422b, miR-497	miR-17-5p, miR-18a, miR-19a, miR-19b, miR-20a, miR-21, miR-25, miR-29a, miR-29b, **miR-31**, miR-34a, miR-93, miR-95, miR-96, **miR-106a**, miR-106b, miR-130b, **miR-181b**, miR-182, miR-183, miR-203, **miR-224**
Slattery, et al, 2011	miR-143, miR-145, miR-192, miR-215	miR-21, miR-21*, miR-183, miR-92a, miR-17, miR-18a, miR-19a, miR-34a

Table 3.

9. The use of circulating satellite MicroRNA for colorectal cancer detection

Recent work by Mitchell & Gilad (Mitchell, et al, 2008 & Gilad, et al, 2008) has identified the presence of cancer related miRNAs in the body fluids of patients with different body organ cancers. These tumour-derived miRNAs are present in human serum or plasma in a remarkably stable form and are protected from endogenous ribonuclease activity. Given that aberrantly expressed miRNAs in CRC tissue are secreted into blood, circulating miRNAs can potentially serve as non-invasive markers for CRC detection. In 2008, Chen and colleagues used high-throughput sequencing technique and compared the miRNA expression profiles of patient with CRC and healthy controls (Chen, et al, 2008). MiRNA expression profiles of CRC and healthy controls were significantly different. However, more than 75% of the aberrantly expressed miRNAs, detected in the serum of CRC patients were also present in the serum of patients with lung cancer. A similar trend was also observed in another study where expression profiles generated from plasma of breast cancer patients were compared with colorectal cancer and other solid organ cancers (Heneghan, et al, 2010). Identification and quantification of cancer related circulating miRNAs are associated with challenges in terms of sample preparation, experimental design, and pre-analytic variation, selection of diagnostic miRNAs, data normalization and data analysis. Meyer & Kroch (Meyer, et al, 2010 & Kroh, et al, 2010) have recently addressed many of these obstacles and provided a guide for effective strategies to overcome these issues.

Preliminary studies (Ng, et al, 2009, Pu, et al, 2010 & Cheng, et al, 2011) suggest that colorectal tumour derived miRNAs are present in the circulation at detectable levels and can used as potential biomarkers for colorectal neoplasia detection. These studies used either whole plasma or total RNA extracted from a defined amount of plasma samples collected from healthy controls and diseased patients. QRT-PCR based detection systems were applied to detect selected circulating miRNAs. Selection of miRNAs was based either on results of plasma miRNA expression profiling experiments performed on relatively small cohorts of healthy and diseased patients or highly up regulated miRNAs in CRC tissue. Table 4 summarizes the sensitivity and specificity of different miRNAs investigated for their utility as biomarkers. Results of these studies are very encouraging due to the high sensitivity for detection of CRCs and adenomas. The accuracy of miRNA based detection modalities is much higher than stool based detection modalities and may be comparable with endoscopic modalities. Furthermore, the ability to detect adenomas highlights the potential role of circulating miRNAs in bowel cancer screening. Therefore, in addition to a stand alone blood test for CRC, a miRNA based blood assay can be used as a replacement of FOBT in bowel cancer screening programmes. With its higher sensitivity and specificity, it may prove cost effective and help reduce the need for unnecessary colonic investigations. Table 4 shows the comparison of sensitivity and specificity of different miRNAs for their utility as biomarkers for detection of adenocarcinoma and adenoma*. QRT-PCR based quantification of miRNAs has been the preferred method of study in the majority of these studies.

Though the analysis of circulating miRNAs in CRC patients has identified several diagnostic miRNAs, their diagnostic accuracy is still questionable. This is due to overlapping miRNA expression with other cancers, non-cancerous conditions and variability of individual miRNA expression with stage and grade of tumour. It is possible that common carcinogenesis-related miRNAs are shared by different types of tumours and investigators

Tissue Type	Studies	Participants	Target MiRNAs	Diagnostic Accuracy	
				Sensitivity %	Specificity %
Whole Plasma	Pu, et al, 2010	CRC (n=103) Controls (n=37)	miR-221	86	41
Plasma RNA	Cheng , et al, 2011	CRC I-IV (n=102) Controls (n=48)	miR-141	66.7	80.8
	Ng, et al, 2009	CRC (n=90)	miR-17-3p	64	70
		Controls (n=40)	miR-92	89	70
	Huang, et al , 2010	CRC (n=100) Adenomas* (n=37)	miR-29	69 62.2*	89.1 84.7*
		Controls (n=59)	miR-92a	84 64.9*	71 81.4*

Table 4.

are detecting cancer-related but not tissue specific miRNAs. Another explanation of the findings is that the detection of miRNAs released into the circulation originates in immune cells which occur as a result of a systemic immune response generated by the tumour causing abnormal proliferation of colonic cells (Dong, et al, 2011). This might also explain the finding of commonly dysregulated miRNAs in patients with CRC and Ulcerative Colitis (Pekow, et al, 2011). Furthermore, studies to date have focused on measuring the circulating levels of either single miRNAs or a subset of the known miRNAs. Due to the above reasons, a single miRNA based detection strategy would be rather ineffective whereas a CRC tissue specific expression signature generated from plasma or serum of patients with CRC and adenoma could be more informative and accurate.

The recent discovery of exosome mediated transport of cancer related miRNAs into the circulation, has shifted the focus of miRNA studies towards the isolation of tissue specific circulating exosomes and their encompassed miRNAs. Exosomes are membrane bound small vesicles (20 to 100 nm in diameter) of endocytic origin and are released by a variety of cells in both healthy and disease conditions (Théry, et al, 2002 & Keller, et al, 2006). Exosomes correspond to the internal vesicles of multivesicular bodies (MVBs) and are released in the extracellular environment upon fusion of MVBs with the plasma membrane (Théry, et al, 2002 & Cocucci, et al, 2009). Since exosome formation includes two inward budding processes, exosomes maintain the same topological orientation as the cell, with membrane proteins on the outside and some cytosol on the inside. Exosomes contain cytoplasmic proteins, miRNAs and mRNA transcripts (Valadi, et al, 2007).

The topical orientation of exosomal membrane may help in identification of their source by using surface antigen directed antibodies e.g. anti-MHCII. One drawback of this isolation method is that unless all the exosomes contain the specific surface antigen used for the

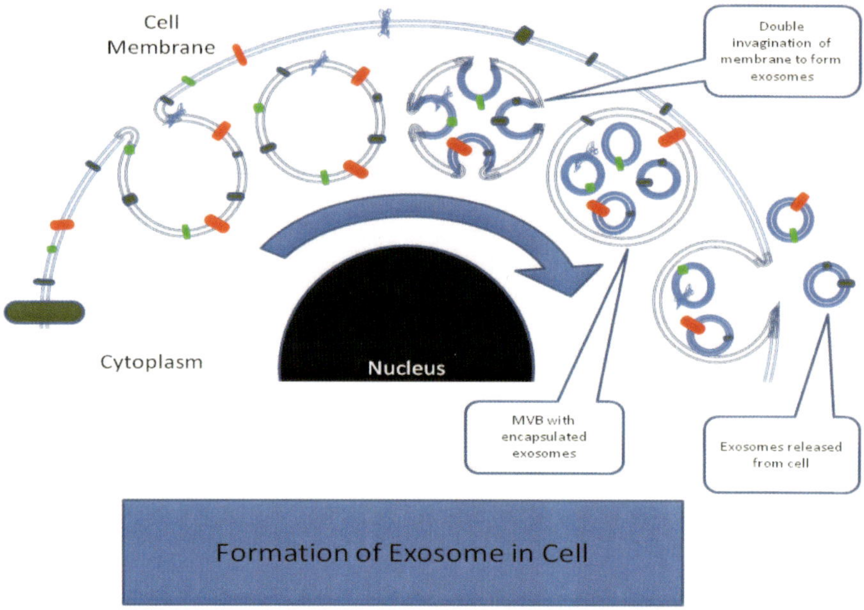

Fig. 2.

isolation, only a fraction of the exosomes will be isolated. Circulating exosomes can also be isolated based on their size, density and surface proteins. A commonly used method of purifying exosomes involves removal of cells and debris with either a filtration process or by a series of centrifugations (differential centrifugation), followed by a final high speed centrifugation (ultracentrifugation) to pellet the exosomes. Exosomes have a specific density and can be purified by floatation in a sucrose density gradient or by sucrosedeuterium oxide (D2O) cushions. Another purification method is based on exosome size and utilizes chromatography. The size and characterisation of exosomes is performed by using transmission electron microscopy, immune-electronmicroscopy, flow cytometry and dynamic light scattering. Table 5 summarizes the exosome isolation and characterisation methods used by different groups to analyse exosomes specific to colorectal cancer cells and methods of isolation of circulating exosomes for miRNAs analysis for other cancers (Simpson, et al, 2009). There is, however, a growing need for a fast and reliable method that yields a highly purified exosome fraction.

Based on this immunoaffinity strategy, several groups have isolated exosomes from the blood of patients with different cancers and have performed miRNA expression profiles on the total RNA isolated from these purified and probably tumour specific exosomes (Taylor, et al, 2008, Logozzi, et al, 2009 & Rabinowits, et al, 2009). Patients with cancer are found to have relatively higher quantities of exosome and encompassed miRNAs in the circulation Rabinowits, et al, 2009). The analysis of miRNAs extracted from circulating exosomes in patients with ovarian cancer, has been proven to be equivalent to ovarian tissue biopsies Taylor, et al, 2008). By using a similar approach of isolation and analysis, exosomal miRNAs in colorectal cancer can be evaluated for their diagnostic accuracy and may prove a breakthrough diagnostic modality.

Isolation and Characterisation of Colorectal Cancer Cell line Exosomes			
Studies	Colorectal Cancer Cell lines	Isolation method	Characterisation and Validation of Exosome
Huber, et al, 2005[69]	SW403 1869col CRC28462	Differential Centrifugation	Transmission Electron Microscopy Immune Electron Microscopy Fluorescence-activated cell sorting (FACS) Western Blotting
Mathivanan, et al, 2010[70]	LIM1215	Filtration, Diafiltration (5K) Ultracentrifugation Immuoaffinity	Transmission Electron Microscopy Immune Electron Microscopy Western Blotting
Choi, et al, 2007[71]	HT29	Differential Centrifugation Diafiltration(100k) Density Gradient	Transmission Electron Microscopy, Western Blotting
van Nigel, et al, 2001[72]	HT29-19A T84-DRB1*0401/CIITA	Differential Centrifugation Density Gradient	Transmission Electron Microscopy, Immune Electron Microscopy Western Blotting
Isolation and Characterisation of Circulating Exosomes for MicroRNA Analysis			
Studies	Cancer Type	Isolation Method	Specific Method/ Technique
Logozzi, et al, 2009[73]	Malignant Melanoma	Ultracentrifugation and filtration	400x g 20 min isolate plasma 1,200x g20 min 10,000x g 30 min and filter through 0.22um filter 1,00,000x g 60 min
Rabinowits, et al, 2009[74]	Lung Cancer	Immunoaffinity Ultracentrifugation	anti-EpCAM coated Immunobead
Taylor , et al, 2008[75]	Ovarian Cancer	Immunoaffinity Ultracentrifugation	anti-EpCAM antibody coated Immunobead

Table 5.

10. The use of stool MicroRNAs for detection of colorectal neoplasia

Colonic epithelium is the most dynamic cell population of the human organism. Highly differentiated colonocytes are continuously shed into the colon of healthy individuals and patients with CRC (Brittan, et al, 2004 & Loktionov, et al, 2007) . It is presumed that exfoliated colonocytes from healthy colon and neoplastic lesions carry important genetic and epigenetic information that could be utilized for subsequent testing, such as the detection of mutant genes or dysregulated mRNAs, proteins and miRNAs (Loktionov, et al, 2009). It is proposed that even small neoplastic loci can alter colonic cell exfoliation rate and may lead to early detection of these lesions (Loktionov, et al, 2007). The effectiveness of an exfoliated colonocyte based detection system requires an efficient isolation of colonocytes while minimizing the amount of background faecal debris. In order to achieve maximum retrieval of colonocytes, strategies that have been employed include density gradient centrifugation and/or immunoaffinity on either homogenized stool samples or scrapings from the stool surface (Loktionov, et al, 2007). However, cell yields are generally very low, often with conspicuous background debris, which makes cell identification difficult and time consuming (Deuter, et al, 1995). Consequently, such preparations would be unsuitable for high-throughput population screening programs (White, et al, 2009). Furthermore, colonocytes shed from a proximal colonic region travel a longer distance and are more exposed to cytolytic agents, thus making them less likely to be preserved and sampled. If this does prove to be a common problem, stool miRNA markers for right-sided CRC will be less effective. There is evidence, from the work of Koga and Colleagues (Koga, et al, 2010) that this is indeed the case. In this study immunomagnetic beads were conjugated with EpCAM monoclonal antibody to isolate colonocytes from stool. Despite the selection of two highly up regulated miRNAs in CRC cells, the sensitivity of detection was approximately 70% as shown in table 6. However, the detection rate for left sided colonic and rectal tumour was significantly higher, suggesting the potential utility of exfoliated colonocytes based miRNA assay as an alternative to flexible sigmoidoscopy. It is well established that profound deregulation of apoptosis is a characteristic feature of cancer. As a result of apoptosis, tumour specific proteins and genetic information i.e. DNA, RNA and miRNA are released into the lumen of colon (Ahlquist, et al, 2010). Stool environment is much more complex and hostile than plasma, and human RNA are rapidly degraded and only constitute <1% of total stool RNA (Ahlquist, et al, 2010). In contrast with the fast degradation of mRNA, human miRNAs are packed in micro vesicles and are well protected from degradation. The available data indicates that stool miRNA analysis can distinguish

Tissue Type	**Studies**	**Participants**	**Target MiRNAs**	**Diagnostic Accuracy**	
				Sensitivity %	**Specificity %**
Exfoliated Colonocytes	Koga , et al, 2010	CRC (n= 197) Control (n=119)	miR-17-92	69.5	81.5
			miR-135	46.2	95
Faeces	Link , et al, 2010	CRC (n=10) Adenoma (n=9) Control (n=10)	miR-21 miR-106	Distinguished adenomas and carcinomas from healthy controls P<0.05	

Table 6.

adenoma and carcinoma from healthy controls (Link, et al, 2010). The detection of miRNAs in stool specimens requires efficient protocols for stool preparation, stool miRNA extraction and quantitative analysis (Ahmed, et al, 2009). The utility of stool miRNAs as a biomarker is still in its infancy; further studies of stool miRNA are needed on larger cohorts to validate its diagnostic accuracy.

In summary, systemic and faecal miRNAs can accurately correlate with disease status and can potentially be used for colorectal cancer detection and screening. Detection of colorectal cancer based on miRNA expression analysis requires extensive pre analytical considerations for sample selection & processing, isolation of miRNAs, the method of expression analysis, selection of endogenous controls for normalisation and data analysis. Studies performed so far have shown great promise for miRNA based detection of colorectal carcinoma and adenoma. There is, however, a further need to develop and evaluate miRNA based assays before their clinical application.

11. References

Ahlquist DA. Molecular detection of colorectal neoplasia. Gastroenterology.2010;138: 2127–2139

Ahmed FE, Jeffries CD, Vos PW, Flake G, Nuovo GJ, Sinar DR, Naziri W, Marcuard SP. Diagnostic microRNA markers for screening sporadic human colon cancer and active ulcerative colitis in stool and tissue. Cancer Genomics Proteomics. 2009;6(5):281-95.

Akao Y, Nakagawa Y, Naoe T.let-7 microRNA functions as a potential growth suppressor in human colon cancer cells. Biol Pharm Bull. 2006;29(5):903-6.

Akao Y, Nakagawa Y, Naoe T. MicroRNAs 143 and 145 are possible common onco-microRNAs in human cancers. Oncol Rep. 2006;16(4):845-50

Bandrés E, Cubedo E, Agirre X, Malumbres R, Zárate R, Ramirez N, Abajo A, Navarro A, Moreno I, Monzó M, García-Foncillas J. Identification by Real-time PCR of 13 mature microRNAs differentially expressed in colorectal cancer and non-tumoral tissues. Mol Cancer. 2006.19;5:29

Bartel DP. MicroRNAs: genomics, biogenesis, mechanism, and function. Cell. 2004 23;116(2):281-97

Bartel DP. MicroRNAs: target recognition and regulatory functions.Cell: 2009;136, 215–233.

Bohnsack M T, Czaplinski K & Gorlich D. Exportin 5 is a RanGTP-dependent dsRNA-binding protein that mediates nuclear export of pre-miRNAs. RNA: 2004(10);185–191

Boyle P, Langman J. ABC of colorectal cancer Epidemiology.BMJ.2000; 321:805-808.

Bray F, Atkin W. International cancer patterns in men: geographical and temporal variations in cancer risk and the role of gender. JMHG.2004;1(1):38-46

Brittan M, Wright NA. Stem cell in gastrointestinal structure and neoplastic development. Gut 2004;53:899–910

Casey G, Lindor NM, Papadopoulos N, Thibodeau SN, Moskow J, Steelman S, Buzin CH, Sommer SS, Collins CE, Butz M, Aronson M, Gallinger S, Barker MA, Young JP, Jass JR, Hopper JL, Diep A, Bapat B, Salem M, Seminara D, Haile R; Colon Cancer Family Registry.Conversion analysis for mutation detection in MLH1 and MSH2 in patients with colorectal cancer. JAMA. 2005.16;293(7):799-809

Chendrimada TP, Gregory RI, Kumaraswamy E, Norman J, Cooch N, Nishikura K, Shiekhattar R. TRBP recruits the Dicer complex to Ago2 for microRNA processing and gene silencing. Nature. 2005;436(7051):740-4.

Chen C, Ridzon DA, Broomer AJ, Zhou Z, Lee DH, Nguyen JT, Barbisin M, Xu NL, Mahuvakar VR, Andersen MR, Lao KQ, Livak KJ, Guegler KJ.Real-time quantification of microRNAs by stem-loop RT-PCR. Nucleic Acids Res.2005; 33:e179

Chen X, Ba Y, Ma L, Cai X, Yin Y, Wang K, Guo J, Zhang Y, Chen J, Guo X, Li Q, Li X, Wang W, Zhang Y, Wang J, Jiang X, Xiang Y, Xu C, Zheng P, Zhang J, Li R, Zhang H, Shang X, Gong T, Ning G, Wang J, Zen K, Zhang J, Zhang CY.Characterization of microRNAs in serum: a novel class of biomarkers for diagnosis of cancer and other diseases. Cell Res. 2008;18(10):997-1006.

Cheng H, Zhang L, Cogdell DE, Zheng H, Schetter AJ, Nykter M, Harris CC, Chen K, Hamilton SR, Zhang W. Circulating plasma MiR-141 is a novel biomarker for metastatic colon cancer and predicts poor prognosis. PLoS One. 2011.17;6(3):e17745

Choi DS, Lee JM, Park GW, Lim HW, Bang JY, Kim YK, Kwon KH, Kwon HJ, Kim KP, Gho YS. Proteomic analysis of microvesicles derived from human colorectal cancer cells. J Proteome Res. 2007;6(12):4646-55

Cocucci E, Racchetti G, Meldolesi J. Shedding microvesicles: artefacts no more. Trends Cell Biol. 2009;19(2):43-51

Coleman MP, Estève J, Damiecki P, Arslan A, Renard H. Trends in cancer incidence and mortality. IARC Sci Publ. 1993; (121):1-806.

Deuter R, Pietsch S, Hertel S, Muller O. A method for preparation of fecal DNA suitable for PCR. Nucleic Acids Res 1995;23:3800–1

Dong Y, Wu WK, Wu CW, Sung JJ, Yu J, Ng SS. MicroRNA dysregulation in colorectal cancer: a clinical perspective. Br J Cancer. 2011.15;104(6):893-8

Eiring AM, Harb JG, Neviani P, Garton C, Oaks JJ, Spizzo R, Liu S, Schwind S, Santhanam R, Hickey CJ, Becker H, Chandler JC, Andino R, Cortes J, Hokland P, Huettner CS, Bhatia R, Roy DC, Liebhaber SA, Caligiuri MA, Marcucci G, Garzon R, Croce CM, Calin GA, Perrotti D. miR-328 functions as an RNA decoy to modulate hnRNP E2 regulation of mRNA translation in leukemic blasts. Cell. 2010.5;140(5):652-65.

Esquela-Kerscher A, Slack FJ. Oncomirs - microRNAs with a role in cancer. Nat Rev Cancer. 2006;6(4):259-69

Ferlay J, Parkin DM, Steliarova-Foucher E. Estimates of cancer incidence and mortality in Europe in 2008. Eur J Cancer. 2010;46(4):765-81.

Ferlay J, Shin HR, Bray F, Forman D, Mathers C, Parkin DM. Estimates of worldwide burden of cancer in 2008: GLOBOCAN 2008. Int J Cancer.2010;127(12): 2893-2917

Flood DM, Weiss NS, Cook LS, Emerson JC, Schwartz SM, Potter JD. Colorectal cancer incidence in Asian migrants to the United States and their descendants. Cancer Causes Control. 2000;11(5):403-11

Friedman RC, Farh KK, Burge CB, Bartel DP. Most mammalian mRNAs are conserved targets of microRNAs. Genome Res. 2009;19(1):92-105.

Gilad S, Meiri E, Yogev Y, Benjamin S, Lebanony D, Yerushalmi N, Benjamin H, Kushnir M, Cholakh H, Melamed N, Bentwich Z, Hod M, Goren Y, Chajut A. Serum microRNAs are promising novel biomarkers. PLoS One. 2008.5; 3(9):e3148

Graser A, Stieber P, Nagel D, Schafer C, Horst D, Becker CR, Nikolaou K, Lottes A, Geisbüsch S, Kramer H, Wagner AC, Diepolder H, Schirra J, Roth HJ, Seidel D, Göke B, Reiser MF, Kolligs FT. Comparison of CT colonography, colonoscopy, sigmoidoscopy and faecal occult blood tests for the detection of advanced adenoma in an average risk population. Gut. 2009; 58(2):241-8.

Guo L, Lu Z. The fate of miRNA* strand through evolutionary analysis: implication for degradation as merely carrier strand or potential regulatory molecule? PLoS One. 2010.30; 5(6):e11387

Hammond SM, Bernstein E, Beach D, Hannon GJ. An RNA-directed nuclease mediates post-transcriptional gene silencing in Drosophila cells. Nature. 2000.16; 404(6775):293-6.

Heneghan HM, Miller N, Kelly R, Newell J, Kerin MJ. Systemic miRNA-195 differentiates breast cancer from other malignancies and is a potential biomarker for detecting noninvasive and early stage disease. Oncologist. 2010; 15(7):673-82

Hewitson P, Glasziou P, Irwig L, Towler B, Watson E. Screening for colorectal cancer using the faecal occult blood test Hemoccult. Cochrane Database Syst Rev.2007; 24(1):CD001216.

Huang Q, Gumireddy K, Schrier M, le Sage C, Nagel R, Nair S, Egan DA, Li A, Huang G, Klein-Szanto AJ, Gimotty PA, Katsaros D, Coukos G, Zhang L, Puré E, Agami R. The microRNAs miR-373 and miR-520c promote tumour invasion and metastasis. Nat Cell Biol. 2008; 10(2):202-10.

Huang Z, Huang D, Ni S, Peng Z, Sheng W, Du X Plasma microRNAs are promising novel biomarkers for early detection of colorectal cancer. Int J Cancer. 2010.1; 127(1):118-26

Huber V, Fais S, Iero M, Lugini L, Canese P, Squarcina P, Zaccheddu A, Colone M, Arancia G, Gentile M, Seregni E, Valenti R, Ballabio G, Belli F, Leo E, Parmiani G, Rivoltini. Human colorectal cancer cells induce T-cell death through release of proapoptotic microvesicles: role in immune escape. Gastroenterology. 2005; 128(7):1796-804

Keller, S, Sanderson, MP, Stoeck, A. Altevogt, P. Exosomes: from biogenesis and secretion to biological function. Immunol Lett. 2006; 107: 102–108

Khraiwesh B, Arif MA, Seumel GI, Ossowski S, Weigel D, Reski R, Frank W. Transcriptional control of gene expression by microRNAs. Cell. 2010.8; 140(1):111-22.

Koga Y, Yasunaga M, Takahashi A, Kuroda J, Moriya Y, Akasu T, Fujita S, Yamamoto S, Baba H, Matsumura Y MicroRNA expression profiling of exfoliated colonocytes isolated from feces for colorectal cancer screening. Cancer Prev Res (Phila). 2010; 3(11):1435-42

Kroh EM, Parkin RK, Mitchell PS, Tewari M. Analysis of circulating microRNA biomarkers in plasma and serum using quantitative reverse transcription-PCR (qRT-PCR).Methods. 2010; 50(4):298-301.

Lanza G, Ferracin M, Gafà R, Veronese A, Spizzo R, Pichiorri F, Liu CG, Calin GA, Croce CM, Negrini M mRNA/microRNA gene expression profile in microsatellite unstable colorectal cancer. Mol Cancer. 2007. 23; 6:54

Lee RC, Feinbaum RL, Ambros V. The C. elegans heterochronic gene lin-4 encodes small RNAs with antisense complementarity to lin-14. Cell. 1993.3; 75(5):843-54.

Lee Y, Ahn C, Han J, Choi H, Kim J, Yim J, Lee J, Provost P, Rådmark O, Kim S, Kim VN. The nuclear RNase III Drosha initiates microRNA processing.Nature. 2003.25; 425(6956):415-9.

Lee DY, Deng Z, Wang CH, Yang BB. MicroRNA-378 promotes cell survival, tumor growth, and angiogenesis by targeting SuFu and Fus-1 expression. Proc Natl Acad Sci U S A. 2007.18; 104(51):20350-5

Link A, Balaguer F, Shen Y, Nagasaka T, Lozano JJ, Boland CR, Goel A. Fecal MicroRNAs as novel biomarkers for colon cancer screening. Cancer Epidemiol Biomarkers Prev. 2010;19(7):1766-74

Liu M, Lang N, Qiu M, Xu F, Li Q, Tang Q, Chen J, Chen X, Zhang S, Liu Z, Zhou J, Zhu Y, Deng Y, Zheng Y, Bi F. miR-137 targets Cdc42 expression, induces cell cycle G1 arrest and inhibits invasion in colorectal cancer cells. Int J Cancer. 2011.15; 128(6):1269-79.

Loktionov A. Cell exfoliation in the human colon: myth, reality and implications for colorectal cancer screening. Int J Cancer. 2007.1; 120(11):2281-9.

Loktionov A, Bandaletova T, Llewelyn AH, Dion C, Lywood HG, Lywood RC, Rockall TA, Stebbing JF, Broughton M, Caffarey S, Marks CG. Colorectal cancer detection by measuring DNA from exfoliated colonocytes obtained by direct contact with rectal mucosa. Int J Oncol. 2009; 34(2):301-11.

Logozzi M, De Milito A, Lugini L, Borghi M, Calabrò L, Spada M, Perdicchio M, Marino ML, Federici C, Iessi E, Brambilla D, Venturi G, Lozupone F, Santinami M, Huber V, Maio M, Rivoltini L, Fais S. High levels of exosomes expressing CD63 and caveolin-1 in plasma of melanoma patients. PLoS One. 2009; 4(4):e5219

Marchand L. Combined influence of genetic and dietary factors on colorectal cancer incidence in Japanese Americans. J Natl Cancer Inst Monogr, 1999. 26: p. 101-105.

Mathivanan S, Lim JW, Tauro BJ, Ji H, Moritz RL, Simpson RJ. Proteomics analysis of A33 immunoaffinity-purified exosomes released from the human colon tumor cell line LIM1215 reveals a tissue-specific protein signature. Mol Cell Proteomics. 2010 Feb;9(2):197-208

Meyer SU, Pfaffl MW, Ulbrich SE. Normalization strategies for microRNA profiling experiments: a 'normal' way to a hidden layer of complexity? Biotechnol Lett. 2010 ;32(12):1777-88

Michael MZ, O' Connor SM, van Holst Pellekaan NG, Young GP, James RJ. Reduced accumulation of specific microRNAs in colorectal neoplasia. Mol Cancer Res. 2003 ;1(12):882-91.

Mitchell PS, Parkin RK, Kroh EM, Fritz BR, Wyman SK, Pogosova-Agadjanyan EL, Peterson A, Noteboom J, O'Briant KC, Allen A, Lin DW,Urban N, Drescher CW, Knudsen BS, Stirewalt DL, Gentleman R,Vessella RL, Nelson PS, Martin DB, Tewari M (2008) Circulating microRNAs as stable blood-based markers for cancer detection. Proc Natl Acad Sci USA 105: 10513–10518

Monzo M, Navarro A, Bandres E, Artells R, Moreno I, Gel B, Ibeas R, Moreno J, Martinez F, Diaz T, Martinez A, Balagué O, Garcia-Foncillas J. Overlapping expression of microRNAs in human embryonic colon and colorectal cancer. Cell Res. 2008;18(8):823-33.

Nakajima G, Hayashi K, Xi Y, Kudo K, Uchida K, Takasaki K, Yamamoto M, Ju J. Non-coding MicroRNAs hsa-let-7g and hsa-miR-181b are Associated with hemoresponse to S-1 in Colon Cancer. Cancer Genomics Proteomics. 2006;3(5):317-324

National Cancer Institute. Surveillance, Epidemiology and End Results (SEER) 2006.

Ng EK, Chong WW, Jin H, Lam EK, Shin VY, Yu J, Poon TC, Ng SS, Sung JJ. Differential expression of microRNAs in plasma of patients with colorectal cancer: a potential marker for colorectal cancer screening. Gut. 2009;58(10):1375-81

Okamura K, Phillips MD, Tyler DM, Duan H, Chou YT, Lai EC. The regulatory activity of microRNA* species has substantial influence on microRNA and 3' UTR evolution. Nat Struct Mol Biol. 2008;15(4):354-63

Ørom UA, Nielsen FN, & Lund AH. MicroRNA-10a binds the 5'UTR of ribosomal protein mRNAs and enhances their translation. Mol. Cell: 2008(4); 460–471

Pekow JR, Dougherty U, Mustafi R, Zhu H, Kocherginsky M, Rubin DT, Hanauer SB, Hart J, Chang EB, Fichera A, Joseph LJ, Bissonnette M. miR-143 and miR-145 are downregulated in ulcerative colitis: Putative regulators of inflammation and protooncogenes. Inflamm Bowel Dis. 2011. doi: 10.1002/ibd.21742

Pradervand S, Weber J, Lemoine F, Consales F, Paillusson A, Dupasquier M, Thomas J, Richter H, Kaessmann H, Beaudoing E, Hagenbuchle O, Harshman K. Concordance among digital gene expression, microarrays, and qPCR when measuring differential expression of microRNAs. Biotechniques.2010;48:219–222

Pu XX, Huang GL, Guo HQ, et al. Circulating miR-221 directly amplified from plasma is a potential diagnostic and prognostic marker of colorectal cancer and is correlated with p53 expression. J Gastroenterol Hepatol. 2010;25(10):1674-80

Rabinowits G, Gerçel-Taylor C, Day JM, Taylor DD, Kloecker GH. Exosomal microRNA: a diagnostic marker for lung cancer. Clin Lung Cancer. 2009;10(1):42-6

Rossi L, Bonmassar E, Faraoni I.Modification of miR gene expression pattern in human colon cancer cells following exposure to 5-fluorouracil in vitro. Pharmacol Res. 2007;56(3):248-53

Schepeler T, Reinert JT, Ostenfeld MS, Christensen LL, Silahtaroglu AN, Dyrskjøt L, Wiuf C, Sørensen FJ, Kruhøffer M, Laurberg S, Kauppinen S, Ørntoft TF, Andersen CL. Diagnostic and prognostic microRNAs in stage II colon cancer. Cancer Res. 2008.1;68(15):6416-24.

Schetter AJ, Leung SY, Sohn JJ, Zanetti KA, Bowman ED, Yanaihara N, Yuen ST, Chan TL, Kwong DL, Au GK, Liu CG, Calin GA, Croce CM, Harris CC. MicroRNA expression profiles associated with prognosis and therapeutic outcome in colon adenocarcinoma. JAMA. 2008.30;299(4):425-36

Segditsas S, Tomlinson I. Colorectal cancer and genetic alterations in the Wnt pathway. Oncogene. 2006.4;25(57):7531-7

Simpson RJ, Lim JW, Moritz RL, Mathivanan S. Exosomes: proteomic insights and diagnostic potential. Expert Rev Proteomics. 2009;6(3):267-83

Slaby O, Svoboda M, Fabian P, Smerdova T, Knoflickova D, Bednarikova M, Nenutil R, Vyzula R.Altered expression of miR-21, miR-31, miR-143 and miR-145 is related to clinicopathologic features of colorectal cancer. Oncology. 2007;72(5-6):397-402

Slattery ML, Wolff E, Hoffman MD, Pellatt DF, Milash B, Wolff RK MicroRNAs and colon and rectal cancer: differential expression by tumor location and subtype. Genes Chromosomes Cancer. 2011;50(3):196-206

Spring KJ, Zhao ZZ, Karamatic R, Walsh MD, Whitehall VL, Pike T, Simms LA, Young J, James M, Montgomery GW, Appleyard M, Hewett D, Togashi K, Jass JR, Leggett BA. High prevalence of sessile serrated adenomas with BRAF mutations: a prospective study of patients undergoing colonoscopy. Gastroenterology.2006; 131(5):1400-7.

Stark A, Kheradpour P, Parts L, Brennecke J, Hodges E, Hannon GJ, Kellis M. Systematic discovery and characterization of fly microRNAs using 12 Drosophila genomes. Genome Res. 2007;17(12):1865-79

Taylor DD, Gercel-Taylor C. MicroRNA signatures of tumor-derived exosomes as diagnostic biomarkers of ovarian cancer. Gynecol Oncol. 2008;110(1):13-21

Théry, C, Zitvogel, L and Amigorena, S. Exosomes: composition, biogenesis and function. Nat Rev Immunol. 2002; 2: 569–579

Valadi H, Ekström K, Bossios A, Sjöstrand M, Lee JJ, Lötvall JO. Exosome-mediated transfer of mRNAs and microRNAs is a novel mechanism of genetic exchange between cells. Nat Cell Biol. 2007; 9(6):654-9

van Niel G, Raposo G, Candalh C, Boussac M, Hershberg R, Cerf-Bensussan N, Heyman M. Intestinal epithelial cells secrete exosome-like vesicles. Gastroenterology. 2001 ;121(2):337-49

Vogelstein B, Fearon ER, Hamilton SR, Kern SE, Preisinger AC, Leppert M, Nakamura Y, White R, Smits AM, Bos JL. Genetic alterations during colorectal-tumor development. N Engl J Med. 1988; 319(9):525-32

Volinia S, Calin GA, Liu CG, Ambs S, Cimmino A, Petrocca F, Visone R, Iorio M, Roldo C, Ferracin M, Prueitt RL, Yanaihara N, Lanza G, Scarpa A, Vecchione A, Negrini M, Harris CC, Croce CM. A microRNA expression signature of human solid tumors defines cancer gene targets.Proc Natl Acad Sci U S A. 2006.14;103(7):2257-61

Wang H, Ach RA, Curry B. Direct and sensitive miRNA profiling from low-input total RNA. RNA. 2007;13:151–159.

White V, Scarpini C, Barbosa-Morais NL, Ikelle E, Carter S, Laskey RA, Miller R, Coleman N. Isolation of stool-derived mucus provides a high yield of colonocytes suitable for early detection of colorectal carcinoma. Cancer Epidemiol Biomarkers Prev. 2009 ;18(7):2006-13

Xi Y, Formentini A, Chien M, Weir DB, Russo JJ, Ju J, Kornmann M, Ju J. Prognostic Values of microRNAs in Colorectal Cancer . Biomark Insights. 2006;2:113-121

Zhou H, Huang X, Cui H, Luo X, Tang Y, Chen S, Wu L, Shen N. miR-155 and its star-form partner miR-155* cooperatively regulate type I interferon production by human plasmacytoid dendritic cells. Blood. 2010.23;116(26):5885-94.

3

Epigenetics in Cancer: The Myelodysplastic Syndrome as a Model to Study Epigenetic Alterations as Diagnostic and Prognostic Biomarkers

Teresa de Souza Fernandez[1],
André Mencalha[1] and Cecília de Souza Fernandez[2]
[1]*National Cancer Institute (INCA),*
Bone Marrow Transplantation Center (CEMO) Laboratory Division,
Rio de Janeiro, RJ,
[2]*Mathematics and Statistics Institute,*
Federal Fluminense University (UFF), Niterói, RJ,
Brazil

1. Introduction

Epigenetics is characterized as hereditary changes in gene activity and expression that occur without alteration in DNA genomic sequence. It is known that epigenetics corresponds basically by two majority modifications: DNA methylation and histone modifications. Epigenetics events are reversible without primary DNA base sequence changes, resulting in possible modulation of the gene expression. The accurate DNA modifications and chromatin changes are important to normal embryonic development, to correct tissue cells differentiation, to precise cell cycle progression and cell death control. However, since epigenetics is also crucial to regulate gene expression, uncontrolled and/or incorrect modifications can unbalance the genetic expression profile and result in cellular transformation from normal to malignant cells.

The development of cancer cell is frequently associated with sequential of genetic and/or epigenetics hits, resulting in loss- or gain-of-function in genes, which leads to cell transformation. At a glance, aberrant global levels of histone modifications as well as incorrect methylation gene promoter may lead to the silencing of tumor suppressor genes and the activation of proto-oncogenes. Recently, many studies have revealed how epigenetics regulation has an implication in the identification of new biomarkers and the development of new therapies at several types of cancers. Moreover, nowadays, a series of identified epigenetics changes have been used as markers for cancer progression and for given prognostic value.

The field of cancer epigenetics is evolving rapidly in many aspects. In myelodysplastic syndrome (MDS), some research groups have been showed the importance to study epigenetic alterations as new diagnostic, prognostic and risk stratification biomarkers. The

MDS comprises a heterogeneous group of clonal bone marrow disorders characterized by varying degrees of pancytopenia, morphological and functional abnormalities of hematopoietic cells and increased risk of transformation into acute myeloid leukemia. This hematologic malignancy became a model to study the genetics and epigenetics changes involved in development stages of leukemia and it is considered a model study to tumorigenesis. MDS is viewed as a disease of adults, particularly the elderly. Pediatric MDS is an uncommon disorder, accounting for less than 5% of hematopoietic malignancies. Some studies in children showed that MDS appears with distinct clinical and laboratory characteristics when compared with adults, which may reflect special biological issues of MDS during childhood. There are different pathways involved in the pathogenesis of MDS. Due to the MDS heterogeneity, little is known about the molecular basis of MDS in adults and mainly in pediatric patients. Identification of the underlying genetic and epigenetic alterations in MDS may promote proper classification and prognostication of disease and, eventually, the development of new therapies. An important point in the epigenetic studies is the introduction of new forms of treatment for MDS patients. It is well documented that hematopoetic stem cell transplantation (HSCT) is, until now, the only curative treatment for MDS, both in adults and in children, but relapse after HSCT is the major cause of treatment failure in advanced stages. Other important factors in HSCT are the necessity of histocompatibility of donor cells and the age of the patients, sometimes limiting the use of this treatment. Thus, it is extremely important detecting biomarkers of disease evolution, especially those involved in epigenetic modifications, because news forms of treatment, as the use of hypomethylation agents, can be introduced as a better treatment option.

This chapter will review the advances in the study of epigenetics in cancer, the discovery of new epigenetic biomarkers and the development of therapeutic strategies using hypomethylation drugs. We will focus the advances in the epigenetic field using the myelodysplastic syndrome as a model, since it was demonstrated the importance of epigenetics alterations in the pathogenesis of this disease. Finally, we will describe the importance of statistical methods to aid the analysis of new diagnostic and prognostic epigenetic biomarkers.

2. The role of epigenetics in cancer

Epigenetics alterations have been growing as a promisor tool to understand cancer development, for better clinical therapy management, to identify new cancer biomarkers, which can help in monitoring disease evolution. It is known that epigenetics corresponds basically by two majority modifications: DNA methylation and chromatin modifications.

DNA methylation is a covalent modification of the cytosine ring 5′ position of a CpG dinucleotide, whereby a methyl group is deposited on carbon 5 of that ring using S-adenosyl methionine as a methyl donor. This transfer of methyl group is a replication-dependent reaction catalyzed by DNA methyltrasferases (DNMTs) (Figure 1).

Humans DNA methyltransferases are represented basically by three proteins: DNMT1, DNMT3A and DNMT3B. In general, DNMT1 are preferentially responsible for the methylation of one strand of DNA using as reference the other strand already methylated, mechanisms known as *de novo* methylation. This DNA hemi-methylation activity is important to maintain the methylation profile of genomic DNA cells during cellular

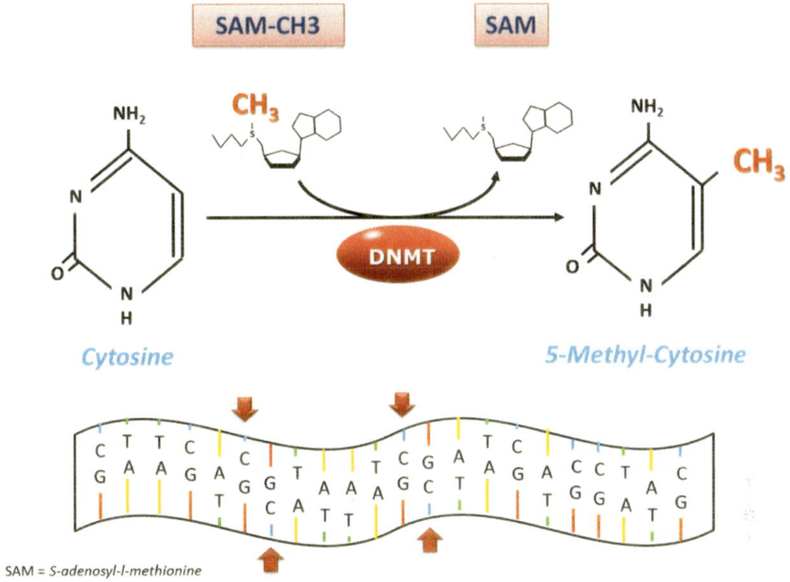

Fig. 1. DNA methylation. (A) Methyl radical transference from SAM (S-adenosyl-l-methionine) to 5th carbon of aromatic ring of cytosine nucleotide mediated by DNMT (DNA methyltransferase). (B) DNA sequence indicating that only cytosines before guanine will be methylate (red arrows). This cytosine/guanine in the methylation studies is also known as CpG and the concentration of CpG in some region of DNA sequence is known as CpG Island.

division. DNA hemi-methylation promoted by DNMT1 is crucial for initial stages of embryonic development and cell survival. In other hand, DNMT3A and DNMT3B play essential role for DNA hemi-methylation or unmethylated with the same level. Catalytic methyl-transferase of DNMT3A or DNMT3B is mainly promoted in cytosine preceded by guanine at the CpG dinucleotide. DNA methylation is a no random phenomenon. It normally occurs at the CG rich DNA sequences (the CpG islands) at promoter regions (Robertson et al., 1999; Tabby & Issa, 2010; Worn & Gulberg, 2002).

DNA methylation is frequently associated to transcriptional gene repression. It has been suggested that repression occurs by physically interfering in transcriptional factors binding at gene promoter regions, modified by 5'-methylcitosine or by recruiting methylated-DNA binding domain (MBD) proteins that block an original site of transcriptional factor. In addition, MBD proteins are frequently found associated with histone deacetylases. Physiological DNA methylation has been shown important to regulate genetic expression during embryonic development, genomic imprinting, X chromosome inactivation and cancer (Worn & Gulberg, 2002).

Chromatin is defined by a DNA and DNA-associated proteins, known as histones, in which genomic eukaryotic DNA is packaged. The basic unit of chromatin is called nucleosome, which is composed of a small DNA sequence, approximately 147 bases pairs, wrapped on protein octamer of the four core Histones (H2A, H2B, H3, and H4) and linker Histone H1. Epigenetics regulation involving chromatin comprises the post-translational modifications of histone protein tails. Depending on the kind of histone alteration, chromatin becomes compressed or weakens, which results in repression or permission to gene expression respectively. The histone complexes can be heterogeneous post-translational modified; it comprises methylation, acetylation, phosphorylation and ubiquitinylation. These distinct levels of combinatory histone modifications possibilities lead to regulation of gene transcription, a process called "histone coding". These histone changes are promoted by a series of distinct proteins, such as histone acetyl transferases (HAT), histone deacetylases (HDAC) and Polycomb group (PcG) proteins (Marks & Dokmanovic, 2005). The HAT and HDAC catalyze the transference of acetyl radical to histone tails (Kleff et al., 1995). Commonly, chromatin acetylation promotes the transcription factors access to DNA consensus sequences. Therefore, chromatin acetylation is frequently related to increase of transcriptional gene activity (Figure 2). Acetylation is not a random event and occurs in H3 and H4 tails, mainly on lysine residue, such as H3K4 and H3K14 (Agalioti et al., 2002).

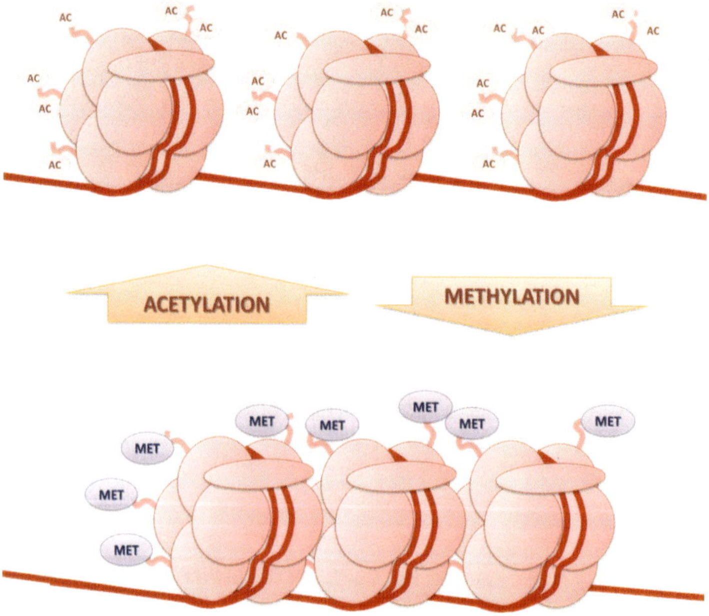

Fig. 2. Chromatin structure and histone tails modifications. Two mainly chromatin modifications, acetylation (AC) and methylation (MET). Acetylation is direct related to loose of chromatin compression which allows transcriptional factors access to DNA molecule and transcript its target gene. Methylation of histone tails is associated to chromatin compression and, as consequence, block the transcriptional factors access.

Among chromatin modifiers, Polycomb Group (PcG) proteins have been established as classical players of epigenetics regulation. PcG genes were discovered at experiments of mutations in *Drosophila* development (Lewis, 1978). In these studies, PcG proteins were found to control the activities of homeotic genes, which determine segmentation and structures body during development (Ingham, 1985). Several PcG orthologues genes were found in humans (van Lohuizen et al., 1991). PcG proteins are subdivided into two classes designed as Polycomb Repressive Complex: PRC1 and PRC2. The number of PcG proteins suggests a greater complexity of functions on the chromatin regulating. In this context, PcG have been reported to act in a myriad of histone modifications such as, ubiquitylation, sumoylation and methylation (Margueron & Reinberg, 2005). PcG proteins perform a critical role in gene regulation. PCR2 and PCR1 are considered to be involved in the initialization and maintenance of the repression of the gene transcription, respectively. PCR2 comprises the core components enhancer of zeste-2 (EZH2), embryonic ectoderm development (EED), and suppressor of zeste 12 (SUZ12), while PCR1 consists in a ring finger protein 1 (RING1), B lymphoma Mo-MLV insertion region 1 (BMI1) and chromobox homologue 2/4/8 (CBX2/4/8). EZH2 is the catalytic subunit of PRC2. It is a highly conserved histone methyltransferase that targets lysine 27 of histone H3. This methylated H3-K27 is usually associated with silencing of genes involved in differentiation. In addition, EZH2 is required for DNA methylation of EZH2- target promoters, serving as a recruitment platform DNA methyltransferases. SUZ12 is a recently identified PcG protein that, together with EED, is essential to maintaining the repressive function of PRC2. RING1 catalyzes the mono ubiquitylation of histone H2A at lysine 119. The H2AK 119 ubiquitylation likely increases chromatin compaction and, thus, interferes with the access or action of transcription factors. BMI 1 is mostly detected in stem cells and progenitors and takes part in stem cell proliferation and self-renewal (Bantignies & Cavalli, 2006; Levine et al., 2004; Rajasekhar & Begemann, 2007).

Cancer development is a consequence of multi-step molecular and cellular events that transform normal to malignant cell. During this process genetic and epigenetic alterations are involved. In recent years, several studies have indicated how epigenetics regulation has an implication in the identification of new biomarkers and the development of new therapies in a majority of cancers. Several evidences of oncogenes and tumor supressor genes DNA methylation indicated the importance of these epigenetics changes under expression control. DNA hypomethylation was directly related to the overexpression of *Raf*, *c-Myc*, *c-Fos*, *c-H-Ras* and *c-K-ras* oncogenes and tumor liver formation (Rao et al., 1989). Hypermethylation of tumor suppressor genes has also been demonstrated. For example, DNA methylation interferes in the expression of key cell cycle checkpoints genes: $p16^{INK4A}$, $p15^{INK4B}$, *Rb*, $p14^{ARF}$. These are the most studied genes used to correlate methylation and cell cycle control in several cancer types (Esteller, 2011). DNA or chromatin epigenetic alterations have been directly related to molecular changes to cancer development. Some epigenenetic modifications have been usefulness as biomarkers to aid in the clinical-therapeutic decision. For instance, *APC* and *GSTP1* gene methylation and H3K4me/H3K4me2/H3K18Ac chromatin modifications have been used to predict response to therapy and prognostic information in prostate cancer (Henrique & Jerónimo, 2004; Jerónimo et al., 2011).

The potential reversibility of epigenetics states offers exciting opportunities for new cancer drugs that can reactivate epigenetically silenced tumor-suppressor genes. Blocking either DNA methyltransferases or histone deacetylase activity could potentially inhibit or reverse the process of epigenetic silencing (Kelley et al., 2010). DNA demethylating drugs (DMI), as

5-azacytidine and 5-aza-2'-deoxycytidine, have been indicated as a promising new treatment for cancer (Streseman & Lyko, 2008). Histone deacetylase inihibitors (HDACs) have also been analyzed at clinical protocols for solid tumors (breast, non-small lung cells, prostatic cancer) and mainly for hematological malignancies (myelomas, leukemias and myelodysplastic syndrome) (Ellis et al., 2009; Graham et al., 2009; Hrebackova et al., 2010; Razak et al., 2011). In figure 3, we can see that the epigenetic therapy can "re-programmed" gene expression patterns.

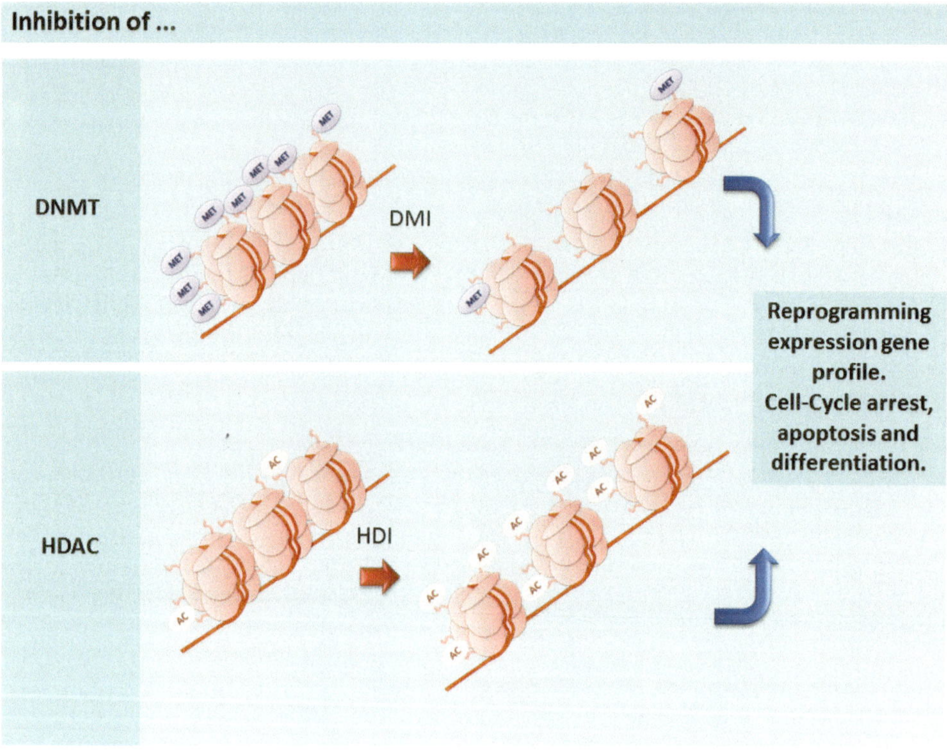

Fig. 3. Epigenetic therapy acting in the effects of DNMT or HDAC. Inhibitors of DNMT (*DNA methyltransferase*) or HDAC (*histone deacetylases*), as DMI (*DNMT inhibitor*) and HDI (*Histone Deacetylase Inhibitor*), respectively, induce the reprogramming expression by chromatin decompression. In summary, these inhibitors act mainly cell-cycle, apoptosis and differentiation related genes.

3. Myelodysplastic syndrome

The primary myelodysplastic syndrome (MDS) comprises a heterogeneous group of clonal bone marrow disorders, characterized by abnormal cellular morphology (dysplasias) and defects in the normal differentiation and prolileration of hematopoietic precursors. These defects result in ineffective hematopoiesis (bone marrow failure) and an increased risk of transformation into acute myeloid leukemia (AML) (Davids & Steensma, 2010; Jadersten & Hellström-Lindberg, 2008). MDS is viewed as a disease of adults, particularly the elderly. Pediatric MDS is an uncommon disorder, accounting for less than 5% of hematopoietic malignancies (Elghetany, 2007; Niemeyer & Baumann, 2008). The primary MDS presents a natural history since an indolent disease with long time of duration to a rapid progression to AML in few months (Nishino & Chang, 2005). The diagnosis is done initially by the hemogram indicating one or more cytopenias in peripheral blood like anemia, neutropenia and thrombocytopenia. The analysis is performed by the myelogram and bone marrow biopsy to identify dysplastic cells, the possible presence of blasts, characterizing later stages of the disease, and the presence of abnormal localization of immature precursors (ALIP). The bone marrow of MDS patients is usually hypercellular or normocellular, but there are a small number of cases with hypocellular bone marrow. In cases where bone marrow is hypocellular, it is recommended to perform differential diagnosis of severe aplastic anemia (SAA) and paroxysmal nocturnal hemoglobinuria (PNH). In these cases, important diagnostic tools, like the cytogenetics and the immunophenotyping, aid this diagnosis (Bennett & Orazi, 2009; Wong & So, 2002). The apparent paradox of hypercellular bone marrow and peripheral blood cytopenias was clarified by studies showing that MDS patients have increased rates of apoptosis in bone marrow in early stages of the disease (Parker et al., 2000).

The primary MDS diagnosis is considered a difficult clinical practice, because there are several clinical manifestations which may present a clinical and histological picture quite similar to MDS, such as nutritional deficiencies, infections and congenital conditions. It is necessary a differential diagnosis, where the presence of cytogenetic clonality helps in the diagnosis of primary MDS and contributes for the prognosis (Haase et al., 2007; Olney & Le Beau, 2009; Solé et al., 2005; Tiu et al., 2011). Nevertheless, there are cases with normal karyotype, so it is important to characterize molecular biomarkers to aid the MDS diagnosis. Because the primary MDS is a disease extremely heterogeneous, the definition of prognostic factors are often difficult. Thus, in the later years, it has been extensively discussed the classifications and prognostic scales for adult and pediatric patients.

3.1 Classifications and prognostic scores systems in myelodysplastic syndrome

Until 1980, the MDS included a variety of hematologic abnormalities classified as syndromes or pre-leukemic states. However, these denominations were unsatisfactory, not grouping all the patients who showed an ineffective hematopoiesis and not progressed to acute leukemia, occurring complications because of the cytopenias leading to death. The term "pre-leukemia" disappeared and the term myelodysplstic syndrome became widely accepted in 1982 with the FAB classification.

3.1.1 FAB classification

In 1982, the FAB group (French, American and British group) proposed a classification for primary MDS into five subgroups: refractory anemia (RA), refractory anemia with ringed sideroblasts (RARS), refractory anemia with excess blasts (RAEB), refractory anemia with excess blasts in transformation (RAEB-t) and chronic myelomonocytic leukemia (CMML).

This classification was based on morphological characteristics and the percentage of blasts in the bone marrow and peripheral blood (Table 1) (Bennett et al., 1982).

Subgroup	Monocytes (µl) peripheral blood	Ringed Sideroblasts (%) bone marrow	Blast cells (%)		Auer rods bone marrow
			peripheral blood	bone marrow	
RA	No	< 15	< 1	< 5	No
RARS	No	> 15	< 1	< 5	No
RAEB	No	No	< 5	5 - 20	No
RAEB-t	No	No	> 5	20 - 30	Yes or No
CMML	> 1000	No	< 5	< 20	No

Table 1. Classification of Myelodysplastic Syndrome according to the FAB Group in 1982.

As we can notice, this classification suggests multiple steps during the evolution from MDS to acute leukemia, being the initial stages the RA and RARS and the advanced stages the RAEB, RAEB-t and CMML. Since it was introduced, several studies have shown the usefulness of the FAB classification, both for monitoring a large number of patients with primary MDS, allowing comparisons between different studies, as for the treatment of patients. However, to determine a precise prognosis this classification still has some problems especially within initial subgroups, RA and RARS. The term "refractory anemia" is not always adequate, and anemia is only one of the three cytopenias in MDS. The CMML presents features of MDS and myeloproliferative diseases, so their inclusion in MDS classification has been discussed in more recent classifications like the World Health Organization (WHO) (Harris et al., 2000; Malcovati & Nimer, 2008).

3.1.2 WHO classification

The classification of the World Health Organization (WHO) was established in 2000 and used many concepts and definitions of the FAB classification and also the knowledge of the cytogenetic and molecular features to improve the definition of subgroups, as well as clinical relevance in order to improve diagnostic criteria and improve the prognosis definition (Harris et al., 2000). The main difference between the two classifications is the disappearance of the subgroup RAEB-t, considered the evolution to AML from 20%of blasts in the bone marrow. The classification system proposed by WHO was reviewed in 2008 and consider the subgroups described in Table 2. In this new classification the subgroup CMML is regarded as a myeloproliferative disorder. The WHO categories have several important clinical implications (Brunning et al., 2008). Patients with unilineage dysplasia have a favorable outcome compared to patients with multilineage dysplasia (Jadersten & Hellstrom, 2008). The presence of del(5q) strongly correlates to the probability of response to lenalidomide (Oliva et al., 2010).

Subgroup	**Peripheral Blood**	**Bone marrow**
Refractory cytopenias with unilineage dysplasia (**RCUD**)	Unicytopenia or bicytopenia; No or rare blasts (<1%)	Unilineage dysplasia; ≥10% of the cells of the affected lineage are dysplastic; <5% blasts; <15% ring sideroblasts
Refractory anemia with ring sideroblasts (**RARS**)	Anemia; No blasts	Erythroid dysplasia only; <5% blasts; ≥15% ringed sideroblasts
Refractory cytopenia with multilineage dysplasia (**RCMD**)	Cytopenia(s); or rare blasts (<1%); No Auer rods; monocytes <1 x 10^9/ L	Dysplasia in ≥10% of cells in two or more myeloid lineages; <5% blasts; No Auer rods; ±15% ring sideroblasts
Refractory anemia with excess blasts-1 (**RAEB-1**)	Cytopenias; <5% blasts; No Auer rods; monocytes <1 x 10^9/ L	Unilineage or multilineage dysplasia; 5-9% blasts; No Auer rods
Refractory anemia with excess blasts-2 (**RAEB-2**)	Cytopenias; 5-19% blasts; ± Auer rods; monocytes <1 x 10^9/ L	Unilineage or multilineage dysplasia; 10–19% blasts; ± Auer rods
Syndrome 5q-	Anemia; No or rare blasts (<1%); Platelet count usually normal or increased	Normal to increased megakaryocytes with hypolobated nuclei; <5% blasts; Isolated del(5q) cytogenetic abnormality; No Auer rods
Myelodysplastic syndrome, unclassified (MDS-U)	Cytopenias; Blasts ≤1%	Dysplasia in <10% of the cells in one or more myeloid lineages; <5% blasts; No Auer rods

Table 2. The WHO 2008 Classification of MDS.

3.1.3 Classification of myelodysplastic syndrome in childhood

Some studies have shown differences in morphological, cytogenetic, molecular and clinical manifestations of primary MDS in childhood that affect their inclusion in traditional classification systems (FAB and WHO), based mainly on adult patients. The rarity of childhood MDS and the heterogeneous nature of the disease have further contributed to the difficulties in classifying this disease (Hasle &Niemeyer, 2011). In 2003, Hasle and colleagues proposed a pediatric approach to the WHO classification of myelodysplastic syndrome: 1- MDS occurring both "de novo" and secondary, including the subtypes refractory cytopenia (RC), RAEB, and RAEB-t.; 2- a group of myelodysplastic/ myeloproliferative disorders with Juvenile Myelomonocytic Leukemia (JMML) as the most common disorder of this category; 3- myeloid leukemia of Down syndrome (DS), a disease with distinct clinical and biological features, encompassing both MDS and AML. In this classification, the minimal diagnostic criteria are: unexplained cytopenia (neutropenia, thrombocytopenia or anemia), at least bilineage morphologic myelodysplasia, acquired clonal cytogenetic abnormality in hematopoietic cells and blast cells number ≥5%. However, this classification has also been widely discussed because not all patients have chromosomal abnormalities, especially in the early stages of the disease (Niemeyer & Baumann, 2008). And in 2009, JMML was considered a myeloproliferative disorder (Hebeda & Fend, 2009).

3.1.4 Prognostic score system in myelodysplastic syndrome

Parallel to the improvement of classification systems, due to the large variability in survival within the same subgroup of primary MDS, it was necessary to develop score systems for prognostic stratification of risk groups, assisting the choice of treatment. The score system for risk groups most widely used for primary MDS is the International Prognostic Score System (IPSS) (Greenberg et al., 1997). The IPSS considers the percentage of bone marrow blasts, the number of peripheral blood cytopenias and the cytogenetic, the prognostic factors most important in relation to survival time and about the rate of leukemic transformation. The IPSS recognized four risk groups: low risk, intermediate 1, intermediate 2 and high risk. This system considers three categories for cytogenetic analysis: low risk [normal karyotypes, -Y, del(5q) and del(20q)]; high risk (alterations involving chromosome 7 and complex karyotypes) and intermediate risk (other chromosome abnormalities) .

The IPSS has gained prominence for its clinical utility due to the fact that it allows the prediction of disease progression in independent series of previously untreated patients. However, despite its importance, this system has some limitations like the risk groups in relation to karyotype. In some studies, trisomy 8, for example, is often associated with disease progression (Fernandez et al., 2000; Garcia-Manero, 2010; Solé et al., 2000). However, the IPSS classifies this chromosomal alteration with intermediate prognosis. Other important point is related to normal karyotypes that are associated, in some cases, to shorter survival when compared to some chromosomal alterations like: -X, del(5q), del(20q), +21 (Haase, 2008). So, the introduction of molecular data will help to characterize new prognostic factors and use these biomarkers to contribute in understanding the development of MDS and its evolution to AML.

3.2 Pediatric and adult myelodysplastic syndrome

Although the pediatric MDS shows dysplastic features and ineffective hematopoiesis, such as MDS in adults, clinical characteristics, the presence of constitucional genetic associated abnormalities and characterization of chromosomal changes have reflected a different biological question of MDS in childhood (Elghetany, 2007; Polychronopoulou et al., 2004). The main differences between childhood and adult MDS are: the incidence of RARS cases are extremely rare in pediatric patients and in adults consists of about 25% of cases; the monosomy 7 is the chromosomal alteration most frequent in pediatric patients and in adults is the deletion of the long arm of chromosome 5; the therapeutic possibilities in adult patients is generally limited due to advanced age and usually it is indicated a palliative therapy, whereas, in children with MDS, the main therapy indicated is curative; the allogeneic hematopoetic stem cell transplantation (Halse & Niemeyer, 2002). Some clinical features are different between adults and children with MDS and the factors that predict survival or progression in adults are of little value to children. So, the IPSS has limited value for pediatric MDS (Hasle et al., 2004).

In relation to cytogenetic studies, they showed a key role in the diagnosis of the suspected cases of pediatric MDS, being used to confirm the clonal nature of this disease (Sasaki et al., 2001). The monosomy 7 is the most common chromosomal abnormality in these patients (Figure 4). This alteration is associated with poor prognosis and a rapid progression to AML (Aktas et al., 2006; Fernandez et al., 2000; Sasaki et al., 2001).

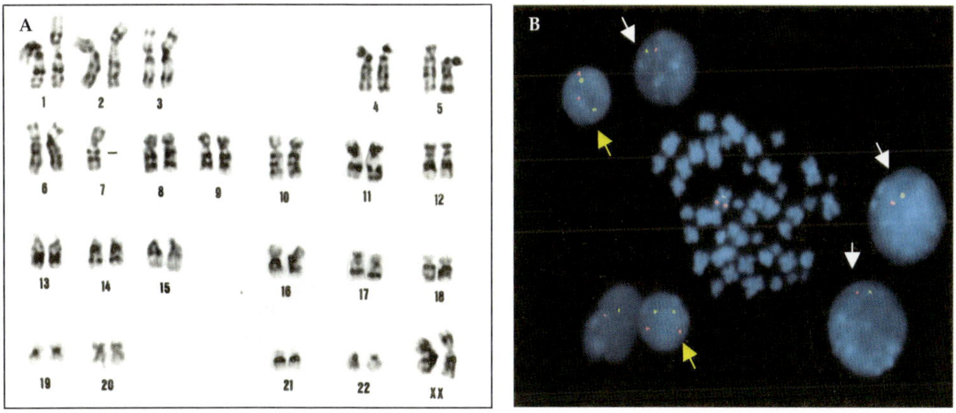

Fig. 4. (A) Karyotype of bone marrow cell by GTG-banding showing: Monosomy 7. (B) FISH analysis showing monosomy 7 using the probe: LSI D7S486 spectrum orange/ CEP 7 spectrum green, Vysis, Inc. Downers Grove, USA. It may be observed in the interphases nucleus four signals characterizing normal cells (yellow arrows) and others interphases nucleus showing two signals (white arrows), confirming the loss of the chromosome 7.

The molecular mechanisms involved in MDS mainly, in childhood, are not well defined. A recent molecular study of *TP53* and *c-fms* genes showed no mutations in children with MDS. The presence of mutations in onocogene *N-ras* also occurs in a very low frequency in childhood MDS. However, mutations in *TP53, c-fms* and *N-ras* genes are involved in the development and evolution from MDS to AML in adult patients (Fernandez et al., 1998; Jekic et al., 2004, 2006). These results suggest that some molecular mechanisms involved in the pathogenesis of MDS in children are different from those seen in adults. It has been observed the importance of epigenetic alterations in the pathogenesis of MDS, but the majority of these studies is focused in adult patients. Few studies showed the epigenetic alterations in children (Hasegawa et al., 2005; Rodrigues et al., 2010; Vidal et al., 2007). Rodrigues and colleagues, 2010, suggested that methylation of $p15^{INK4B}$ and $p16^{INK4A}$ genes are epigenetic alterations in pediatric MDS patients and, as in adult patients, are later events associated with the leukemogenesis process in MDS.

3.3 Cytogenetics and epigenetics alterations in myelodysplastic syndrome

The discovery of non-random chromosomal abnormalities in primary MDS confirmed the clonality, providing a way to identify the malignant clone and point out some oncogenes and tumor suppressor genes possibility involved in the development and progression of disease. The cytogenetics evaluation of a bone marrow sample from patients with MDS has become an integral part of clinical care. The clonal cytogenetic alterations can be detected in 30-50% of adult patients with primary MDS. In pediatric patients this incidence is 50-70% of the cases. These changes range from a single numerical or structural changes to complex genomic lesions involving three or more different chromosomes. The most frequent chromosomal abnormalities in MDS are: del(5q), del(7q)/-7, +8, del(11q), del(12p), del(17p), del(20q) and loss of Y chromosome (Bejar et al., 2011; Fernandez et al., 2000; Haase, 2008).

The frequency of cytogenetic abnormalities increases with the severity of disease as well as the risk of leukemic transformation. In this group, unfavorable chromosomal abnormalities are frequently found as complex abnormalities or karyotypes including monosomy 7 or trisomy 8 (Bacher, 2010; Fernandez et al., 2000). A normal karyotype is found in 30-60% of patients with MDS. This group of patients is almost certainly genetic heterogeneous, probably the leukemogenic alterations occurred at the molecular level and were not detectable with standard cytogenetic methods (Greenberg et al., 1997; Onley & Le Beau, 2009).

In MDS, some studies suggest some genes involved with specific chromosome alterations, as the del(5q). The 5q syndrome represents a distinct clinical entity characterized by a del(5q) as the sole karyotypic abnormality. The 5q syndrome occurs commonly in women. The initial laboratory findings are usually a macrocytic anemia with a normal or elevated count. The diagnosis is usually RA. On bone marrow examination, abnormalities in the megakaryocytic lineage (particularly micromegakaryocytes) are prominent. These patients have a favorable prognosis, with low rates of leukemic transformation and a relatively long survival of several years. The loss of a single copy of the RPS14 gene may be involved in the MDS 5q- pathogenesis. The RPS14 is an essential component of the 40S subunit of ribosomes and ribosomes synthesis is impaired in CD34 + cells from 5q syndrome patients (Onley & Le Beau, 2009).

The role of cytogenetic analysis in MDS is an important factor for establishing the diagnosis, prognosis and therapeutic plan and the follow up of altered clinical behavior of the disease. The chromosomal abnormalities have not only provided insights into prognosis but also into the molecular pathogenesis of this heterogeneous disease. The type of chromosomal abnormality (unbalanced, most commonly the result of the loss of a whole chromosome or a deletion of a part of a chromosome) in primary MDS indicates that the main class of genes involved in the pathogenesis of this disease is the tumor suppressor genes. The mechanism involved in the inactivating tumor suppressor genes are deletions, mutations and epigenetic alterations as the DNA methylation.

Three main epigenetic events regulate tumor-associated genes: 1) the aberrant hypermethylation of tumor suppressor genes, 2) post-translational modifications of histones and 3) post-transcriptional modifications by regulatory miRNA. The underlying causes of the pathogenesis of MDS remain to be fully elucidated. Knudson model of the "two hits" provides the basis of the concept of a multistep pathogenesis in the development of MDS, where loss or inactivation of only one allele is not sufficient to result in the development of tumors or expansion of a malignant clone. In fact, MDS in early stages with its relatively slow (but with increased tendency) to AML progression represents a prototype of the multistep concept in leukemogenesis with accumulation of cellular and molecular defects during the initiation and disease progression (Vigna et al., 2011).

Recent studies have revealed that DNA methylation and histone modification may be controlled by Polycomb-group (PcG) proteins, which may give new clues toward understanding the epigenetic mechanisms of MDS. PcG family members, such as EZH2, RING1 and BMI-1, are essential for the self-renewal and proliferation of normal cells. However, the induced over expression of these proteins can drive tumorigenesis. In MDS patients, the expression of EZH2, RING1 and BMI 1 were positively correlated with the IPSS prognostic scoring system, suggesting that the over expression of each of these three genes is a negative prognostic indicator (Xu et al., 2011). The EZH2 expression level was positively correlated with a reduction of peripheral blood cells, which was likely to reflect the severity of ineffective hematopoiesis. Molecular analyses of EZH2 showed that deletions, missense and frameshift mutations strongly suggest that EZH2 is a tumor suppressor gene in MDS pathogenesis (Nikoloski et al., 2010). Other mutations have been identified in the genes that regulate endogenous methylation networks within cells including IDH1/2, TET2 and DNMT3. The relevance of these lesions in being able to predict response to epigenetic modulators and their correlation with epigenetic signatures in MDS are beginning to emerge (Tan & Wei, 2011).

In MDS, aberrant silencing due to promoter hypermethylation involves genes encoding cell adhesion molecules, cell cycle regulation and tumor suppressor genes possibly leading to dysregulation of hematopoiesis. It has been shown in MDS a high prevalence of methylation for the tumor suppressor genes $p15^{INK4B}$, cadherin 1 (CDH1), death associated protein kinase (DAPK) and suppressor of cytokine signaling (SOCS-1). Some methylation patterns in specific genes in MDS can predict poor prognosis even in early stage of the disease (Aggerholm et al., 2006; Bejar et al., 2011; Vigna et al., 2011). Hence, epigenetic changes have been implicated as potential mechanisms in the pathogenesis and progression of MDS, which has already resulted in promising therapeutic approaches in a subset of patients.

3.4 Methylation changes in myelodysplastic syndrome: Diagnostic and therapeutical implications

Different studies in MDS showed the importance of methylation changes during the clinical evolution of disease to AML. So, the identification in the diagnosis of these alterations is important for risk group stratification. Aberrant DNA methylation is view as a poor prognostic feature in MDS. For example, p15^{INK4B} and p16^{INK4A} genes are members of cyclin dependent kinase inhibitors family which controls the progression of cell cycle from G1 to S phase. The products of these genes regulate RB function by modulating the complexes of cyclin D-CDK4/6 which can phosphorylate and inactive the RB protein, and set up an important pathway for inhibiting cell growth (Serrano et al., 1996; Shimamoto et al., 2005). In addition, p15^{INK4B} has been suggested to act as a regulator of proliferation and differentiation in myelo-monocytic and megakaryocytic lineages by arresting the cell cycle (Sakashita et al., 2001; Teofili et al., 2000). Therefore, the silencing of these genes via aberrant methylation is a critical event in leukaemogenesis. In MDS, aberrant methylation of p15^{INK4B}

gene has been related to more aggressive subtypes of disease and it is a possible biomarker of disease evolution (Quesnel et al., 1998; Rodrigues et al., 2010).

Another gene methylated in MDS is the death-associated protein kinase (DAP-kinase), a proapoptotic serine/threonine kinase. The analysis of the methylation status of DAP-kinase in bone marrow samples from patients with MDS at the time of initial diagnosis showed that hypermethylation of DAP-kinase was significantly correlated to loss of DAP-kinase expression. Alteration in the apoptotic response due to the loss of DAP-kinase function may be an early event in the transformation pathway to secondary leukemia via myelodysplasia (Wu et al., 2011).

The mechanistic bases of CIMP (CpG island methylator phenotype) in MDS remains unknown. One proposed mechanisms involves aberrant recruitment of DNA methyltransferases to CpG islands and/or loss of methylation protection. Another possible explanation is that hypermethylation may not be directly linked to the methylation machinery, but rather reflects environmental exposures (Shen et al., 2010).

The reversible character of epigenetic alterations (in contrast to genetic changes) was an important point for the development of therapeutic strategies evolving various epigenetic components for anticancer therapy. So, in MDS, the characterization in the diagnosis of epigenetic biomarkers of disease evolution may indicate the use of hypomethylating drugs in this group of patients.

A large number of treatments has been used in adults and children with primary MDS, with the goal of eliminating the cytopenias as well as to recover hematopoiesis. One of the therapies used is the support that involves blood transfusions, antibiotics, growth factors alone or in combination, cyclosporin or anti-lymphocyte globulin (ATG) are also used in patients with hypocellular bone marrow. In more advanced MDS subtypes (RAEB, RAEB-t), in some cases, it has been used the chemotherapy. The allogeneic hematopoietic stem cell transplantation (HSCT) is the only curative therapeutic option for patients with MDS, however, its use is limited to patients up to 55 years old and patients who have histocompatible donors (Giralt et al., 2005; Kindwall-Keller & Isola, 2009). For children with MDS, allogeneic HSCT is considered as the best treatment option (Niemeyer & Kratz, 2008).

With the delineation of the characteristics that drive the biological phenotype of MDS, new drugs introduced in the treatment of this disease have shown a great therapeutic potential, such as the hypomethylant agents, called methyltransferase inhibitors (IMT). The representatives of this class include azacitidine (5-azacytidine) and decitabine (5-aza 2 'deoxycytidine). Both are incorporated into DNA and then irreversibly bind and inhibit the action of DNA methyltransferase. This interaction results initially in a semi-methylated DNA. However, after further cell cycles, it becomes completely unmethylated. The action of these drugs leads to reactivation of epigenetically repressed genes, such as tumor suppressor genes. Initial results showed that patients with higher-risk MDS have an increased time to AML transformation and an increase of survival time (Atallah et al., 2007; Fenaux et al., 2009; Silverman & Mufti, 2005). The decitabine and azacytidine are approved for treatment of patients with int-2 and high-risk MDS. Demethylating agents seem to be the best choice for elderly patients with MDS, even in case of high risk cytogenetic changes in karyotype, like monosomy 7 (Gurion et al., 2010; Szmigielska-Kaplon & Robak, 2011).

Some studies have shown that reduced methylation overtime was correlated with better clinical response for patients during decitabine treatment. But, further studies of methylation dynamics, both before and after treatment, will be useful to determine the ability of epigenetic biomarkers to direct the treatment and may predict for the success (Shen et al., 2010). However, in some clinical trials, it was found that a number of patients does not respond to decitabine initially (primary resistance) and most patients, who initially respond to decitabine treatment, eventually relapse (secondary resistance) despite continued therapy. Clinical response to hypomethylating drugs *in vivo* is complex and may involve differentiation and immune activating components. Cytogenetic analysis showed that MDS patients after relapse using decitabine showed evolution in 20% patients with abnormalities such -7, del(16q) and +8 (Qin et al., 2011).

The understanding of the epigenetic changes characteristic of the malignant phenotype also permit the development of drugs that are able to target other regulators of chromatin conformation that contribute to aberrant gene transcription and dysregulated cell growth. The histone deacetylase inhibitors (HDAC) belong to one class of therapeutics developed using this paradigm. HDAC inhibitors modulate gene expression by inhibiting the deacetylation of histone lysine tails, relaxing the chromatin structure by decreasing the interaction between positively charged lysine tails of histones and negatively charged DNA. Although responses using HDAC inhibitors alone in MDS have been modest, preclinical data drives clinical trials in which they are utilized in combination with DNA methyltransferase inhibitors. Combination therapy offers the possibility of hematologic improvement and remission to MDS patients with previously untreatable disease (Vigna et al., 2011).

DNA methyltransferase inhibitors (hypomethylating agents) have emerged as options for the treatment of patients with MDS. These drugs lead to the progressive loss of methylation and reversal of gene silencing. In addition to their differentiation-inducing activity, these agents also have direct cytotoxic effects (Gurion et al., 2009). Currently available DNA methylation blocks all DNMTs. One of the main problems in using DNMT-Is in therapy is activation of cancer-promoting genes as well as other disease-promoting genes by hypomethylation. Recent studies suggest that there might be differences in the target specificity of different DNMTs. It is important to characterize the cancer related genes regulated by each of the DNMTs and develop DNMT gene-specific inhibitors. Moreover, treatment duration and maintenance therapy of using these agents require further investigation (Vigna et al., 2011).

3.5 DNA methylation alterations as diagnostic and prognostic biomarkers

Epigenetic transcriptional silencing of genes required for proliferation and differentiation of the hematopoetic cells are likely to contribute to the leukemogenic event underlying MDS. Altered DNA methylation patterns of some genes are not only of importance to our understanding of the molecular pathogenesis of the MDS, but may also serve as novel indicators for the diagnosis, the prognosis and the prediction of response to therapy. We can see in table 3 some genes that are methylated in MDS and are suggested as possible biomarkers that may aid the diagnosis and the prognosis.

Genes	Function	MDS Incidence of aberrant methylation	Role in MDS Pathogenesis / Prognosis
p15^INK4B *p16^INK4A*	Members of the cyclin-dependent kinase (CDK) inhibitor family. They play an important pathway for inhibiting cell growth. Localization: 9p21	p15^INK4 - adult patients : 61% (25/41); pediatric patients: 32% (15/47) ; p16^INK4A - adult patients : 37% (15/41) pediatric patients: 8% (4/47)	High incidence in RAEB and RAEB-t. Hypermethylation in both genes are involved in evolution from MDS to AML and confers a poor prognosis. (Rodrigues et al., 2010)
CDH-1 (E-cadherin)	Homotypic cell-cell adhesion protein, involved in cell-proliferation. Localization: 16q22	adult patients : 39% (16/41)	Occurs in the various subgroups of MDS with higher incidence in RAEB and RAEB-t. (Solomon et al., 2008)
SOCS-1 (suppressor of cytokine sinaling)	Member of stat-induced STAT inhibitor (SSI), also known as a suppressor of cytokine signaling (SOCS) family. Localization: 16p13	adult patients : 31% (27/86)	Higher risk of leukemic transformation. (Brakensiek et al., 2005)
DAPK1 (death associated protein kinase)	DAPK1 is a serine/threonine kinase, a positive mediator of gamma-interferon induced programmed cell death. Localization: 9q34.1	adult patients : 42,3% (33/78)	Associated with unfavorable cytogenetic risk group. Poor prognosis. (Xu et al., 2011)
FHIT (fragile histidine triad)	Fragile histidine triad gene member of a superfamily HIT of nucleotide binding proteins. Localization: 3p14.2	adult patients : 47,2% (26/55)	Advanced stages of MDS (RAEB, RAEB-t). Disease progression. (Lin et al., 2008)
RIZ-1 (retinoblastoma protein-interacting zinc finger gene)	Induce cell cycle arrest, apoptosis. Localization: 1p36	adult patients: 50% (17/34)	No statistically differences in low and high risk, it is relatively early event in MDS. (Mori et al., 2011)

Table 3. Methylation alterations in genes involved in the pathogenesis of MDS.

4. Statistical analysis of epigenetics biomarkers

Biomarkers have become important tools for diagnosis and treatment of a wide range of illnesses, including cancer. Early detection of cancer through biomarkers will allow for the development of new therapeutic procedures in order to increase survival rate of patients diagnosed with cancer. To help the evaluation of new biomarkers for medical practice, we use statistical methods. In this section, we shall discuss statistical techniques for biomarkers evaluation in the myelodysplastic syndrome (MDS). While the application of the methods presented is on biomarkers in MDS, the content of this section can be applied to any medical research.

The main mathematical concept necessary to understand statistical methods is *probability*. Although earlier work on the subject was done by the Italian mathematician Giralamo Cardano (1501-1576), the investigation of probability as a branch of Mathematics sprang about 1654 with two great French mathematicians: Blaise Pascal (1623-1662) and Pierre Fermat (1601–1665). Both Pascal and Fermat were interested in predicting outcomes in the games of chance popular among the French nobility of the mid-seventeenth century. Of course, we shall not do a discourse on probability. But we need to say that the theory of probability underlies the procedures in inferential statistics, which is very useful to medicine and other disciplines in the health field. In our exposition, we will try to avoid mathematical formulas and theorems.

4.1 Descriptive statistics and inferential statistics

Statistics is a branch of Mathematics. The word "statistics" derives from the Latin word *status*, meaning "manner of standing" or "position". Statistics were first used by tax assessors to collect information for determining assets and assessing taxes. Nowadays, the application of statistics is broad and includes business, marketing, economics, agriculture, education, medicine and others. Statistics applied to medicine and other health disciplines is called biostatistics or biometrics. For those who would like to review or study this subject we recommend the book of Zar, 2010.

Statistics is divided into two branches: descriptive and inferential. The goal of descriptive statistics is to organize and summarize data. And the goal of inferential statistics is to draw inferences and reach conclusions about a population, when only a sample from the population has been studied. A population is a complete set of observations, patients, measurements, and so forth. A sample is a subset of a certain population.

To organize data and summarize their main characteristics we can use *tables, graphs* and *quantitative indices*. Tables are often used to present qualitative and quantitative data. Graphs are used widely to provide a visual display data. The bar diagram, histogram and frequency polygon are three graphic formats that are commonly used to present medical data. A table or a graph in which all values of a variable of interest are displayed with their corresponding frequency is called a *frequency distribution,* or simply a *distribution*. We shall see in the next subsection that in inferential statistics we are interested in a special type of distribution: a probability distribution.

Quantitative indices are numbers that describe the center and the variation of a distribution. Quantitative indices that describe the center of a distribution are referred to as *measures of central tendency*. The mean, known also as the arithmetic mean, median and mode are three common measures of central tendency. Quantitative indices that describe the variation or dispersion of a distribution are referred to as *measures of dispersion*. The range, variance and standard deviation are three common measures of dispersion. In medicine we usually work with other quantitative indices as risk difference, relative risk and odds ratio. To draw inferences and reach conclusions about a population, when only a sample from that population has been studied, we need to know probability, because we use *statistical hypothesis testing* and *estimates*.

Statistical hypothesis tests can be *parametric* or *nonparametric*. Surveys of statistical methods used in journals indicate that the *t test* is one of the most commonly used statistical tests. The percentages of articles that use the t test range from 10% to more than 60%. Williams and colleagues (1997) noted a number of problems in using the t test. Welch and Gabbe (1996) found a number of errors in using the t test when a nonparametric procedure is called for. Thus, being able to use these techniques needs some skills in order to choose the correct statistical test.

4.2 Parametric and nonparametric tests

Combining the notion of a frequency distribution (descriptive statistics) and probability, we can explain what means a probability distribution. A *probability distribution* is a table or a graph that describes the probability of an event occurs. It describes what probably will happen instead of describing what really happened.

A probability distribution can be discrete or continuous. An important example of a discrete probability distribution is the *binomial distribution* and an important example of a continuous distribution is the *normal distribution*.

The binomial distribution is generated from a series of Bernoulli trials, named in honor of James Bernoulli (1654-1705). The binomial distribution is used when we have only two possible outcomes, which are mutually exclusive. For example, survived/died, male/female, adequate/inadequate, and others.

The normal distribution is known also as the Gaussian distribution, in honor of Carl F. Gauss (1777-1855), who made significant contributions in the beginning of the 19th century to its development. The geometric representation of such a distribution is a symmetric and bell-shaped curve, known as the normal curve. The most important characteristic of the normal curve is the following: if perpendiculars are erected at the distance of one standard deviation above and one standard deviation below the mean, approximately 68% of the total area is between these perpendiculars, the x-axis and the curve. If perpendiculars are constructed at a distance of two standard deviations above and below the mean, approximately 95% of the total area is enclosed. If perpendiculars are set at a distance of three standard deviations to the left and right of the mean, approximately 99,7% of the total area is included, as shown in Figure 5. Since there is a correspondence between area and probability, we have information about the probability of data be located k standard deviation around the mean, for k = 1, 2 or 3.

Comparing the above information with the information obtained by the Chebyshev theorem, we note that we can obtain more accurate results when data present a normal distribution. The Chebyshev theorem claims that, for any probability distribution, the probability of data be located k standard deviation around the mean is, at least, $1-1/k^2$, where k is a positive number greater than 1. Table 4 compares the Chebyshev's proportions with the proportions of a normal distribution, assuming k = 1, 2, 3 or 4.

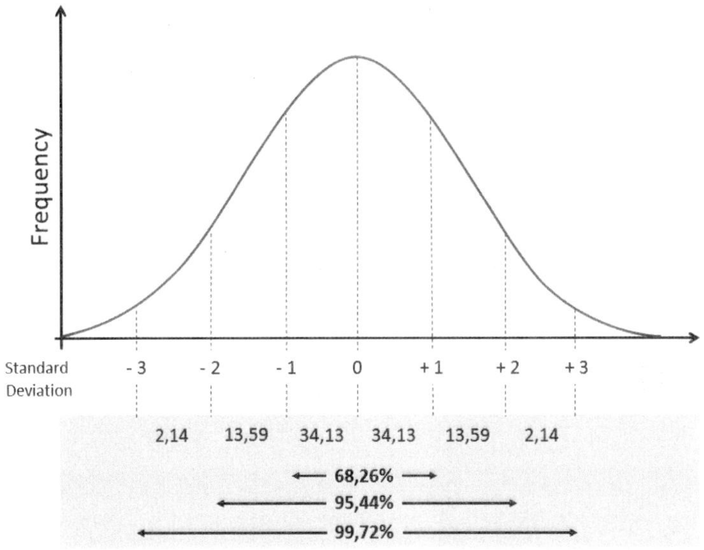

Fig. 5. Gaussian distribution.

k	Any distribution	Normal distribution
1	no information	68%
2	≥ 75%	95%
3	≥ 88%	99,7%
4	≥ 93,75 %	99,9%

Table 4. Chebyshev'proportions compared with proportions of a normal distribution.

If we decide to approximate clinical measurements by a normal curve, we are deciding to use a parametric hyphotesis test. A *hypothesis test* asks if an effect (difference) exists or not using statistics tests to verify the *hypothesis that there is no difference*. This is the *null hypothesis* and designated H_0. The hypothesis that contradicts H_0 is the *alternative hypothesis* and written H_A. In the null hypothesis we use the words *no difference* or *equal to* and in the alternative hypothesis we use the words *different from, less than* or *greater than*. But let us mention that, in fact, we should say *no statistical difference, statistically equal to, statistically different from, statistically less than* or *statistically greater than*, because we are dealing with the probabilities of an event happens or not. When we retain H_A (equivalently reject H_0), we say the results are significant and when we retain H_0 (equivalently reject H_A), we say the results are not significant. Because we are dealing with probabilities, this implies in making two possible errors from four possible relations between statistical conclusions and real situations, as shown in Table 5.

		Real difference	
		Presence	Absence
Conclusion of the statistical test	Results are significant	True	Type I error
	Results are not significant	Type II error	True

Table 5. Relations between statistical conclusions and real situations.

The two errors mentioned in the previous paragraph are known as Type I error and Type II error. A Type I error leads to a *false positive* conclusion. The probability of such an error occurs is noted by $\boldsymbol{\alpha}$. Mathematically, $\boldsymbol{\alpha}$ is a conditional probability: $\boldsymbol{\alpha}$ is the probability of reject H_0 when there is no real difference. A Type II error leads to a *false negative* conclusion. The probability of such an error occurs is noted by $\boldsymbol{\beta}$. Mathematically, $\boldsymbol{\beta}$ is a conditional probability: $\boldsymbol{\beta}$ is the probabilities of retain H_0 when there is a real difference.

Statistical tests are used to estimate the probability of a Type I error. In the literature, we usually use $\boldsymbol{\alpha} < 0.05$. This means we are assuming a probability less than 0.05 of rejecting H_0 when there is no real difference between treatments, drugs or procedures. In other words, if the study were repeated one-hundred times, we *probably* would find five outcomes showing H_0 should be accepted.

There are several tests commonly used in the medical literature; they are resumed in Table 6. Investigators should decide by using a parametric or a nonparametric test. This choice depends on the purpose of the study, the size of the sample, the type of the variables involved at the study, for instance. To use a parametric test we need to guarantee that the sampling distribution is normal or approximately normal. Because normal distribution has nice mathematical properties (bell-shaped, symmetric, and so on), using a parametric test leads to better statistical results compared with a nonparametric test. In other words, we say that nonparametric tests are less powerful, in the sense that they lead to a small probability to reject H_0, when H_0 is false.

To test the statistical significance of the difference between ...		
Two or more proportions	Chi-square	nonparametric
Two proportions	Fisher's exact	parametric
Two medians	Mann-Whitney	nonparametric
Two means	t-Student	parametric
More than two means	Kruskal-Wallis (one-factor)	nonparametric
More than two means	ANOVA (one-factor)	parametric
More than two means	ANOVA (more-factors)	parametric

Table 6. Statistical tests usually used in the medical literature.

When we use a statistic test we compute a *p-value*. The *p-value* is the probability of obtaining a result as extreme or more extreme than the sample value, assuming that the null hypothesis is true. The sample value is calculated. Depending on the test we use, there is a specific formula to calculate the sample value. Appropriate computer software can do such a calculation.

An increasing number of journals require that investigators include p-values in their manuscripts. When p-values are given, we are able to compare this probability to our own decision rule, which is the value of **α**. If the p-value is less than **α**, we say that the results are significant statistically. If the p-value is greater than **α**, we say that the results are not significant statistically.

4.3 Statistical methods for evaluation of biomarkers in myelodysplastic syndrome

Biostatistics gives us important tools to evaluate biomarkers in myelodysplastic syndrome and other diseases. Quantitative indices, estimates, hypothesis tests and survival tables are useful to point out biomarkers. We already discussed about quantitative indices and hypothesis tests. Let us make few comments about estimates and survival tables.

In many situations, populations are so large that it is impossible to describe their central tendency and dispersion by studying 100% of their members, or by studying a sufficiently large portion of population to justify treating sample statistics as population parameters. In other situations, clinicians may study a new phenomenon with little basis to determine a population parameter. In these cases, we use estimates. Two types of estimates of a population parameter can be used: a point estimate and an interval estimate. A point estimate is a single numerical value of a sample statistic used to estimate the corresponding population parameter. Point estimates are not used widely because the value of some statistic, such as the sample mean, varies from sample to sample. So, an interval estimative is typically used. An interval estimate is a range of values which the parameter is likely to occur. Interval estimates are also called confidence intervals.

Survival tables are used to describe prognosis. Prognosis is a prediction of the future course of a disease following its onset (Fletcher et al., 1988). We can describe the prognosis of a disease considering a fixed period of time (measures or taxes) or considering varying periods of time (survival tables). Table 7 shows the common measures used to describe prognosis when we consider a fixed period of time.

Measure	Definition
Five-year survival	Percentage of patients who survive for five years from a certain time of the course of the disease
Response	Percentage of patients who show some evidence of improvement after a procedure or an intervention
Remission	Percentage of patients who start a period in which the disease is not detectable
Recurrence	Percentage of patients who present reappearance of the disease after a free period

Table 7. Common measures that describe prognosis.

Survival tables can handle situations in which patients enter in some trial at different times and are followed for varying periods. We usually consider the length of time in a certain trial as being days, weeks or months and the end point may be, in the MDS case, death or the reappearance of the disease. The usual method used to construct a survival table is the Kaplan-Meier method. The curve obtained from the data presented in a survival table is called a survival curve.

The survival tables can allow us to compare two or more groups of patients. In this case, the first thing we should do is draw the survival curves for the two (or more) groups on the same graph. Statistical methods are important here, because we cannot make judgments simply on the basis of the amount of separation between the curves; a small difference may be statistically significant if the sample size is large, and a large difference may not if the sample size is small. We have mainly two methods to determine if the differences are statistically significant: the Wilcoxon rank sum test and the log rank test. Figure 6 shows comparative survival curves for pediatric and adult patients diagnosed with MDS treated with allogeneic hematopoietic stem cell transplantation (HSCT).

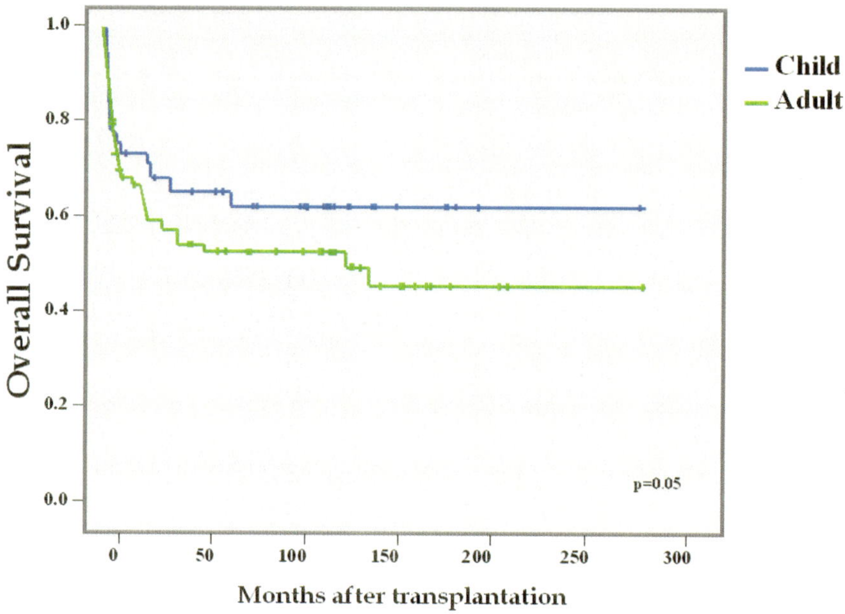

Fig. 6. Overall survival of primary MDS patients treated with allogeneic HSCT, pediatric patients versus adult patients.

In the Rodrigues et al (2010) study, the authors studied the methylation status of the $p15^{INK4B}$ and $p16^{INK4A}$ genes in 47 pediatric patients with MDS, its correlation with subtype, and the role of $p15^{INK4B}$ and $p16^{INK4A}$ in the evolution of MDS toward AML. The results obtained suggest that methylation of these genes is an epigenetic biomarker of pediatric disease evolution. The authors used some statistical tools presented here. For example, the correlation between $p15^{INK4B}$ gene methylation status and subtypes of pediatric primary MDS, considering initial stage RC, and later stages RAEB and RAEB-t, was assessed by the chi-square test, which is a nonparametric test. The statistical analysis suggested that the frequency of $p15^{INK4B}$ gene methylation was significantly higher in later stages of disease compared with the initial stage, with p-value < 0.003. The correlation between $p16^{INK4A}$ gene methylation status and subtypes of pediatric primary MDS was also assessed by the chi-square test, with a slight modification. In fact, it is a correction factor, which is necessary when we have a small number of data. This is known as chi-square with continuity correction or chi-square with Yates'correction. The results obtained suggested that the frequency of $p16^{INK4A}$ gene methylation was found more frequently in subtypes characterizing the advanced stages of MDS, with p-value < 0.05.

Quantitative analysis to evaluate whether there was a correlation between percentage of $p15^{INK4B}$ methylation and MDS subtypes was performed in (Rodrigues et al., 2010). The percentage of $p15^{INK4B}$ methylation was higher in RAEB and RAEB-t compared to RC. The authors used ANOVA (one-factor) and obtained a p-value $< 0{,}0001$. The same result was obtained for the $p16^{INK4A}$ gene. The authors used ANOVA (more-factors) to verify that QMS-PCR method was more sensitive than COBRA method, obtaining a p-value < 0.0001, although both methods were accurate in showing a correlation between the subtypes of disease and the level of methylation.

The Mann-Whitney test was also used. The authors calculated the mean time of disease evolution in patients who had $p15^{INK4B}$ methylation and in patients with no $p15^{INK4B}$ methylation. The results were 4.6 months and 14.6 months, respectively. The mean time of disease evolution for patients who had $p15^{INK4B}$ methylation, therefore, was three times less than the mean time of evolution for patients who had no $p15^{INK4B}$ methylation, which was statistically significant by using Mann-Whitney (p-value < 0.02).

Many concepts and theorems that are not familiar to medical professionals are used in Statistics, as null hypothesis, regression, parametric tests, the central limit theorem, Bayes theorem and so on. Of course, medical professionals should put away the complexity of such concepts and the mathematics is behind all this theory, although only mathematics could explain *rigorously* why these techniques really work. Nevertheless we must say that Statistics is an important tool that *can help* making decisions and must be used if the statistics outcomes are clinically meaningful. Accumulated experience and specific knowledge must be combined with results from statistical tests to assess the usefulness of a particular outcome or medical decision.

5. Conclusion

The field of cancer epigenetics is evolving rapidly. Advances in the understanding of chromatin structure, histone modifications, DNA methylation and transcriptional activity have resulted in an increasingly integrated view of epigenetics. These discoveries lead to the development of new treatments in cancer using epigenetic therapies. The MDS comprises a complex spectrum of hematopoietic stem cell disorders, where the study of epigenetics has brought new knowledge about the development and evolution of this disease to AML. Other important points in epigenetics studies in MDS were the introduction of the treatments using hypomethylant drugs and histone deacethylases inhibitors. The MDS may be considered a good model to study the epigenetics in the cancer pathogenesis research and the applicability in clinical. The identification of biomarkers of diagnosis and prognosis in MDS will possibility the elaboration of new classification and score prognostic systems and will help to understand the different pathways involved in the MDS pathogenesis. With the advance of the technologies involving epigenome projects, future research in the epigenetic therapies will be the development of inhibitors with specificity to particular biomarkers.

6. Acknowledgments

This work was supported by grants from Rio de Janeiro State Research Support Foundation (FAPERJ) (project nº E-26/102.235/2009), Brazil; Brazilian Ministry of Health, National Cancer Institute (INCA).

7. References

Agalioti, T.; Chen, G. & Thanos, D. (2002). Deciphering the transcriptional histone acetylation code for a human gene. *Cell*, vol.111, pp. 381-392.

Aggerholm, A.; Holm, M.S.; Gulberg, P.; Olesen, L.H. & Hokland, P. (2006). Promoter hypermethylation of p15Ink4B, HIC1, CDH1 and ER is frequent in myelodysplastic syndrome and predicts poor prognosis in early-stage patients. Eur J Haematol, vol.76, pp.23-32.

Akatas, D. & Tuncbilek, E. (2006). Myelodysplastic syndrome associated with monosomy 7 in chuildhood: a retrospective study. *Cancer Genets and Cytogen*, vol.171, pp.72-75.

Atalhah, E.; Kantarjian, H. & Garcia Manero G. (2007). The role of decitabine in the treatment of myelodysplastic syndromes. *Exp O. Pharmac*, vol.8, pp.65-73.

Bacher, U.; Haferlach, C.; Krogher, N.; Schnittger, S.; Kern, W.; Wiedemann, B.; Zander, A.R. & Haferlach, T. (2010). Diagnostic tools in the indicators for allogeneic stem cell tranplantation in myelodysplastic syndromes. Biol Blood Marrow Transplant, vol.16, pp.1-11.

Bantignies, F. & Cavalli, G. (2006). Cellular memory and dynamic regulation of polycomb group proteins. *Curr Opin Cell Biol*, vol.18, pp.275-283.

Bejar, R.; Levine, R. & Ebert, B.L. (2011). Unraveling the molecular Pathophysiology of Myelodysplastic Syndrome. *Journal of Clinical Oncology*, vol.29, pp.504-515.

Bennett, J. & Orazi, A. (2009). Diagnostic criteria to distinguish hypocellular acute leukemia from hypocellular myelodysplastic syndrome and aplastic anemia: recomendations for standardized approach. *Haematologica*, vol.94, pp.264-268.

Bennett, J.M.; Catovsky, D.; Daniel, M.T.; Flandrin, G.; Galton, D.A.; Gralnick, H.R. & Sultan, C. (1982). Proposals for the classification of the myelodysplastic syndromes. *British Journal of Haematology*, vol.51, pp.189-199.

Brakensiek, K.; Länger, F.; Schlegelberger, B.; Kreipe, H. & Lehmann, U. (2005). Hypermethylation of the suppressor of cytokine signalling-1 (SOCS-1) in myelodysplastic syndrome. *Br J Haematol*, vol.130, pp.209-17.

Brunning, R.D.; Orazi, A.; Germing, U.; Le Beau, M.M., Porwit, A.; Baumann, I.; Vardimann, J.W. & Hellstrom-Lindberg, E. (2008). Myelodysplastic syndromes. In: Swedlow, S.H.; Campo, E.; Harris, N. L. ed. WHO classification of Tumors of Haematopoietic and Lymphoid Tissues. 4th ed. Lyon, France: IARC Press; pp:88-107.

Davids, M.S. & Steensma, D.P. (2010). The molecular pathogenesis of myelodysplastic syndromes. *Cancer Biology & Therapy*, vol.10, pp.309-319.

Elghetany, M.T. (2007). Myelodysplastic Syndromes in Children: A Critical Review of Issues in the Diagnosis and Classification of 887 Cases from 13 Published Series. *Arch Pathol Lab Med*, vol.131, pp.1110-1116.

Ellis, L.; Atadja, P.W. & Johnstone, R.W. (2009). Epigenetics in cancer. Targeting chromatin modifications. Mol Cancer Ther, vol.8, pp.1409-1420.

Esteller, M. (2011). Cancer Epigenetics for the 21st Century: What's Next? *Genes Cancer*, vol.2, pp.604-606.

Fenaux,P.; Mufti, G.J., Hellstrom-Lindberg, E.; Santini, V.; Finelli, C.; Giagounidis, A.; Schoch, R.; Gatterman, N.; Sanz, G.; List, A.; Gore, S.D.; Seymour, JF.; Bennett, J.M.; Byrd, J.; Backstrom, J.; Zimmerman, L.; McKenzle, D.; Beach, C.; Silverman, L.R. (2009). Efficacy of azacitidine compared with that of conventional care regimens in the treatment of higher risk myelodysplastic syndromes: a randomized, open-label, phase III study. Lancet Oncol, vol. 10, pp.223-232.

Fernandez, T.S.; Ornellas, M.H.; Carvalho, L.O.; Tabak, D. & Abdelhay, E. (2000). Chromosomal alterations associated with evolution from myelodysplastic syndrome to acute myeloid leukemia. *Leuk Res*, vol.24, pp.839-848.

Fernandez, T.S.; Souza, J.; Silva, M.L.; Tabak, D. & Abdelhay, E. (1998). Correlation of N-ras point mutation with specific chromosomal abnormalities in primary myelodysplastic syndrome. Leuk Res, vol.22, pp.225-134.

Fletcher, R.; Fletcher, S. & Wagner, E. (1988). Clinical Epidemiology: The Essentials. 2nd (Ed.). In: *Williams & Wilkins*.

Garcia-Manero, G. (2010). Prognosis of Myelodysplastic Syndromes. *Hematology Am Soc Hematol Educ Program*, pp.330-337.

Giralt, S. (2005). Bone marrow transplant in myelodysplastic syndromes: new technologies, same questions. *Curr hematol Rep*, vol.4, pp.200-207.

Graham, J.S.; Kaye, S.B. & Brown, R. (2009). The promises and pitfalls of epigenetic therapies in solid tumours. *Eur J Cancer*, vol.45, No.7, pp.1129-36.

Greenberg, P.; Cox, C.; Le Beau, M.M.; Fenaux, P.; Morel, P.; Sanz, G.; Sanz, M.; Vallespi, T.; Hamblin, T.; Oscier, D.; Ohyashiki, K.; Toyama, K.; Aul, C.; Mufti, G. & Bennett, J. (1997). International Scoring System for Evaluating Prognosis in Myelodysplastic Syndromes. *Blood*, vol.89, pp.2079-2088.

Gurion, R.; Vidal, L.; Gafter-Gvili, A.; Belnik, Y.; Yeshurun, M.; Raanani, P. & Shpilberg, O. (2010). 5-azacitidine prolongs overall survival in patients with myelodysplastic syndrome- a systematic review and meta-anlaysis. *Haematologica*, vol. 95, pp.303-3010.

Haase, D. (2008). Cytogenetics features in myelodysplastic syndromes. *Annals of Hematology*, vol.87, pp.515-526.

Haase, D.; Germing, U., Schanz, J.; Pfeilstöcker, M.; Nösslinger, T.; Hildebrandt, B.; Kundgen, A.; Lübbert, M.; Kunzmann, R.; Giagounidis, A.A.; Aul, C.; Trümper, L.; Krieger, O.; Stauder, R.; Müller, T.H.; Wimazal, F.; Valent, P.; Fonatsch, C. & Steidl, C. (2007). New insights into the prognostic impact of the karyotype in MDS and correlation with subtypes: evidence from a core dataset of 2124 patients. *Blood*, vol.110, pp.4385-4395.

Harris, N.L.; Jaffe, E.S.; Diebold, J.; Flandrin, G.; Muller-Hermelink, H.K.; Vardiman, J.; Lister, T.A. & Bloomfield, C.D. (2000). The World Health Organization classification of hematological malignancies report of the Clinical Advisory Committee Meeting, Airlie House, Virginia. *Mod Pathol*, vol.13, pp.193-207.

Hasegawa, D.; Manabe, A.; Kubota, T.; Kawasaki, H.; Hirose, I.; Ohtsuka, Y.; Tsuruta, T.; Ebihara, Y.; Goto, Y.; Zhao, X.Y.; Sakashita, K.; Koike, K.; Isomura, M.; Kojima, S.; Hoshika, A.; Tsuji, K. & Nakahata, T. (2005). Methylation status of p15 and p16 genes inpediatric myelodysplastic síndrome and juvenile myelomonocytic leukemia. *Br J Haematol*, vol.128, pp. 805-812.

Hasle, H.; Baumann, I.; Bergsträsser, E.; Fenu, S.; Fischer, A.; Kardos, G.; Kerndrup, G.; Locatelli, F.; Rogge, T.; Schultz, K.R.; Starý, J.; Trebo, M.; van den Heuvel-Eibrink, M.M.; Harbott, J.; Nöllke, P. & Niemeyer, C.M. (2004). The international prognostic scoring system (IPSS) for childhood myelodysplastic syndrome (MDS) and juvenile myelomonocytic leukemia (JMML). *Leukemia*, vol.18, pp.2008–2014.

Hasle, H. & Niemeyer, C.M. (2002). Myelodysplastic syndrome and Juvenile Myelomonocytic leukemia in children. In: The Myelodysplastic syndromes: Pathobiology and Clinical Management. (Ed.) Bennett JM & Dekker, Inc, Ney York, Basel, pp.299-344.

Hasle,H. & Niemeyer, C. (2011). Advances in the prognostication and management of advanced MDS in children. Br J Haematol, vol. 154, pp.185-195.

Hasle, H.; Niemeyer, C.M.; Chessels, J.M.; Baumann, I.; Bennett, J.M.; Kerndrup, G. & Head, D.R. (2003). A pediatric approach to the WHO classification of myelodysplastic and myeloproliferative diseases. *Leukemia*, vol.17, pp.277-282.

Hebeda, K.M. & Fend, F. (2009). Changed concepts and definitions of myeloproliferative neoplasms (MPM), myelodysplastic syndromes (MDS) and myelodysplastic/myeloproliferative neoplasms (MDS/MPM) in the updated 2008 WHO classification. *J Hematopathol*, vol.2, pp.205-210.

Henrique, R. & Jerônimo, C. (2004). Molecular detection of prostate cancer: a role for GSTP1 hypermethylation. *Eur Urol*, vol.46, No.5, pp.660-669.

Hrebackova, J.; Hrabeta, J. & Eckschlager, T. (2010). Valproic acid in the complex therapy of malignant tumors. *Curr Drug Targets*, vol.11, No.3, pp.361-379.

Ingham, P.W. (1985). A clonal analysis of the requirement for the trithorax gene in the diversification of segments in Drosophila. *J Embryol Exp Morphol*, vol.89, pp.349-365.

Jädersten, M. & Hellström-Lindberg, E. (2008). Myelodysplastic syndromes: biology and treatment. *Journal of Internal Medicine*, vol.265, pp.307-328.

Jekic, B.; Novakovic, I.; Lukovic, L.; Kuzmanovic, M.; Popovic, B.; Pastar, I.; Milasin, J.; Bunjevacki, G. & Bunjevacki, V. (2004). Low frequency of N-ras and K-ras gene mutations. Cancer Genet Cytogenet, vol.154, No.2, pp.180-182.

Jekic, B.; Novakovic, I.; Lukovic, L.; Kuzmanovic, M.; Popovic, B.; Milasin, J.; Bunjevacki, G.; Damnjanovic, T.; Cvjeticanin, S. & Bunjevacki V. (2006). Lack of TP53 and FMS gene mutations in children with myelodysplastic syndrome. Cancer Genet Cytogenet, vol.166, No.2, pp.163-165.

Jerónimo, C.; Bastian, P.J.; Bjartell, A.; Carbone, G.M.; Catto, J.W.; Clark, S.J.; Henrique, R.; Nelson, W.G. & Shariat, S.F. (2011). Epigenetics in prostate cancer: biologic and clinical relevance. *Eur Urol*, vol.60. No.4, pp.753-766.

Katz, V. J. (1993). A History of Mathematics, In: An Introduction. Harper Collins College Publishers, New York.

Kelly, T.K.; De Carvalho, D.D. & Jones, P.A. (2010). Epigenetic modifications as therapeutic targets. Nat Biotechnol, vol.28, No.10, pp.1069-1078.

Kindwall-Keller, T. & Isola, L.M. (2009). The evolution of hematopoietic SCT in myelodysplastic syndrome. *Bone Marrow Transplantation*, vol.43, pp.597-609.

Kleff, S.; Andrulis, E.D.; Anderson, C.W. & Sternglanz, R. (1995). Identification of a gene encoding a yeast histone H4 acetyltransferase. *Journal of Biological Chemistry,* vol.270, No.42, pp.24674–24677.

Levine, S.S.; King, I.F. & Kingston, R.E. (2004). Division of labor in polycomb group repression. *Trends Biochem Sci*, vol.29, pp.478-485.

Lewis, E.B. (1978). A gene complex controlling segmentation in Drosophila. *Nature*, vol.276, No.5688, pp.565-570.

Lin, J.; Yao, D.M.; Qian, J.; Wang, Y.L.; Han, L.X.; Jiang, Y.W.; Fei, X.; Cen, J.N. & Chen, Z.X. (2008). Methylation status of fragile histidine triad (FHIT) gene and its clinical impact on prognosis of patients with myelodysplastic syndrome. *Leuk Res,* vol.32, pp.541-1545.

Malcovati, L. & Nimer, S.D. (2008). Myelodysplastic Syndromes: diagnosis and staging. *Cancer Control*, vol.15, pp.4-13.

Margueron, R. & Reinberg, D. (2005). The Polycomb complex PRC2 and its mark in life. Nature, vol.2011, pp.343-349.

Marks, P.A. & Dokmanovic, M. (2005). Histone deacetylase inhibitors: discovery and development as anticancer agents. *Expert Opin Investig Drugs,* vol.14, pp.1497-1511.

Mori, N.; Yoshinaga, K.; Tomita, K.; Ohwashi, M.; Kondoh, T.; Shimura, H.; Wang, Y.H.; Shiseki, M.; Okada, M. & Motoji, T. (2011). Aberrant methylation of the RIZ gene in myelodysplastic syndrome and acute myeloid leukemia. Leuk Res, vol.35, No.4, pp.516-21.

Niemeyer, C.M. & Baumann, I. (2008). Myelodysplastic Syndrome in Children and Adolescents. *Semin Hematol*, vol.45, pp.60-70.

Niemeyer, C.M. & Kratz, C.P. (2008). Pediatric myelodysplastic syndromes and juvenile myelomonocytic leukemia: molecular classification and treatment options. *Br J haematol*, vol.140, pp.610-624.

Nikoloski, G.; Langemeijer, S.M.; Kuiper, R.; Knops, R.; Massop, M.; Tönnissen, E.R.; van der Heijden, A.; Scheele, T.N.; Vandenberghe, P.; de Witte, T.; van der Reijden, B.A. & Jansen, J.H. (2010). Somatic mutations of the histone methyltransferase gene EZH2 in myelodysplastic syndromes. Nat Genet, vol.42, No.8, pp.665-667.

Nishino, H.T. & Cahng, C.C. (2005). Myelodysplastic syndromes: Clinicopathologic features, pathobiology and molecular pathogenesis. *Arch Pathol Lab Med,* vol. 129, pp.1299-1310.

Oliva, E.M.; Cuzzola, M.; Nobile, F.; Ronco, F.; D'Errigo, M.G.; Lagana, C.; Morabito, F.; Galimberti, S.; Cortelezzi, A.; Aloe Spiriti, M.A.; Specchia, G.; Poloni, A.; Breccia, M.; Ghio, R.; Finelli, C.; Iacopino, P.; Alimena, G. & Latagliata, R. (2010). Changes in RPS14 expression levels during lenalidomide treatment in low and intermediate-1 risk myelodysplastic syndromes with chromosome 5q deletion. Eur J Haematol, vol.85, No.3, pp.231-235.

Olney, H.J. & Le Beau, M.M. (2009). *The Cytogenetics and Molecular Biology of the Myelodysplastic Syndromes.* In: Myelodysplastic Syndromes: Pathobiology and Clinical Management . (Ed.) 2nd Edition.,pp. 49-86.

Onley, H.J. & Le Beau, M.M. (2009). Myelodysplastic Syndromes. In: *Cancer Cytogenetics.* (Ed.) Heim S and Mitelman F. ed. Wiley-Blackwell, pp.141-178.

Parker, J.E.; Mufti, G.J.; Rasoll, F.; Mijovic, A.; Devereux, S. & Pagliuca, A. (2000). The role of apoptosis, proliferation, and the Bcl-2-related proteins in the myelodysplastic syndromes and acute myeloid leukemia secondary to MDS. *Blood*, vol. 96, pp.3932-3938.

Polychronopoulou, S.; Panagiotou, J.P.; Kossiva, L.; Mavrou, A.; Anagnostou, D. & Haidas, S. (2004). Clinical and morphological features of pediatric myelodysplastic syndromes: a review of 34 cases. *Acta pediatric*, vol.93, pp.1015-1023.

Qin, T.; Castoro, R.; El Ahdab, S.; Jelinek, J.; Wang, X.; Si, J.; Shu, J.; He, R.; Zhang, N.; Chung, W.; Kantarjian, H.M.& Issa, J.P. (2011). Mechanisms of Resistance to Decitabine in the Myelodysplastic Syndrome. *PloS One*, vol.6, pp.1-10.

Quesnel, B.; Guillerm, G.; Vereecque, R.; Wattel, E.; Preudhomme, C.; Bauters, F.; Vanrumbeke, M. & Fenaux, P. (1998). Methylation of the p15(INK4b) gene in myelodysplastic syndromes is frequent and acquired during disease progression. Blood, vol.91, No.8, pp.2985-90.

Rajasekhar, V.K. & Begemann, M. (2007). Concise review: roles of polycomb group proteins in development and disease: a stem cell prospective. *Stem Cells*, vol.25, pp.2498-2510.

Rao, P.M.; Antony, A.; Rajalakshmi, S. & Sarma, D.S. (1989). Studies on hypomethylation of liver DNA during early stages of chemical carcinogenesis in rat liver. *Carcinogenesis*, vol.10, pp.933–37.

Razak, A.R.; Hotte, S.J.; Siu, L.L.; Chen, E.X.; Hirte, H.W.; Powers, J.; Walsh, W.; Stayner, L.A.; Laughlin, A.; Novotny-Diermayr, V.; Zhu, J. & Eisenhauer, E.A. (2011). Phase I clinical, pharmacokinetic and pharmacodynamic study of SB939, an oral histone deacetylase (HDAC) inhibitor, in patients with advanced solid tumours. *Br J Cancer*, vol.104, No.5, pp.756-762.

Robertson, K.D.; Uzvolgyi, E.; Liang, G.; Talmadge, C.; Sumegi, J.; Gonzales, F.A. & Jones, P.A. (1999). The human DNA methyltransferases (DNMTs) 1, 3a and 3b: coordinate mRNA expression in normal tissues and overexpression in tumors. Nucleic Acids Res, vol.27, No.11, pp.2291-2298.

Rodrigues, E.F.; Santos-Rebouças, C.B.; Pimentel, M.M.G.; Mencalha, A.L.; Dobbin, J.; Costa, E.S.; Fernandez, C.S.; Bouzas, L.F.; Abdelhay, E. & Fernandez, T.S. (2010). Epigenetic alterations of $p15^{Ink4B}$ and $p16^{Ink4A}$ genes in pediatric primary myelodysplastic syndrome. *Leukemia & Lymphoma*, vol.51, pp.1887-94.

Sakashita, K.; Koike, K.; Kinoshita, T.; Shiohara, M.; Kamijo, T.; Taniguchi, S. & Kubota, T. (2001). Dynamic DNA methylation change in the CpG island region of p15 during human myeloid development. J Clin Invest, vol.108, No.8, pp.1195-1204.

Sasaki, H.; Manabe, A.; Kojima, S.; Tsuchida, M.; Hayashi, Y.; Ikuta, K.; Okamura, I.; Koike, K.; Ohara, A.; Ishii, E.; Komada, Y.; Hibi, S. & Nakahata, T. (2001). MDS Committee of the Japanese Society of Pediatric Hematology, Japan. Myelodysplastic syndrome in childhood: a retrospective study of 189 patients in Japan. Leukemia, vol.15, No.11, pp.1713-1720.

Serrano, M.; Lee, H.; Chin, L.; Cordon-Cardo, C.; Beach, D. & DePinho, R.A. (1996). Role of the Ink4a locus in tumor suppression and cell mortality. *Cell*, vol.85, pp.27-37.

Shen, L.; Kantarjian, H.; Guo, Y.; Lin, E.; Shan, J.; Huang, X.; Berry, D.; Ahmed, S.; Zhu, W.; Pierce, S.; Kondo, Y.; Oki, Y.; Jelinek, J.; Saba, H.; Estey, E. & Issa, J.P. (2010). DNA methylation predicts survival and response to therapy in patients with myelodysplastic syndromes. J Clin Oncol, vol.28, No.4, pp.605-613.

Shimamoto, T.; Ohyashiki, J.H. & Ohyashiki, K. (2005). Methylation of p15Ink4B and E-caherin genes is independently correlated with poor prognosis in acute myeloid leukemia. *Leuk Res*, vol.29, pp.653-659.

Silverman, L.R. & Mufti, G. (2005). Methylation inhibitor therapy in the treatment of myelodysplastic syndrome. *Nat Clin Pract Oncol*, vol.2, pp.12-23.

Solé, F.; Espinet, B.; Sanz, G.F.; Cervera, J.; Calasanz, M.J.; Luño, E.; Prieto, F.; Granada, I.; Hernández, J.M.; Cigudosa, J.C.; Diez, J.L.; Bureo, E.; Marqués, M.L.; Arranz, E.; Ríos, R.; Martínez-Climent, J.A.; Vallespí, T.; Florensa, L. & Woessner, S. (2000). Incidence, characterization and prognostic significance of chromosomal abnormalities in 640 patients with primary myelodysplastic syndromes. Grupo Cooperativo Español de Citogenética Hematológica. Br J Haematol, vol.108, No.2, pp.346-356.

Solé, F.; Luno, E.; Sanzo, C.; Espinet, B.; Sanz, G.F.; Cervera, J.; Calasanz, M.J.; Cigudosa, J.C.; Milla, F.; Ribera, J.M.; Bureo, E.; Marquez, M.L.; Arranz, E. & Florensa, L. (2005). Identification of novel cytogenetic markers with prognostic significance in a series of 968 patients with primary myelodysplastic syndromes. *Haematologica*, vol.90, pp.1168-1178.

Solomon, P.R.; Munirajan, A.K.; Tsuchida, N.; Muthukumarasamy, K.; Rathinavel, A.; Selvam, G.S. & Shanmugam, G. (2008). Promoter hypermethylation analysis in myelodysplastic syndromes: diagnostic & prognostic implication. *Indian J Med Res*, pp.127:52-7.

Stresemann, C. & Lyko, F. (2008). Modes of action of the DNA methyltransferase inhibitors azacytidine and decitabine. *Int J Cancer*, vol.123, No.1, pp.8-13.

Szmigielska-Kapłon, A. & Robak, T. (2011). Hypomethylating Agents in the Treatment of Myelodysplastic Syndromeas and Myeloid Leukemia. *Curr Cancer Drug Targets*. (Jun 15). In: PubMed PMID: 21762079.

Tabby, R. & Issa, J.P. (2010). Cancer Epigenetics. *CA Cancer J Clin*, vol.60, pp.376-392.

Tan, P.T. & Wei, A.H. (2011). The epigenomics revolution in myelodysplasia: a clinico-pathological perspective. Pathology, vol.43, pp.536-546.

Teofili, L.; Morosetti, R.; Martini, M.; Urbano, R.; Putzulu, R.; Rutella, S.; Pierelli, L.; Leone, G. & Larocca, L.M. (2000). Expression of cyclin-dependent kinase inhibitor p15(INK4B) during normal and leukemic myeloid differentiation. Exp Hematol, vol.28, No.5, pp.519-526.

Tiu, R.V.; Visconte, V.; Traina, F.; Schwandt, A. & Maciejewski, J.P. (2011). Updates in Cytogenetics and Molecular Markers in MDS. *Curr Hematol Malig Rep*, vol.6, pp.126-35.

van Lohuizen, M.; Frasch, M.; Wientjens, E. & Berns, A. (1991). Sequence similarity between the mammalian bmi-1 proto-oncogene and the Drosophila regulatory genes Psc and Su(z)2. *Nature*, vol.26, No.353(6342), pp.353-355.

Vidal, D.O.; Paixão, V.A.; Brait, M.; Souto, E.X.; Caballero, O.L.; Lopes, L.F. & Vettore, A.L. (2007). Aberrant methylation in pediatric myelodysplastic syndrome. Leuk Res, vol.31, No.2, pp.175-181.

Vigna, E.; Recchia, A.G.; Madeo, A.; Gentile, M.; Bossio, S.; Mazzone, C.; Lucia, E.; Morabito, L.; Gigliotti, V.; Stefano, L.D.; Caruso, N.; Servillo, P.; Franzese, S.; Fimognari, F.; Bisconte, M.G.; Gentile, C. & Morabito, F. (2011). Epigenetic regulation in myelodysplastic syndromes: implications for therapy. Expert Opin Investig Drugs, vol.20, No.4, pp.465-493.

Welch, G.E. & Gabbe, S.G. (1996). Review of statistics usage in the American Journal of Obstetrics and Gynecology. *Am J Obstet Gynecol,* vol.175, pp.1138-1141.

Williams, J.L.; Hathaway, C.A.; Kloster, K.L. & Layne, B.H. (1997). Low power, type II errors, and other statistical problems in recent cardiovascular research. *Am J Physiol,* vol.273, pp.4487-4493.

Wong, K.F. & So, C.C. (2002). Hypoplastic Myelodysplastic Syndrome - a Clinical, Morphologic, or Genetic Diagnosis? *Cancer Genetics and Cytogenetics*; vol.138, pp.85-88.

Worn, J. & Gulberg, P. (2002). DNA methylation: an epigenetic pathway to cancer and promising target for anticancer therapy. *J Oral Pathol Med,* vol.31, pp.443-449.

Wu, X.; Liu, W.; Tian, Y.; Xiao, M.; Wu, Y. & Li, C. (2011). Aberrant methylation of death-associated protein kinase 1 CpG islands in myelodysplastic syndromes. *Acta Haematol,* vol.125, pp.179-85.

Xu, F.; Li, X.; Wu, L.; Zhang, Q.; Yang, R.; Yang, Y.; Zhang, Z.; He, Q. & Chang, C. (2011). Overexpression of the EZH2, RING1 and BMI1 genes is common in myelodysplastic syndromes: relation to adverse epigenetic alteration and poor prognostic scoring. Ann Hematol, vol.90, No.6, pp.643-53.

Zar, J.H. (2010). Biostatistical Analysis. 5th ed. Prentice Hal, New Jersey.

4

Urinary Water-Soluble Vitamins as Nutritional Biomarker to Estimate Their Intakes

Tsutomu Fukuwatari and Katsumi Shibata
The University of Shiga Prefecture, Japan

1. Introduction

The traditional approach of nutritional assessment is to survey the amount of nutrients consumed by dietary assessment. Although this method can provide approximate intake, this approach often makes misreporting, and can't determine nutritional status. Especially, to determine micronutrient intake by dietary assessment is difficult because of high variations in habitual micronutrient intake. A nutritional biomarker can be an indicator of nutritional status with respect to intake or metabolism of dietary constituents. The nutritional biomarkers can be designated into one or more of three categories, 1) a means of validation of dietary instruments, 2) surrogate indicators of dietary intakes, or 3) integrated measures of nutritional status for a nutrient (Potischman & Freudenheim, 2003). Recent validation studies have developed the urinary compounds as nutritional biomarkers to estimate nutrient intakes. For example, 24-hr urinary nitrogen has been established as a biomarker for protein intake (Bingham, 2003), same as urinary potassium and potassium intake (Tasevska et al., 2006), and urinary sugars for sugar intake (Tasevska et al., 2005).

Water-soluble vitamins are absorbed from the digestive tract after ingestion, stored in the liver, delivered to peripheral, and then excreted to urine (Food and Nutrition Board, Institute of Medicie, 1998). Urinary water-soluble vitamins or their metabolites decrease markedly as vitamin status declines, and they are affected by recent dietary intake (Food and Nutrition Board, Institute of Medicie, 1998). Urinary excretion of water-soluble vitamins such as thiamin, riboflavin and niacin has been used for setting Dietary Reference Intakes (DRIs) in USA and Japan (Food and Nutrition Board, Institute of Medicie, 1998; The Ministry of Health, Labour, and Welfare, 2009). Although pharmacological dose of water-soluble vitamin intake such as vitamin B_2 (Zempleni et al., 1996), nicotinamide (Shibata & Matsuo, 1990) and biotin (Zempleni & Mock, 1999) dramatically increase urinary vitamin levels, a few study had studied about the relationship between several oral dose correspond to dietary intake and urinary excretion of vitamin C (Levine et al., 1996, 2001). Thus, little attention had been paid to assess the quantitative relationships between intakes and urinary excretion of water-soluble vitamins. However, only a single study had investigated urinary vitamin as a possible marker for intake until 2007. Individuals' 30-day means of thiamin intake are highly correlated with their mean 24-hr urine thiamin levels under strictly controlled condition, showing 24-hr urinary thiamin as a useful marker for thiamin intake under strictly controlled conditions (Tasevska et al., 2007).

In the present review, recent findings from our intervention and cross-sectional studies are described to contribute to the establishment and effective use of urinary water-soluble vitamins as potential nutritional biomarkers. Furthermore, we propose the reference values for urinary water-soluble vitamins to show adequate nutritional status based on the findings. Our findings suggest that urinary water-soluble vitamins can be used as nutritional biomarkers to assess their mean intakes in groups. More accurate estimation of individuals' water-soluble vitamin intakes based on urinary excretion requires additional, precise biological information such as the bioavailability, absorption rate, and turnover rate.

2. Intervention studies

2.1 Factors affecting the urinary excretion of water-soluble vitamins

Urinary excretion of water-soluble vitamins varied among subjects more than blood levels did (Shibata et al., 2009). One possible explanation is that one or more of several factors such as nutrient requirements, energy expenditure, tissue turnover, intestinal absorption, kidney reabsorption, and physical characteristics differ between individuals. In fact, urinary excretion of vitamin B_1 is varied with the urine volume (Ihara et al., 2008), and furosemide-induced diuresis increases vitamin B_1 excretion rate (Rieck et al., 1999). Physical characteristics also affect the amount of urinary compounds. For example, individuals excreting higher urinary nitrogen had greater weight and body mass index (BMI) than those excreting average or lower nitrogen (Bingham et al., 1995), and creatinine clearance is positively correlated with BMI (Gerchman, 2009). In this context, the physical characteristics and urine volume may affect urinary excretion of B-group vitamins. We measured urinary excretion of B-group vitamins in free-living, healthy human subjects, and determined the correlations between each of the urinary B-group vitamins and factors such as physical characteristics and urine volume (Fukuwatari, 2009).

Twenty four-hr urine samples were collected from 186 free-living Japanese females aged 19–21 years, and 104 free-living Japanese elderly aged 70–84 years, and correlations were determined between urinary output of each B-group vitamin and body height, body weight, body mass index, body surface area, urine volume, and urinary creatinine. Only urinary excretion of vitamin B_{12} showed strong correlation with urine volume in both young female and elderly subjects ($r = 0.683$, $p < 0.001$ and $r = 0.523$, $p < 0.001$, respectively). All factors such as urine volume, urinary creatinine and physical characteristics such as body height, body weight, BMI and body surface area showed weak or no correlations with other 7 urinary B-group vitamins including thiamin, riboflavin, pyridoxal metabolite 4-pyridoxic acid, sum of nicotinamide metabolites, pantothenic acid, folate and biotin. To determine how urinary vitamin B_{12} is affected by its intake and urine volume, healthy Japanese adults (10 men; mean age, 25.9 ± 1.0 years; 10 women; mean age, 23.5 ± 6.4 years) orally administrated 1.5 mg cyanocobalamin, which is 500-fold higher daily intake. The Twenty Japanese adults consumed similar foods for 3 days and took a 1.5-mg cyanocobalamin tablet after breakfast on day 2. The 24-hour urine sample was collected for 3 successive days, and Pearson correlation coefficients between urinary vitamin B_{12} and urine volume on each day were determined.

Pharmacologic dose of cyanocobalamin increased Urinary vitamin B_{12} only 1.3-fold, and its concentration was not affected (Fig. 1A). Urinary vitamin B_{12} was always strongly correlated with urine volume even on the day before, the day of, and the day after intake (Fig. 1B-D). These results clearly showed that urinary excretion of vitamin B_{12} was dependent uponurine volume, but not on intake of vitamin B_{12}.Vitamin B_{12} is different from other B-group vitamins with respect to main excretion route, which is through the bile, and <10% of the total loss of vitamin B_{12} from the body is through urine (Shinton, 1972). These results suggest that the change in the level of urinary vitamin B_{12} is too small to evaluate intake of vitamin B_{12}, and thus urinary vitamin B_{12} was unavailable to be used as biomarker for estimation of its intake. To excrete vitamin B_{12} into urine, vitamin B_{12} binds to carrier protein transcobalamin (TC) in serum (Allen, 1975), the TC–vitamin B_{12} complex is filtered in the glomeruli, and the proximal convoluted tubule reabsorbs this complex via a receptor-mediated system (Birn, 2006). Megalin is an essential receptor for reabsorption of the TC–vitamin B_{12} complex in the proximal tubule (Birn et al., 2002), binds to the TC–vitamin B_{12} complex with an estimated affinity (K_d) of ~183 nmol/L (Moestrup et al., 1996). This high affinity may explain why urinary loss of vitamin B_{12} is very low. However, little is known about how water regulation mediated by regulatory factors such as aquaporin, vasopressin and angiotensin is linked to reabsorption of vitamin B_{12}.

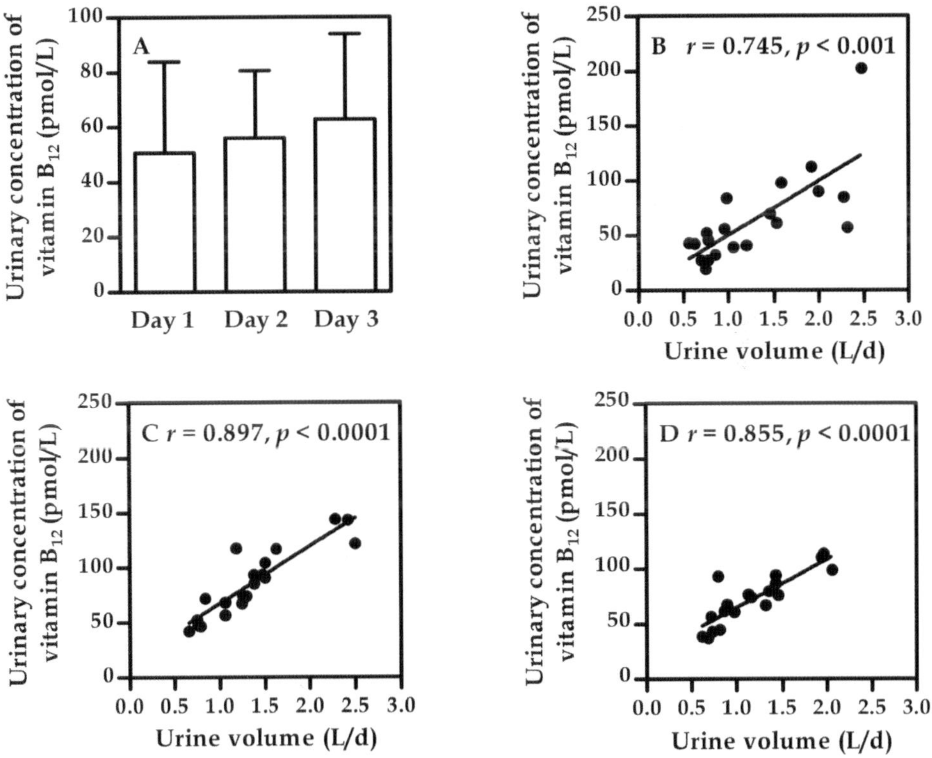

Fig. 1. Effect of administration of a pharmacologic dose of cyanocobalamin on urinary concentration of vitamin B_{12} (A) and the correlations between urinary vitamin B_{12} and urine volume on the day before cyanocobalamin intake (B), the day of intake (C) and the day after intake (D) (Fukuwatari et al., 2009).

2.2 Determination of urinary water-soluble vitamins as biomarkers for evaluating its intakes under strictly controlled conditions

As mentioned above, it is well known that pharmacological dose of water-soluble vitamin intake dramatically increase urinary vitamin levels, but a few study had studied about the relationship between several oral dose correspond to dietary intake and urinary excretion of vitamin C (Levine et al., 1996, 2001). We also determined whether urinary levels of water-soluble vitamins and their metabolites can be used as possible markers for estimating their intakes in the intervention study (Fukuwatari & Shibata, 2008). Six female Japanese college students participated to the intervention study, and their age, body weight, height and BMI (mean ± SD) were 21.0 ± 0.0 years old, 161.7 ± 1.7 cm, 51.2 ± 2.8 kg and 19.6 ± 1.2, respectively. They were given a standard Japanese diet in the first week, same diet with synthesized water-soluble vitamin mixture as the diet as approximately one-fold vitamin mixture based on DRIs for Japanese in the second week, with three-fold vitamin mixture in the third week, and six-fold mixture in the fourth week. The 24-hr urine was collected on each week, and the relationships were determined between oral dose and urinary vitamin levels. All urinary vitamin and their metabolites levels except vitamin B_{12} increased linearly in a dose-dependent manner, and highly correlated with vitamin intake (r = 0.959 for vitamin B_1, r = 0.927 for vitamin B_2, r = 0.965 for vitamin B_6, r = 0.957 for niacin, r = 0.934 for pantothenic acid, r = 0.907 for folic acid, r = 0.962 for biotin, and r = 0.952 for vitamin C; Fig. 2). These findings show that water-soluble vitamin and their metabolite levels in 24-hr urine reflect the vitamin intakes under strictly controlled conditions.

Humans can synthesize the vitamin nicotinamide from tryptophan in the liver, and the resultant nicotinamide is distributed to non-hepatic tissues. The purpose of the synthetic pathway in the liver is not the supply of NAD^+ but the supply of nicotinamide for non-hepatic tissues. The conversion pathway of nicotinamide from tryptophan is affected by various nutrients (Shibata et al., 1995, 1997a, 1998; Kimura et al., 2005), hormones (Shibata, 1995; Shibata & Toda, 1997), exercise (Fukuwatari et al., 2001) and drugs (Shibata et al., 1996, 1997b, 2001; Fukuwatari et al., 2004), based on data concerning the urinary excretion of metabolic intermediates in the tryptophan–nicotinamide pathway. However, the intervention study showed that administration of nicotinamide did not affect de novo nicotinamide synthesis from tryptophan (Fukuwatari & Shibata, 2007).

3. Cross-sectional studies: Determination of urinary water-soluble vitamins as biomarkers for evaluating its intakes in free-living subjects

The intervention study showed that urinary water-soluble vitamin levels are correlated highly with their intake in a strictly controlled environment (Fukuwatari & Shibata, 2008). Performance of a study under a free-living environment without any interventions is the next step to confirm the applicability of methods using a biomarker. Thus, we conducted the Values are individual points of six subjects in each dose. 4-PIC signifies 4-pyridoxic acid, a catabolite of pyridoxal, and the Nam metabolites signify the total amount of nicotinamaide metabolites, N^1-methylnicotinamide (MNA), N^1-methyl-2-pyridone-5-carboxamide (2-Py) and N^1-methyl-4-pyridone-3-carboxamide (4-Py).

Cross-sectional studies, and free-living healthy subjects who were 216 university dietetics students aged 18-27 years, 114 Japanese elementary school children aged 10-12 years and 37

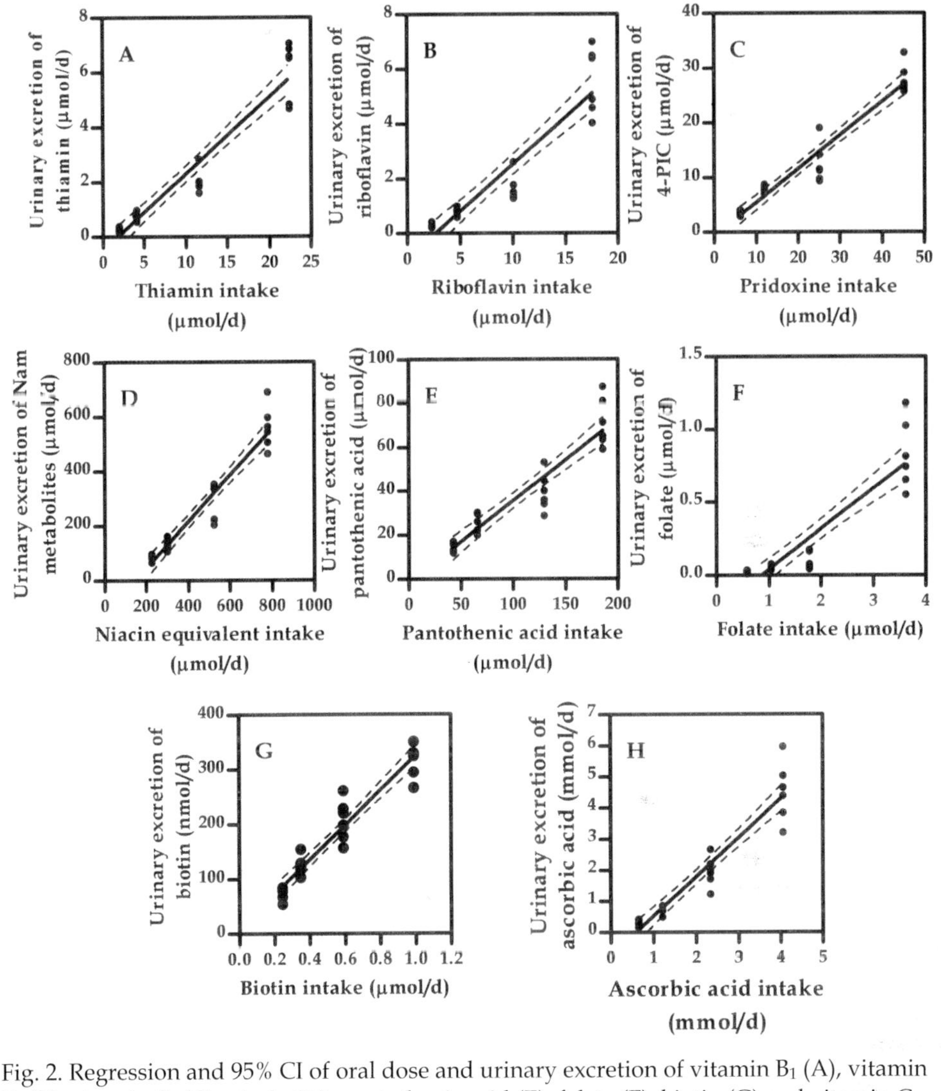

Fig. 2. Regression and 95% CI of oral dose and urinary excretion of vitamin B_1 (A), vitamin B_2 (B), vitamin B_6 (C), niacin (D), pantothenic acid (E), folate (F), biotin (G) and vitamin C (H) (Fukuwatari et al., 2008).

Japanese elderly females aged 70–84 years were participated (Tsuji et al., 2010a, 2010b, 2011). The subjects performed 4-day dietary assessment by recording all food consumed during the consecutive 4-day period with a weighed food record, and collected 24-hr urine samples on the fourth day. The results showed that the correlation between the urinary excretion and the dietary intake on the same day as urine collection was highest compared with the correlations on other days in each generation (Table 1-3). Moreover, the correlations between the urinary excretion and the mean dietary intakes during the recent 2–4 days

Vitamins	24-h urinary excretion of vitamin[a]	Vitamin intake at Day 4		Vitamin intake at Day 3		Vitamin intake at Day 2		Vitamin intake at Day 1	
	mean ± SD	mean ± SD	r^b	mean ± SD	r^b	mean ± SD	r^b	mean ± SD	r^b
Vitamin B_1	0.425 ± 0.286 (μmol/d)	2.27 ± 0.92 (μmol/d)	0.29§	2.46 ± 1.06 (μmol/d)	0.35§	2.46 ± 1.00 (μmol/d)	0.27§	2.09 ± 0.84 (μmol/d)	0.12
Vitamin B_2	0.382 ± 0.321 (μmol/d)	3.32 ± 1.09 (μmol/d)	0.32§	3.47 ± 1.35 (μmol/d)	0.28§	3.43 ± 1.35 (μmol/d)	0.31§	3.17 ± 1.46 (μmol/d)	0.11
Vitamin B_6	3.68 ± 1.31 (μmol/d)	5.30 ± 2.15 (μmol/d)	0.26‡	5.62 ± 2.38 (μmol/d)	0.37§	5.83 ± 2.14 (μmol/d)	0.21‡	5.25 ± 2.37 (μmol/d)	0.21‡
Vitamin B_{12}	0.028 ± 0.018 (nmol/d)	2.88 ± 3.42 (nmol/d)	0.05	3.59 ± 3.86 (nmol/d)	0.01	3.49 ± 5.16 (nmol/d)	-0.06	3.05 ± 5.69 (nmol/d)	0.10
Niacin	---	90.8 ± 39.4 (μmol/d)	0.32§	96.5 ± 45.7 (μmol/d)	0.26‡	98.8 ± 39.5 (μmol/d)	0.17*	93.4 ± 49.0 (μmol/d)	0.22‡
Niacin equivalent	84.5 ± 28.1 (μmol/d)	184 ± 65 (μmol/d)	0.29§	191 ± 70 (μmol/d)	0.24‡	196 ± 63 (μmol/d)	0.20*	184 ± 74 (μmol/d)	0.21*
Pantothenic acid	16.5 ± 5.2 (μmol/d)	23.6 ± 8.2 (μmol/d)	0.33§	23.9 ± 8.5 (μmol/d)	0.44§	24.3 ± 9.6 (μmol/d)	0.28§	22.7 ± 11.2 (μmol/d)	0.10
Folate	23.1 ± 8.8 (nmol/d)	569 ± 338 (nmol/d)	0.15	591 ± 321 (nmol/d)	0.24‡	610 ± 423 (nmol/d)	0.19*	569 ± 515 (nmol/d)	0.07
Vitamin C	139 ± 131 (μmol/d)	425 ± 362 (μmol/d)	0.29§	476 ± 354 (μmol/d)	0.34§	546 ± 435 (μmol/d)	0.16	388 ± 276 (μmol/d)	0.22‡

[a]Urinary excretion for each vitamin corresponds to thiamin for vitamin B_1, riboflavin for vitamin B_2, 4-PIC for vitamin B_6, the sum of nicotinamide, MNA, 2-Py and 4-Py for niacin equivalent, the sum of reduced and oxidized ascorbic acid and 2,3-diketogluconic acid for vitamin C.
[b]r means a correlation between urinary excretion and dietary intake of vitamin, for which values are denoted as *P<0.05, ‡P<0.01, §P<0.001

Table 1. Measured values for 24-hr urinary excretion collected on Day 4 and daily vitamin intake for each water-soluble vitamin, and correlation between 24-hr urinary excretion and daily vitamin intake in young Japanese (n=148) (Tsuji et al., 2010a).

showed higher correlations, except for vitamin B_{12}, than those for daily intakes (Table 4-6). However, these correlations ranged from 0.27 to 0.59, and these modest correlations were not enough to use urinary vitamins as biomarkers to estimate their intakes in individuals. Several factors are known to affect water-soluble vitamin metabolism. For example, alcohol, carbohydrate and physical activity are expected to affect vitamin B_1 metabolism (Hoyumpa et al., 1977; Manore, 2000; Elmadfa et al., 2001); bioavailability of pantothenic acid in food is half that of free pantothenic acid (Tarr et al., 1981); and the single nucleotide polymorphism of methylenetetrahydrofolate reductase (MTHFR) gene affects folate metabolism (Bagley & Selhub, 1998). When estimated intake of water-soluble vitamins was calculated using mean recovery rate and urinary excretion values, estimated water-soluble vitamin intakes except vitamin B_{12} were correlated with 3-day mean intakes, and showed 91–107% of their 3-day mean intakes, except vitamin B_{12} (61-79%) (Table 2). These findings showed that urinary water-soluble vitamins reflected their dietary intake over the past few days, and could be used as biomarkers to assess their intakes in groups.

Vitamins	24-h urinary excretion of vitamin[a]	Vitamin intake at Day 4		Vitamin intake at Day 3		Vitamin intake at Day 2		Vitamin intake at Day 1	
	mean ± SD	mean ± SD	r^b	mean ± SD	r^b	mean ± SD	r^b	mean ± SD	r^b
Vitamin B_1	0.766 ± 0.383 (μmol/d)	3.13 ± 1.01 (μmol/d)	0.41§	2.90 ± 0.85 (μmol/d)	0.25‡	2.60 ± 0.74 (μmol/d)	0.22*	2.75 ± 0.92 (μmol/d)	0.07
Vitamin B_2	0.290 ± 0.209 (μmol/d)	3.47 ± 0.94 (μmol/d)	0.36§	3.75 ± 1.13 (μmol/d)	0.36§	3.59 ± 1.00 (μmol/d)	0.33§	3.60 ± 1.17 (μmol/d)	0.23*
Vitamin B_6	2.36 ± 0.92 (μmol/d)	5.93 ± 1.86 (μmol/d)	0.42§	5.96 ± 1.65 (μmol/d)	0.32§	5.97 ± 1.69 (μmol/d)	0.36§	6.00 ± 2.41 (μmol/d)	0.17
Vitamin B_{12}	0.026 ± 0.015 (nmol/d)	3.15 ± 1.97 (nmol/d)	0.18	4.85 ± 5.93 (nmol/d)	0.14	4.76 ± 4.29 (nmol/d)	-0.02	4.64 ± 3.37 (nmol/d)	0.11
Niacin	---	97.0 ± 32.3 (μmol/d)	0.28§	101.7 ± 38.2 (μmol/d)	0.11	105.3 ± 31.3 (μmol/d)	0.21*	101.4 ± 32.5 (μmol/d)	0.23*
Niacin equivalent	65.6 ± 27.6 (μmol/d)	214 ± 56 (μmol/d)	0.28‡	218 ± 56 (μmol/d)	0.23‡	218 ± 52 (μmol/d)	0.16	218 ± 56 (μmol/d)	0.25‡
Pantothenic acid	11.6 ± 5.5 (μmol/d)	27.6 ± 6.9 (μmol/d)	0.23*	30.1 ± 7.4 (μmol/d)	0.20*	27.0 ± 6.3 (μmol/d)	0.31§	28.7 ± 7.8 (μmol/d)	0.25‡
Folate	16.8 ± 6.6 (nmol/d)	575 ± 170 (nmol/d)	0.27‡	615 ± 423 (nmol/d)	0.12	491 ± 123 (nmol/d)	0.18	532 ± 164 (nmol/d)	0.24*
Vitamin C	161 ± 221 (μmol/d)	477 ± 225 (μmol/d)	0.35§	448 ± 313 (μmol/d)	0.23*	403 ± 289 (μmol/d)	0.26‡	445 ± 328 (μmol/d)	0.18

[a]Urinary excretion for each vitamin corresponds to thiamin for vitamin B_1, riboflavin for vitamin B_2, 4-PIC for vitamin B_6, the sum of nicotinamide, MNA, 2-Py and 4-Py for niacin equivalent, the sum of reduced and oxidized ascorbic acid and 2,3-diketogluconic acid for vitamin C.
[b]r means a correlation between urinary excretion and dietary intake of vitamin, for which values are denoted as *$P<0.05$, ‡$P<0.01$, §$P<0.001$

Table 2. Measured values for 24-hr urinary excretion collected on Day 4 and daily vitamin intake for each water-soluble vitamin, and correlation between 24-hr urinary excretion and daily vitamin intake in Japanese school children (n=114) (Tsuji et al., 2010b).

Vitamins	24-h urinary excretion of vitamin[a]	Vitamin intake at Day 4		Vitamin intake at Day 3		Vitamin intake at Day 2		Vitamin intake at Day 1	
	mean ± SD	mean ± SD	r^b	mean ± SD	r^b	mean ± SD	r^b	mean ± SD	r^b
Vitamin B_1	0.459 ± 0.494 (μmol/d)	2.51 ± 0.91 (μmol/d)	0.47‡	2.50 ± 0.73 (μmol/d)	0.54§	2.62 ± 0.85 (μmol/d)	0.28	2.37 ± 0.74 (μmol/d)	0.42*
Vitamin B_2	0.852 ± 0.828 (μmol/d)	3.47 ± 1.22 (μmol/d)	0.49‡	3.60 ± 1.08 (μmol/d)	0.46‡	3.69 ± 1.12 (μmol/d)	0.52§	3.54 ± 1.14 (μmol/d)	0.34*
Vitamin B_6	4.45 ± 2.26 (μmol/d)	7.06 ± 2.78 (μmol/d)	0.37*	7.04 ± 2.35 (μmol/d)	0.13	7.57 ± 2.71 (μmol/d)	0.34*	7.45 ± 2.41 (μmol/d)	0.16
Vitamin B_{12}	0.034 ± 0.035 (nmol/d)	5.81 ± 4.91 (nmol/d)	0.15	5.89 ± 5.31 (nmol/d)	-0.07	4.95 ± 4.31 (nmol/d)	0.12	6.75 ± 8.43 (nmol/d)	-0.03
Niacin	---	113 ± 49 (μmol/d)	0.35*	127 ± 57 (μmol/d)	0.38*	129 ± 65 (μmol/d)	0.39*	121 ± 47 (μmol/d)	0.32
Niacin equivalent	89.7 ± 30.8 (μmol/d)	213 ± 72 (μmol/d)	0.37*	232 ± 73 (μmol/d)	0.45‡	239 ± 94 (μmol/d)	0.39*	223 ± 71 (μmol/d)	0.26
Pantothenic acid	15.1 ± 6.2 (μmol/d)	26.1 ± 8.9 (μmol/d)	0.59§	25.5 ± 8.9 (μmol/d)	0.49‡	25.6 ± 6.4 (μmol/d)	0.46‡	24.5 ± 7.1 (μmol/d)	0.30
Folate	36.6 ± 16.9 (nmol/d)	792 ± 305 (nmol/d)	0.55§	845 ± 360 (nmol/d)	0.24	854 ± 301 (nmol/d)	0.48‡	818 ± 366 (nmol/d)	0.28
Vitamin C	214 ± 271 (μmol/d)	627 ± 310 (μmol/d)	0.46‡	620 ± 407 (μmol/d)	0.43‡	722 ± 423 (μmol/d)	0.39*	642 ± 356 (μmol/d)	0.53§

[a]Urinary excretion for each vitamin corresponds to thiamin for vitamin B_1, riboflavin for vitamin B_2, 4-PIC for vitamin B_6, the sum of nicotinamide, MNA, 2-Py and 4-Py for niacin equivalent, the sum of reduced and oxidized ascorbic acid and 2,3-diketogluconic acid for vitamin C.
[b]*r* means a correlation between urinary excretion and dietary intake of vitamin, for which values are denoted as $^*P<0.05$, $^‡P<0.01$, $^§P<0.001$

Table 3. Measured values for 24-hr urinary excretion collected on Day 4 and daily vitamin intake for each water-soluble vitamin, and correlation between 24-hr urinary excretion and daily vitamin intake in elderly Japanese (n=35) (Tsuji et al., 2011).

Vitamins	2 days mean vitamin intake (Days 3–4)		3 days mean vitamin intake (Days 2–4)		4 days mean vitamin intake (Days 1–4)		Recovery rate[c] (%)	Mean estimated vitamin intake[d]		
	mean ± SD	r^a	mean ± SD	r^a	mean ± SD	r^a	mean ± SD	mean ± SD	r^e	% ratio[f]
Vitamin B_1	2.37 ± 0.79 (μmol/d)	0.40§	2.40 ± 0.73 (μmol/d)	0.42§	2.32 ± 0.63 (μmol/d)	0.39§	17.8 ± 11.4	2.38 ± 1.61 (μmol/d)	0.40§	100 %
Vitamin B_2	3.04 ± 0.87 (μmol/d)	0.39§	3.05 ± 0.83 (μmol/d)	0.43§	3.00 ± 0.81 (μmol/d)	0.39§	12.4 ± 10.0	3.08 ± 2.59 (μmol/d)	0.38§	101 %
Vitamin B_6	5.46 ± 1.85 (μmol/d)	0.40§	5.58 ± 1.62 (μmol/d)	0.40§	5.50 ± 1.54 (μmol/d)	0.39§	69.6 ± 28.6	5.29 ± 1.88 (μmol/d)	0.40§	95%
Vitamin B_{12}	3.24 ± 2.62 (nmol/d)	0.06	3.32 ± 2.60 (nmol/d)	0.02	3.23 ± 2.84 (nmol/d)	0.07	1.4 ± 1.5	2.04 ± 1.33 (nmol/d)	0.06	61%
Niacin	93.6 ± 33.7 (μmol/d)	0.35§	95.4 ± 28.7 (μmol/d)	0.33§	94.9 ± 28.7 (μmol/d)	0.33§	---	---	---	---
Niacin equivalent	189 ± 54 (μmol/d)	0.33§	192 ± 47 (μmol/d)	0.32§	190 ± 47 (μmol/d)	0.32§	45.8 ± 16.0	184 ± 61 (μmol/d)	0.33§	96%
Pantothenic acid	23.7 ± 7.0 (μmol/d)	0.47§	23.9 ± 6.7 (μmol/d)	0.46§	23.6 ± 7.0 (μmol/d)	0.41§	71.6 ± 23.3	23.0 ± 7.3 (μmol/d)	0.47§	96%
Folate	583 ± 243 (nmol/d)	0.24‡	593 ± 243 (nmol/d)	0.27‡	588 ± 273 (nmol/d)	0.24‡	4.3 ± 1.9	540 ± 206 (nmol/d)	0.24‡	91%
Vitamin C	446 ± 285 (μmol/d)	0.44§	478 ± 267 (μmol/d)	0.42§	455 ± 244 (μmol/d)	0.41§	31.3 ± 29.6	446 ± 420 (μmol/d)	0.44§	93%

[a]Mean dietary intake was calculated using daily dietary intake for each individual.
[b]*r* means a correlation between 24-h urinary excretion and mean dietary intake.
[c]Recovery rate was derived from 24-h urinary excretion/3-Days mean intake.
[d]Mean estimated intake was calculated using 24-hr urinary excretion and recovery rate.
[e]*r* means a correlation between 3-day mean dietary intake and mean estimated intake.
[f]% ratio means a ratio between 3-day mean intake and mean estimated intake.
*P<0.05, ‡P<0.01, §P<0.001.

Table 4. Correlations between 24-hr urinary excretion and mean vitamin intakes, recovery rates, and mean estimated intakes in young Japanese (n=148) (Tsuji et al., 2010a).

Vitamins	2 days mean vitamin intake (Days 3–4)		3 days mean vitamin intake (Days 2–4)		4 days mean vitamin intake (Days 1–4)		Recovery rate[c] (%)	Mean estimated vitamin intake[d]		
	mean ± SD	r^a	mean ± SD	r^a	mean ± SD	r^a	mean ± SD	mean ± SD	r^e	% ratio[f]
Vitamin B_1	3.02 ± 0.77 (μmol/d)	0.42§	2.88 ± 0.63 (μmol/d)	0.42§	2.85 ± 0.58 (μmol/d)	0.35§	27.6 ± 12.2	2.83 ± 1.42 (μmol/d)	0.37§	100%
Vitamin B_2	3.61 ± 0.85 (μmol/d)	0.41§	3.60 ± 0.79 (μmol/d)	0.43§	3.60 ± 0.78 (μmol/d)	0.42§	7.9 ± 5.2	3.66 ± 2.63 (μmol/d)	0.26‡	102%
Vitamin B_6	5.94 ± 1.41 (μmol/d)	0.45§	5.95 ± 1.29 (μmol/d)	0.49§	5.96 ± 1.35 (μmol/d)	0.43§	39.8 ± 14.0	5.90 ± 2.30 (μmol/d)	0.41§	100%
Vitamin B_{12}	4.00 ± 3.14 (nmol/d)	0.19*	4.25 ± 2.55 (nmol/d)	0.10	4.35 ± 2.10 (nmol/d)	0.10	0.7 ± 0.6	3.72 ± 2.14 (nmol/d)	0.06	79%
Niacin	99 ± 26 (μmol/d)	0.24*	101 ± 21.7 (μmol/d)	0.29‡	101 ± 20.4 (μmol/d)	0.32§	---	---	---	---
Niacin equivalent	216 ± 48 (μmol/d)	0.29‡	217 ± 43 (μmol/d)	0.29‡	217 ± 39 (μmol/d)	0.32§	30.7 ± 12.6	215 ± 91 (μmol/d)	0.20*	99%
Pantothenic acid	28.8 ± 6.0 (μmol/d)	0.26‡	28.2 ± 5.6 (μmol/d)	0.32§	28.3 ± 5.7 (μmol/d)	0.32§	41.4 ± 19.5	28.1 ± 13.3 (μmol/d)	0.27‡	99%
Folate	595 ± 236 (nmol/d)	0.23*	560 ± 174 (nmol/d)	0.24*	553 ± 147 (nmol/d)	0.27‡	3.1 ± 1.3	536 ± 211 (nmol/d)	0.09	97%
Vitamin C	462 ± 200 (μmol/d)	0.39§	442 ± 183 (μmol/d)	0.39§	443 ± 170 (μmol/d)	0.39§	36.4 ± 50.3	447 ± 613 (μmol/d)	0.39§	100%

[a]Mean dietary intake was calculated using daily dietary intake for each individual
[b]*r* means a correlation between 24-h urinary excretion and mean dietary intake.
[c]Recovery rate was derived from 24-h urinary excretion/3-Days mean intake.
[d]Mean estimated intake was calculated using 24-hr urinary excretion and recovery rate.
[e]*r* means a correlation between 3-day mean dietary intake and mean estimated intake
[f]% ratio means a ratio between 3-day mean intake and mean estimated intake.
*$P<0.05$, ‡$P<0.01$, §$P<0.001$.

Table 5. Correlations between 24-hr urinary excretion and mean vitamin intakes, recovery rates, and mean estimated intakes in Japanese school children (n=114) (Tsuji et al., 2010b).

Vitamins	2 days mean vitamin intake (Days 3–4)		3 days mean vitamin intake (Days 2–4)		4 days mean vitamin intake (Days 1–4)		Recovery rate[c] (%)	Mean estimated vitamin intake[d]		
	mean ± SD	r^a	mean ± SD	r^a	mean ± SD	r^a	mean ± SD	mean ± SD	r^e	% ratio[f]
Vitamin B_1	2.51 ± 0.66 (μmol/d)	0.62§	2.55 ± 0.62 (μmol/d)	0.58§	2.50 ± 0.59 (μmol/d)	0.59§	16.9 ± 17.7	2.71 ± 2.92 (μmol/d)	0.58§	107 %
Vitamin B_2	3.53 ± 1.03 (μmol/d)	0.53§	3.59 ± 0.99 (μmol/d)	0.57§	3.57 ± 0.95 (μmol/d)	0.55§	23.1 ± 22.9	3.69 ± 3.58 (μmol/d)	0.52§	103 %
Vitamin B_6	7.05 ± 2.17 (μmol/d)	0.30	7.22 ± 2.01 (μmol/d)	0.35*	7.58 ± 1.95 (μmol/d)	0.33	64.2 ± 31.7	6.93 ± 3.5 (μmol/d)2	0.35*	96 %
Vitamin B_{12}	5.85 ± 3.55 (nmol/d)	0.01	5.55 ± 3.16 (nmol/d)	0.01	5.85 ± 3.16 (nmol/d)	-0.03	0.9 ± 1.6	3.62 ± 3.73 (nmol/d)	0.12	65 %
Niacin	120 ± 42 (μmol/d)	0.46‡	123 ± 37 (μmol/d)	0.54§	122 ± 36 (μmol/d)	0.52§	---	---	---	---
Niacin equivalent	222 ± 58 (μmol/d)	0.50‡	228 ± 56 (μmol/d)	0.54§	227 ± 55 (μmol/d)	0.49‡	40.1 ± 12.3	224 ± 77 (μmol/d)	0.54§	98 %
Pantothenic acid	25.8 ± 8.1 (μmol/d)	0.58§	25.8 ± 7.1 (μmol/d)	0.57§	25.4 ± 6.5 (μmol/d)	0.56§	59.6 ± 24.2	25.3 ± 10.4 (μmol/d)	0.46‡	98 %
Folate	819 ± 279 (nmol/d)	0.42*	831 ± 257 (nmol/d)	0.47‡	828 ± 266 (nmol/d)	0.43‡	4.5 ± 2.0	805 ± 372 (nmol/d)	0.48‡	97 %
Vitamin C	624 ± 337 (μmol/d)	0.50‡	657 ± 339 (μmol/d)	0.50‡	653 ± 334 (μmol/d)	0.53§	32.0 ± 39.3	682 ± 847 (μmol/d)	0.51‡	101 %

[a]Mean dietary intake was calculated using daily dietary intake for each individual.
[b]r means a correlation between 24-h urinary excretion and mean dietary intake.
[c]Recovery rate was derived from 24-h urinary excretion/3-Days mean intake.
[d]Mean estimated intake was calculated using 24-hr urinary excretion and recovery rate.
[e]r means a correlation between 3-day mean dietary intake and mean estimated intake.
[f]% ratio means a ratio between 3-day mean intake and mean estimated intake.
*$P<0.05$, ‡$P<0.01$, §$P<0.001$.

Table 6. Correlations between 24-hr urinary excretion and mean vitamin intakes, recovery rates, and mean estimated intakes in elderly Japanese (n=35) (Tsuji et al., 2011).

Relatively low correlations were found between urinary folate and dietary intake in the cross-sectional studies, whereas a high correlation was found in the intervention study (Fukuwatari & Shibata, 2008). The relatively low correlation of folate in free-living subjects may be explained by several reasons. Urinary folate excretion responds slowly to change in dietary folate intake, and is reduced significantly in people who consume a low-folate diet (Kim & Lim, 2008). Some Japanese subjects consumed Japanese green tea and liver well, and these foods contain 16 μg/100 g and 1000 μg/100 g folate, respectively, in the Japanese Food Composition Table (The Ministry of Education, Culture, Sports, Science and Technology, 2007). The composition of Japanese tea may vary depending on whether the extract of tea was made personally or whether it was a bottled tea beverage, because the present Japanese Food Composition Table cannot differentiate such products. Similarly, since the Food

Composition Table only describes the composition of raw liver, an error exists between the quantity of vitamin intake obtained from the Food Composition Table and the actual intake from cooked liver. Nutrient intakes were calculated using this Food Composition Table which did not take account of cooking loss for the above foods, and thus this might cause potential low level of accuracy. There might be also a technical issue. Urinary intact folates were measured by a microbiological assay in the cross-sectional studies. However, folates are catabolized into *p*-aminobenzoylglutamate and the acetylated form, *p*-acetamidobenzoylglutamate, which are excreted into the urine (Wolfe et al., 2003).

4. Reference values for urinary water-soluble vitamins

Urinary water-soluble vitamins can be used as potential biomarker not only for estimation of its intake but also evaluation for its nutritional status. The intervention study comprehensively investigated urinary water-soluble vitamin values in subjects consuming semi-purified diet with vitamin mixture for 7 days (Shibata et al., 2005). The study revealed the mean values and ranges for each water-soluble vitamin except vitamin B_{12} in the subjects with vitamin mixture based on DRIs for Japanese. Based on these results, we propose the reference values for urinary water-soluble vitamins to show adequate nutritional status in Table 7. When urinary excretion of some vitamins is lower than the lower reference value, subject may not intake its vitamin enough for DRIs. When urinary vitamin is higher than the upper value, subject may intake its vitamin supplement. These reference values may be useful for first screening to check one's vitamin nutritional status and vitamin supplement intake.

Vitamins[a]	Reference values
Vitamin B_1	300-2400 (nmol/d)
Vitamin B_2	200-1800 (nmol/d)
Vitamin B_6	3.0-16.0 (μmol/d)
Vitamin B_{12}	---
Niacin	50-300 (μmol/d)
Pantothenic acid	10-60 (μmol/d)
Folate	15-80 (nmol/d)
Biotin	50-300 (nmol/d)
Vitamin C	150-2400 (μmol/d)

[a]Urinary excretion for each vitamin corresponds to thiamin for vitamin B_1, riboflavin for vitamin B_2, 4-PIC for vitamin B_6, the sum of nicotinamide, MNA, 2-Py and 4-Py for niacin equivalent, the sum of reduced and oxidized ascorbic acid and 2,3-diketogluconic acid for vitamin C.

Table 7. Proposed reference values for urinary water-soluble vitamins in adults.

5. Conclusion

Recent studies have induced great advances for urinary water-soluble vitamins as biomarkers for its intakes. Measuring urinary water-soluble vitamin levels can be the good approach for assessing dietary vitamin intake in groups, and for simply evaluation of its nutritional status in individuals. However, there is limitation for its use; urinary vitamins have not been suitable biomarker to estimate its intake in individuals yet. More accurate estimation of the dietary intake of water-soluble vitamins based on urinary excretion requires additional, precise biological information such as the bioavailability, absorption rate, and turnover rate. Next step in this type of study will be to determine whether vitamin contents in spot urine sample is used to assess water-soluble vitamin intakes in groups.

6. Acknowledgement

The preparation of this manuscript was supported by a Research Grant for Comprehensive Research on Cardiovascular and Lifestyle Related Diseases from the Ministry of Health, Labour and Welfare of Japan (Principal Investigator, Katsumi Shibata).

7. References

Allen, RH. (1975). Human vitamin B_{12} transport proteins. *Prog Hematol*, Vol.9, pp. 57-84.

Bagley, PJ & Selhub, J. (1998). A common mutation in the methylenetetrahydrofolate reductase gene is associated with an accumulation of formylated tetrahydrofolates in red blood cells. *Proc Natl Acad Sci U S A*, Vol.95, pp. 13217-13220.

Bingham, SA.; Cassidy, A. Cole, TJ. Welch, A. Runswick, SA. Black, AE. Thurnham, D. Bates, C. Khaw, KT. Key, TJ. & Day, NE. (1995). Validation of weighed records and other methods of dietary assessment using the 24 h urine nitrogen technique and other biological markers. *Br J Nutr*, Vol.73, pp. 531-550.

Bingham, SA. (2003). Urine nitrogen as a biomarker for the validation of dietary protein intake. *J Nutr*, Vol.133, pp. 921S-924S.

Birn, H.; Willnow, TE. Nielsen, R. Norden, AG. Bonsch, C. Moestrup, SK. Nexø, E. & Christensen, EI. (2002). Megalin is essential for renal proximal tubule reabsorption and accumulation of transcobalamin-B_{12}. *Am J Physiol Renal Physiol*, Vol.282, pp. F408-F416.

Birn, H. (2006). The kidney in vitamin B_{12} and folate homeostasis: characterization of receptors for tubular uptake of vitamins and carrier proteins. *Am J Physiol Renal Physiol*, Vol.291, pp. F22-F36.

Elmadfa, I.; Majchrzak, D. Rust, P. & Genser, D. (2001). The thiamine status of adult humans depends on carbohydrate intake. *Int J Vitam Nutr Res*, Vol.71, pp. 217–221.

Food and Nutrition Board, Institute of Medicine (1998). Dietary Reference Intakes for Thiamin, Riboflavin, Niacin, Vitamin B_6, Folate, Vitamin B_{12}, Pantothenic Acid, Biotin, and Choline. Washington, DC: National Academy Press.

Fukuwatari, T.; Shibata, K. Ishihara, K. Fushiki, T. & Sugimoto, E. (2001). Elevation of blood NAD level after moderate exercise in young women and mice. *J Nutr Sci Vitaminol*, Vol.47, pp. 177-179.

Fukuwatari, T.; Ohta, M. Sugimoto, E. Sasaki, R. & Shibata, K. (2004). Effects of dietary di(2-ethylhexyl)phthalate, a putative endocrine disrupter, on enzyme activities involved in the metabolism of tryptophan to niacin in rats. *Biochim Biophys Acta*, Vol.1672, pp. 67-75.

Fukuwatari, T. & Shibata, K. (2007). Effect of nicotinamide administration on the tryptophan-nicotinamide pathway in humans. *Int J Vitam Nutr Res*, Vol.77, pp. 255-262.

Fukuwatari, T. & Shibata, K. (2008) Urinary water-soluble vitamin and their metabolites contents as biomarkers for evaluating vitamin intakes in young Japanese women. *J Nutr Sci Vitaminol*, Vol.54, pp. 223-229.

Fukuwatari, T.; Sugimoto, E. Tsuji, T. Hirose, J. Fukui, T. & Shibata, K. (2009). Urinary excretion of vitamin B_{12} depends on urine volume in female university students and elderly subjects in Japan. *Nutr Res*, Vol.29, pp. 839-845.

Gerchman, F.; Tong, J. Utzschneider, KM. Zraika, S. Udayasankar, J. Udayasankar, J. McNeely, MJ. Carr, DB. Leonetti, DL. Young, BA. de Boer, IH. Boyko, EJ. Fujimoto, WY. & Kahn, SE. (2009). Body mass index is associated with increased creatinine clearance by a mechanism independent of body fat distribution. *J Clin Endocrinol Metab,* Vol.94, pp. 3781-3788.

Hoyumpa, Jr. AM.; Nichols, SG. Wilson, FA. & Schenker, S. (1977). Effect of ethanol on intestinal (Na, K) ATPase and intestinal thiamine transport in rats. *J Lab Clin Med*, Vol.90, pp. 1086–1095.

Ihara, H.; Matsumoto, T. Kakinoki, T. Shino, Y. Hashimoto, R. & Hashizume, N. (2008). Estimation of vitamin B_1 excretion in 24-hr urine by assay of first-morning urine. *J Clin Lab Anal,* Vol.22, pp. 291-294.

Kim, HA. & Lim, HS. (2008). Dietary folate intake, blood folate status, and urinary folate catabolite excretion in Korean women of childbearing age. *J Nutr Sci Vitaminol*, Vol.54, pp. 291-297.

Kimura, N.; Fukuwatari, T. Sasaki, R. & Shibata, K. (2005). The necessity of niacin in rats fed on a high protein diet. *Biosci Biotechnol Biochem*, Vol.69, pp. 273-279.

Levine, M.; Conry-Cantilena, C. Wang, Y. Welch, RW. Washko, PW. Dhariwal, KR. Park, JB. Lazarev, A. Graumlich, JF. King, J. & Cantilena, LR. (1996). Vitamin C pharmacokinetics in healthy volunteers: evidence for a recommended dietary allowance. *Proc Natl Acad Sci USA*, Vol.93, pp. 3704-3709.

Levine, M.; Wang, Y. Padayatty, SJ. & Morrow, J. (2001). A new recommended dietary allowance of vitamin C for healthy young women. *Proc Natl Acad Sci USA*, Vol.98, pp. 9842-9846.

Manore, MM. (2000). Effect of physical activity on thiamine, riboflavin, and vitamin B_6 requirements. *Am J Clin Nutr*, Vol.72, pp. 598S–606S.

Moestrup, SK.; Birn, H. Fischer, PB. Petersen, CM. Verroust, PJ. Sim, RB. Christensen, EI. & Nexø, E. (1996). Megalin-mediated endocytosis of transcobalamin-vitamin-B_{12} complexes suggests a role of the receptor in vitamin-B_{12} homeostasis. *Proc Natl Acad Sci U S A*, Vol.93, pp. 8612-8617.

Potischman, N. & Freudenheim, JL. (2003). Biomarkers of nutritional exposure and nutritional status: an overview. *J Nutr*, Vol.133, pp. 873S-874S.

Rieck, J.; Halkin, H. Almog, S. Seligman, H. Lubetsky, A. Olchovsky, D. & Ezra D. (1999). Urinary loss of thiamine is increased by low doses of furosemide in healthy volunteers. *J Lab Clin Med,* Vol.134, pp. 238-243.

Shibata, K. & Matsuo, H. (1990). Changes in blood NAD and NADP levels, and the urinary excretion of nicotinamide and its metabolism in women student after nicotinamide administration. *Vitamins*, Vol.64, pp. 301-306.

Shibata, K.; Mushiage, M. Kondo, T. Hayakawa, T. & Tsuge, H. (1995). Effects of vitamin B_6 deficiency on the conversion ratio of tryptophan to niacin. *Biosci Biotechnol Biochem*, Vol.59, pp. 2060-2063.

Shibata, K. (1995). Effects of adrenalin on the conversion ratio of tryptophan to niacin in rats. *Biosci Biotechnol Biochem*, Vol.59, pp. 2127-2129.

Shibata, K.; Kondo, T. Marugami, M. & Umezawa, C. (1996). Increased conversion ratio of tryptophan to niacin by the administration of chlofibrate, a hypolipidemic drug, to rats. *Biosci Biotechnol Biochem*, Vol.60, pp. 1455-1459.

Shibata, K.; Kondo, T. & Yonezima, M. (1997a). Conversion ratio of tryptophan to niacin in rats fed a vitamin B_1-free diet. *J Nutr Sci Vitaminol*, Vol.43, pp. 479-483.

Shibata, K.; Ishikawa, A. & Kondo, T. (1997b). Effects of dietary pyrazinamide on the metabolism of tryptophan to niacin in streptozotocin-diabetic rats. *Biosci Biotechnol Biochem*, Vol.61, pp. 1679-1683.

Shibata, K. & Toda, S. (1997). Effects of sex hormones on the metabolism of tryptophan to niacin and to serotonin in male rats. *Biosci Biotechnol Biochem*, Vol.61, pp. 1200-1202.

Shibata, K.; Kondo, T. & Miki, A. (1998). Increased conversion ratio of tryptophan to niacin in severe food restriction. *Biosci Biotechnol Biochem*, Vol.62, pp. 580-583.

Shibata, K.; Fukuwatari, T. Enomoto, A. & Sugimoto, E. (2001). Increased conversion ratio of niacin by dietary di-n-butylphthalate. *J Nutr Sci Vitaminol*, Vol.47, pp. 263-266.

Shibata, K.; Fukuwatari, T. Ohta, M. Okamoto, H. Watanabe, T. Fukui, T. Nishimuta, M. Totani, M. Kimura, M. Ohishi, N. Nakashima, M. Watanabe, F. Miyamoto, E. Shigeoka, S. Takeda, T. Murakami, M. Ihara, H. & Hashizume, N. (2005). Values of water-soluble vitamin in blood and urine of Japanese young men and women consuming a semi-purified diet based on the Japanese Dietary Reference Intakes. *J Nutr Sci Vitaminol*, Vol.51, pp. 319-328.

Shibata, K.; Fukuwatari, T. Watanabe, T. & Nishimuta, M. (2009) Intra- and inter-individual variations of blood and urinary water-soluble vitamins in Japanese young adults consuming a semi-purified diet for 7 Days. *J Nutr Sci Vitaminol*, Vol.55, pp. 459-70.

Shinton, NK. (1972) Vitamin B_{12} and folate metabolism. *Br Med J*, Vol.1, pp. 556-559.

Tarr, JB.; Tamura, T. & Stokstad, ELR. (1981). Availability of vitamin B_6 and pantothenate in an average American diet in man. *Am J Clin Nutr*, Vol.34, pp. 1328-1337.

Tasevska, N.; Runswick, SA. McTaggart, A. & Bingham, SA. (2005). Urinary sucrose and fructose as biomarkers for sugar consumption. *Cancer Epidemiol Biomarkers Prev*, Vol.14, pp. 1287-1294.

Tasevska, N.; Runswick, SA. & Bingham, SA. (2006). Urinary potassium is as reliable as urinary nitrogen for use as a recovery biomarker in dietary studies of free living individuals. *J Nutr*, Vol.136, pp. 1334-1340.

Tasevska, N.; Runswick, SA. McTaggart, A. & Bingham, SA. (2007). Twenty-four-hour urinary thiamine as a biomarker for the assessment of thiamine intake. *Eur J Clin Nutr*, Vol.62, pp. 1139-1147.

The Ministry of Education, Culture, Sports, Science and Technology (2007). Standard Tables of Food Composition in Japan Fifth Revised and Enlarged Edition. Tokyo.

The Ministry of Health, Labour, and Welfare (2009). Dietary Reference Intakes for Japanese, 2010, Tokyo.

Tsuji, T.; Fukuwatari, T. Sasaki, S. & Shibata, K. (2010a). Twenty-four-hour urinary water-soluble vitamin levels correlate with their intakes in free-living Japanese university students. *Eur J Clin Nutr*, Vol.64, pp. 800-807.

Tsuji, T.; Fukuwatari, T. Sasaki, S. & Shibata, K. (2010b). Urinary excretion of vitamin B_1, B_2, B_6, niacin, pantothenic acid, folate, and vitamin C correlates with dietary intakes of free-living elderly, female Japanese. *Nutr Res*, Vol.30, pp. 171-178.

Tsuji, T.; Fukuwatari, T. Sasaki, S. & Shibata, K. (2011). Twenty-four-hour urinary water-soluble vitamin levels correlate with their intakes in free-living Japanese school children. *Public Health Nutr*, Vol.14, pp. 327-333.

Zempleni, J.; Galloway, JR. & McCormick, DB. (1996). Pharmacokinetics of orally and intravenously administered riboflavin in healthy humans. *Am J Clin Nutr*, Vol.63, pp. 54-66.

Zempleni, J. & Mock, DM. (1999). Bioavailability of biotin given orally to humans in pharmacologic doses. *Am J Clin Nutr*, Vol.69, pp. 504-508.

Wolfe, JM.; Bailey, LB. Herrlinger-Garcia, K. Theriaque, DW. Gregory, JF III. & Kauwell, GPA. (2003). Folate catabolite excretion is responsible to changes in dietary folate intake in elderly women. *Am J Clin Nutr*, Vol.77, pp. 919-923.

Potential Muscle Biomarkers of Chronic Myalgia in Humans – A Systematic Review of Microdialysis Studies

Björn Gerdle and Britt Larsson
Rehabilitation Medicine, Faculty of Health Sciences, Linköping University, Linköping, and Pain and Rehabilitation Centre, University Hospital, Linköping, Sweden

1. Introduction

1.1 Epidemiology

Approximately 20% of the European population report severe chronic pain (Breivik et al., 2006), with higher prevalences in women and in lower income groups (Gerdle et al., 2004; Larsson et al., 2007). Common chronic pain conditions are localized neck-shoulder pain including trapezius myalgia (prevalence in population 10-20%) (Lidgren, 2008), chronic whiplash associated disorders (WAD) (prevalence in the population 1.5%) (Guez et al., 2002), and chronic widespread pain (CWSP) (prevalence in population 5-10%) (Gerdle et al., 2008a). Chronic pain is associated with disability, low quality of life, and substantial socioeconomic costs (Breivik et al., 2006; Phillips, 2006; SBU, 2006).

1.2 Development of chronic myalgia – Chronic trapezius myalgia as an example

There is a connection between physical demands, psychosocial demands, and the risk of persistent muscle pain (Bernard, 1997; Punnett & Wegman, 2004); however, the mechanisms behind chronic myalgia are poorly understood. Myalgia usually starts with a feeling of tiredness and stiffness. At the beginning, the initial intermittent stage, pain can be alleviated for short or long periods. Chronic regional myalgia (CRM) in the neck-shoulder area often gradually becomes more easily triggered and more diffuse and can be spread to include most of the body (CWSP). CWSP includes fibromyalgia, a subgroup characterized by widespread hyperalgesia. The risk factors for the transition from a local/regional pain condition to CWSP are poorly understood (Larsson et al., in press). The diagnoses CRM (e.g., chronic trapezius myalgia) and CWSP are settled by careful anamnesis and clinical examinations that reveal tender muscle at palpation corresponding to the reported painful areas.

1.3 Neurobiological alterations in chronic pain

Acute pain results from a complex integrated series of events at peripheral and central levels. In healthy subjects, mechanisms related to acute pain might not necessarily be valid in subjects with subchronic, intermittent, or chronic pain.

Pace et al. suggested two types of persistent chronic pain: 1) nociceptive/inflammatory pain and 2) neuropathic pain (Pace et al., 2006). The present study mainly discusses nociceptive/inflammatory pain. Chronic pain is more complex than acute pain as extensive short-term and long-term plastic and sometimes permanent changes (including peripheral and/or central hyperexcitability/sensitization) of the pain transmission system can occur at different levels (Kuner, 2010; Reichling & Levine, 2009) and by the modification of psychological (e.g., attentional, emotional, and anticipation status) and context factors (Grachev et al., 2000; Hunt & Mantyh, 2002; Petersen-Felix & Curatolo, 2002; Schmidt-Wilcke, 2008; Wilder-Smith et al., 2002; Woolf & Salter, 2000). Different structures in the brain – vaguely labelled as the pain matrix (Iannetti & Mouraux, 2010; Lee & Tracey, 2010; Legrain et al., 2011) – are dynamically involved in processing of nociception and pain (including emotions, cognitions, and motivation) (Ossipov et al., 2010). In patients with chronic pain conditions, a pain matrix shows different types of alterations including morphological changes (Apkarian, 2008; Schweinhardt & Bushnell, 2010), indicating that different chronic pain conditions exhibit unique anatomical "brain signatures" (Baliki et al., 2011).

Descending supraspinal control of spinal nociception originates from many brain regions (Heinricher et al., 2009; Ossipov et al., 2010). The descending supraspinal control includes a dynamic balance between inhibiting and facilitating mechanisms that can be altered due to behavioural, emotional, and pathological states (Heinricher et al., 2009; Ossipov et al., 2010). When the system shifts towards inhibition, hyposensibility or lack of pain in spite of inputs from peripheral tissue may result (Heinricher et al., 2009; Kuner, 2010; Porreca et al., 2002; Ren & Dubner, 2002; Robinson & Zhuo, 2002; Wilder-Smith et al., 2002). The evolutionary value of this is that the organism can ignore pain during critical situations, e.g., flight or fight scenarios (Kuner, 2010). A facilitating shift of the descending system has been reported for different groups of patients with persistent pain (Heinricher et al., 2009; Julien et al., 2005; Kuner, 2010; Porreca et al., 2002; Ren & Dubner, 2002; Robinson & Zhuo, 2002; Wilder-Smith et al., 2002).

Decreased production of substances such as endorphins or gamma-aminobutyric acid (GABA), the most common inhibitory neurotransmitter in the central nervous system, may contribute to disturbances in pain inhibition. Animal and human studies have confirmed that the endogenous opioid system and GABA play a role in the modulation of pain. However, the understanding of the mechanisms, including the peripheral balances between nociceptive and anitinociceptive processes, behind chronic myalgia is incomplete. The analgesic properties of *exogenous* cannabinoids have been recognized for many years. Data clearly implicate endocannabinoids as endogenous tonic pain controlling molecules (Agarwal et al., 2007; Richardson et al., 1998; Walker & Huang, 2002), but little is known as to whether *peripheral* endocannabinoid signalling is disturbed in human pain.

1.4 Muscle nociception and peripheral sensitization

Neurophysiological studies have indicated that small-diameter, slowly conducting afferent nerve fibres from skeletal muscle –free nerve endings of group III (Aδ) and IV afferent (C) fibres – have to be excited to elicit pain (Mense, 2003). The nociceptor is specialized to respond to noxious stimuli and communicate this information to the CNS. Nociceptors or noxious stimulus detectors (Woolf & Ma, 2007) are sensitive to chemical substances released from damaged or overloaded cells and excessive tissue deformation (Coutaux et al., 2005; Mense, 1993). Nociceptors respond to single or combinations of stimuli: noxious mechanical stimuli, temperature, and chemical substances such as serotonin H^+, (5-HT), bradykinin (BKN), glutamate, prostaglandin E_2 (PGE_2), substance P, nerve growth factor (NGF), ATP, and potassium (Coutaux et al., 2005; Mense, 1993; 2009). Administration of any of these substances, alone or in combination, results in excitation of nociceptors (Mense, 1993). The relative effectiveness of these substances is unknown. In a pathophysiological situation due to trauma or inflammation, a combination of substances acts on the nociceptors (the inflammatory "soup" or "cocktail")(Mense, 2009). The nociceptor is not a static detector as plastic changes can occur such as peripheral sensitization (Woolf & Ma, 2007). A sensitized nociceptor has a lowered threshold for activation and can thus be activated by stimuli that are normally innocuous (Coutaux et al., 2005; Mense, 1993). Several substances - e.g., H^+, NO, K^+, ATP, bradykinin (BKN), PGE_2, NGF, TNF-α, IL-6, and glutamate - are known to cause peripheral sensitization (Coutaux et al., 2005; Mense, 2009; Momin & McNaughton, 2009). The action of these substances is mediated by their specific receptors mainly found in three classes: 1) G protein coupled receptors; 2) receptor tyrosine kinases; and 3) ionotropic receptors/ion channels (Linley et al., 2010). Sensitization is often accompanied by an increase in the sensitive area (Mense, 1993). In addition, other alterations of the nociceptors, including activation of silent nociceptors, have been found as the result of injury or inflammation (Schaible et al., 2009). When persistent alterations in the nociceptors as the result of induced gene transcription and protein synthesis drive pain in the absence of noxious stimuli these alterations represent a pathological condition (Woolf & Ma, 2007).

1.5 The bio-psycho-social model of chronic pain

The net result of the above mentioned and other alterations are clinically registered as pain hypersensitivity - an increased responsiveness to nociception and sometimes to innocuous stimuli. In clinical management of chronic pain, a bio-psycho-social model (Gatchel et al., 2007) is preferred since the above mentioned complex blend of factors - neurobiological, psychological (e.g., depression, catastrophizing, and anxiety), coping styles, and contextual factors - contribute to the development and maintenance of chronic pain (Alonso et al., 2004; Asmundson & Katz, 2009; Börsbo et al., 2008; Dersh et al., 2001; Ericsson et al., 2002; Means-Christensen et al., 2008; Ocañez et al., 2010; Sofat et al., 2011; Sullivan et al., 2001).

1.6 Central versus peripheral causes for chronic pain

One of the consequences of the discovery of central sensitization is that CNS can change pain -e.g., amplification, duration, degree, and spatial extent - so that pain no longer directly reflects the peripheral noxious situation (Woolf, 2011). It is unknown whether a chronic pain condition can be driven by established central alterations such as central hyperexcitability, alterations in pain matrix, and alterations in descending mechanisms (facilitation) with very little or no peripheral stimuli or nociception. However, there are several indications that central alterations in nociceptive processing are driven by peripheral tissue alterations (Gerdle et al., 2008c) and peripheral nociceptive input (Schneider et al., 2010; Staud, 2010; Staud et al., 2009; Woolf, 2011).

1.7 The microdialysis technique

Concerns have been expressed at the lack of success in translating basic science data using animals into clinical analgesics (Lascelles & Flecknell, 2010). Microdialysis may be able to replace animal experiments (Langley et al., 2008). The microdialysis technique offers a well-established *in vivo* method for studying the local biochemistry of individual tissues in the body (Ungerstedt, 1991), e.g., nociceptive and metabolic mechanisms. This technique has been used in neuroscience to monitor neurotransmitter release, but has also found application in monitoring the biochemistry of peripheral tissues in both animals and humans (Ungerstedt, 1991).

Microdialysis mimics the function of a capillary blood vessel by perfusing a thin dialysis tube (catheter) implanted into the tissue with a physiological saline solution. Through simple diffusion, substances can move across the dialysis membrane along the concentration gradient. The chemical analysis of the dialysate reveals the composition of the extracellular fluid. Thus microdialysis allows for continuous sampling of compounds in the interstitial space of the muscle, where nociceptor free nerve endings terminate close to the muscle fibres, providing accurate information on regional biochemical changes before such compounds are diluted and cleared by the circulatory system. The trapezius muscle has been used as a *human model muscle* for chronic myalgia both due to its clinical importance and to its accessibility for invasive investigations. Some studies use the masseter, vastus lateralis, and gastrocnemius muscles to examine myalgia.

To determine the concentrations of small molecules such as lactate, pyruvate, glutamate, and glucose, a catheter with a 20 kDa cut-off is usually used (Waelgaard et al., 2006). To determine the concentrations of larger molecules such as cytokines, a catheter with a 100 kDa cut-off is usually used (Waelgaard et al., 2006).

A crucial parameter in microdialysis is relative recovery (RR): the ratio between substance concentrations in the dialysate to that in the perfusate (Afinowi et al., 2009; Dahlin et al., 2010 ; Ungerstedt, 1991). RR is used to determine the true concentration of extracellular fluid. Because the perfusate constantly flows across the membrane, a state of equilibrium will never be achieved and as a result the dialysate will only represent a certain percentage of the actual concentration of the extracellular fluid (Afinowi et al., 2009; Hamrin et al., 2002). Therefore, the final concentration in the dialysate partially depends on the flow rate of the perfusate. Low flow rate results in higher RR; high flow rates, result in lower RR. At a very low flow (i.e., $\leq$ 0.3μl/min), the recovery is near 100%, but factors such as alterations in the osmotic pressure, temperature, weight cut-off, area of the membrane, concentration gradient, and composition of the perfusate can influence RR (Dahlin et al., 2010 ; Hamrin et al., 2002 ; Plock & Kloft, 2005). Between cytokines have been reported marked variation in RR; molecular weight correlated negatively with RR (Helmy et al., 2009).

1.8 Aim

Microdialysis has several important advantages, but studies with patients are expensive and time consuming. Hence a systematic review of the literature is needed. Systematic knowledge of the results of such studies might help provide new assessment approaches of patients with chronic myalgia, new treatments, and new rehabilitation techniques for patients with chronic myalgia. Most research on muscle pain has been conducted on animals; however, this review will primarily focus on human studies of neck and shoulder myalgia, for which the frequently affected trapezius muscle often serves as a model muscle. This study systematically reviews studies in the literature that have investigated alterations in metabolic substances, pain-related substances (algesics), and anti-analgesics in different chronic muscle pain conditions (mainly myalgia) in humans using microdialysis. This systematic review was done to identify potential biomarkers - an objectively measured and evaluated indicator of, e.g., normal pathogenic processes (Ptolemy & Rifai, 2010).

2. Methods

2.1 Inclusion and exclusion criteria

Studies that focused on chronic pain conditions affecting human muscles (myalgias) were included. To be included, the studies had to use microdialysis and had to use a patient group and a healthy control group, so articles concerning only healthy subjects have been excluded.

2.2 Search strategy

This review identified the studies fulfilling the above criteria in the systematic review of Larsson et al. (Larsson et al., 2007). Furthermore, we modified their search strategy in the following ways: ((muscle OR pain) AND microdialysis) OR (muscle AND pain AND induced) AND (Humans[Mesh] AND (Clinical Trial[ptyp] OR Meta-Analysis[ptyp] OR Review[ptyp]) AND English[lang] AND adult[MeSH] AND "last 10 years"[PDat]).

Using this strategy, PubMed was searched. From this search, the titles and abstracts were scrutinized. If the articles were relevant and necessary, they were read for further evaluation. We also checked reference lists of these articles. If the article was relevant according to our aim and inclusion criteria, we listed the results in tables. The tables of the different conditions reported the statistics concerning comparisons between the patient group and control group with respect to baseline data or corresponding data for all investigated substances. Moreover, we listed gender, flow rate, number of subjects in each group, and if and how the authors handled RR.

2.3 Positive outcome with respect to potential biomarker

A specific substance was classified as a potential biomarker if the majority of studies (including the majority of subjects) showed significantly lower or significantly higher concentrations in the patient group compared to the controls.

3. Results

Using the modified search strategy, we had 441 hits after searching PubMed. After screening, we identified 17 articles that fulfilled our inclusion criteria. Thirteen of these were not mentioned by Larsson et al. (Larsson et al., 2007). After scrutinizing these 13 articles and the articles selected by Larsson et al., we found 22 articles concerning different chronic pain conditions involving muscle. These articles are summarized in **Tables 1-7**. Moreover, we identified three articles concerning chronic tendinosis (**Table 8**).

3.1 Chronic trapezius myalgia

For chronic trapezius myalgia, we identified seven groups of patients reported in ten studies (**Table 1**). The majority of the studies reported increases in the interstitial concentrations of lactate (Flodgren et al., 2010; Flodgren et al., 2006; Larsson et al., 2008; Rosendal et al., 2004b; Sjogaard et al., 2010). However, the studies conducted by Flodgren et al. (Flodgren et al., 2010; Flodgren et al., 2006) did not compensate for relative recovery despite the fact that the flow rate was relatively high (2μl/min) compared to a flow rate associated with full recovery (0.3μ l/min).

Study	Condition Number of Subjects, % women (W) Muscles	Substances investigated Flow rate	Results (Comparisons between patients and HC; p-values)	Comments (Compensated for RR (Y/N) or low flow rate* (NA or Y/N)
Flodgren et al. (Flodgren et al., 2005)	Chronic shoulder pain (CSP; n=9), 100% W HC (n=9), 100%W Trapezius	Glutamate PGE_2 0.3μl/min	Glutamate-trapezius: ns PGE_2-trapezius: ns	Compensated for RR: N Low flow: Y
Flodgren et al. (Flodgren et al., 2010)	Chronic trapezius myalgia (MYA; n=14), 100% W HC (compared with healthy subjects (n=20) in (Flodgren et al., 2006)), 100% W Trapezius	Lactate Pyruvate Glutamate PGE_2 2μl/min	Lactate-trapezius: ns Pyruvate-trapezius: Glutamate-trapezius: MYA<HC, significant PGE_2-trapezius: not reported.	Compensated for RR: N Low flow: N
Rosendal et al. (Rosendal et al., 2004b)	Chronic trapezius myalgia (MYA; n=19), 100%W HC (n=20), 100%W Trapezius	Lactate Pyruvate Glutamate 5-HT 5μl/min	Lactate-trapezius: MYA > HC; P=0.001 Pyruvate-trapezius: MYA > HC; P=0.001 Glutamate-trapezius: MYA > HC; P=0.05 5-HT-trapezius: MYA > HC; P=0.01	Compensated for RR: Y Low flow: NA
Rosendal et al. (Rosendal et al., 2005)	Chronic trapezius myalgia (MYA; n=19), 100%W HC (n=20), 100%W Trapezius	K^+ LDH IL-6 Collagen turnover 5μl/min	K^+-trapezius: MYA > HC; P=significant LDH-trapezius: ns IL-6-trapezius: ns Collagen turnover-trapezius: ns	Compensated for RR: Y Low flow: NA

Study	Condition Number of Subjects, % women (W) Muscles	Substances investigated Flow rate	Results (Comparisons between patients and HC; p-values)	Comments (Compensated for RR (Y/N) or low flow rate* (NA or Y/N)
Gerdle et al. (Gerdle et al., 2008b)	Chronic trapezius myalgia (MYA; n=19), 100%W Chronic whiplash associated disorders (WAD; n=22), 100%W HC (n=20), 100%W Trapezius	BKN Kallidin 5µl/min	BKN-trapezius: No group differences. Kallidin-trapezius: MYA>HC; P=0.018 No other group differences for this substance.	Compensated for RR: Y Low flow: NA
Larsson et al. (Larsson et al., 2008)	Chronic trapezius myalgia (MYA; n=20), 100%W HC (n=20), 100%W Trapezius	Lactate Pyruvate Glutamate 5-HT K^+ BKN GM-CSF IL-1β IL-6 IL-8 TNF-α IL-2 IL-4 IL-5 IL-10 5µl/min	Lactate-trapezius: ns Pyruvate-trapezius: MYA > HC; P=0.032 Glutamate-trapezius: MYA > HC; P=0.005 5-HT-trapezius: MYA > HC; P=0.023 K^+-trapezius: ns BKN- trapezius: ns GM-CSF- trapezius: ns IL-1β-trapezius: ns IL-6-trapezius: ns IL-8-trapezius: ns TNF-α-trapezius: ns IL-2-trapezius: ns IL-4-trapezius: ns IL-5-trapezius: ns IL-10-trapezius: ns	Compensated for RR: Y Low flow: NA
Ghafouri et al. (Ghafouri et al., 2010)	Chronic trapezius myalgia, (MYA; n=18), 100%W HC (n=30), 100%W Trapezius	5-HT 5µl/min	5-HT- trapezius: MYA>HC, P=0.044	Compensated for RR: Y Low flow: NA

Study	Condition Number of Subjects, % women (W) Muscles	Substances investigated Flow rate	Results (Comparisons between patients and HC; p-values)	Comments (Compensated for RR (Y/N) or low flow rate* (NA or Y/N)
Ghafouri et al. (Ghafouri et al., 2011)	Chronic trapezius myalgia, (MYA; n=11), 100%W HC (n=11), 100%W Trapezius	PEA SEA 5μl/min	PEA-trapezius: MYA>HC, P=0.011 SEA-trapezius: MYA>HC, P=0.002 (The statistics are for dialysate concentrations, but significant differences were found when compensated for RR)	Compensated for RR: Y Low flow: NA
Sjøgaard et al (Sjogaard et al., 2010)	Chronic trapezius myalgia (MYA; n=43), 100%W HC (n=19), 100%W Trapezius	Lactate Pyruvate Glucose K^+ 5μl/min	Lactate-trapezius: MYA>HC, significant Pyruvate-trapezius: MYA>HC, significant Glucose-trapezius: ns K^+-trapezius: ns	Compensated for RR: Y Low flow: NA
Shah et al (Shah et al., 2005)	Myofascial trapezius pain with active trigger point (MFactive; n=3) HC with latent trigger point (HClatent; n=3) HC without trigger point (HC;n=3) Trigger points of Trapezius	BKN CGRP Substance P IL-1β TNF-α 5-HT Norepinephrine H^+ 1and 2 μl/min	BKN-trapezius: MFactive>two other groups; P<0.01 CGRP-trapezius: MFactive>two other groups; P<0.01 Substance P- trapezius: MFactive>two other groups; P<0.01 IL-1β-trapezius: MFactive>two other groups; P<0.01 TNF-α-trapezius: MFactive>two other groups; P<0.01 5-HT-trapezius: MFactive>two other groups; P<0.01 Norepinephrine-trapezius: MFactive>two other groups; P<0.01 H^+-trapezius: MFactive>two other groups; P<0.01	Compensated for RR: Y Low flow: NA

Study	Condition Number of Subjects, % women (W) Muscles	Substances investigated Flow rate	Results (Comparisons between patients and HC; p-values)	Comments (Compensated for RR (Y/N) or low flow rate* (NA or Y/N)
Shah et al. (Shah et al., 2008)	Myofascial trapezius pain with active trigger point (MFactive; n=3) HC with latent trigger point (HClatent; n=3) HC without trigger point (HC; n=3) Trigger points of Trapezius Gastrocnemius medialis without trigger points	BKN CGRP Substance P IL-1β TNF-α IL-6 IL-8 5-HT Norepinephrine H^+ 1 and 2μl/min	BKN-gastrocnemius: MFactive>2 other groups; Sign CGRP-gastrocnemius: MFactive>2 other groups; Sign Substance P-gastrocnemius: MFactive>2 other groups; Sign IL-1β-gastrocnemius: MFactive>2 other groups; Sign TNF-α-gastrocnemius: MFactive>2 other groups; Sign 5-HT-gastrocnemius: MFactive>2 other groups; Sign Norepinephrine-trapezius: MFactive>2 other groups; Sign H^+-gastrocnemius: MFactive>2 other groups; Sign Comparisons between trapezius (T) and gastrocnemius (G) in MFactive: BKN: T>G; Sign CGRP: T>G; Sign Substance P: T>G; Sign IL-1β: T>G; Sign TNF-α: T>G; Sign IL-6: T>G; Sign IL-8: T>G; Sign 5-HT: T>G; Sign Norepinephrine: T>G; Sign H^+:ns Comparisons between trapezius (T) and gastrocnemius (G) in MFlatent: BKN, IL-1β, IL-6, IL-8, 5-HT, Norepinephrine, H^+: ns CGRP: T>G; Sign	Compensated for RR: Y Low flow: NA

Study	Condition Number of Subjects, % women (W) Muscles	Substances investigated Flow rate	Results (Comparisons between patients and HC; p-values)	Comments (Compensated for RR (Y/N) or low flow rate* (NA or Y/N)
			Substance P: T>G; Sign TNF-α: T>G; Sign Comparisons between trapezius (T) and gastrocnemius (G) in HC: BKN: T>G; Sign Other substances: ns	

*Low flow rate associated with 100% relative recovery was defined as 0.3μl/min.

Table 1. Studies of chronic trapezius myalgia. The results of the different substances are baseline data. Healthy controls are abbreviated as HC. The bold horizontal lines indicate different patient groups.

A similar pattern was noted for the majority of studies reporting increased interstitial concentrations of pyruvate (Flodgren et al., 2010; Flodgren et al., 2006; Larsson et al., 2008; Rosendal et al., 2004b; Sjogaard et al., 2010). Flodgren et al. did not show any significant differences for pyruvate (Flodgren et al., 2010; Flodgren et al., 2006).

Three studies that focused on chronic trapezius myalgia investigated the interstitial muscle concentration of glutamate (Flodgren et al., 2005; Larsson et al., 2008; Rosendal et al., 2004b). In two of these studies (Larsson et al., 2008; Rosendal et al., 2004b), which were markedly larger than the third study (Flodgren et al., 2005), revealed significant increases in the interstitial concentrations of glutamate. In all the studies investigating glutamate, the interstitial muscle concentration of 5-HT was significantly increased (Ghafouri et al., 2010; Larsson et al., 2008; Rosendal et al., 2004b; Shah et al., 2008; Shah et al., 2005). Furthermore, glutamate was also increased in patients with chronic WAD (**Table 2**) (Gerdle et al., 2008c).

Four studies examined the interstitial concentrations of BKN and/or Kallidin (Gerdle et al., 2008b; Larsson et al., 2008; Shah et al., 2008; Shah et al., 2005). Shah et al. (Shah et al., 2008; Shah et al., 2005) found increased levels of BKN in subjects with active trigger points and the levels were higher in the trapezius (with pain) than in a pain-free distant muscle. In contrast, two studies - a field study and a laboratory study - found no differences between patients and controls (Gerdle et al., 2008b; Larsson et al., 2008). Kallidin was only investigated in one study and this study reported significantly higher interstitial levels in patients with chronic trapezius myalgia (Gerdle et al., 2008b).

Several studies have investigated cytokines, but only Shah et al. found significant differences for active trigger points (Shah et al., 2008; Shah et al., 2005). These authors also have compared the levels of cytokines in the myalgic trapezius (trigger points) with a muscle without pain and found higher levels in the aching muscle. These studies, however, are limited because their sample size was small. Larger studies have not found elevated levels of cytokines (Larsson et al., 2008; Rosendal et al., 2005). In three relatively large studies, potassium revealed no consistent pattern (Larsson et al., 2008; Rosendal et al., 2005; Sjogaard et al., 2010). PGE_2 was not increased in two groups of patients (Flodgren et al., 2005; Flodgren et al., 2010; Flodgren et al., 2006), but the first of these groups was relatively small (Flodgren et al., 2005) and the other had possible methodological drawbacks related to RR (Flodgren et al., 2010; Flodgren et al., 2006).

Study	Condition Number of Subjects, % women (W) Muscles	Substances investigated Flow rate	Results (Comparisons between patients and HC; p-values)	Comments (Compensated for RR (Y/N) or low flow rate* (NA or Y/N)
Gerdle et al. (Gerdle et al., 2008c)	Chronic whiplash associated disorders (WAD; n=22), 100% W HC (n=20), 100% W Trapezius	Lactate Pyruvate Glutamate K^+ 5-HT IL-6 5μl/min	Lactate-trapezius: ns Pyruvate-trapezius: ns Glutamate-trapezius: ns K^+ trapezius: ns 5-HT-trapezius: WAD>HC; P=0.05 IL-6-trapezius: WAD>HC; P=0.008	Compensated for RR: Y Low flow: NA
Gerdle et al. (Gerdle et al., 2008b)	Chronic trapezius myalgia (MYA; n=19), 100% W Chronic whiplash associated disorders (WAD; n=22), 100% W HC (n=20), 100%W Trapezius	BKN Kallidin 5μl/min	BKN- trapezius: No group differences. Kallidin-trapezius: MYA>HC; P=0.018 No other group differences for this substance.	Compensated for RR: Y Low flow: NA

*Low flow rate associated with 100% relative recovery was defined as 0.3μl/min.

Table 2. Studies of chronic WAD. The results of the different substances are baseline data. Healthy controls are abbreviated as HC.

In two studies, Shah et al. investigated P and CGRP (Shah et al., 2008; Shah et al., 2005). They found significant increases in active trigger points in the trapezius and found that these levels were higher in the aching trapezius than in a distant pain-free muscle.

Substances only reported in single studies/patient groups were glucose (no difference) (Sjogaard et al., 2010), norepinephrine (significant difference) (Shah et al., 2008; Shah et al., 2005), and H^+ (significant difference) (Shah et al., 2008; Shah et al., 2005).

3.2 Chronic WAD

We identified two studies (**Table 2**) using the same material concerning patients with chronic WAD (Gerdle et al., 2008b; Gerdle et al., 2008c), and 5-HT and IL-6 were significantly higher in WAD than in HC. No differences were found in the concentrations of investigated metabolites, potassium, glutamate, BKN, or kallidin compared with healthy controls.

3.3 Fibromyalgia

Two studies investigated fibromyalgia patients (**Table 3**). In the larger study investigating the painful trapezius muscle of fibromyalgia patients, significantly higher interstitial concentrations of lactate and pyruvate were found compared to healthy controls (Gerdle et al., 2010). In the other study, the vastus lateralis muscle was investigated in eight patients with fibromyalgia and the authors reported no differences in concentrations of lactate compared to controls (McIver et al., 2006). It is unclear from this study if the vastus lateralis was habitually painful and/or painful at palpation (e.g., tender point examination). Moreover, no compensation for RR was done despite a relatively high flow rate.

Study	Condition Number of Subjects, % women (W) Muscles	Substances investigated Flow rate	Results (Comparisons between patients and HC; p-values)	Comments (Compensated for RR (Y/N) or low flow rate* (NA or Y/N)
Gerdle et al. (Gerdle et al., 2010)	Fibromyalgia (FM; n=19), 100% W HC (n=19), 100% W Trapezius	Lactate Pyruvate Glutamate 0.3μl/min	Lactate-trapezius: FM>HC; P=0.039 Pyruvate-trapezius: FM>HC; P=0.001 Glutamate-trapezius: ns.	Compensated for RR: N Low flow: Y
McIver et al (McIver et al., 2006)	Fibromyalgia (FM; n=8), 100%W HC (n=8), 100% W Vastus lateralis	Lactate 2μl/min	Lactate-vastus: ns	Compensated for RR: N Low flow: N

*Low flow rate associated with 100% relative recovery was defined as 0.3μl/min

Table 3. Studies of fibromyalgia. The results of the different substances are baseline data. Healthy controls are abbreviated as HC.

3.4 Temporomandibular pain disorders

Compared to the healthy controls, fibromyalgia patients had increased 5-HT in the masseter muscle (Ernberg et al., 1999). Compared to the healthy controls, myofascial temporomandibular disorder patients had significantly higher glutamate levels (Castrillon et al., 2010) (**Table 4**).

Study	Condition Number of Subjects, % women (W) Muscles	Substances investigated Flow rate	Results (Comparisons between patients and HC; p-values)	Comments (Compensated for RR (Y/N) or low flow rate* (NA or Y/N)
Ernberg et al (Ernberg et al., 1999)	Fibromyalgia (FM; n=18), 100%W Localized myalgia of the temporomandibular system (LM; n=17), 76% W HC (n=10), 60%W Masseter	5-HT (corrected for S-5-HT) 7μl/min	5-HT (corrected for S-5-HT)-trauma-masseter: FM>HC: P=0.05 5-HT (corrected for S-5-HT)-baseline-masseter: no group differences	Compensated for RR: N, but corrected for S-5-HT Low flow:N
Hedenberg-Magnusson et al (Hedenberg-Magnusson et al., 2001)	Fibromyalgia (FM; n=19), 89%W Localized myalgia of the temporomandibular system (LM; n=19), 74%W HC (n=11), 64% W Masseter	PGE_2 Leukotriene B_4(LTB4) 7μl/min	PGE_2-masseter: ns LTB4-masseter: FM>LM; P=0.05	Compensated for RR: N Low flow: N
Castrillon (Castrillon et al., 2010)	Myofascial temporomandibular disorder pain (TMD; n=13), 77%W HC (n=10), 80%W Masseter	Glutamate 2μl/min	Glutamate-masseter: TMD> HC; P=0.023	Compensated for RR: Low flow:

*Low flow rate associated with 100% relative recovery was defined as 0.3μl/min.

Table 4. Studies of temporomandibular pain disorders. The results of the different substances are baseline data. Healthy controls are abbreviated as HC.

3.5 Chronic tension type headaches

In two studies of one group of patients (Ashina et al., 2002; Ashina et al., 2003) with chronic tension headaches, no differences were found in metabolites and some algesic substances (e.g., BKN and PGE2) in the trapezius muscle (**Table 5**).

3.6 Polymyalgia rheumatica

We found two studies of polymyalgia rheumatica based on the same groups of subjects (Kreiner & Galbo, 2011; Kreiner et al., 2010) (**Table 6**). These two studies reported marked alterations in cytokines but also to some extent in algesic substances such as glutamate in two muscles. These two studies also reported 5-HT in one muscle and in BKN in one muscle. Interestingly, all alterations were normalized after prednisolone treatment.

Study	Condition Number of Subjects, % women (W) Muscles	Substances investigated Flow rate	Results (Comparisons between patients and HC; p-values)	Comments (Compensated for RR (Y/N) or low flow rate* (NA or Y/N)
Ashina et al. (Ashina et al., 2003)	Chronic tension-type Headache (CTTH; n=16), 63% W HC (n=17), 71% W Trapezius	Pyruvate Glucose Urea Glutamate K^+ BKN PGE_2 ATP 2μl/min	Pyruvate-trapezius: ns Glucose-trapezius: ns Urea-trapezius: ns Glutamate-trapezius: ns K^+-trapezius: ns BKN-trapezius: ns PGE_2-trapezius: ns ATP-trapezius: ns	Compensated for RR: Y Low flow: NA
Ashina et al. (Ashina et al., 2002)	Chronic tension-type Headache (CTTH; n=16), 63% W HC (n=17), 71% W Trapezius	Lactate 2μl/min	Lactate- trapezius: ns	Compensated for RR: Y Low flow: NA

*Low flow rate associated with 100% relative recovery was defined as 0.3μl/min.

Table 5. Studies of chronic tension type headaches. The results of the different substances are baseline data. Healthy controls are abbreviated as HC.

3.7 Mitochondrial myopathy

In a study of mitochondrial myopathy that included four patients, no significant differences were found for metabolites, glutamate, hypoxanthine, urate, and aspartate (**Table 7**).

3.8 Chronic tendinosis

We also found three studies that focused on chronic tendinosis (**Table 8**). These three studies are small and have investigated different tendons with pain. The interstitial concentrations of glutamate, PGE_2, and lactate were investigated, but no consistent pattern with respect to these substances was found.

Study	Condition Number of Subjects, % women(W) Muscles	Substances investigated Flow rate	Results (comparisons between patients and HC; p-values)	Comments (Compensated for RR (Y/N) or low flow rate* (NA or Y/N)
Kreiner & Galbo (Kreiner & Galbo, 2011)	Polymyalgia rheumatica (PMR)(n=20), 60%W Healthy controls (HC) (n=20), 65%W Trapezius Vastus lateralis	Lactate Pyruvate Glutamate 5-HT BKN PGE2 K+ ATP 3μl/min	Lactate -trapezius: PMR >HC; P=0.05 Pyruvate -trapezius: ns Glutamate–trapezius: PMR >HC; P=0.05 5-HT–trapezius: ns BKN–trapezius: ns PGE2–trapezius: ns K+–trapezius: ns ATP–trapezius: ns Lactate–vastus: ns Pyruvate–vastus: ns Glutamate–vastus: PMR >HC; P=0.05 5-HT–vastus: PMR >HC; P=0.05 BKN–vastus: ns PGE2–vastus: PMR >HC; P=0.05 K+–vastus: ns ATP–vastus: ns	Compensated for RR: Y Low flow: NA
Kreiner et al. (Kreiner et al., 2010)	Polymyalgia rheumatica (PMR)(n=20), 60%W Healthy controls (HC) (n=20), 65% W Trapezius Vastus lateralis	IL-1α/β IL-1 receptor antagonist (IL-1Ra) IL-6 IL-8 TNF-α Monocyte chemoattractant protein 1(MCP-1) 3μl/min	IL-1α–trapezius: PMR >HC; P=0.001 IL-1β–trapezius: PMR >HC; P=0.01 IL-1Ra–trapezius: PMR >HC; P=0.01 IL-6–trapezius: PMR >HC; P=0.01 IL-8–trapezius: PMR >HC; P=0.05 TNF-α–trapezius: PMR >HC; P=0.05 MCP-1–trapezius: PMR >HC; P=0.05 IL-1α–vastus: PMR >HC; P=0.01 IL-1β–vastus: PMR >HC; P=0.05 IL-1Ra–vastus: PMR >HC; P=0.05 IL-6–vastus: PMR >HC; P=0.05 IL-8–vastus: PMR >HC; P=0.05 TNF-α–vastus: PMR >HC; P=ns MCP-1–vastus: PMR >HC; P=0.05	Compensated for RR: Y Low flow: NA

*Low flow rate associated with 100% relative recovery was defined as 0.3μl/min.

Table 6. Studies of Polymyalgia rheumatica. The results of the different substances are baseline data. Healthy controls are abbreviated as HC.

Study	Condition Number of Subjects, % women(W) Muscles	Substances investigated Flow rate	Results (Comparisons between patients and HC; p-values)	Comments (Compensated for RR (Y/N) or low flow rate* (NA or Y/N)
Axelson et al (Axelson et al., 2002)	Mitochondrial Myopathy (MM; n=4); 50% W HC (n=11), 36% W Tibialis anterior	Lactate Pyruvate Glutamate Hypoxanthine Urate Aspartate 0.3µl/min	Lactate-tibialis: ns Pyruvate-tibialis: ns Glutamate-tibialis: ns Hypoxanthine-tibialis: ns Urate-tibialis: ns Aspartate-tibialis: ns	Compensated for RR: N Low flow: Y

*Low flow rate associated with 100% relative recovery was defined as 0.3µl/min.

Table 7. Studies of mitochondrial myopathy. The results of the different substances are baseline data. Healthy controls are abbreviated as HC.

Study	Condition Number of Subjects, % women(W) Tendon	Substances investigated	Results (Comparisons between patients and HC; p-values)	Comments (Compensated for RR (Y/N) or low flow* (NA or Y/N))
Alfredson et al (Alfredson et al., 2000)	Tennis Elbow (TE; n=4), 25% W HC (n=4), 50%W Extensor carpi radialis brevis tendon	Glutamate PGE_2	Glutamate: ns PGE_2:TE>HC;P< 0.001	Compensated for RR: N Low flow: Y
Alfredson et al (Alfredson et al., 2001)	Jumpers' knee (JK; n=5), 20%W HC (n=5), 20%W Patellar tendon	Glutamate PGE_2	Glutamate: JK>HC; P=0.01 PGE_2: ns	Compensated for RR: N Low flow: Y
Alfredson et al (Alfredson, 2005)	Chronic Achilles tendinosis (CAT; n=4), 0%W HC (n=5), 0%W Achilles tendon	Lactate	Lactate: CAT>HC; P=0.05	Compensated for RR: N Low flow: Y

*Low flow was defined as 0.3µl/min.

Table 8. Studies of tendons with chronic pain. The results of the different substances are baseline data. Healthy controls are abbreviated as HC.

4. Discussion

4.1 Metabolites

The majority of studies concerning the trapezius in chronic trapezius myalgia have reported increases in the interstitial concentrations of lactate and pyruvate (Flodgren et al., 2010; Flodgren et al., 2006; Larsson et al., 2008; Rosendal et al., 2004b; Sjogaard et al., 2010). However, Flodgren et al. (Flodgren et al., 2010; Flodgren et al., 2006) did not compensate for RR and their results might be biased.

There are several possible explanations for the generally higher interstitial levels of pyruvate levels in chronic trapezius myalgia and in the trapezius of patients with FMS. For example, changes in the lactate-pyruvate metabolism via lactate dehydrogenase isoforms may result in higher pyruvate levels (Philip et al., 2005). Another explanation is a reduction in tissue oxygenation in FMS (Bengtsson, 2002) and chronic trapezius myalgia (Larsson et al., 2004), reductions that may result in higher pyruvate and higher lactate concentrations due to a shift towards an anaerobic state. A lower fitness level is a third explanation as a low fitness level means more frequent reliance on anaerobic metabolism. However, it is unknown if a general deconditioning in these two pain conditions involves the postural trapezius. The aerobic capacity of a muscle is largely governed by the number of mitochondria and their enzymes (Weibel & Hoppeler, 2005). The mitochondrial density increases as result of exercise and this increased density affects the level of metabolites (i.e., enhanced aerobic capacity) (Norrbom, 2008). Lower capillary density and/or enzymes associated with aerobic metabolism have been reported in FMS and in chronic trapezius myalgia (Larsson et al., 2004; Lindh et al., 1995). For FMS and chronic trapezius myalgia, the trapezius muscle fibres can appear with alterations in mitochondrial content and distribution, e.g., moth-eaten fibres and ragged red-fibres (Bengtsson, 2002; Bengtsson et al., 1986; Larsson et al., 2000; Larsson et al., 2004).

The role of lactate is complex. Lactate may assist in the detection of exercise stress before tissue damage occurs and can be exchanged rapidly among tissue compartments where it may be oxidized as a fuel or reconverted to form pyruvate or glucose (Gladden, 2004; Kim et al., 2007; Philip et al., 2005; Robergs et al., 2004). Lactate is also involved in peripheral nociception and it appears to facilitate the response of the acid-sensing ion channel 3 (ASIC-3) to low pH (Kim et al., 2007). Such ASIC channels are considered to be molecular transducers for nociception and mechanosensation (Kim et al., 2007).

To summarize, most studies of myalgic trapezius muscles show significant increases in interstitial levels of lactate and pyruvate. These results might be explained by decreased fitness level, reduced tissue oxygenation, increased muscle activation, and/or damaged mitochondria.

4.2 Pain-related substances

4.2.1 Glutamate

Two of the studies of chronic trapezius myalgia (Larsson et al., 2008; Rosendal et al., 2004b), which are markedly larger than the third study (Flodgren et al., 2005), found significant increases in the interstitial concentrations of glutamate. A possible difference between subjects of these studies may contribute to the inconsistent glutamate finding. The myalgic subjects studied by Larsson et al. and Rosendal et al. (Larsson et al., 2008; Rosendal et al., 2004b) comprised subjects reporting considerable pain and had distinct current muscular signs confirmed at clinical examination. The pain history, the present pain, and clinical muscular neck status of the subjects are very sparsely presented in the Flodgren study (Flodgren et al., 2005). Moreover, one study found the painful masseter was significantly associated with increased glutamate (Castrillon et al., 2010).

Glutamate, a pain modulator in the human central nervous system, acts via the N-methyl-D-aspartate (NMDA) receptor (Coggeshall & Carlton, 1997) (Hudspith, 1997) and influences peripheral pain processing (Carlton, 2001; Varney & Gereau, 2002), e.g., muscle inflammation and delayed onset muscle soreness (Cairns et al., 2001a; Cairns et al., 2001b; Cairns et al., 2003; Svensson et al., 2003; Svensson et al., 2005; Tegeder et al., 2002). Glutamate is released from peripheral afferent nerve terminals (Miller et al., 2011). Studies of animals have shown that glutamate receptors are located on the peripheral ends of small-diameter primary afferents in several tissues such as muscle (Coggeshall & Carlton, 1998). Inflammatory animal models reveal increased levels of glutamate in peripheral tissues and nociceptive behaviours (Miller et al., 2011). Several studies have demonstrated that injections of glutamate increase pain intensity (Cairns et al., 2003; Gazerani et al., 2006). A review from 2008 concluded that elevation of interstitial glutamate in skeletal muscle alters pain sensitivity in healthy humans and is associated with pain symptoms in some chronic non-inflammatory muscle pain conditions (Cairns & Dong, 2008), which are probably mediated through activation of peripheral excitatory amino acid receptors located on the terminal ends of nociceptors. The present review mainly supports the conclusions of that review. However, the interstitial concentrations of glutamate were not increased in the trapezius of patients with chronic WAD (Gerdle et al., 2008c) or in patients with fibromyalgia (Gerdle et al., 2010). One difference between chronic trapezius myalgia and the two other conditions might be the more widespread (spatial) hyperalgesia in the two latter conditions (Arendt-Nielsen & Graven-Nielsen, 2003; Wallin et al., 2011).

4.2.2 Serotonin

Serotonin (5-hydroxtryptamine, 5-HT) is involved in the central and peripheral modulation of nociceptive pain and hyperalgesia (Sommer, 2004). 5-HT is synthesized in brain neurons from the essential amino acid tryptophan and released from platelets and mast cells in the periphery due to tissue damage (Mense, 1993). Whether 5-HT has an analgesic or hyperalgesic action depends on the cell type and type of receptor it targets. Currently, seven receptor families have been identified. These receptors are cell-surface proteins that bind 5-HT and trigger intracellular changes that influence the behaviour of cells and explain the broad physiological actions and distribution of this biochemical mediator. According to animal studies, the 5-HT receptor classes currently identified, the 5-HT_1 and the 5-HT_2, may be involved in mainly chemical and thermal hyperalgesia (Ernberg, 2008). 5-HT activates the descending endogenous pain system and this inhibits centrally mediated pain transduction (Sommer, 2006; Suzuki et al., 2004). In the periphery, 5-HT sensitizes afferent nerve fibres, contributing to hyperalgesia in inflammation and nerve injury (Giordano & Rogers, 1989; Sommer, 2004; Taiwo & Levine, 1992). Intramuscular administration of 5-HT into the human masseter muscle has been demonstrated to induce pain (Ernberg et al., 2006). The studies identified in this systematic review concerning chronic trapezius myalgia (**Table 1**) clearly indicate significantly increased levels of 5-HT in the whole spectrum of severity of chronic trapezius myalgia and these findings agree with other studies of muscle pain conditions such as myalgic masseter muscle (Ernberg et al., 1999) (**Table 4**) and chronic whiplash associated pain including trapezius pain (Gerdle et al., 2008c) (**Table 2**). The finding that there are higher interstitial levels of 5-HT in chronic trapezius myalgia than in controls at rest agrees with other studies that also found that 5-HT is a peripheral pro-nociceptive substance activated by afferents and by the release of other substances (Saria et al., 1990; Sommer, 2004). The results of the present systematic review clearly indicate that 5-HT can be a potential biomarker of different types and severity of chronic myalgia.

4.2.3 Bradykinin (BKN) and Kallidin (KAL)

BKN and KAL are kinins - a group of structurally related 9-11 amino acid peptides that are produced by kallikrein-mediated enzymatic cleavage of kininogen (Coutaux et al., 2005; Riedel & Neeck, 2001; Wang et al., 2006). Kinins mediate their effects via two different G protein coupled receptors, B_1 and B_2, that provoke an increase in intracellular Ca^{2+} (Meyer et al., 2006; Zubakova et al., 2008). In normal tissue in the acute situation, BKN and KAL act via the B_2 receptor. In the chronic phase of the response of tissue injury and infection, B_1 receptors are expressed by BKN and KAL via this receptor (Calixto et al., 2004; Coutaux et al., 2005; Couture et al., 2001; Graven-Nielsen & Mense, 2001; McMahon et al., 2006). Interstitial muscle BKN and KAL have been suggested as algesic kinins involved in muscle pain. BKN was the first inflammatory mediator recognized to have potent hyperalgesic properties (Levine & Reichling, 1999). BKN induces pain and modifies the receptive fields of dorsal horn neurons to noxious stimuli in humans when administered in different ways (Boix et al., 2005; Meyer et al., 2006). BKN and cytokines are central factors in the link between tissue damage and inflammatory responses (Coutaux et al., 2005). Moreover, BKN is a potent vasodilatator and is increased in the interstitium of muscle during exercise (Clifford & Hellsten, 2004; Schmelz et al., 2003; Stewart & Rittweger, 2006). Animal studies have shown that BKN can both excite (i.e., algogenic) and sensitize nociceptors (Levine & Reichling, 1999; Wang et al., 2006). The present review identified four studies investigating the interstitial concentrations of BKN and/or Kallidin (Gerdle et al., 2008b; Larsson et al., 2008; Shah et al., 2008; Shah et al., 2005). The relatively small studies conducted by Shah et al. (Shah et al., 2008; Shah et al., 2005) clearly indicated that BKN was involved since increased levels of BKN in subjects with active trigger points and the levels were higher in the trapezius (with pain) than in a pain-free distant muscle. In contrast no significant differences in BKN were found between patients and controls in a field study and a laboratory study, (Gerdle et al., 2008b; Larsson et al., 2008) The difference in results between the above mentioned studies could be due to the fact that alterations in BKN might be very localized (i.e., in the trigger points) and not generally found in the aching trapezius muscle. KAL was only investigated in one study and increased in chronic trapezius myalgia but not in the trapezius of chronic WAD compared to controls (Gerdle et al., 2008b). Clearly, more pathophysiological *in vivo* studies are necessary in order to understand the roles of BKN and KAL for nociception and pain in patients with chronic pain.

4.2.4 Potassium

Increased interstitial potassium levels may be related to muscle pain (Graven-Nielsen et al., 1997). Green et al., however, did not find potassium related to acute ischaemic myalgia in healthy subjects (Green et al., 2000). Repetitive work in healthy subjects may increase potassium levels (Rosendal et al., 2004a), although in the present systematic review no consistent pattern of increased potassium was found in patients with chronic trapezius myalgia (Larsson et al., 2008; Rosendal et al., 2005; Sjogaard et al., 2010) (**Table 1**) or with chronic WAD (**Table 2**).

4.2.5 Cytokines

There are several direct and indirect pathways that link cytokines with nociception or hyperalgesia (Coutaux et al., 2005; Sommer & Kress, 2004; Uceyler et al., 2009). Four studies investigated cytokines in chronic trapezius myalgia, but significant differences were only found for active trigger points (Shah et al., 2008; Shah et al., 2005). These studies, however, used very few subjects, an obvious limitation. Larger studies have not found elevated levels of cytokines (Larsson et al., 2008; Rosendal et al., 2005). On the other hand, these studies might have had some technical problems due to the catheters used, also a limitation. However, the chronic WAD study found increased IL-6 (Gerdle et al., 2008c).

4.3 Anti-analgesic substances

As is obvious from the above, most studies concern metabolites and algesic substances. Little is known about changes in the pain-inhibitory signalling molecules. One interesting group of such molecules is the *N*-acylethanolamines (NAEs), which is a family of endogenous lipid mediators that have several roles including the regulation of inflammation and pain (Pacher et al., 2006). Examples of NAEs are *N*-palmitoylethanolamine (PEA), N-stearoylethanolamine (SEA), N-oleoylethanolamine (OEA), and N-arachidonoylethanolamine (anandamide, AEA). The most thoroughly studied of the NAEs is AEA, which interacts with cannabinoid receptors. At higher concentrations, AEA also targets transient receptor potential (vanilloid-1) receptors and has been shown to have anti-nociceptive actions in a number of animal models of pain (Calignano et al., 1998). The present review also includes one study of SEA and PEA (Ghafouri et al., 2011), which reported significantly increased levels of two NAEs.

4.4 Other pain conditions identified

According to our review, microdialysis of painful muscles have also been investigated, but these studies have only been based on one group of patients of each condition: polymyalgia rheumatic, chronic tension-type headache, and mitochondrial myopathy. Hence no definite conclusions concerning potential biomarkers can be drawn for these conditions. The results concerning polymyalgia rheumatic were prominent for several algesics including cytokines. Kreiner et al. investigated the presence of muscle alterations (Kreiner & Galbo, 2011; Kreiner et al., 2010), and they found that the biochemical alterations were normalized after treatment with prednisolone. Although more studies are needed, their results suggest that intramuscular mechanisms are important.

In the studies of different chronic tendinosis, the number of patients was low and no consistent patterns were seen. Larger studies are needed to identify biochemical alterations.

4.5 Suggestions with respect to future studies

The fact that most studies of chronic trapezius myalgia, chronic WAD, and temporomandibular pain disorders included women is expected, as the prevalence of these conditions are higher in women. Future studies should also include groups of men with chronic muscle pain conditions. In addition, it is important to describe the patient group in detail with respect to clinically relevant examination parameters. Furthermore, systematic descriptions of the patient groups are needed that reflect pain intensity and psychological distress as well as consequences such as work participation and sick leave. A systematic description will allow a more accurate characterization of pain severity in a broad context. Most studies rely on bivariate correlations between pain descriptors such as pain intensity or pressure pain thresholds and the concentration of a certain substance. Multivariate correlation analyses and regression analyses are methods that can be used to investigate how groups of clinical examination variables, several simultaneous symptoms, and the concentrations of several biochemical substances intercorrelate. To better understand the potentially complex biochemical situation of the muscle in chronic pain conditions, it is necessary to also investigate the multivariate interrelationships between the concentrations of the investigated substances. According to ICD, the clinically used pain diagnoses are symptom diagnoses based on temporal and anatomical characteristics (e.g., chronic lumbago). Hence a certain diagnosis may include patients with different activated pathophysiological mechanisms. To identify subgroups of patients with identical pathophysiological mechanisms, it is important to use large patient groups and appropriate statistical methods (e.g., cluster analysis and principal component analysis).

5. Conclusion

This systematic review found that most of the studies focused on trapezius myalgia (seven patient groups reported in ten studies), temporomandibular pain syndromes (two patient groups reported in three studies), and fibromyalgia (two patient groups but different muscles). Relatively strong scientific support identifies 5-HT as a potential biomarker in chronic myalgia. Moderately strong scientific support identifies glutamate, pyruvate, and lactate as potential biomarkers in chronic trapezius myalgia. There is a need for larger studies of well-characterized patient groups with respect to perceived situations, symptoms, and signs so as to investigate several substances simultaneously in order to improve the understanding of peripheral nociceptive processes in myalgia.

6. Acknowledgements

There are no conflicts of interest. No financial or personal relationships have inappropriately influenced this work. This study was supported by the Swedish Council for Working Life and Social Research (2010-0683, 2007-0760) and the Swedish Research Council (2010-2893). The funders had no role in study design, data collection and analysis, decision to publish, or preparation of the manuscript.

7. References

Afinowi, R., Tisdall, M., Keir, G., Smith, M., Kitchen, N., & Petzold, A. (2009). Improving the recovery of S100B protein in cerebral microdialysis: implications for multimodal monitoring in neurocritical care. *Journal of neuroscience methods*, 181, pp. 95-99.

Agarwal, N., Pacher, P., Tegeder, I., Amaya, F., Constantin, CE., Brenner, GJ., Rubino, T., Michalski, CW., Marsicano, G., Monory, K., Mackie, K., Marian, C., Batkai, S., Parolaro, D., Fischer, MJ., Reeh, P., Kunos, G., Kress, M., Lutz, B., Woolf, CJ., & Kuner, R. (2007). Cannabinoids mediate analgesia largely via peripheral type 1 cannabinoid receptors in nociceptors. *Nat Neurosci*, 10, pp. 870-879.

Alfredson, H. (2005). The chronic painful Achilles and patellar tendon: research on basic biology and treatment. *Scandinavian journal of medicine & science in sports*, 15, pp. 252-259.

Alfredson, H., Forsgren, S., Thorsen, K., & Lorentzon, R. (2001). In vivo microdialysis and immunohistochemical analyses of tendon tissue demonstrated high amounts of free glutamate and glutamate NMDAR1 receptors, but no signs of inflammation, in Jumper's knee. *J Orthop Res*, 19, pp. 881-886.

Alfredson, H., Ljung, BO., Thorsen, K., & Lorentzon, R. (2000). In vivo investigation of ECRB tendons with microdialysis technique--no signs of inflammation but high amounts of glutamate in tennis elbow. *Acta Orthop Scand*, 71, pp. 475-479.

Alonso, J., Angermeyer, MC., Bernert, S., Bruffaerts, R., Brugha, TS., Bryson, H., de Girolamo, G., Graaf, R., Demyttenaere, K., Gasquet, I., Haro, JM., Katz, SJ., Kessler, RC., Kovess, V., Lepine, JP., Ormel, J., Polidori, G., Russo, LJ., Vilagut, G., Almansa, J., Arbabzadeh-Bouchez, S., Autonell, J., Bernal, M., Buist-Bouwman, MA., Codony, M., Domingo-Salvany, A., Ferrer, M., Joo, SS., Martinez-Alonso, M., Matschinger, H., Mazzi, F., Morgan, Z., Morosini, P., Palacin, C., Romera, B., Taub, N., & Vollebergh, WA. (2004). 12-Month comorbidity patterns and associated factors in Europe: results from the European Study of the Epidemiology of Mental Disorders (ESEMeD) project. *Acta Psychiatr Scand Suppl*, pp. 28-37.

Apkarian, AV. (2008). Pain perception in relation to emotional learning. *Curr Opin Neurobiol*, 18, pp. 464-468.

Arendt-Nielsen, L., & Graven-Nielsen, T. (2003). Central sensitization in fibromyalgia and other musculoskeletal disorders. *Current Pain and Headache Reports*, 7, pp. 355-361.

Ashina, M., Stallknecht, B., Bendtsen, L., Pedersen, JF., Galbo, H., Dalgaard, P., & Olesen, J. (2002). In vivo evidence of altered skeletal muscle blood flow in chronic tension-type headache. *Brain*, 125, pp. 320-326.

Ashina, M., Stallknecht, B., Bendtsen, L., Pedersen, JF., Schifter, S., Galbo, H., & Olesen, J. (2003). Tender points are not sites of ongoing inflammation -in vivo evidence in patients with chronic tension-type headache. *Cephalalgia*, 23, pp. 109-116.

Asmundson, GJG., & Katz, J. (2009). Understanding the co-occurrence of anxiety disorders and chronic pain: state-of-the-art. *Depress Anxiety*, 26, pp. 888-901.

Axelson, HW., Melberg, A., Ronquist, G., & Askmark, H. (2002). Microdialysis and electromyography of experimental muscle fatigue in healthy volunteers and patients with mitochondrial myopathy. *Muscle Nerve*, 26, pp. 520-526.

Baliki, M., Schnitzer, T., Bauer, W., & Apkarian, A. (2011). Brain morphological Signatures for chronic Pain. *PLoS One*, 6, pp. e26010.

Bengtsson, A. (2002). Editorial, The muscle in fibromyalgia. *Rheumatol* 41, pp. 721-724.

Bengtsson, A., Henriksson, KG., & Larsson, J. (1986). Muscle biopsy in primary fibromyalgia. Light-microscopical and histochemical findings. *Scand J Rheumatol*, 15, pp. 1-6.

Bernard, BP. Musculosceletal disorders and workplace factors. In: A critical review of epidemiological evidence for work-related musculosceletal disorders of the neck, upper extremity, and low back.NIOSH: DHHS; 1997.

Boix, F., Roe, C., Rosenborg, L., & Knardahl, S. (2005). Kinin peptides in human trapezius muscle during sustained isometric contraction and their relation to pain. *Journal of applied physiology*, 98, pp. 534-540.

Breivik, H., Collett, B., Ventafridda, V., Cohen, R., & Gallacher, D. (2006). Survey of chronic pain in Europe: prevalence, impact on daily life, and treatment. *Eur J Pain*, 10, pp. 287-333.

Börsbo, B., Peolsson, M., & Gerdle, B. (2008). Catastrophizing, depression, and pain: Correlation with and influence on quality of life and health - A study of chronic whiplash-associated disorders. *J Rehabil Med*, 40, pp. 562-569.

Cairns, BE., & Dong, X. (2008). The role of peripheral glutamate and glutamate receptors in muscle pain. *J Musculoskelet Pain*, 16, pp. 85-91.

Cairns, BE., Hu, JW., Arendt-Nielsen, L., Sessle, BJ., & Svensson, P. (2001a). Sex-related differences in human pain and rat afferent discharge evoked by injection of glutamate into the masseter muscle. *J Neurophysiol*, 86, pp. 782-789.

Cairns, BE., Sessle, BJ., & Hu, JW. (2001b). Characteristics of glutamate-evoked temporomandibular joint afferent activity in the rat. *J Neurophysiol*, 85, pp. 2446-2445.

Cairns, BE., Wang, K., Hu, JW., Sessle, BJ., Arendt-Nielsen, L., & Svensson, P. (2003). The effect of glutamate-evoked masseter muscle pain on the human jaw-stretch reflex differs in men and women. *Journal of orofacial pain*, 17, pp. 317-325.

Calignano, A., La Rana, G., Giuffrida, A., & Piomelli, D. (1998). Control of pain initiation by endogenous cannabinoids. *Nature* 394, pp. 277-281.

Calixto, JB., Medeiros, R., Fernandes, ES., Ferreira, J., Cabrini, DA., & Campos, MM. (2004). Kinin B1 receptors: key G-protein-coupled receptors and their role in inflammatory and painful processes. *Br J Pharmacol*, 143, pp. 803-818.

Carlton, SM. (2001). Peripheral excitatory amino acids. *Curr Opin Pharmacol*, 1, pp. 52-56.

Castrillon, EE., Ernberg, M., Cairns, BE., Wang, K., Sessle, BJ., Arendt-Nielsen, L., & Svensson, P. (2010). Interstitial glutamate concentration is elevated in the masseter muscle of myofascial temporomandibular disorder patients. *J Orofac Pain*, 24, pp. 350-360.

Clifford, PS., & Hellsten, Y. (2004). Vasodilatory mechanisms in contracting skeletal muscle. *J Appl Physiol*, 97, pp. 393-403.

Coggeshall, RE., & Carlton, SM. (1997). Receptor localization in the mammalian dorsal horn and primary afferent neurons. *Brain research Brain research reviews*, 24, pp. 28-66.

Coggeshall, RE., & Carlton, SM. (1998). Ultrastructural analysis of NMDA, AMPA, and kainate receptors on unmyelinated and myelinated axons in the periphery. *J Comp Neurol*, 391, pp. 78-86.

Coutaux, A., Adam, F., Willer, JC., & Le Bars, D. (2005). Hyperalgesia and allodynia: peripheral mechanisms. *Joint Bone Spine*, 72, pp. 359-371.

Couture, R., Harrisson, M., Vianna, RM., & Cloutier, F. (2001). Kinin receptors in pain and inflammation. *Eur J Pharmacol*, 429, pp. 161-176.

Dahlin, A., Wetterhall, M., Caldwell, K., Larsson, A., Bergquist, J., Hillered, L., & Hjort, K. (2010). Methodological aspects on microdialysis protein sampling and quantification in biological fluids: an in vitro study on human ventricular CSF. *Anal Chem*, 82, pp. 4376-4385.

Dersh, J., Gatchel, RJ., & Polatin, P. (2001). Chronic spinal disorders and psychopathology: research findings and theoretical considerations. *The Spine Journal*, 1, pp. 88-94.

Ericsson, M., Poston, W., Linder, J., Taylor, J., Haddock, C., & Foreyt, J. (2002). Depression predicts disability in long-term chronic pain patients. *Disabil Rehabil*, 24, pp. 334-340.

Ernberg, M. Serotonergic Receptor involvement in Muscle pain and hyperalgesia. In: Fundamentals of Musculoskeltal Pain. 1th. Seattle: IASP Press; 2008; 139-153.

Ernberg, M., Hedenberg-Magnusson, B., Alstergren, P., & Kopp, S. (1999). The level of serotonin in the superficial masseter muscle in relation to local pain and allodynia. *Life sciences*, 65, pp. 313-325.

Ernberg, M., Hedenberg-Magnusson, B., Kurita, H., & Kopp, S. (2006). Effects of local serotonin administration on pain and microcirculation in the human masseter muscle. *J Orofac Pain*, 20, pp. 241-248.

Flodgren, GM., Crenshaw, AG., Alfredson, H., Fahlstrom, M., Hellstrom, FB., Bronemo, L., & Djupsjobacka, M. (2005). Glutamate and prostaglandin E2 in the trapezius muscle of female subjects with chronic muscle pain and controls determined by microdialysis. *European journal of pain*, 9, pp. 511-515.

Flodgren, GM., Crenshaw, AG., Hellstrom, F., & Fahlstrom, M. (2010). Combining microdialysis and near-infrared spectroscopy for studying effects of low-load repetitive work on the intramuscular chemistry in trapezius myalgia. *J Biomed Biotechnol*, 2010, pp. 513803.

Flodgren, GM., Hellstrom, FB., Fahlstrom, M., & Crenshaw, AG. (2006). Effects of 30 versus 60 min of low-load work on intramuscular lactate, pyruvate, glutamate, prostaglandin E(2) and oxygenation in the trapezius muscle of healthy females. *European journal of applied physiology*, 97, pp. 557-565.

Gatchel, R., Peng, Y., Peters, M., Fuchs, P., & Turk, D. (2007). The biopsychosocial approach to chronic pain: scientific advances and future directions. *Psychol Bull*, 133, pp. 581-624.

Gazerani, P., Wang, K., Cairns, BE., Svensson, P., & Arendt-Nielsen, L. (2006). Effects of subcutaneous administration of glutamate on pain, sensitization and vasomotor responses in healthy men and women. *Pain*, 124, pp. 338-348.

Gerdle, B., Bjork, J., Coster, L., Henriksson, KG., Henriksson, C., & Bengtsson, A. (2008a). Prevalence of widespread pain and associations with work status: a population study. *Bmc Musculoskeletal Disorders*, 9, pp.

Gerdle, B., Bjork, J., Henriksson, C., & Bengtsson, A. (2004). Prevalence of current and chronic pain and their influences upon work and healthcare-seeking: A population study. *Journal of Rheumatology*, 31, pp. 1399-1406.

Gerdle, B., Hilgenfeldt, U., Larsson, B., Kristiansen, J., Sogaard, K., & Rosendal, L. (2008b). Bradykinin and kallidin levels in the trapezius muscle in patients with work-related trapezius myalgia, in patients with whiplash associated pain, and in healthy controls - A microdialysis study of women. *Pain*, 139, pp. 578-587.

Gerdle, B., Lemming, D., Kristiansen, J., Larsson, B., Peolsson, M., & Rosendal, L. (2008c). Biochemical alterations in the trapezius muscle of patients with chronic whiplash associated disorders (WAD) - A microdialysis study. *European Journal of Pain*, 12, pp. 82-93.

Gerdle, B., Soderberg, K., Salvador Puigvert, L., Rosendal, L., & Larsson, B. (2010). Increased interstitial concentrations of pyruvate and lactate in the trapezius muscle of patients with fibromyalgia: a microdialysis study. *J Rehabil Med*, 42, pp. 679-687.

Ghafouri, B., Larsson, BK., Sjors, A., Leandersson, P., & Gerdle, BU. (2010). Interstitial concentration of serotonin is increased in myalgic human trapezius muscle during rest, repetitive work and mental stress - an in vivo microdialysis study. *Scand J Clin Lab Invest*, 70, pp. 478-486.

Ghafouri, N., Ghafouri, B., Larsson, B., Turkina, M., Karlsson, L., Fowler, C., & Gerdle, B. (2011). High levels of N-palmitoylethanolamide and N-stearoylethanolamide in microdialysate samples from myalgic trapezius muscle in women. *PLOS One*, 6 (11), pp e27257; doi:10.1371/journal.pone.0027257.

Giordano, J., & Rogers, LV. (1989). Peripherally administered serotonin 5-HT3 receptor antagonists reduce inflammatory pain in rats. *European journal of pharmacology*, 170, pp. 83-86.

Gladden, LB. (2004). Lactate metabolism: a new paradigm for the third millenium. *J Physiol (Lond)*, 558, pp. 5-30.

Grachev, ID., Fredrickson, BE., & Apkarian, AV. (2000). Abnormal brain chemistry in chronic back pain: an in vivo proton magnetic resonance spectroscopy study. *Pain*, 89, pp. 7-18.

Graven-Nielsen, T., McArdle, A., Phoenix, J., Arendt-Nielsen, L., Jensen, TS., Jackson, MJ., & Edwards, RH. (1997). In vivo model of muscle pain: quantification of intramuscular chemical, electrical, and pressure changes associated with saline-induced muscle pain in humans. *Pain*, 69, pp. 137-143.

Graven-Nielsen, T., & Mense, S. (2001). The peripheral apparatus of muscle pain: evidence from animal and human studies. *Clin J Pain*, 17, pp. 2-10.

Green, S., Langberg, H., Skovgaard, D., Bulow, J., & Kjaer, M. (2000). Interstitial and arterial-venous [K+] in human calf muscle during dynamic exercise: effect of ischaemia and relation to muscle pain. *The Journal of physiology*, 529 Pt 3, pp. 849-861.

Guez, M., Hildingsson, C., Nilsson, M., Toolanen, G., & Aug;():. (2002). The prevalence of neck pain: a population-based study from northern Sweden. *Acta Orthop Scand*, 73, pp. 455-459.

Hamrin, K., Rosdah, lH., Ungerstedt, U., & Henriksson, J. (2002). Microdialysis in human skeletal muscle: effects of adding a colloid to the perfusate. *J Appl Physiol*, 92, pp. 385-393.

Hedenberg-Magnusson, B., Ernberg, M., Alstergren, P., & Kopp, S. (2001). Pain mediation by prostaglandin E2 and leukotriene B4 in the human masseter muscle. *Acta odontologica Scandinavica*, 59, pp. 348-355.

Heinricher, MM., Tavares, I., Leith, JL., & Lumb, BM. (2009). Descending control of nociception: Specificity, recruitment and plasticity. *Brain Res Rev*, 60, pp. 214-225.

Helmy, A., Carpenter, KL., Skepper, JN., Kirkpatrick, PJ., Pickard, JD., & Hutchinson, PJ. (2009). Microdialysis of cytokines: methodological considerations, scanning electron microscopy, and determination of relative recovery. *J Neurotrauma*, 26, pp. 549-561.

Hudspith, MJ. (1997). Glutamate: a role in normal brain function, anaesthesia, analgesia and CNS injury. *Br J Anaesth*, 78, pp. 731-747.

Hunt, SP., & Mantyh, PW. Understanding the neurobiology of chronic pain: molecular and cellular biology. In: Pain 2002- An updated Review: Refresher Course Syllabus.Seattle: IASP Press; 2002; 237-247.

Iannetti, GD., & Mouraux, A. (2010). From the neuromatrix to the pain matrix (and back). *Exp Brain Res*, 205, pp. 1-12.

Julien, N., Goffaux, P., Arsenault, P., & Marchand, S. (2005). Widespread pain in fibromyalgia is related to a deficit of endogenous pain inhibition. *Pain*, 114, pp. 295-302.

Kim, TJ., Freml, L., Park, SS., & Brennan, TJ. (2007). Lactate concentrations in incisions indicate ischemic-like conditions may contribute to postoperative pain. *J Pain*, 8, pp. 59-66.

Kreiner, F., & Galbo, H. (2011). Elevated muscle interstitial levels of pain-inducing substances in symptomatic muscles in patients with polymyalgia rheumatica. *Pain*, 152, pp. 1127-1132.

Kreiner, F., Langberg, H., & Galbo, H. (2010). Increased muscle interstitial levels of inflammatory cytokines in polymyalgia rheumatica. *Arthritis Rheum*, 62, pp. 3768-3775.

Kuner, R. (2010). Central mechanisms of pathological pain. *Nat Med*, 16, pp. 1258-1266.

Langley, CK., Aziz, Q., Bountra, C., Gordon, N., Hawkins, P., Jones, A., Langley, G., Nurmikko, T., & Tracey, I. (2008). Volunteer studies in pain research--opportunities and challenges to replace animal experiments: the report and recommendations of a Focus on Alternatives workshop. *Neuroimage*, 42, pp. 467-473.

Larsson, B., Bjork, J., Henriksson, KG., Gerdle, B., & Lindman, R. (2000). The prevalences of cytochrome c oxidase negative and superpositive fibres and ragged-red fibres in the trapezius muscle of female cleaners with and without myalgia and of female healthy controls. *Pain*, 84, pp. 379-387.

Larsson, B., Bjork, J., Kadi, F., Lindman, R., & Gerdle, B. (2004). Blood supply and oxidative metabolism in muscle biopsies of female cleaners with and without myalgia. *Clin J Pain*, 20, pp. 440-446.

Larsson, B., Björk, J., Börsbo, B., & Gerdle, B. (in press). A systematic review of risk factors associated with transitioning from regional musculoskeletal pain to chronic widespread pain. *Eur J Pain*, pp.

Larsson, B., Rosendal, L., Kristiansen, J., Sjogaard, G., Sogaard, K., Ghafouri, B., Abdiu, A., Kjaer, M., & Gerdle, B. (2008). Responses of algesic and metabolic substances to 8 h of repetitive manual work in myalgic human trapezius muscle. *Pain*, 140, pp. 479-490.

Larsson, B., Sogaard, K., & Rosendal, L. (2007). Work related neck-shoulder pain: a review on magnitude, risk factors, biochemical characteristics, clinical picture and preventive interventions. *Best Pract Res Clin Rheumatol*, 21, pp. 447-463.

Lascelles, B., & Flecknell, P. (2010). Do animal models tell us about human pain? *Pain Clinical Updates*, 18, pp. 1-6.

Lee, MC., & Tracey, I. (2010). Unravelling the mystery of pain, suffering, and relief with brain imaging. *Curr Pain Headache Rep*, 14, pp. 124-131.

Legrain, V., Iannetti, GD., Plaghki, L., & Mouraux, A. (2011). The pain matrix reloaded: a salience detection system for the body. *Prog Neurobiol*, 93, pp. 111-124.

Levine, JD., & Reichling, DB. Peripheral mechanisms of inflammatory pain. In: Textbook of Pain, 4th ed.Edinburgh: Churchill Livingstone; 1999; 59-84.

Lidgren, L. (2008). Preface: Neck pain and the decade of the Bone and Joint 2000-2010. *Spine*, 33, pp. S1-S2.

Lindh, M., Johansson, G., Hedberg, M., Henning, GB., & Grimby, G. (1995). Muscle fiber characteristics, capillaries and enzymes in patients with fibromyalgia and controls. *Scand J Rheumatol*, 24, pp. 34-37.

Linley, JE., Rose, K., Ooi, L., & Gamper, N. (2010). Understanding inflammatory pain: ion channels contributing to acute and chronic nociception. *Pflugers Arch*, 459, pp. 657-669.

McIver, KL., Evans, C., Kraus, RM., Ispas, L., Sciotti, VM., & Hickner, RC. (2006). NO-mediated alterations in skeletal muscle nutritive blood flow and lactate metabolism in fibromyalgia. *Pain*, 120, pp. 161-169.

McMahon, SB., Bennett, DLH., & Bevan, S. Inflammatory mediators and modulators of pain. In: Texbook of Pain, 5th ed. Elsevier; 2006; 49-72.

Means-Christensen, AJ., Roy-Byrne, PP., Sherbourne, CD., Craske, MG., & Stein, MB. (2008). Relationships among pain, anxiety, and depression in primary care. *Depression & Anxiety (1091-4269)*, 25, pp. 593-600.

Mense, S. (1993). Nociception from skeletal muscle in relation to clinical muscle pain. *Pain*, 54, pp. 241-289.

Mense, S. (2003). The pathogenesis of muscle pain. *Current pain and headache reports*, 7, pp. 419-425.

Mense, S. (2009). Algesic agents exciting muscle nociceptors. *Exp Brain Res*, 196, pp. 89-100.

Meyer, RA., Ringkamp, M., Campbell, JN., & Raja, SN. Peripheral mechanisms of cutaneous nociception. In: Textbook of Pain , 5th ed. Elsevier; 2006; 3-34.

Miller, KE., Hoffman, EM., Sutharshan, M., & Schechter, R. (2011). Glutamate pharmacology and metabolism in peripheral primary afferents: physiological and pathophysiological mechanisms. *Pharmacol Ther*, 130, pp. 283-309.

Momin, A., & McNaughton, PA. (2009). Regulation of firing frequency in nociceptive neurons by pro-inflammatory mediators. *Exp Brain Res*, 196, pp. 45-52.

Norrbom, J.Exercise and Regulation of Mithochondrial Biogenesis Factors in Human Skeletal Muscle. Stockholm: Karolinska Institute; 2008; 61.

Ocañez, KLS., Kathryn McHugh, R., & Otto, MW. (2010). A meta-analytic review of the association between anxiety sensitivity and pain. *Depression and Anxiety*, 27, pp. 760-767.

Ossipov, MH., Dussor, GO., & Porreca, F. (2010). Central modulation of pain. *J Clin Invest*, 120, pp. 3779-3787.

Pace, MC., Mazzariello, L., Passavanti, MB., Sansone, P., Barbarisi, M., & Aurilio, C. (2006). Neurobiology of pain. *J Cell Physiol*, 209, pp. 8-12.

Pacher, P., Batkai, S., & Kunos, G. (2006). The endocannabinoid system as an emerging target of pharmacotherapy. *Pharmacol Rev*, 58, pp. 389-462.

Petersen-Felix, S., & Curatolo, M. (2002). Neuroplasticity--an important factor in acute and chronic pain. *Swiss Med Wkly*, 132, pp. 273-278.

Philip, A., Macdonald, AL., & Watt, PW. (2005). Lactate - a signal coordnating cell and systemic function. . *Exp Biol*, 208, pp. 4561-4575.

Phillips, CJ. (2006). Economic burden of chronic pain. *Expert Rev Pharmacoecon Outcomes Res*, 6, pp. 591-601.

Plock, N., & Kloft, C. (2005). Microdialysis--theoretical background and recent implementation in applied life-sciences. *Eur J Pharm Sci*, 25, pp. 1-24.

Porreca, F., Ossipov, MH., & Gebhart, GF. (2002). Chronic pain and medullary descending facilitation. *Trends Neurosci*, 25, pp. 319-325.

Ptolemy, AS., & Rifai, N. (2010). What is a biomarker? Research investments and lack of clinical integration necessitate a review of biomarker terminology and validation schema. *Scand J Clin Lab Invest Suppl*, 242, pp. 6-14.

Punnett, L., & Wegman, DH. (2004). Work-related musculoskeletal disorders: the epidemiologic evidence and the debate. *J Electromyogr Kinesiol*, 14, pp. 13-23.

Reichling, DB., & Levine, JD. (2009). Critical role of nociceptor plasticity in chronic pain. *Trends Neurosci*, 32, pp. 611-618.

Ren, K., & Dubner, R. (2002). Descending modulation in persistent pain: an update. *Pain*, 100, pp. 1-6.

Richardson, JD., Kilo, S., & Hargreaves, KM. (1998). Cannabinoids reduce hyperalgesia and inflammation via interaction with peripheral CB1 receptors. *Pain*, 75, pp. 111-119.

Riedel, W., & Neeck, G. (2001). Nociception, pain, and antinociception: current concepts. *Z Rheumatol*, 60, pp. 404-415.

Robergs, RA., Ghiasvand, F., & Parker, D. (2004). Biochemistry of exercise-induced metabolic acidosis. *American Journal of Physiology Regulatory, Integrative and Comparative Physiology*, 287, pp. R502-R516.

Robinson, DA., & Zhuo, M. (2002). Genetic analysis of pain mechanisms. *Crit Rev Eukaryot Gene Expr*, 12, pp. 275-295.

Rosendal, L., Blangsted, AK., Kristiansen, J., Sogaard, K., Langberg, H., Sjogaard, G., & Kjaer, M. (2004a). Interstitial muscle lactate, pyruvate and potassium dynamics in the trapezius muscle during repetitive low-force arm movements, measured with microdialysis. *Acta physiologica Scandinavica*, 182, pp. 379-388.

Rosendal, L., Kristiansen, J., Gerdle, B., Sogaard, K., Peolsson, M., Kjaer, M., Sorensen, J., & Larsson, B. (2005). Increased levels of interstitial potassium but normal levels of muscle IL-6 and LDH in patients with trapezius myalgia. *Pain*, 119, pp. 201-209.

Rosendal, L., Larsson, B., Kristiansen, J., Peolsson, M., Sogaard, K., Kjaer, M., Sorensen, J., & Gerdle, B. (2004b). Increase in muscle nociceptive substances and anaerobic metabolism in patients with trapezius myalgia: microdialysis in rest and during exercise. *Pain*, 112, pp. 324-334.

Saria, A., Javorsky, F., Humpel, C., & Gamset, R. (1990). 5-HT3, receptor antagonists inhibit sensory neuropeptide release from the rat spinal cord. *Neuroreport*, 1, pp. 104-106.

SBU. Metoder för behandling av långvarig smärta. En systematisk litteraturöversikt. Stockholm: Statens beredning för medicinsk utvärdering. 2006.

Schaible, HG., Richter, F., Ebersberger, A., Boettger, MK., Vanegas, H., Natura, G., Vazquez, E., & Segond von Banchet, G. (2009). Joint pain. *Exp Brain Res*, 196, pp. 153-162.

Schmelz, M., Schmidt, R., Weidner, C., Hilliges, M., Torebjork, HE., & Handwerker, HO. (2003). Chemical response pattern of different classes of C-nociceptors to pruritogens and algogens. *J Neurophysiol*, 89, pp. 2441-2448.

Schmidt-Wilcke, T. (2008). Variations in brain volume and regional morphology associated with chronic pain. *Curr Rheumatol Rep*, 10, pp. 467-474.

Schneider, GM., Smith, AD., Hooper, A., Stratford, P., Schneider, KJ., Westaway, MD., Frizzell, B., & Olson, L. (2010). Minimizing the source of nociception and its concurrent effect on sensory hypersensitivity: An exploratory study in chronic whiplash patients. *BMC Musculoskelet Disord*, 11, pp. 29.

Schweinhardt, P., & Bushnell, MC. (2010). Pain imaging in health and disease--how far have we come? *J Clin Invest*, 120, pp. 3788-3797.

Shah, JP., Danoff, JV., Desai, MJ., Parikh, S., Nakamura, LY., Phillips, TM., & Gerber, LH. (2008). Biochemicals associated with pain and inflammation are elevated in sites near to and remote from active myofascial trigger points. *Arch Phys Med Rehabil*, 89, pp. 16-23.

Shah, JP., Phillips, TM., Danoff, JV., & Gerber, LH. (2005). An in vivo microanalytical technique for measuring the local biochemical milieu of human skeletal muscle. *Journal of applied physiology*, 99, pp. 1977-1984.

Sjogaard, G., Rosendal, L., Kristiansen, J., Blangsted, AK., Skotte, J., Larsson, B., Gerdle, B., Saltin, B., & Sogaard, K. (2010). Muscle oxygenation and glycolysis in females with trapezius myalgia during stress and repetitive work using microdialysis and NIRS. *Eur J Appl Physiol*, 108, pp. 657-669.

Sofat, N., Ejindu, V., & Kiely, P. (2011). What makes osteoarthritis painful? The evidence for local and central pain processing. *Rheumatology (Oxford)*, pp.

Sommer, C. (2004). Serotonin in pain and analgesia. *Mol Neurobiol*, 30, pp. 117-125.

Sommer, C. (2006). Is serotonin hyperalgesic or analgesic? *Curr Pain Headache Rep*, 10, pp. 101-106.

Sommer, C., & Kress, M. (2004). Recent findings on how proinflammatory cytokines cause pain: peripheral mechanisms in inflammatory and neuropathic hyperalgesia. *Neuroscience Letters*, 361, pp. 184-187.

Staud, R. (2010). Is it all central sensitization? Role of peripheral tissue nociception in chronic musculoskeletal pain. *Curr Rheumatol Rep*, 12, pp. 448-454.

Staud, R., Nagel, S., Robinson, ME., & Price, DD. (2009). Enhanced central pain processing of fibromyalgia patients is maintained by muscle afferent input: a randomized, double-blind, placebo-controlled study. *Pain*, 145, pp. 96-104.

Stewart, CE., & Rittweger, J. (2006). Adaptive processes in skeletal muscle: molecular regulators and genetic influences. *J Musculoskelet Neuronal Interact*, 6, pp. 73-86.

Sullivan, M., Thorn, B., Haythornthwaite, J., Keefe, FJ., Martin, M., Bradley, L., & Lefebvre, J. (2001). Theoretical perspectives on the relation between catastrophizing and pain. *Clin J Pain*, 17, pp. 52-64.

Suzuki, R., Rygh, LJ., & Dickenson, AH. (2004). Bad news from the brain: descending 5-HT pathways that control spinal pain processing. *Trends Pharmacol Sci*, 25, pp. 613-617.

Svensson, P., Cairns, BE., Wang, K., Hu, JW., Graven-Nielsen, T., Arendt-Nielsen, L., & Sessle, BJ. (2003). Glutamate-evoked pain and mechanical allodynia in the human masseter muscle. *Pain*, 101, pp. 221-227.

Svensson, P., Wang, K., Arendt-Nielsen, L., Cairns, BE., & Sessle, BJ. (2005). Pain effects of glutamate injections into human jaw or neck muscles. *J Orofac Pain*, 19, pp. 109-118.

Taiwo, YO., & Levine, JD. (1992). Serotonin is a directly-acting hyperalgesic agent in the rat. *Neuroscience*, 48, pp. 485-490.

Tegeder, L., Zimmermann, J., Meller, S., & Geisslinger, G. (2002). Release of algesic substances in human experimental muscle pain. *Inflamm Res*, 51, pp. 393-402.

Uceyler, N., Schafers, M., & Sommer, C. (2009). Mode of action of cytokines on nociceptive neurons. *Exp Brain Res*, 196, pp. 67-78.

Ungerstedt, U. (1991). Microdialysis--principles and applications for studies in animals and man. *Journal of internal medicine*, 230, pp. 365-373.

Waelgaard, L., Pharo, A., Tonnessen, TI., & Mollnes, TE. (2006). Microdialysis for monitoring inflammation: efficient recovery of cytokines and anaphylotoxins provided optimal catheter pore size and fluid velocity conditions. *Scand J Immunol*, 64, pp. 345-352.

Walker, JM., & Huang, SM. (2002). Endocannabinoids in pain modulation. *Prostaglandins Leukot Essent Fatty Acids*, 66, pp. 235-242.

Wallin, M., Liedberg, G., Börsbo, B., & Gerdle, B. (2011). Thermal detection and pain thresholds but not pressure pain thresholds are correlated with psychological factors in women with chronic whiplash associated pain. *Clin J Pain*, Jul 11. [Epub ahead of print], pp.

Wang, H., Ehnert, C., Brenner, GJ., & Woolf, CJ. (2006). Bradykinin and peripheral sensitization. *Biol Chem*, 387, pp. 11-14.

Varney, MA., & Gereau, RW. (2002). Metabotropic glutamate receptor involvement in models of acute and persistent pain: prospects for the development of novel analgesics. *Curr Drug Targets CNS Neurol Disord*, 1, pp. 283-296.

Weibel, ER., & Hoppeler, H. (2005). Exercise-induced maximal metabolic rate scales with muscle aerobic capacity. *J Exp Biol*, 208, pp. 1635-1644.

Wilder-Smith, OH., Tassonyi, E., & Arendt-Nielsen, L. (2002). Preoperative back pain is associated with diverse manifestations of central neuroplasticity. *Pain*, 97, pp. 189-194.

Woolf, CJ. (2011). Central sensitization: implications for the diagnosis and treatment of pain. *Pain*, 152, pp. S2-15.

Woolf, CJ., & Ma, Q. (2007). Nociceptors--noxious stimulus detectors. *Neuron*, 55, pp. 353-364.

Woolf, CJ., & Salter, MW. (2000). Neuronal Plasticity: increasing the gain in pain. *Science*, 288, pp. 1765-1768.

Zubakova, R., Gille, A., Faussner, A., & Hilgenfeldt, U. (2008). Ca2+ signalling of kinins in cells expressing rat, mouse, and human B1/b2 receptor. *Intern Immunopharmacology*, 8, pp. 276-281.

6

Inorganic Signatures of Physiology: The X-Ray Fluorescence Microscopy Revolution

Lydia Finney
Advanced Photon Source,
Argonne National Laboratory,
USA

1. Introduction

1.1 Metals as an essential, yet potentially toxic part of cellular chemistry

Metals are vital to nearly all the life processes within the cell. It is estimated that nearly a third of cellular proteins bind metals. Yet, the very same properties of these metal ions which make them so useful, also makes them potentially hazardous within the cell. Endogenous metals, such as copper, zinc, and iron are also potentially toxic, performing deleterious redox chemistry if not carefully controlled and regulated(Finney and O'Halloran 2003). The intricate cellular machinery that manages these metals are collectively known as the metal homeostasis and trafficking proteins of the cell. While we have learned much with respect to how the cell partitions and allocates metals, and at times attempted to define the 'concentration' in various compartments of the cell, instead we have begun to see how ill-defined a 'resting' condition really is, and how much the partitioning of cellular metals can change (Dodani, Leary et al. 2011; Qin, Dittmer et al. 2011).

What is it about metals which make them so critical, and so useful? Unlike other elements, biological metals, and particularly the first row of transition metals in the periodic table, have a partially filled d-shell of orbitals. This gives them multiple semi-stable oxidation states under ambient conditions. And the changes between these states provide reduction and oxidation potential for the chemistry of the cell (Bertini, Gray et al. 2007). For example, iron, as part of hemoglobin, shuffles between a (II) and (III) oxidation state to perform the vital act of delivering oxygen throughout the body. However, the same element, iron, if it were a 'free' aquo- ion in the cytoplasm of the cell would likely undergo Fenton chemistry, and these same changes in oxidation state would give rise to the generation of radicals that would damage the cell.

Still, biology manages, most of the time, to work. The efficient chemistry of these life processes often exceeds our own ability to accomplish their work synthetically. Unraveling the ways in which the chemistry of these metals is controlled promises not only to improve what we know about chemistry, accomplishing important reactions such as the oxidation of methane or the fixation of nitrogen in new and more efficient ways, but also to remarkably improve our understanding of biology, and our ability to manipulate it as well.

1.2 The location of metals, and bioavailability, within the cell regulates cell function

Metals serve roles in thousands of proteins and enzymes, and are found in various species throughout the mammalian cell. Good recent reviews of biological copper (Boal and Rosenzweig 2009; Banci, Bertini et al. 2010; Lutsenko 2010), iron (Kosman 2010), and zinc (Eide 2006; Tomat and Lippard 2010) exist. Our understanding of the location and bioavailability of metals, until rather recently, was mainly accessible by studying the properties of the proteins that bind them.

For example, one role of copper is as an important component of cytochrome c oxidase, which performs respiration in mitochondrion (Tsukihara, Aoyama et al. 1995; Tsukihara, Aoyama et al. 1996). From this as well as other examples, we know copper to be an important component in the mitochondrion. Among its many roles, zinc is a critical structural component of zinc-finger proteins, which regulate transcription in the nucleus. A significant reference of zinc-binding proteins is available for understanding the compartments of the cell where zinc may be found (Vallee and Auld 1990). Taken together, this kind of indirect knowledge leads to a coordinated, systems-based approach to understanding the location of cellular metals, as has been recently applied in the case of copper (Banci, Bertini et al. 2010).

These indirect approaches are also useful in understanding bioavailability of metals. For example, based upon the measurement of the metal-binding constant of superoxide dismutase we have been able to extrapolate that there is no free copper in the cytoplasm of yeast (Rae, Schmidt et al. 1999). Additionally, measurement of the zinc-binding potential of the CueR copper regulatory protein demonstrated that there was no 'free' copper in the cytoplasm of E. *coli* bacteria (Changela, Chen et al. 2003), setting the window of such ions at less than one atom per cell.

In addition to achieving the chemistry vital to the cell, metalloproteins open up a new avenue of cellular regulation. Not only can their activity be up- or down-regulated by changes in the expression level, but also by changes in the availability of their metal cofactors. An elegant illustration of this is the work of Tottey et al., which found, in examining the periplasm of the bacteria *Synechocystis* PCC 6803 that compartmentalization can be used to keep competitive metals out of the 'wrong' nascent proteins (Tottey, Waldron et al. 2008). In another, more clinical example, it has long been known that copper availability can modulate the growth of tumors in the body (Pan, Kleer et al. 2002). When copper is depleted by adminstering copper-chelating compounds such as tetrathiomolybdate to the patient, the growth of new blood vessels as well as the tumors that rely on them is inhibited.

1.3 We can now visualize changes in cellular metal distributions, and their signature patterns, during physiological changes

Recent technological advances have also made it possible to directly visualize metals within cells at the sub-cellular level. As early as the 1980's, advances in microanalysis were enabling the development of electron microscopy capable of compositional analysis – or the ability to distinguish the chemical composition of samples at the cellular or subcellular level. An excellent example of this is the work of Peter Ingram and Ann Le Furgey (Ingram, Shelburne et al. 1999). One of the limitations of electron microscopy is the thickness of samples, which generally must be no more than 100 nm thick, requiring specialized sample preparation.

On the other hand, hard X-ray microscopy (~10 keV or greater incident energy), generally does not face this limitation. The focal depth is on the order of 200 – 300 microns, and anything thinner than this will simply appear as 2-D projection of the volume. Thus, as zone plate technology and third generation synchrotron sources have developed, the minimal sample preparation required has made X-ray fluorescence microscopy a very accessible technique.

The accessibility of X-ray fluorescence microscopy, with relatively simple sample preparation and publically available synchrotron facilities, has facilitated its application – even to areas quite clinical and far removed from the physics of the synchrotron facilities that support it. The findings, some of which are highlighted below, have at times been startling. Could 80% of the cell's copper simply be exported during the angiogenic process of tubulogenesis (Finney, Mandava et al. 2007)? Isn't this a drastic commitment of energy? Despite clinical findings regarding chelation, as mentioned earlier, it is doubtful any scientist would have predicted this. But, it is precisely the directness of these methods which makes such surprising findings possible.

1.4 Are these signatures diagnostic?

According to the National Cancer Institute, a biomarker is "A biological molecule found in blood, other body fluids, or tissues that is a sign of a normal or abnormal process, or of a condition or disease. A biomarker may be used to see how well the body responds to a treatment for a disease or condition. Also called molecular marker and signature molecule". In this sense, a biomarker is something that is diagnostic – serving as an indicator of a physiological state or disease condition.

The cellular distributions of metals clearly have the potential to fulfill this role. As we learn more about the distributions and compartmentalization of cellular metals, and how these change in various conditions, it is increasingly clear that signatures should exist.

2. Overview of X-ray fluorescence imaging

2.1 Prinicples of biological X-ray fluorescence imaging

Fluorescence exists in many familiar forms. It is the absorption of light at one wavelength, and its re-emission as light of a longer wavelength (with less energy). It can be seen when you put certain laundry detergents under a simple black-light, which you cannot see with your eyes, and watch optical light come back out, making it 'glow'. Optical fluorescence like this is also a critical tool in almost all of biology, where even the most complex optical fluorescence microscopes still use monochromatic light and emission filters to image optically-fluorescent dyes and protein labels, revealing information about cellular structures. X-ray fluorescence imaging is fundamentally no different from this. However, unlike optical light which excites vibrational states, X-rays are of such energy that, for metals, they excite the electrons bound to the atom directly.

2.1.1 Basics of X-ray fluorescence

The energy and wavelength of light are inversely related, as follows from Equation 1, where E is energy, h is Planck's constant, c is the speed of light, and λ is the wavelength.

$$E = h \times c / \lambda \quad (1)$$

Looking at this equation, it is simple to see that if the energy of an incoming photon is decreased, such as might happen when it runs into an electron, the photon is not only reduced in energy but its wavelength will increase, changing its 'color'. In fact, the photon may excite the electron into a higher energy state. When this happens, it leaves behind an opening, or 'hole' in the electron shell. Since the spacing of orbitals, or the difference in energy between them, is constant for a particular metal atom, when an electron 'falls' back down in energy, into the 'hole' that was left behind, it emits light at a very characteristic energy - much like a pipe of a particular length on an organ plays a very specific note. It is this property of X-ray fluorescence, the fact that each element - zinc, copper, iron - will emit fluorescence at characteristic energies with specific relative intensities that are intrinsic to the metal itself, that makes it possible to distinguish the emission spectrum of iron from that of copper, for example. Or to distinguish how much of either one is present in a mixture.

2.1.2 Special considerations for biological samples

Critical to the success of biological X-ray fluorescence imaging is preparation of samples which are both structurally and compositionally intact. At the same time, the samples must be preserved such that they can withstand the damaging potential of a focused X-ray beam. The most ideal way of ensuring this is to prepare samples which are frozen in a vitreous glass of ice. This avoids creating crystalline ice, which would break cellular structures and membranes and is not a simple task. Also, to keep the sample completely frozen without any recrystallization of the ice is not straight-forward. Current research is attempting to achieve both of these.

Yet, much interesting and useful research has been done on dry samples. Recent studies examine either flash-frozen and freeze-dried samples, or chemically fixed and dried samples (McRae, Bagchi et al. 2009).

Another consideration in examining biological samples is that the emission peaks of most common biological metals overlap quite strongly in the emission spectrum generated by energy-dispersive detectors. Thus, proper fitting of the data, including de-convolution of these peaks, is critical to correct assignment of intensity to a metal of interest. The development of software, particularly MAPS, has been of paramount importance in this field (Vogt 2003). Likewise, the selection and use of reference standards, to convert emitted intensity to a calculated quantity, is also critical to proper analysis.

3. The revolution: Peering into the unseen

3.1 Case 1: The biology of selenium

3.1.1 Overview of selenium biochemistry

Selenium exists, in mammals, primarily as part of selenomethionine or selenocystine, and less abundantly as selenite, selenide, monomethylselenol, dimethylselenide, trimethylselenonium, L-selenomethionine (SM), Se-methyl-L-selenocysteine. Because of its chemical similarity, it is utilized by the body in many of the same pathways as sulphur. Some controversy has surrounded its use as a nutritional supplement in the prevention of cancer - where it has been purported to function in an anti-oxidative capacity.

3.1.2 What XFM has revealed

X-ray fluorescence has shed light on the biological roles of selenium in biochemistry. Kehr et al. obtained beautiful images, the first of their kind, of the selenium in sperm (Kehr, Malinouski et al. 2009). It had long been known that selenium is essential for sperm production and therefore fertility in mammals (Maiorino, Roveri et al. 2006). By directly imaging the selenium in the sperm at various stages of development, scientists found that a high and specific accumulation of selenium occurs during spermatid development. Further, they determined that it related to an increased need for the plasma selenoprotein SelP in order to produce additional mGPx4 protein. This work not only expanded the current understanding of selenium biology, but also demonstrated the utility of direct imaging of selenium at the subcellular level for better understanding of mammalian biology.

In another example, the effects of GPx1 deficiency were explored in mice. GPx1 is the major mammalian selenoprotein and it is expressed at a particularly high level in the liver (Malinouski, Kehr et al. 2011). The uniform distribution of Se in hepatocytes is consistent with the concept that XFM largely detects GPx1. In this work, it was found that in addition to homogenous signal from GPx1, the kidney also showed highly localized circular structures of Se surrounding proximal tubules. It was reported that this signal represents GPx3, which was secreted from these tubules and remained bound to the basement membrane. It represented approximately 20% of the Se pool in mouse kidney, and an even higher fraction in the kidney of the naked mole rat. This observation supports the postulate that the production of these two proteins, and their sources of selenium, are separate. The authors also postulate that advances in X-ray fluorescence imaging, increasing its resolution and sensitivity, will lead to a greater understanding of selenium biology.

3.2 Case 2: A role for zinc in cell fertilization, differentiation, lactation

3.2.1 A historical perspective on the cell biology of zinc

Zinc has long been known to play an important role in biology. Studies of the biochemistry of zinc may well have first begun in the 1950's, with the study of metallothionein. We now know that zinc plays both structural roles, such as in zinc finger proteins, and catalytic roles such as it does in carbonic anhydrase. Yet, there remains much to learn about this metal. Results from direct X-ray fluorescence imaging of this element in cells may indeed have revealed that there is still much to learn.

3.2.2 A new view of zinc from XFM

One of the first findings regarding zinc (utilizing sub-micron X-ray fluorescence imaging) was that it may be involved in cell differentiation, particularly looking at HL-60 cells (Glesne, Vogt et al. 2006). In examining the growth of human embryonic stem cells, taking a systems biology approach to examining entire colonies of cells and all the first row transition metals, we also found that the amount of zinc present in cells directly correlated with their differentiation (Wolford, Chishti et al. 2010). The images in Figure 1, of stem cells differentiated with retinoic acid, are particularly illustrative. Loss of Oct4 (pink) is associated with higher zinc (red in 'Zn' panel). This was found to be true regardless of the method of differentiation, or whether the cells at the outer edge or at the center of the colony were the ones to differentiate first. This exciting finding brings us to a new understanding of how little we know about the majority of nuclear zinc, as well as the roles of metals during differentiation.

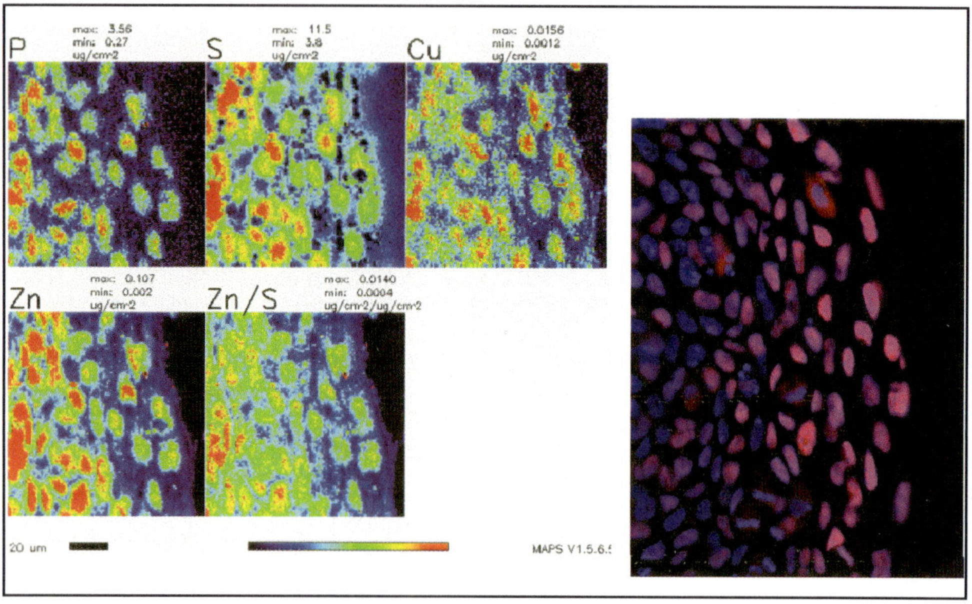

Fig. 1. Correlating XRF and immuno-fluorescence images of human embryonic stem cells.

At the same time, zinc plays many roles in the cell, as well as roles even outside of the cell. An elegant example of work utilizing X-ray fluorescence to better understand zinc physiology is reported by the Kelleher group in their studies of lactation (McCormick, Velasquez et al. 2010). In contrast to the coordination of zinc throughout much of the cell, zinc in milk is significantly associated with lower molecular weight molecules - at relatively high concentration relative to other essential metals. And it is not known how the mammary gland regulates the transfer of zinc into milk. By directly imaging the zinc in mammary tissue of both lactating and non-lactating mice, the researchers were able to demonstrate that zinc associates with a distinct peri-nuclear pool. Further, through experiments utilizing the chemical indictor Fluo-zin-3, which is a zinc indicator, together with dyes for the endoplasmic reticulum, mitochondrion, and Golgi, optical fluorescence microscopy indicated that this zinc was 'labile' on account with its ability to bind the zinc dye, and at least partially associated with the Golgi complex. This work represents some of the first X-ray fluorescence imaging of mammary tissue at the sub-micron scale, and suggests that the pathways for zinc export during lactation likely are similar to those utilized in the prostate.

Another particularly surprising finding from direct X-ray fluorescence imaging of metals in cells relates to fertilization. Work by a team of scientists from Northwestern University has recently shown that the accumulation of zinc is essential for fertilization (Kim, Vogt et al. 2010). In this work, single-cell elemental analysis of mouse oocytes by X-ray fluorescence microscopy revealed a 50% increase in total zinc content within the 12-14-h period of meiotic maturation. While the reason for this is still unclear, the team has recently reported that experiments utilizing extra-cellular optically-fluorescent zinc indicators have shown that some of this zinc is exported upon fertilization (Kim, Bernhardt et al. 2011). This may be an example of the cell using metal bioavailability to regulate protein function.

3.3 Case 3: The potential of copper as a dynamic, signaling molecule

3.3.1 Established, enzymatic roles for copper

Copper is widely used in biology for enzymatic chemistry. Its ability to cycle between (I) and (II) oxidation states makes it particularly useful for reduction and oxidation chemistry. It is used to activate oxygen, detoxify radicals, and in mitochondrial function. Yet, for as much as is known about copper, direct X-ray fluorescence imaging is revealing new roles, and changes in distributions that may have the potential to serve as biomarkers of the future.

3.3.2 Viewing copper differently – Dramatic fluxes of copper

It was reported in 2006 by Gitlin et al. that copper in hippocampal neurons appeared to be exported following NMDA-receptor stimulation (Schlief, Craig et al. 2005). The use of Cu-64 to try to measure this export made it somewhat difficult to determine exactly how much of the cellular copper was exported, or image exactly where the copper was. But, clearly, new roles for copper were emerging.

Shortly after this, Finney et al. reported that a dramatic efflux of copper occurs during the angiogenic process of tubulogenesis, or the process by which new capillaries are formed. As mentioned earlier, copper had long been known to be important to angiogenesis, and thus also to the growth of cancerous tumors that rely upon a growing blood supply. By directly imaging the tubulogenesis process, at fixed points, using X-ray fluorescence microscopy scientists found that between 80-90% of the cell's copper was exported at early points, and then taken back up later in the growth of capillary-like structures (Finney, Mandava et al. 2007). Exactly why this happens remains a mystery, and has sparked new efforts in the development of tools for metalloproteomics (Finney, Chishti et al. 2010). From this, one might speculate that a role for copper in intercellular signaling, of some sort, may exist.

Taking this technique, and applying it back to the same sort of systems which Gitlin et al. had examined, leads to another remarkable finding. As shown in Figure 2, a typical SH-sy5y cell, the majority of cellular copper is typically localized in the perinuclear area in neuronal cells. Upon stimulation, the copper may be seen to relocalize such that a significant increase in the fraction of cellular copper that is along the dendrites of the cell is seen. Not only can fluxes of copper be seen in hippocampal neurons, but they are dependent on calcium, and induced by extracellular stimulation (Dodani, Domaille et al. 2011). Clearly, undiscovered roles for copper as an important part of cell signaling exist. And X-ray fluorescence imaging is enabling our further understanding of them. As roles for metals such as this are further defined, they hold the potential to reveal patterns and signatures that may become the biomarkers of the future.

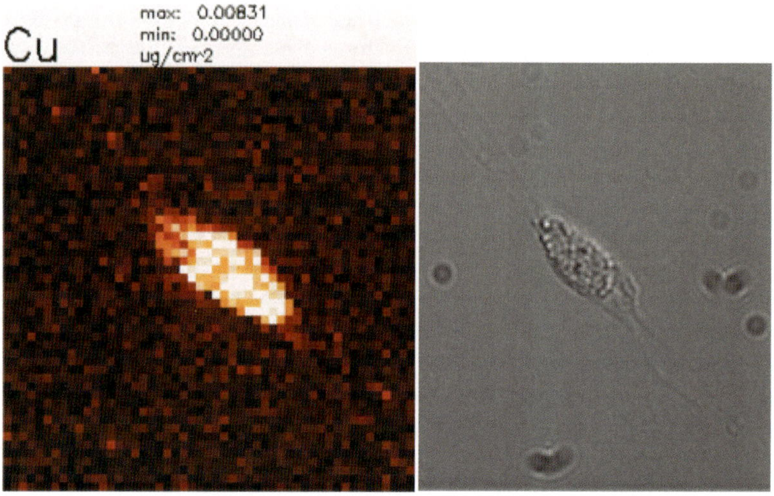

Fig. 2. Copper localizes peripherally to the nucleus in a cell

4. Inorganic signatures of life: Can metal ion distributions be biomarkers of physiological state?

4.1 A need to link metal ion fluxes with other biomolecules

The key to more insightful interpretations from much of this imaging is linking it to known physiological pathways. Much of what we know about cell function, and many therapeutic targets, is because of the specificity of proteins. Unleashing the potential of this tool calls for matching our developing understanding of the role of metal ions themselves in biology with our greater understanding of physiology in general.

Can the distribution of metal ions be diagnostic? Can these metal ions, or at least their signature distribution and quantity in subcellular compartments, serve as biomarkers? Consider this:

- Metal ions are essential to many processes
- Inorganic signatures can identify specific physiological processes
- Intervention, clinical diagnostics require targeting associated proteins

Thus, while it seems entirely possible that the distributions of metals may be used as a signature diagnostic of a pathological state in the future, the development of metalloproteomics and other methods of identifying their partner biomolecules is essential to therapeutic intervention in these metal-related disease processes.

4.2 Need for higher resolution imaging to better define subcellular compartments

A need exists for higher-resolution X-ray fluorescence imaging, to better identify the specific cellular compartments where metals are distributed. Many examples highlighted here look at changes in metal distributions that are either 'in' vs. 'out' of the cell, 'near' or 'away' from the nucleus. At the advent of the age of nano-scale imaging of biological samples, imaging cells at the scale of 10's of nanometers, where we can begin to see within the mitochondrion, for example, will reveal many new and exciting things about the cell biology of metals.

4.3 Need for other data acquisition schemes to improve statistics

Another important consideration in the context of biomarkers is speed. X-ray fluorescence imaging is currently quite slow. Samples are raster-scanned through an X-ray beam with dwell times of 1s or more per pixel. With potentially hours of scan time required for imaging a single cell, good statistical sampling is difficult to achieve. What is needed for this? Some current areas of development may help, particularly the development of fast fly-scanning data acquisition, where samples are raster scanned continuously and fluorescence information is recorded 'on-the-fly'. Another area with promise for speed is the development of microfluidic devices that will enable X-ray fluorescence spectra of whole cells to be individually captured while flowing in a stream, thus allowing measurement of at least the total metals in individual cells over populations of hundreds of cells. As techniques like these emerge, the promise of X-ray fluorescence imaging for diagnostics comes closer to a reality.

5. Acknowledgment

This work was supported by the DOE Office of Science under contract DE-AC02-06CH11357. The author thanks all of her collaborators, especially those cited here, for sharing the excitement of their research.

6. References

Banci, L., I. Bertini, et al. (2010). "Cellular copper distribution: a mechanistic systems biology approach." *Cellular and Molecular Life Sciences* 67(15): 2563-2589.

Bertini, I., H. B. Gray, et al., Eds. (2007). *Biological Inorganic Chemistry: Structure and Reactivity*. Sausalito, CA, University Science Books.

Boal, A. K. and A. C. Rosenzweig (2009). "Structural biology of copper trafficking." *Chemical Reviews* 109(10): 4760-4779.

Dodani, S. C., D. W. Domaille, et al. (2011). "Calcium-dependent copper redistributions in neuronal cells revealed by a fluorescent copper sensor and X-ray fluorescence microscopy." *Proceedings of the National Academy of Sciences of the United States of America* 108(15): 5980-5985.

Dodani, S. C., S. C. Leary, et al. (2011). "A targetable fluorescent sensor reveals that copper-deficient SCO1 and SCO2 patient cells prioritize mitochondrial copper homeostasis." *Journal of the American Chemical Society* 133(22): 8606-8616.

Eide, D. J. (2006). "Zinc transporters and the cellular trafficking of zinc." *Biochimica et Biophysica Acta* 1763(7): 711-722.

Finney, L., Y. Chishti, et al. (2010). "Imaging metals in proteins by combining electrophoresis with rapid X-ray fluorescence mapping." *ACS Chem Biol* 5(6): 577-587.

Finney, L., S. Mandava, et al. (2007). "X-ray fluorescence microscopy reveals large-scale relocalization and extracellular translocation of cellular copper during angiogenesis." *Proceedings of the National Academy of Sciences of the United States of America* 104(7): 2247-2252.

Finney, L. A. and T. V. O'Halloran (2003). "Transition metal speciation in the cell: Insights from the chemistry of metal ion receptors." *Science* 300(5621): 931-936.

Glesne, D., S. Vogt, et al. (2006). "Regulatory properties and cellular redistribution of zinc during macrophage differentiation of human leukemia cells." *Journal of Structural Biology* 155(1): 2-11.

Ingram, P., J. Shelburne, et al. (1999). *Biomedical Applications of Microprobe Analysis*. San Diego, CA, Academic Press.

Kehr, S., M. Malinouski, et al. (2009). "X-ray fluorescence microscopy reveals the role of selenium in spermatogenesis." *Journal of Molecular Biology* 389(5): 808-818.

Kim, A. M., M. L. Bernhardt, et al. (2011). "Zinc sparks are triggered by fertilization and facilitate cell cycle resumption in mammalian eggs." *ACS Chem Biol* 6(7): 716-723.

Kim, A. M., S. Vogt, et al. (2010). "Zinc availability regulates exit from meiosis in maturing mammalian oocytes." *Nat Chem Biol* 6(9): 674-681.

Kosman, D. J. (2010). "Redox cycling in iron uptake, efflux, and trafficking." *Journal of Biological Chemistry* 285(35): 26729-26735.

Lutsenko, S. (2010). "Human copper homeostasis: a network of interconnected pathways." *Current Opinion in Chemical Biology* 14(2): 211-217.

Maiorino, M., A. Roveri, et al. (2006). Selenium and male reproduction. *Selenium: Its Molecular Biology and Role in Human Health*. D. L. Hatfield, M. J. Berry and V. N. Gladyshev. New York, Springer Science+Business Media, LLC.

Malinouski, M., S. Kehr, et al. (2011). "High-Resolution Imaging of Selenium in Kidneys: a Localized Selenium Pool Associated with Glutathione Peroxidase 3." *Antioxid Redox Signal*.

McCormick, N., V. Velasquez, et al. (2010). "X-ray fluorescence microscopy reveals accumulation and secretion of discrete intracellular zinc pools in the lactating mouse mammary gland." *PLoS One* 5(6): e11078.

McRae, R., P. Bagchi, et al. (2009). "In situ imaging of metals in cells and tissues." *Chemical Reviews* 109(10): 4780-4827.

Pan, Q., C. G. Kleer, et al. (2002). "Copper deficiency induced by tetrathiomolybdate suppresses tumor growth and angiogenesis." *Cancer Research* 62(17): 4854-4859.

Qin, Y., P. J. Dittmer, et al. (2011). "Measuring steady-state and dynamic endoplasmic reticulum and Golgi Zn2+ with genetically encoded sensors." *Proceedings of the National Academy of Sciences of the United States of America* 108(18): 7351-7356.

Rae, T. D., P. J. Schmidt, et al. (1999). "Undetectable intracellular free copper: the requirement of a copper chaperone for superoxide dismutase." *Science* 284(5415): 805-808.

Schlief, M. L., A. M. Craig, et al. (2005). "NMDA receptor activation mediates copper homeostasis in hippocampal neurons." *Journal of Neuroscience* 25(1): 239-246.

Tomat, E. and S. J. Lippard (2010). "Imaging mobile zinc in biology." *Current Opinion in Chemical Biology* 14(2): 225-230.

Tottey, S., K. J. Waldron, et al. (2008). "Protein-folding location can regulate manganese-binding versus copper- or zinc-binding." *Nature* 455(7216): 1138-1142.

Tsukihara, T., H. Aoyama, et al. (1995). "Structures of metal sites of oxidized bovine heart cytochrome c oxidase at 2.8 A." *Science* 269(5227): 1069-1074.

Tsukihara, T., H. Aoyama, et al. (1996). "The whole structure of the 13-subunit oxidized cytochrome c oxidase at 2.8 A." *Science* 272(5265): 1136-1144.

Vallee, B. L. and D. S. Auld (1990). "Zinc coordination, function, and structure of zinc enzymes and other proteins." *Biochemistry* 29(24): 5647-5659.

Vogt, S. (2003). "MAPS: A set of software tools for analysis and visualization of 3D X-ray fluorescence data sets." *J Phys IV France* 104: 635-638.

Wolford, J. L., Y. Chishti, et al. (2010). "Loss of pluripotency in human embryonic stem cells directly correlates with an increase in nuclear zinc." *PLoS One* 5(8): e12308.

7

Biomarkers and Therapeutic Drug Monitoring in Psychiatry

R. Lozano, R. Marin, A. Pascual, MJ. Santacruz, A. Lozano and F. Sebastian
Pharmacy and Psychiatry Services, Hospital Real Ntra. Sra. De Gracia, Zaragoza, Spain

1. Introduction

The World Health Organization, WHO, reported in 2010 that there were approximately 490 million (7%) of people suffering from mental disorders, such as abuse of alcohol and other substances, major depression, bipolar disorder, schizophrenia and dementia, recommending research the pathophysiology of these disorders in order to improve their understanding and to develop more efficient and cost-effective interventions (WHO 2001, 2005).

The diagnosis of mental disorders, should be based on objectively measurable parameters and, also, should help us to establish therapeutic guidelines, based on the etiology of the diseases, and their adaptation to each individual. The absence of an objective biological test for the diagnosis of mental disorders which would constitute the Gold Standard for this task, along with the frequent psychiatric comorbidity, heterogeneity and, polygenic and multifactorial etiology, requires the search for Biomarkers that facilitated the diagnosis and treatment of the psychiatric illnesses. The Convergent Functional Genomics has revealed that proteins, compounds of biochemical nature related to different physiological functions, genetic tests for diagnosis or, even, different functional tests such as, for example, the dexamethasone suppression test, DEX, used to study the function of the hypothalamic-pituitary-adrenal axis, HPA, can be candidates (Avissar & Schreiber 2003; Kemperman 2007; Russell 2004).

The use of Biomarkers, that is, a physical characteristic, or a biochemical or biological parameter, objectively measurable and quantifiable, that report the evolution and condition of certain normal physiological processes or pathological, or response to a therapeutic intervention, pharmacological or otherwise, is relatively new but this field has gained much interest in recent decades among clinicians and researchers. A Biomarker, as a measurable biological entity that points the presence or absence of a disease, a toxin, a biological condition, a genetic pattern, or a therapeutic response to a drug, must be related quantitatively with the disease progression and/or therapy (http://www.gaba-network.org; Biomarkers Definitions Working Group, BDWG, 2001).

Biomarkers, are utilized in psychiatry not only as tools that aid us in the diagnosis and treatment of various diseases, facilitating the use of therapies aimed at specific groups or individuals, but also, as Surrogate Markers or Clinical Surrogate Endpoints for PK, PD and

PG modelling in drug response, and to investigate the biological mechanisms of action and the efficacy and safety profile of the target drug, being this last point developed along this chapter (Riggs 1990).

The search of a Biomarker begins with the selection of the groups of patients and controls, continous with the selection of the type of sample to use and, finally, the selection of the statistical analysis that allowed us to demonstrate differences between both groups, such as the multivariate analysis of cross-sectional data and multivariate correlation analysis of longitudinal data, so that, there was clear evidence that these Biomarkers are able to distinguish between controls and affected individuals. To complete the validation, we have to check this on a large group of patients following Food and Drugs Administration guidelines (FDA 2008). In the case of Biomarkers used to monitor pharmacological therapies, the choice and validation of these should be supported, in addition, on studies of the etiology of the disease being treated and mechanism of drug action, as well as provide data on its cost-effectiveness and its side effects (Kemperman 2007).

In the other hand, a Surrogate Marker, defined as a laboratory measurement, physical sign or symptom, is used in therapy as a direct measure of how patient feels, functions, or survives and is expected was able to predict the effect of a treatment, ie, it is a test that is used as measure of the effect of a given specific treatment. It is a candidate Biomarker if it can be validated, taking this atribute when the evidence has proven that the predicted effect induced by drugs or other therapy, on the Surrogate Marker, produces the outcomes desired on the clinical characteristic of interest, such as blood pressure, serum cholesterol, intraocular pressure, etc, while Clinical Surrogate Endpoint refers to the final desirable value that we want to achieve for a specific Surrogate Marker, which is related to the level of disease progression, intensity of a symptom or sign, or a laboratory test, that constitute the desired target and that reflect the expected clinical outcome (BDWG 2001).

To validate a Surrogate Marker as a Biomarker, we need to understand the biological relationship between the Surrogate Marker that predicts the desired clinical benefit and the clinical outcome achieved. For pharmacological treatments, we have to know, moreover, all therapeutic actions, if we want to conclude that the effect obtained on the Surrogate Marker will result in the beneficial clinical outcomes desired. (Buckley & Schatzberg 2009; Russell 2004).

In short, at the present time the biological causality of most psychiatric illnesses and the intimate mechanism of action of most psychotropic drugs are unknown. However, it is possible to modulate pharmacologically a large number of neuroreceptors, using this tool as target of drug therapies and utilizing to control of psychiatric disorders symptoms. We will review in this chapter, the role and potential use of Biomarkers and / or Surrogate Markers to optimize the pharmacological treatments of most common psychiatric illnesses, with emphasis on schizophrenia and depression, in order to use them in the dosage regimen calcualtion and choosing a particular therapeutic drug strategy (Noll 2006; Shaheen 2010).

2. Models for therapeutic drug monitoring

After the administration of a drug, several processes occur leading to the pharmacological effect, so that we can define Pharmacokinetics, PK, as "what the body does to a drug" and pharmacodynamics, PD, as " what the drug does to the body " (Geldof 2007).

There are three unitary models for the therapeutic drug monitoring:

1. Pharmacokinetic models, PK. They are used to describe control processes of drug concentration in biological fluids at any time after its administration, being absorption, distribution, metabolism and excretion, the main stages that determine the evolution of the drug concentration versus time, so the PK-models, determine the overall course of the process (Perez-Urizar 2000).
2. Pharmacodynamic models, PD. They are used to describe the relationship between the drug concentration and/or active metabolites and the magnitude of the pharmacological effect obtained such as, eg, blood pressure, heart rate, etc (Geldof 2007; Holford & Sheiner 1981; Rowland & Tozer 1995; Sheiner et al 1997) .
3. Pharmacogenetic models, PG. They are used to describe the influence of interindividual genetic variations in the response to a drug in terms of efficacy and safety. They use genotype-phenotype, gene-concentration and gene-dose correlations for predicting the phenotype of a individual and provide support to achieve a optimal pharmacotherapy.

As important part of the construction of these models, a Surrogate Marker or Biomarker is defined as measure that characterizes, in a strictly quantitative manner, the various processes and stages that occur between the administration of a drug and its pharmacological effect, and can be used in clinical practice for the individualization of drug therapy, from the viewpoint of dosage regimen calculation and therapeutic strategy. In fact, there is a growing interest in the use of biomarkers in drug development, as is reflected in the publication of numerous reviews and comments, appeared recently, on this topic. As well as, the recent increase in the number of publications about PK-PD models in journals of Clinical Pharmacology and Clinical Pharmacy, concerning to theoretical models and their implementation. Despite the continued increase in the number of articles, there are still, a large number of publications that contain pharmacokinetic and pharmacodynamic data without PK-PD modeling studies (Francheteau 1993; Geldof 2007; Mandem & Wada 1995; Zuideveld 2001).

Optimization of pharmacologic treatment is usually done by monitoring serum drug concentrations, in PK models, or by the direct or indirect pharmacological response, represented by Biomarkers or Surrogate Markers, in PD models, combined with pharmacogenetic and environmental characteristics, in PG models.

PK models can be non-parametric or compartimental. Non-parametric models provide an empirical description of the temporal evolution of drug concentration in terms of the maximum concentration, Cmax, and time needed to reach it, Tmax, and area under the concentration versus time curve, AUC. While compartmental models provide a description of concentration profile versus time of the drug in a body fluid compartment (Csajka & Vérotte 2006; Geldof 2007; Holford & Sheiner 1982; Perez-Urizar et al 2000).

Binary models PK-PD, PK-PG and PD-PG, as a result of the union of simple models, are aimed to find out the suitable therapeutic dose, body "clearance" and other kinetic parameters related to plasma drug concentration or pharmacological effect, establish an adequate dosage scheme to achieve the desired therapeutic goal, as well as know the time evolution of the pharmacological effect, using the appropiate model and the individual genotype of the different populations to which treatment is targeted, by using the following mathematical tools:

1. General equation of the dose-response relationship, receptor mediated, which relates the intensity of the pharmacological effect, E, with the concentration of the drug, D, and of the receptor, R, presents in the body:

$$\frac{\partial^2 E}{\partial D^2} = \left(\frac{dD}{dR}\right)^2 \frac{\partial^2 E}{\partial R^2} \quad \text{Where} \quad \frac{dD}{dR} = K(cons\tan t) \tag{1}$$

Once the steady-state and a pharmacological response, ranging between the 20-80% of maximal effect, is reached we can estimate the optimal dose required to achieve the desired Clinical Surrogate Endpoint, using the following expression, an approximation of the equation 1:

$$\frac{[\Delta CSE]_1}{[\Delta CSE]_2} = 2^{\left[\frac{(DD)_1}{(DD)_2}\right]-1} \tag{2}$$

Where $[\Delta CSE]_1$ is the Clinical Surrogate Endpoint of the drug, equivalent to the average increase (delta, Δ) value obtained for CSE in the patients drug treated, $[\Delta\ CSE]_2$ is the experimental delta value obtained for CSE in a individual, $(DD)_2$ is the dose of drug with which has been obtained a $[\Delta\ CSE]_2$ value equal to 10 and $(DD)_1$ is the drug target dose (Lozano et al 2007,2008a,2008b, 2009b,2010a,2010b,2010c, 2011a).

2. Hill`s equation, equation 3, a partial solution of the above equation 1, from which comes, which relates the intensity of the pharmacological effect, E, on the Biomarker with the concentration of drug in the body, C, (Hill 1910):

$$E = \frac{C^{\gamma} E_{max}}{C^{\gamma} + EC_{50}^{\gamma}} \tag{3}$$

3. Kernel density estimation, Kernel`s test, used for poblational analysis, performed in the PK-PG and PD-PG models, which incorporate pharmacogenetic analysis (Wessa 2008).
4. Finally, for interaction-based models, where two or more drugs that interact on the same receptor, the following equation, equation 4, serves to describe the relation between the reaction velocity, d_V/d_C, of a drug, A, with the receptor, , versus to that of another drug, B, on the same receptor:

$$\frac{d_{Va}}{d_{Ca}} = -\frac{d_{Vb}}{d_{Cb}} \tag{4}$$

(Lozano et al 2009a, 2009c, 2010d).

2.1 PK-PD models

Consist of mathematical expressions that describe the quantitative relationships between the response intensity of a Biomarker or Surrogate Marker and drug dose applied. They have three components: a PK model, which characterizes the temporal evolution of the concentration of the drug and/or active metabolites, in blood or plasma, a PD model that characterizes the relationship between a drug concentration and/or possible active metabolites to the pharmacological effect, and finally, an aggregate model that takes into consideration other factors that may affect the pharmacological effect, frequently observed in the models of compartmentalized pharmacological effect and in those of indirect pharmacological response (Breimer & Danhof 1997; Geldof 2007).

The PK-PD models, can be:

1. Mechanistic-based models, which characterize the time course of drug effect, "in vivo", using expressions that describe the biophase drug distribution, target-drug binding, target-drug activation and feedback homeostatic processes and contain elements corresponding to the distribution in the target site , target-drug binding, and activation and transduction. They are based on the principles of receptor theory, that characterizes the interaction of the receptor with the drug in terms of affinity and intrinsic activity. In these models, PK-PD, when steady-state is reached, drug concentration in the biophase is paralell to the plasma concentration and directly proportional to the dose (BDWG 2001; Geldof 2007; Sheiner et al 1979 Van der Graaf & Danhof 1997).

Under stable conditions, relatively simple models, such as those linear or log-linear, can be used to characterize the dose-response relationship. The most used is the sigmoid model, which is an empirical function to describe the nonlinear relationship between drug concentration and the pharmacological effect; this model is mathematically expressed by the general equation for dose-response curve, equation 1, or also by Hill`s equation, equation 3, a partial solution of the previous, where E is the pharmacological effect observed with a given dose , E_0 is the response in the absence of drug, E_{max} is the maximum effect or intrinsic activity of drug, C is the concentration of drug and/or metabolite in plasma and/or biophase, EC_{50} is the concentration of drug and / or metabolites that produce 50% of maximal effect, potency, and γ is the Hill factor, that expresses the sigmoidicity of the curve (Geldof 2007; Hill 1910; Holford & Sheiner 1982; Meibohm & Derendorf, 1997).

Under conditions of non steady-state , the basic models PK-PD are unable to describe the time evolution of the pharmacological effect. Factors such as the compartimiental effect, acute tolerance and sensitization, and indirect response modeling, can explain the dissociation, frequently observed, between the temporal evolution of the drug concentration and pharmacological effect, using, in these cases, the previous model but applied to different doses to simulate the change in concentration along the time (Bauer et al 1997; Dayneko et al 1993; Derendorf & Meibohm 1999; Jusko & Ko 1994; Ragueneau et al 1998; Sheiner et al 1979).

2. Indirect response models, are based on a combination of the inhibitor or stimulant effect, that can produce the drug, and the factors controling the increase or decrease of the pharmacological response, represented by the constants K_{in} and K_{out} (Derendorf & Meibohm 1999, Mager et al 2003; Meibohm & Derendorf 1997; Rowland & Tozer 1995).
3. Drug interaction-based models, are used to describe the influence of two or more drugs among them, acting on the same receptor. Their use are limited to situations in which several drugs are administered together, or when a drug becomes an active metabolite. In theoretical terms refer to the prediction of the combined effects of more than one drug. The general approach to the study of these interactions involves the analysis of changes in the velocity of reaction that occur when the drugs are used combined or separately (Lozano et al 2009a, 2009c, 2010d).

4. Poblational models, are used to solve the problem of inter and intra-individual variability in the therapeutic response to a drug. In PK and PD models, the kinetic parameters of each individual are modeled in terms of the fixed effect observed, and other of random nature, while PK-PD poblational models, based on nonlinear mixed effects analysis, characterize the pharmacokinetic parameters and concentration-effect relationship, in poblational terms more than individual. Thus, in PK and PK-PD poblational models, we need to know in advance the average behaviour of pharmacokinetic parameters in target population, to identify and assess demographic, pathophysiological and environmental factors, affecting population under study and, finally, evaluate the inter and intraindivual variability through the variation coefficient of the PK parameters and their residual components (Dominguez-Gil & Lanao 1999; Schnider et al 1996).

2.2 The PK-PG models

Consist of mathematical expressions that describe the quantitative relationship between the drug dose necessary to achieve the same response intensity of a Biomarker or Surrogate Marker, for each one of the different genotypes phenotypically actives present in a population.

Pharmacogenetic models, PK-PG, are used to adapt the therapeutic use of different drugs to the idiosyncrasy of each patient and their genetic characteristics, increasing its efficiency and minimizing their side effects. Approximately 20-90% of the interindividual variability in drug response is consequence of individual genotype and variants that encode different polymorphs of the enzymes that metabolize and / or transport drugs.

Single Nucleotide Polymorphisms, SNPs, have been associated with substantial changes in the metabolism or in the effect of a drug, and therefore are being used to predict the clinical response to a drug of an individual. For the biotransformation of a drug, there are over 30 families of metabolizers enzymes belonging the family of cytochrome P-450, whose genetic polymorphisms normally lead to a functional changes in the encoded protein, resulting in individuals with different phenotypes:

a. Poor Metabolizers, PM: The encoded enzyme has no activity, the metabolic activity is very reduced or absent and the phenotype is predicted by the presence of two inactive alleles.
b. Intermediate Metabolizers, IM: The encoded enzyme has its activity decreased, the phenotype is predicted by the presence of two alleles with decreased activity, or a combination of a reduced activity allele and a allele with no activity.
c. Extended metabolizers, EM: They are carriers of one active gene copy at least, have a normal metabolic activity and phenotype is predicted from the combination of two active alleles. For some genes, the presence of one active allele combined with one allele with decreased activity or allele with no activity, causes that the metabolic activity was normal.
d. Ultrafast Metabolizers, UM: They have a double metabolic capacity and the phenotype is predicted by the presence of three or more functional alleles or the presence of two inducible alleles http://cpmc.coriell.org/Sections/Medical/DrugsAndGenes_mp.aspx?PgId=216).

Carrier proteins of drugs play an important role in regulating the absorption, distribution and excretion of many drugs. Within the ATP-binding cassette family, P-glycoprotein, encoded by the ABCB1 gene, is one of the best known , being its main function the control of the outflow from inside the cells of certain endogenous and / or exogenous substrates, including several drugs and substances such as bilirubin, so the presence of polymorphisms in this gene, entails changes in the PK and PD of certain drugs.

2.3 The PD-PG models

PD-PG models, consist of mathematical expressions that describe the quantitative relationship between the response intensity of a Biomarker or Surrogate Marker, to a single dose of the drug, and the different genotypes phenotypically actives present in a specific population.

Pharmacogenetic models, PD-PG, are used to adapt the therapeutic use of different drugs to the idiosyncrasy of each patient and their genetic characteristics, increasing its efficiency and minimizing their side effects. Approximately 20-90% of the interindividual variability in drug response is consequence of individual genotype and variants that encode different polymorphs of therapeutic targets.

Genetic polymorphisms with indirect effects on the response to drugs are those that affect to a genes encoding proteins that often are involved in the mechanisms of the drug disposition, producing alterations in the response to treatment only under certain situations.

Therefore, both PK -PG and PD-PG models are used to describe the genotype-phenotype, gene-concentration and gene-dose correlations, necessary to achieve an optimal pharmacotherapy (Brockmöller & Tzvetkov 2008, Tsai & Hoyme 2002; Weinshilboum & Wang 2006).

3. Biomarkers for therapeutic drug monitoring in psychiatry

3.1 Lithium

Bipolar disorder, BD, is characterized by the presence of one or more episodes of mania or, in mild cases, hypomania and additional depressive episodes, concomitants or alternants.

The cause is unknown, although recent studies suggest the presence of an imbalance between excitatory neurotransmitters, mainly glutamate, and inhibitors, principally GABA, as well as alterations in cation pumps, such as of sodium and of calcium, which would explain the pathogenesis of bipolar disorder and another pathologies as epilepsy (Brown & Sherwood 2006).

To explain the action mechanism of Lithium salts there are several proposals, being the most known:

1. Inhibition of the enzyme GSK-3B, whose complete mechanism in relation with BD has not yet been hypothesized (Jonker et al 2003).
2. Blockade of the NMDA/ NO receptor: The Nitric Oxide, NO, plays a crucial role in neuronal plasticity, having shown that the NO system may be involved in the antidepressant effect of lithium amd the increase in antidepressant capacity of lithium by the blockade of NMDA receptor would indicate an involvement of the NMDA/NO receptor in the pharmacological action of lithium (Ghasemi et al. 2008, 2009a, 2009b; Ghasemi & Race 2008).
3. Inhibition of Inositol monophosphatase enzyme (Einat et al 1998).

All the pharmacological activity of lithium salts is carried out by the insolubilization of intracellular inorganic phosphate salts through the formation of inorganic lithium phosphates. These ones have much lower solubility than their sodium salts (eg the solubility of Li_3PO_4 in water is 0.03821 g/dL/20 ° C versus of the Na_3PO_4 that is 8.8 g/dL/25 ° C), which leads to decrease the amount of intracellular inorganic soluble phosphates, P_i, causing, consequently, decrease in intracellular phosphate stored in organic compounds, P_o, and slowdown all metabolic reactions that involve exchange of inorganic phosphates, mainly those using ATP but, also, those using another nucleotides with capacity for the storage of phosphates, as we know now , and affecting in a hierarchically manner to several intracellular pathways of activation and/or inhibition, being those of GSK and inositol-phosphates, among other, the first to be affected (Lozano et al 2009a, 2010a,2010b).

In the case of the thyroid gland, lithium salts cause a dose-dependent decrease in serum free thyroxine, FT_4, due to the very low solubility of inorganic lithium phosphates, formed in the interior of target cells by action of lithium, which leads to a decrease in the intracellular pH and in the tyrosine iodination reaction, pH dependent, with consequent decrease of the FT_4 levels, because the iodination of phenols is a direct reaction of iodine, I_2, on the phenolate ion, very sensitive to changes in pH, decreasing exponentially the rate of iodination when the pH does it (Kessler et al 2008; Lozano et al 2010a, 2010b; Taylor & Evans 1953).

3.1.1 PK-PD model

Mechanistic-model. We can use the FT_4 levels in plasma as a biomarker for quantifying the intraneuronal concentration of Lithium and the dosage regimen calculation in the treatments of bipolar disorder with salts Lithium, increasing o decreasing the daily dosage to reach FT_4 values, in the range of 1.02-1.08 ng/dL, its Clinical Surrogate Endpoint (Lozano et al 2010a, 2010b).

3.1.2 PK-PG model

Due to the Lithium elimination by glomerular filtration, the poblational analisys conducted by Kernel`s test has allowed us to detect two subpopulations related to serum creatinine and therefore with the Lithium Clearance, caused by the presence of MDR1 polymorphisms, altering the aldosterone level and therefore the Creatinine Clearance, obtaining from the application of the equation 2, the following equi-effective dose ratio:

$$\frac{\text{DOSE (genotype:wild type)}}{\text{DOSE (genotype:polimorphic type)}} = 1.5 - 2$$

(Lozano et al 2011b).

3.1.3 PK-PG model

Poblational analysis conducted by Kernel`s test has not detected any subpopulation.

3.2 Escitalopram-SSRI

Depression is a pathological alteration of mood, being Major Depressive disorder the most studied with a prevalence of 10-25%. Its complex origin, is attributed to a defective transmission of noradrenaline and dopamine associated with dysregulation of the hypothalamic-pituitary-adrenal axis , HPA, which is reflected by the alteration of the cortisol escape from suppression by dexamethasone in the Dexamethasone Suppression test, DEX test, and by the increased response of cortisol in the Dexamethasone-Suppressed Corticotropin-Releasing Hormone Stimulation Test, DEX-CRH test. The decrease in serotonergic transmission in the brain and increased secretion of cortisol in patients with major depression have reached the status of an axiom in textbooks, being the cortisol the biological key mediator through which the brain slows down serotonergic transmission that causes depression in vulnerable people (American Psychiatric Association 2000; Dinan, 1996; Goodwin & Post 1983; Noll 2006; Schnider et al 1996).

Deregulation of the hypothalamic-pituitary-adrenal axis is present in a high rate among the patients with depression and its normalization, observed by the response to the DEX-CRH test, is verified when there is a good response to pharmacological treatment. Moreover, the serotonergic system interacts with the hypothalamic-pituitary-adrenal axis and, because of this, the stimulation of this axis can be used as a Surrogate Marker for the pharmacological action of the 5-HT agonist in the CNS (Cowen 1993, 1998; Gartside & Cowen 1990; Meltzer & Maes 1994; Meltzer et al 1991).

The reduced serotonergic neurotransmission is well known feature of the depression and therefore it is not surprising that SSRI drugs were the first line of treatment in depressive disorders. Plasma levels of Escitalopram and another SSRI drugs decrease the HPA-response in the DEX test and there is a good correlation between dose of the SSRI drug and decreasing of plasma cortisol. Cortisol values obtained by Nugent's test, can be used as a Biomarker or Surrogate Marker for dosage regimen calculation of antidepressant drugs that act on serotonergic regulation of the HPA axis. The SSRI drugs whose main action is the activation of serotonergic transmission, produce a decrease of plasma cortisol value obtained by Nugent`s test, in dose-dependent manner and can be used as surrogate marker of SERT-carrier occupation and 5-HT receptor activation by the Escitalopram and/or other SSRI drugs and to serve for their dosage regimen calculation (Bel & Artigas 1992; Berkenbosch et al 1987; Bosker et al 1994; Hsieh et al 2010; Ising et al 2005, 2007; Knorr et al 2011; Maes et al 1993; Meltzer 1985; Nordstrom & Farde 1998; Sasayama et al 2011; Schule et al 2009).

3.2.1 PK-PD model

PK-PD mechanistic-model. Around 50-60% of patients with depression have an increased activity of the hypothalamic-pituitary-adrenal axis and altered its regulation by negative feedback. Escitalopram and other SSRI produce an up-regulation of CRH receptors in a dose-dependent manner that can be measured by Nuggent`s test and this can be used for dosage regimen calculation of escitalopram and other SSRIs.

Once the steady-state and a pharmacological response, ranging between the 20-80% of maximal effect, is reached we can estimate the optimal dose required to achieve cortisol values of 9.0 ± 2.1 mcg/dl, its Clinical Surrogate Endpoint, using equation 2 (Lozano et al 2008a, 2011a).

3.2.2 PK-PG model

Metabolic studies for Escitalopram /Citalopram indicate that CYP3A4 and CYP2C19 are the major isozymes involved in N-demethylation of Escitalopram /Citalopram. The alleles

CYP2C19 * 2, CYP2C19 * 3 and CYP2C19 * 17 CYP2C19 and their combinations lead to phenotypes PM and IM, obtaining from the application of the equation 2, the following equi-effective dose ratios:

$$\frac{\text{DOSE}\left(\text{CYP2C19 phenotype}:\text{EM}\right)}{\text{DOSE}\left(\text{CYP2C19 phenotype}:\text{IM}\right)}=2 \text{ and } \frac{\text{DOSE}\left(\text{CYP2C19 phenotype}:\text{EM}\right)}{\text{DOSE}\left(\text{CYP2C19 phenotype}:\text{PM}\right)}=4$$

Paroxetine, Fluoxetine and Sertraline, which are metabolized by the CYP2D6 whose activity ranges considerably within a population and includes Ultrafast metabolizers, UM, Extensive metabolizers, EM, Intermediate metabolizers,IM, and Poor metabolizers, PM. Among these are fully functional alleles, alleles with reduced function and null, non-functional, alleles, which convey a wide range of enzyme activity, from no activity to ultrarapid metabolism of substrates. Null alleles of CYP2D6 do not encode a functional protein and have no detectable residual enzymatic activity, being responsibles for the PM phenotype in homozygous and for IM phenotype in heterozygous, when to present (Zhou 2008), obtaining from the application of the equation 2, the following equi-effective dose ratios:

$$\frac{\text{DOSE}\left(\text{CYP2D6 phenotype}:\text{EM}\right)}{\text{DOSE}\left(\text{CYP2D6 phenotype}:\text{IM}\right)}=2 \text{ and } \frac{\text{DOSE}\left(\text{CYP2D6 phenotype}:\text{EM}\right)}{\text{DOSE}\left(\text{CYP2D6 phenotype}:\text{PM}\right)}=4$$

(Lozano et al 2008a).

3.3 Antipsychotics

Schizophrenia first described by Benedict Morel in 1853 and with a prevalence of 1% in the general population, represents a group of chronic and severe mental disorders. Although its origin is unknown, there is an increased dopaminergic activity in the mesolimbic pathway of the brain. This biochemical alteration is used as target for the drug treatment of this disease, being the blockade of dopamine D_2 receptors in the limbic system important for the control of the psychotic symptoms and the blockade of $5HT_{2a}$ receptor for the control of negative symptoms.

Despite the unknown action mechanism of antipsychotic drug, is known that all of them act on the dopaminergic system but their affinitiy for dopamin and serotonin receptors,D_2 and 5-HT, are different, being necessary the blockade of these receptors for its pharmacological action, being the combined blockade of the receptors $5\text{-}HT_{2a}$ and D_2 a method that evidence has proposed for the treatment of schizophrenia (Horacek et al 2006).

Prolactin plasma level, PRL, reflects the tuberoinfundibular D_2 blockade and can be used as a Biomarker or Surrogate Marker for drugs affecting dopaminergic system and, in general, for atypical antipsychotics which main action was the blockade of D_2 receptors, since they produce a dose-dependent prolactin increase that can be used as a surrogate for D_2 receptor occupation and to serve at the same time for the dose adjustment and/or, by extension, the absence of prolactin increase levels after antipsychotic treatment could be considered a surrogate of a decrease occupancy of the D_2 receptor, as for Aripiprazole. Eventually, low occupancy of D_2 receptors in the striatum can be used as Surrogate Marker for the likelyhood of motor side effects (Avrantis & Miller 1997; Kapur et al 2000; Meltzer 1985; Nordstrom & Farde 1998).

Prolactin plasma levels are also high in several drug treatments, such as: (a) Those that are expected to increase extracellular 5-HT levels in the brain as L-tryptophan, and 5-hydroxytrytophan, (b) those that acting stimulating different types of 5HT receptors, and some, but not all, $5HT_{1a}$ selective agonists. In all these cases, prolactin plasma level becomes a surrogate of the increase of serotonergic transmission in one or more regions of the brain. The blockade of this effect, by an antagonist drug of the 5-HT receptors, appropriate and specific, can serve, in turn, as a substitute for the ability of a drug for the functional antagonization of the receptor (Goddard 1993; Golden et al 1989; Murphy et al 1996;; Seibyl et al 1991; Seletti et al 1995; Silverstone & Cowen 1994).

3.3.1 Risperidone

Risperidone, an atypical antipsychotic with high affinity for dopamine receptors D_2 and Serotonin $5\text{-}HT_{2a}$, produces a dose-dependent D_2 receptor occupancy in the mesolimbic system, necessary for the control of the disease, while the blockade in the nigrostriatal would be responsible for extrapyramidal side effects and in the tuberoinfundibular of the hiperprolactinemy.

3.3.1.1 PK-PD model

Mechanistic-model. Risperidone produces a blockade of D_2 receptor in the tuberoinfundibular system causing a dose-dependent increase in prolactin that can be used for dosing it. Using the values of serum prolactin, obtained in the morning before administration of Risperidone and not before steady-state plasma levels , minimum concentration in "steady-state", are reached we can construct the dose-response curve of prolactin plasma level versus Risperidone dose, which fits a rectangular modified hyperbola, equation 5, and permit us to establish a maximum value of PRL= 80-90 (40-45) ng/ml and a minimum value of PRL= 40-50 (20-25) ng/ml, for the optimal dose of risperidone, in women and men, in parentheses (Lozano et al 2007, 2010c):

$$PRL = \frac{84 Risp^2}{90 + Risp^2} \tag{5}$$

3.3.1.2 PK-PG model

Risperidone is eliminated by metabolism mainly through the action of citochrome CYP2D6, and to a lesser extent through CYP3A4. Risperidone and its main metabolite, 9-OH-risperidone, constitute the "active fraction" with an elimination half-life of 6 and 24 hours, respectively, in extensive metabolisers, EM, and 20 and 30 h in the case of patients with phenotype "poor metabolizer" PM. The "clearance", Cl, for the active fraction of Risperidone is respectively of 5.0 and 13.7 l/h in EM subjects and 3.2 and 3.3 l/h in individuals PM (Janssen Research Foundation 1994).

The CYP2D6 activity ranges considerably within a population and includes Ultrafast metabolizers, UM, Extensive metabolizers, EM, Intermediate metabolizers,IM, and Poor metabolizers, PM. Among these are fully functional alleles, alleles with reduced function and null, non-functional, alleles, which convey a wide range of enzyme activity, from no activity to ultrarapid metabolism of substrates. Null alleles of CYP2D6 do not encode a functional protein and have no detectable residual enzymatic activity, being responsibles for the PM phenotype in homozygous and for IM phenotype in heterozygous, when to present (Zhou 2008), obtaining from the application of the equation 2, the following equi-effective dose ratios:

$$\frac{\text{DOSE}\left(\text{CYP2D6 phenotype}:\text{EM}\right)}{\text{DOSE}\left(\text{CYP2D6 phenotype}:\text{IM}\right)}=1.5 \quad \text{and} \quad \frac{\text{DOSE}\left(\text{CYP2D6 phenotype}:\text{EM}\right)}{\text{DOSE}\left(\text{CYP2D6 phenotype}:\text{PM}\right)}=3$$

(Lozano et al 2007, 2010c).

3.3.1.3 PD-PG model

The poblational analysis of PRL values, using Kernel`s test, allowed us to detect two subpopulations, sex-linked, and related to an alteration of the dopaminergic and / or serotonergic pathways, caused by a combination of polymorphisms of the genes encoding receptors 5-HT_{2a} , D_2, and SERT, among others, obtaining from the application of the equation 2, the following equi-effective dose ratio:

$$\frac{\text{DOSE}\left(\text{genotype: wild type}\right)}{\text{DOSE}\left(\text{genotype: polimorphic type}\right)}=0.4\,/\,2.5$$

in men and women, respectivily (Lozano et al 2007, 2010c).

3.3.2 Clozapine and olanzapine

Since the HPA axis regulation appears altered in patients with schizophrenia, its modulation may be relevant for the control of symptoms in schizophrenia and antipsychotic treatment response. Otherwise, cortisol can be used as surrogate of the $5HT_{2a}$ receptor blockade, the receptor that has manifested itself as the most important in the serotonergic regulation of HPA axis and, thus, can be used as Surrogate Marker for dosing antipsychotics that act predominantly on the serotonergic pathways (Marx & Lieberman 1998; Meltzer et al 2001; Morrow et al 1995). Moreover, the alteration of the HPA axis, induced by antipsychotic with capacity for serotoninergic antagonism, that bind strongly to receptors 5-$HT_{2a/2c}$, can be used to modulate the response of cortisol and, eventually, to suppress the axis and to cause a decrease of the corticotropin-releasing factor, CRF, and the adrenocorticotropin hormone, ACTH (Morrow et al 1995; Patchev et al 1994).

Clozapine and Olanzapine, a $5HT_{2a}$ antagonists, show strong affinity for some dopamine receptors, but weak ability to antagonize the D_2 receptor, a receptor that modulates the neuroleptic activity. Evidence has shown that cortisol levels achieved in individuals treated with olanzapine and clozapine are dose dependent and directly proportional to the plasma concentrations of these drugs, at the start of antipsychotic treatment and along it.

Not only Olanzapine and Clozapine have shown a dose-dependent effect on the plasma cortisol levels, Risperidone also has significant effects but less pronounced compared with Olanzapine and Clozapine, whereas, Haloperidol has more modest effects. Olanzapine and Clozapine produce a cortisol increases, Δ-delta, up to 4-5 times higher than those produced by Haloperidol, while, risperidone produces a cortisol increases almost 1.5 times greater than observed with Haloperidol. Therefore, antipsychotics dosage are suitable to be monitored by using cortisol plasma levels (Girdler et al 2001).

3.3.2.1 PK-PD model

Mechanistic-model. Clozapine and Olanzapine, among other antipsychotics, cause an increase plasma cortisol levels in a dose-dependent manner, so the daily dosage has to be increased or decreased in order to reach cortisol plasma levels of 19.6 ± 6.6 mcg / dL and 18.3 ± 5.3 mcg / dL, the Clinical Surrogate Endpoint for Clozapine or Olanzapine, respectively (Lozano et al 2007, 2008a, 2010c, 2011a).

Once the steady-state and a pharmacological response, ranging between the 20-80% of maximal effect, is reached, we can estimate the optimal dose required to achieve cortisol values of 19.6 ± 6.6 mcg / dL and 18.3 ± 5.3 mcg / dL, the Clinical Surrogate Endpoints for Clozapine or Olanzapine, respectively, using equation 2 (Lozano et al 2008a, 2011a).

3.3.2.2 PK-PD model

Clozapine and Olanzapine are extensively metabolized in the liver, via the cytochrome P450 system, to polar metabolites suitable for its elimination in the urine and faeces. The CYP1A2 isoenzyme is primarily responsible for metabolism of Clozapine and Olanzapine , but another CYP`s seems to play a role, as well. Inducers agents, e.g. cigarette smoke, or inhibitor agents, e.g. Theophylline, Ciprofloxacin, Fluvoxamine, of the CYP1A2 may increase or decrease, respectively, the metabolism of Clozapine and Olanzapine. For example, the induction of metabolism caused by smoking means, that smokers would require double up the dose of Clozapine and/or Olanzapine compared with non-smokers ir order to achieve an equivalent plasma concentration (Entrez Gene 2011).

3.3.2.3 PD-PG model

The poblational analysis of plasma cortisol levels, using Kernel`s test , allow us to detect 2 populations, sex-linked and related to an alterations of the dopaminergic and/or serotonergic, caused by a combination of the different polymorphisms of genes encoding SERT and 5-HT_{2a} receptor, among others, obtaining from the application of the equation 2, the following equi-effective dose ratio:

$$\frac{\text{DOSE}\ (\text{genotype : wild type})}{\text{DOSE}\ (\text{genotype : polimorphic type})} = 2 \text{ or } 4$$

in dependence of the variant alleles present (Lozano et al 2008a, 2010c).

3.4 Methadone

The reduction of the testosterone levels induced by drugs with opioid activity, seems to be receptor mediated, since the different isomers have different activities: the levorotatory isomers are much more effective than dextrorotatory isomers (Cicero et al 1974, 1975, 1976, 1977; Mendelson et al 1976).

There are many different studies showing that the relative potency of drugs to reduce serum testosterone levels is parallel to its analgesic activity and its affinity for opioid receptors in the brain. So, this ability to decrease plasma testosterone and/or urine can be used as a trial to evaluate the structure-activity relationship, kinetic constants of association-dissociation to receptors, and reach conclusions about their pharmacological potency and its optimal therapeutic dose (Cicero et al 1975, Mendelson et al 1976).

The ability of opioid drugs to reduce serum testosterone levels, also, can be effectively used as a measure to assess the pharmacological activity of Methadone. Therefore, indirect assessment of the Methadone concentration in the biophase, can be accomplished by using the test of depletion of testosterone or test of depletion of LH that, also, seems to be specific for narcotic effect and correlates well with changes in testosterone levels (Kosterlitz & Warp 1968; Lozano et al 2008b, 2009b; Snyder 1975).

3.4.1 PK-PD model

Methadone, among other opiate drugs, causes a decrease in the value of index, testosterone/creatinine in urine, in a dose-dependent manner. We can dose Methadone by increasing o decreasing the daily dosage to reach index values of 20-30 mg / g, the Clinical Surrogate Endpoint. (Lozano et al 2008b, 2009b).

Once the steady-state and a pharmacological response, ranging between the 20-80% of maximal effect, is reached we can estimate the optimal dose required to achieve its Clinical Surrogate Endpoint, using equation 2

3.4.2 PK-PG model

Poblational analysis of the index, testosterone/creatinine in urine, using Kernel`s test , have allowed us to detect 3 different populations, as a result of combination of the different polymorphisms affecting the genes that encode CYP3A, CYP2B6, and NAT2, obtaining from the application of the equation 2, the following equi-effective dose ratio:

$$\frac{\text{DOSE (genotype : wild type)}}{\text{DOSE (genotype : polimorphic type)}} = 2 \text{ or } 4$$

in dependence of the variant alleles present (Lozano et al 2008b, 2009b).

3.5 Lamotrigine

Lamotrigine is a drug specifically used for epilepsy but also is effective as a mood stabilizer in treating bipolar depression, one of the most intractable stages of this disorder. Its iatrogenic effects, rare but extremely serious, such as Stevens-Johnson syndrome or Lyell syndrome, usually appear at 2-8 weeks of starting treatment. With unknown mechanism of action, it is believed that acts on sodium channels, its use is reserved for prevention of depressive episodes in bipolar disorder.

Lamotrigine is eliminated from the body by the action of the UGT1A4 enzyme, competing with bilirubin for the formation of their respective conjugates with glucuronide acid. Taking advantage of this interaction over UGT1A4, we can use bilirubin plasma levels as a indicator of plasma Lamotrigine concentration (French 2004; Lees & Leach 1993; Pellock 1999; Ramsay et al 1991; Rogawski & Löscher 2004).

The influence of bilirubin and other inhibitors of the UGT1A4 enzyme, on plasma concentrations of Lamotrigine, is calculated assuming a Michaelis-Menten kinetics, using equation 4, and a competitive inhibition model, as follows:

$$\Delta[Ltg] = \frac{\Delta[Bil]}{[E_o]^2 K_{M_{Ltg}} K_{M_{Bil}}} \quad (6)$$

(E_o = [UGT], K_M = Michaelis-Menten Constant)
(Bil= Bilirrubina, Ltg= Lamotrigina, Inh= Inhibidor)

allowing us to conclude that the main factors affecting Cp of Lamotrigine are the amount of UGT enzyme (Eo) and K_M values of inhibitors with respect to those of Lamotrigine and Bilirubin, according to the following relation:

$$\frac{\Delta[Ltg]}{\Delta[Inh]} = \frac{K_{M_{Inh}}}{K_{M_{Ltg}}} \quad (7)$$

This method described above allows the analysis of the main factors affecting competitive inhibition between two substrates, such as: UGT enzyme concentration, exponentially, and K_M value of substrates (Lozano et al 2009a, 2009b, 2010d).

3.5.1 PK-PG model

Is based on individual genetic polymorphisms which can alter the enzymatic activity of UGT1A1: The enzyme that conjugates bilirubin is called uridindifosfoglucuronato glucuronosyltransferase,UGT, and its production is regulated by a promoter that can have a mutation that causes decreased production of this enzyme. The amounts of UGT, in Gilbert's syndrome, are reduced until 30% of the normal value. The genetic defect is in the insertion of an extra base pair in the promoter TATA box in the gene encoding the enzyme UGT and that is located on chromosome 2 (Bosma et al 1995). Gilbert's syndrome, therefore, is a disease in which there is a high bilirubin level and the values in these patients ranging between 20 mmol/dl and 80 mmol/dl, obtaining from the application of the equation 6, the following equi-effective dose ratio for Lamotrigine:

$$\frac{\text{DOSE (genotype : wild type)}}{\text{DOSE (genotype : Gilbert`s syndrome)}} = 2$$

(Lozano et al 2009a, 2009c, 2010d).

3.6 New antiepileptics

The new generation of AEDs such as Topiramate, Oxcarbazepine, Gabapentin, and Levetiracetam, acts by enhancing GABAergic neurotransmission: The gamma-aminobutyric acid, GABA, has 2 types of receptors, A and B. When GABA binds to $GABA_A$ receptor, facilitates the passage of chlorine, negatively charged ion, inside the cell through chloride channels. This influx of chloride increases the negativity of the cell (ie, a resting potential more negative membrane) causing it a greater difficulty to reach the action potential resulting, finally, in a cell stabilization (Barnard et al 1998; Kravitz et al 1963; Krnjević & Schwartz 1967; Sieghart & Sperk 2002; Takeuchi & Onodera 1972; Takeuchi & Takeuchi 1967, 1969).

The GABAergic transmission, may be increased or facilitated, by direct binding of an agonist, such as progesterone, benzodiazepines, barbiturates, to the $GABA_A$ receptors and its subsequent activation; by blocking the presynaptic uptake of GABA by Tiagabine; by inhibiting the metabolism of GABA by GABA-transaminase, such as Vigabatrin and Valproate, or by increasing GABA synthesis modulating the enzyme glutamic acid decarboxylase, GAD, responsible for the decarboxylation of glutamate to GABA, as is the case of Gabapentin and other AEDs that enhance the production of GABA and causes a down-regulation of glutamate. For Felbamate, whose exact mechanism is unknown, it is known that exerts its effect on the GABA receptor and by antagonizing the NMDA receptor, while, Topiramato locks the sodium channels of voltage-gated and increases the activity of GABA through the activation of some subtype of GABA receptors, antagonizing some subtype of glutamate receptor and inhibiting the enzyme carbonic anhydrase, particularly isozymes II and IV (Kapetanovic et al 1998; Kume al 1994).

The GH plasma levels, also, have been used as a Surrogate Marker of noradrenergic transmission and, more recently, as evidence of $5HT_{1a}$ and $5HT_{1b/d1}$ receptor activation, being this another example of how one Surrogate Marker serves as measure for very different effects in the CNS (Dinan 1996; Facchinetti et al 1994; Herdman et al 1994; Laakman al 1990; Mota et al 1997).

3.6.1 PK-PD model

The GH plasma levels, can serve as a Surrogate Marker for assessing the GABAergic transmission in the CNS and is therefore a useful tool for dosage regimen calculation of the new antiepileptic drugs and for the right choice of therapeutic strategy, since, the oral administration of drugs that facilitates GABAergic transmission, among them the antiepileptics, cause a rise of growth hormone plasma levels, GH, in a dose-dependent manner, being GH release induced by gamma-aminobutyric acid, GABA, and mediated by a dopaminergic mechanism, via dopamine release at suprapituitary level (Cavagnini et al 1980a, 1980b; Powers et al 2008).

Thus, eg, Diazepam administration causes a dose-dependent rise in GH and the reached plasmatic peak is related to the plasma level of the drug. This highly significant correlation of the serum concentrations, between GH and Diazepam, has been found, also, with other AEDs, that act via the release or facilitation of GABAergic transmission, so we can use the plasma levels of GH as a Biomarker for dose adjustment of Diazepam, Topiramate, Gabapentin, Oxcarbazepine, Valproate and Levetiracetam, being the optimal dose, that which allow us to achieve the Clinical Surrogate Endpoint of GH equal to 15-25 ng/ml (Monteiro et al 1990; Monteleone et al 1987; Syvälahti & Kanto 1975).

Once the steady-state and a pharmacological response, ranging between the 20-80% of maximal effect, is reached we can estimate the optimal dose required to achieve the Clinical Surrogate Endpoint of GH equal to 15-25 ng/ml, using equation 2.

4. Conclusion

In this chapter, we have developed some PK, PD and PG models , in order to study and monitor the effectiveness, dosage regimen calculation and security of drugs used in psychiatry, by means of Biomarkers of drug concentration in biophase and the incorporation of all the most innovative techniques in pharmacokinetics, pharmacodynamics and pharmacogenetics , which allow us to:

1. Estimate their pharmacokinetic and pharmacodynamic parameters, using for this purpose, PK-PD, PK-PD and PG-PG modelling, and quantitative analysis of dose-effect relationships with mathematical covariant techniques.
2. Quantify the effect of different genetic polymorphisms of CYP450, receptors and carriers, in dosage regimen calculation of different drugs above described.
3. Identify, using Kernel`s test, the different phenotypes and subpopulations originated in the different dose-response and metabolic behavior, such as the EM, PM and UM phenotypes.

In conclusion, the use of Biomarkers in PK, PD and PG modelling, in continuos developing, has provided us with the adequate tools to choose the best therapeutic strategy and calculate optimal dose, in order to improve the therapeutic drug monitoring of psychiatric drugs, relapses, drug side effects and clinical outcome of the most common psychiatric diseases. http://cpmc.coriell.org/Sections/Medical/DrugsAndGenes_mp.aspx?PgId=216.

5. References

American Psychiatric Association (2000). *Diagnostic and statistical manual of mental disorders*, APA eds., 4th ed.

Avissar S, Schreiber G (2002). Toward molecular diagnostics of mood disorders in psychiatry. *Trends Mol Med*, 8(6):294-300.

Avrantis LA, Miller BG (1997). Multiple fixed doses of "Seroquel"(quetiapine) in patients with acute exacerbation of schizophrenia:a comparison with haloperidol and placebo: the Seroquel Trial 13 Study Group. *Biol Psychiatry*, 42:233–246.

Barnard EA, Skolnick P, Olsen RW, Mohler H, Sieghart W, Biggio G, Braestrup C, Bateson AN, Langer SZ (1998). International Union of Pharmacology. XV. Subtypes of gamma-aminobutyric acidA receptors: classification on the basis of subunit structure and receptor function. *Pharmaco Rev*, 50 (2): 291–313.

Bauer JA, Balthasar JP, and Fung HL (1997). Application of pharmacodynamic modeling for designing time-variant dosing regimens to overcome nitroglycerin tolerance in experimental heart failure. *Pharm Res*, 14:1140-1145

Bel N and Artigas F (1992). Fluvoxamine preferentially increases extracellular 5-hydroxytryptamine in the raphe nuclei: an in vivo microdialysis study. *Eur J Pharmacol*, 229:101-103.

Berkenbosch F, van Oers J, del Rey A, Tilders F, Besedovsky H (1987). Corticotropin-releasing factor-producing neurons in the rat activated by interleukin-1. *Science*, 238:524-526.

Biomarkers Definitions Working Group (2001). Biomarkers and surrogate endpoints: preferred definitions and conceptual framework. *Clin Pharmacol Ther*, 69:89-95.

Bosker FJ, Donker MG, Klompmakers AA, Kurata K, and Westenberg HG (1994). 5-Hydroxytryptamine release in dorsal hippocampus of freely moving rats: modulation by pindolol. *Prog Neuropsychopharmacol Biol Psychiatry*, 18:765-778.

Bosma PJ, Chowdhury JR, Bakker C, Gantla S, de Boer A, Oostra BA, Lindhout D, Tytgat GN, Jansen PL, Oude Elferink RP, et al (1995).. The genetic basis of the reduced expression of bilirubin UDP-glucuronosyltransferase 1 in Gilbert's syndrome. *New England Journal of Medicine.*

Breimer DD and Danhof M (1997). Relevance of the application of pharmacokinetic-pharmacodynamic modelling concepts in drug development. The "wooden shoe' paradigm. *Clin Pharmacokinet,* 32:259-267.

Brockmöller J, Tzvetkov MV (2008).Pharmacogenetics: data, concepts and tools to improve drug discovery and drug treatment. *Eur J Clin Pharmacol,* 64 (2): pp. 133-57.

Brown, E. Sherwood (2006). Trastorno bipolar. Elsevier, ISBN 8445816489, España.

Buckley TM, Schatzberg AF (2009). A pilot study of the phase angle between cortisol and melatonin in major depression - A potential biomarker?. J Psychiatr Res.

Cavagnini F, Invitti C, Pinto M, Maraschini C, Di Landro A, Dubini A, Marelli A (1980a).Effect of acute and repeated administration of gamma aminobutyric acid (GABA) on growth hormone and prolactin secretion in man. Acta Endocrinol , 93(2):149-54.

Cavagnini F, Benetti G, Invitti C, Ramella G, Pinto M, Lazza M, Dubini A, Marelli A, Müller EE. (1980b).Effect of gamma-aminobutyric acid on growth hormone and prolactin secretion in man: influence of pimozide and domperidone. J Clin Endocrinol Metab, 51(4):789-92.

Cicero TJ , Meyer ER , Bell RD and Wizs'r W (1974). Effects of morphine on the secondary sex organs and plasma testosterone levels of rats. *Res Commun Chem Pathob Phanmacob,* 7: 17-24.

Cicero TJ, Bell RD, Wies'r WG, Allison JH , PoiıKosiu K and Robins E (1975). Function of the male sex ongans in heroin and methadone users. *N Eng J Med,* 292: 882-887.

Cicero TJ , Meyer ER , Bell RD and Koch GA (1976). Effects of morphine and methadone on testosterone, lutoinizing hormone and the secondary sex organs of the male rat. *Endocrinology,* 98: 365-370.

Cicero TJ, Bell RD, Meyer ER and Schweitzer J (1977). Narcotics and the hypothalamicpituitary-gonadal axis: Acute effects on lutoinizmg hormone, testosterone and androgon-dopendont systems. *J Pharmacol Exp Ther,* 201: 76-83.

Cowen PJ (1998). Use of surrogate markers in clinical psychopharmacology.In: Balant LP, Benitez J, Dahl SG, et al., eds. *Clinical pharmacology in psychiatry: finding the right dose of psychotropic drugs.* Brussels: European Commission: 151–160.

Csajka C and Verotta D (2006). Pharmacokinetic-Pharmacodynamic Modelling: History and Perspectives. *J Pharmacokinet Pharmacodyn,* 1-53.

Dayneka NL, Garg V, and Jusko WJ (1993). Comparison of four basic models of indirect pharmacodynamic responses. *J Pharmacokinet Biopharm,* 21:457-478.

Dinan TG (1996). Serotonin and the regulation of hypothalamic-pituitary-adrenal axis function. *Life Sci,* 58:1683–1694.

Dominguez- Gil A, Lanao JM (1999). Population pharmacokinetics of amikacin in patients with haematological malignancies. *J Antimic Chemother,* 44:235- 242.

Einat H, Kofman O, Itkin O, Lewitan RJ, Belmaker RH (1998). Augmentation of lithium's behavioral effect by inositol uptake inhibitors. *J Neural Transm,* 105 (1): 31–8.

Entrez Gene (2011). Cytochrome P450. Available in: http://jura.wi.mit.edu/entrez_gene

Facchinetti F, Nappi RE, Sances G, et al (1994).The neuroendocrine effects of sumatriptan, a specific ligand for 5-HT1-like receptors. *Clin Endocrinol* ,40:211–214.

Food and Drug Administration (2008).*Guidance for Industry: E15 Definitions for Genomic Biomarkers, Pharmacogenomics, Pharmacogenetics, Genomic Data and Sample Coding*

Categories. U.S. Department of Health and Human Services . Food and Drug Administration ed. Rockville USA.

Francheteau P, Steimer JL, Merdjan H, Guerret M, Dubray C (1993) .A mathematical model for dynamics of cardiovascular drug action: application to intravenous dihydropyridines in healthy volunteers. *J Pharmacokinet Biopharm*, 21: 489-514.

French JA, Kanner AM, Bautista J, et al. (2004). Efficacy and tolerability of the new antiepileptic drugs II: treatment of refractory epilepsy: report of the Therapeutics and Technology Assessment Subcommittee and Quality Standards Subcommittee of the American Academy of Neurology and the American Epilepsy Society. *Neurology*. 62 (8): 1261–73.

Gartside SE, Cowen PJ (1990). Mediation of ACTH and prolactin responses to 5-HTP by 5-HT2 receptors. *Eur J Pharmacol*, 173:103-9.

Geldof M (2007).In:*Mechanism-based PK/PD modeling of Selective Serotonin Reuptake Inhibitors Animal Behavioral Models for the Study of Depression*. University of Leyden ed.,Tesis

Ghasemi M, Sadeghipour H, Mosleh A, Sadeghipour HR, Mani AR, Dehpour AR (2008). Nitric oxide involvement in the antidepressant-like effects of acute lithium administration in the mouse forced swimming test. *Eur Neuropsychopharmacol*, 18 (5): 323–32.

Ghasemi M, Raza M, Dehpour AR (2009a). NMDA receptor antagonists augment antidepressant-like effects of lithium in the mouse forced swimming test. *J Psychopharmacol* ,24 (4): 585–94..

Ghasemi M, Sadeghipour H, Poorheidari G, Dehpour AR (2009b). A role for nitrergic system in the antidepressant-like effects of chronic lithium treatment in the mouse forced swimming test. *Behav Brain Res*, 200 (1): 76–82.

Girdler SS, Straneva PA, Light KC, Pedersen CA, Morrow AL (2001). Allopregnanolone levels and reactivity to mental stress in premenstrual dysphoric disorder. *Biological Psychiatry*, 49:788-797.

Goddard AW, Wood SW, Sholomskas DE, et al (1993). Effects of the serotonin reuptake inhibitor fluvoxamine on yohimbineinduced anxiety in panic disorder. *Psychiatry Res*, 3;48: 119–133.

Golden RN, Hsiao J, Lane E, et al (1989). The effects of intravenous clomipramine on neurohormones in normal subjects. *J Clin Endocrinol Metab*, 68:632.

Goodwin FK and Post RM (1983). 5-hydroxytryptamine and depression: a model for the interaction of normal variance with pathology. *Br J Clin Pharmacol* 15 Suppl, 3:393S-405S.

Herdman JRE, Delva NJ, Hockney RA, et al (1994). Neuroendocrine effects of sumatriptan. *Psychopharmacology*, 113:561–564.

Hill AV (1910). The possible effects of the aggregation of the molecules of haemoglobin on its dissociation curves. *J Physio Lond.*

Holford NH and Sheiner LB (1981). Understanding the dose-effect relationship: clinical application of pharmacokinetic-pharmacodynamic models. *Clin Pharmacokinet*, 6:429-453.

Holford NH and Sheiner LB (1982). Kinetics of pharmacologic response. *Pharmacol Ther*, 16:143-166.

Holsboer F (2001). Stress, hypercortisolism and corticosteroid receptors in depression: implications for therapy. *J Affect Disord*, 62:77-91.

Horacek J, Bubenikova-Valeova V, Kopecek M, Palenicek T, Dockery C, Mohr P & Höschl C (2006). Mechanism of Action of Atypical Antipsychotic Drugs and the Neurobiology of Schizophrenia. *Drugs*, 20(5) 389-405.

Hsieh CH, Li HY, Chen JC (2010). Nitric oxide and interleukin-1beta mediate noradrenergic induced corticotrophin-releasing hormone release in organotypic cultures of rat paraventricular nucleus. *Neuroscience*, 165:1191-1202.

http://cpmc.coriell.org/Sections/Medical/DrugsAndGenes_mp.aspx?PgId=216

http://www.gaba-network.org.

Ising M, Horstmann S, Kloiber S, Lucae S, Binder EB, Kern N, Kunzel HE, Pfennig A, Uhr M, Holsboer F (2007). Combined dexamethasone/corticotropin releasing hormone test predicts treatment response in major depression - a potential biomarker?. *Biol Psychiatry*, 62:47-54.

Ising M, Kunzel HE, Binder EB, Nickel T, Modell S, et al (2005). The combined dexamethasone/CRH test as a potential surrogate marker in depression. *Prog Neuropsychopharmacol Biol Psychiatry*, 29: 1085–1093.

Janssen Pharmaceutica (2004). *Risperdal: risperidone, clinical monograph.* Janssen Pharmaceutica. Janssen Research Foundation ed. ISBN 0444019057.

Jonker DM, Vermeij DA, Edelbroek PM, Voskuyl RA, Piotrovsky VK, and Danhof M (2003). Pharmacodynamic analysis of the interaction between tiagabine and midazolam with an Allosteric model that incorporates signal transduction. *Epilepsia*, 44:329-338.

Jusko WJ and Ko HC (1994). Physiologic indirect response models characterize diverse types of pharmacodynamic effects. *Clin Pharmacol Ther*, 56:406-419.

Kapetanovic IM, Torchin CD, Thompson CD, Miller TA, McNeilly PJ, MacdonaldTL, Kupferberg HJ, Perhach JL, Sofia RD, Strong JM (1998). Potentially reactive cycliccarbamate metabolite of the antiepileptic drug felbamate produced by human livertissue in vitro. *Drug Metab Dispos*, 26(11):1089-95.

Kapur S, Zipursky R, Jones C, et al (2000). A positron emission tomography study of quetiapine in schizophrenia: a preliminary finding of an antipsychotic effect with only transiently high dopamine D2 receptor occupancy.**Arch Gen Psychiatry**,57: 553–9.

Kemperman RFJ (2007). *Nutrition and Biomarkers in Psychiatry*. University of Groningen Ed., Groningen. ISBN: 978-90-367-3220-8.

Kemperman RFJ, Kema IP, Knegtering H, Bischoff R, Muskiet FAJ (2007). *Nutrition and Biomarkers in Psychiatry. Biomarker research in mental disorders Linking biomarkers to etiology*. University of Groningen ed. ISBN: 978-90-367-3220-8.

Kessler J, Obinger C Eales, G (2008). Factors Influencing the Study of Peroxidase-Generated Iodine Species and Implications for Thyroglobulin Synthesis. *Thyroid*, 18(7) : 769-74.

Knorr U, Vinberg M, Hansen A, Klose M, Feldt-Rasmussen U, Hilsted L, Hasselstrøm J, Gether U, Winkel P, Gluud C, Wetterslev J, Kessing LV (2011). PLoS One, 6(6):e21224.

Kosterlitz HW and Warp AJ (1968). Kinetic parameters of narcotic agonists and antagonists, with particular reference to N-ablylnoroxymorphino(naboxone). *Brit J Pharmacol*, 33: 266-276.

Kravitz EA, Kuffler SW, Potter DD (1963). Gamma-aminobutyric acid and other blocking compounds in crustacea. III. Their relative concentrations in separated motor and inhibitory axons. *J Neurophysiol*, 26: 739–51.

Krnjević K, Schwartz S (1967). The action of gamma-aminobutyric acid on cortical neurones. *Exp Brain Res*, 3 (4): 320–36.

Kume A, Greenfield LJ, Macdonald RL, Albin RL (1996). Felbamate inhibits [3Ht-butylbicycloorthobenzoate (TBOB) binding and enhances Cl- current at the gamma-aminobutyric AcidA (GABAA) receptor. *J Pharmacol Exp Ther*, 277 (3): 1784–92.

Laakman G, Hinz A, Voderholzer U, et al (1990). The influence of psychotropic drugs and releasing hormones on anterior pituitary hormone secretion in healthy subjects and depressed patients. *Pharmacopsychiatry*,23:18–26

Lakhan SE, Vieira K and Hamlat E (2010) . Biomarkers in psychiatry: drawbacks and potential for misuse. *Int Arch Med*, 3:1.

Lees G, Leach MJ (1993). Studies on the mechanism of action of the novel anticonvulsant lamotrigine (Lamictal) using primary neurological cultures from rat cortex. *Brain Research*, 612 (1-2): 190–9.

Lozano R, Marín R, Andrés I, Pascual A, San Juan P, Pardo C (2007). Utilización de la prolactina como biomarcador en los tratamientos con risperidona parenteral. In: *Libro de ponencias y comunicaciones del 52º congreso de la SEFH*. Tenerife. Available from: http://www.sefh.es/sefhpublicaciones/detallecomunicacion.php?id=2244

Lozano R, Marín R, Andrés I, Pascual A, Orea B, Santacruz M J (2008a). El test de nugent como biomarcador en pacientes tratados con escitalopram. In: Libro de ponencias y comunicaciones del 53º congreso de la SEFH. SEFH eds., Valencia. Available from: http://www.sefh.es/53congreso/documentos/comunicaciones/108.pdf:

Lozano R, Domeque N, Andrés I, González J, Perálvarez C, Torrellas D (2008b). Estudio de la variabilidad posologica de metadona en pacientes incluidos en un programa de mantenimiento de una unidad de conductas adictivas. In: *Libro de ponencias y comunicaciones del 53º congreso de la SEFH*. SEFH eds.,Valencia. Available from : http://www.sefh.es/53congreso/documentos/posters/087.pdf.

Lozano R, Garcia M, Andres I, Sebastian F, Bolea M, De la fuente F (2009a). Uso de la bilirrubinemia como biomarcador de la concentracion plasmatica de rifampicina: implicaciones clinicas. In: *Libro de ponencias y comunicaciones del 54 congreso de La SEFH*. SEFH eds. Zaragoza, Available from:
http://www.congresosefh2009.es/buscarPosters.aspx?idTema=6

Lozano R, Domeque N, Riba V, Perálvarez C, Andrés I, Torrellas D (2009b). Estudio del indice urinario testosterona/creatinina como biomarcador en los tratamientos con metadona y su aplicación al analisis poblacional farmacogenetico. *Farm Hosp*, 33 (Espec Congr):384-385.

Lozano R, Marín R, Pascual A, Santacruz MJ, De Miguel S, Vázquez D (2009c). Influencia de la inhibicion e induccion de la UDP glucuronil transferasa (ugt) en la farmacocinetica de lamotrigina. In: *Libro de ponencias y comunicaciones del 54 congreso de la SEFH*. SEFH eds., Zaragoza, available from:
http://www.congresosefh2009.es/buscarPosters.aspx?idTema=6

Lozano R (2010a).Lithium clearly and directly affects the activity of the thyroid gland in human. *Hum Psychopharmacol*, 25(7-8):586.

Lozano R, Marín R, Pascual A, Vázquez D, Santacruz MJ, Sebastián F, (2010b).¿Es útil la concentración plasmática de tiroxina libre como biomarcador para el cálculo de regímenes posológicos de sales de litio?. *Psiquiatr Biol*, 17:140.

Lozano R, Marín R, Pascual A, Santacruz MJ, Sebastián F (2010c). Is prolactin a useful biomarker for risperidone dosage adjustment?. *Psiquiatria.com*, 14:4.

Lozano R, Apesteguia AF, Martinez A, Lozano A, Velilla A (2010d). Analisis farmacocinetico de la interaccion bilirrubina-lopinavir sobre el transportador OATP1B1. In: *Libro de ponencias y comunicaciones del 55 congreso de la SEFH*. SEFH ed.. Madrid. Available from:Http://55congreso.sefh.es/buscarPosters.aspx?idTema=9

Lozano R, Marín R, Pascual A, Vázquez MD, Santacruz M J, Sebastián F (2011a). Is the nugent test a useful biomarker for the escitalopram dosage?. *ECNP congress*, Paris.

Lozano R, Rebollar E, Morlanes T, Chávez F, Hernandez A y Mesa MP (2011b). Monitorización farmacocinética de digoxina en pacientes geriatricos. In: *Libro de ponencias y comunicaciones del 56 congreso de la SEFH*. SEFH ed., Santiago de Compostela, In press.

Maes M, Bosmans E, Meltzer HY, Scharpe S, Suy E (1993). Interleukin-1 beta: a putative mediator of HPA axis hyperactivity in major depression?. *Am J Psychiatry*, 150:1189-93.

Mager DE, Wyska E, and Jusko WJ (2003). Diversity of mechanism-based pharmacodynamic models. *Drug Metab Dispos*, 31:510-518.

Mandema JW, Tuk B, van Steveninck AL, Breimer DD, Cohen AF, and Danhof M (1992). Pharmacokinetic-pharmacodynamic modeling of the central nervous system effects of midazolam and its main metabolite alpha-hydroxymidazolam in healthy volunteers. *Clin Pharmacol Ther*, 51:715-728.

Mandema, J. W., Wada, D. R. (1995). Pharmacodynamic model for acute tolerance development to the electroencephalographic effects of alfentanil in the rat. *J Pharmacol Exp Ther*, 279: 1035-1042

Marx CE, Lieberman JA (1998). Psychoneuroendocrinology of schizophrenia. *Psychiatr Clin North Am*, 21(2):413-24

Meibohm B and Derendorf H (1997). Basic concepts of pharmacokinetic/pharmacodynamic (PK/PD) modelling. *Int J Clin Pharmacol Ther*, 35:401-413.

Meltzer HY (1985). Long-term effects of neuroleptic drugs on the neuroendocrine system. *Adv Biochem Psychopharmacol*, 40:59–68

Meltzer HY, Kolakowska T, Fang VS, et al (2001). Growth hormone and prolactin response to apomorphine in schizophrenia. *Arch Gen Psychiatry*, 58:1025-1031.

Meltzer HY, Maes M (1994). Effect of pindolol on the L-5-HTPinduced increase in plasma prolactin and cortisol concentrations in man. *Psychopharmacology*, 114:635–643.

Mendelson JH, Ilımtuı1usI CE, Renault P and Sinay EC (1976) Effects of acetylmethadol on plasma testosterone. *Clin Pharmacol Then*, 19:171-374.

Monteiro MG, Schuckit MA, Hauger R, Irwin M, Duthie LA (1990). Growth hormone response to intravenous diazepam and placebo in 82 healthy men. Biol Psychiatr, 1;27(7):702-10.

Monteleone P, Iovino M, Orio F, Steardo L (1987). Psychopharmacology, 91(1):10-3.

Morrow AL. Regulation of GABAa receptor function and gene expresionin the central nervous system. In: Bradley RJ and Harris RA (Eds), *International review of neurobiology*, pp. 1-14. Academic Press, New York.

Mota A, Bento A, Penalva A, et al (1995). Role of the serotonin receptor subtype 5-HT1D on basal and stimulated growth hormone secretion. *J Clin Endocrinol Metab*, 80:1973–77.

Murphy DL, Aulakh CS, Mazzola-Pomietto P, et al (1996). Neuroendocrine responses to serotonergic agonists as indices of the functional status of central serotonin neurotransmission in humans: a preliminary comparative analysis of neuroendocrine endpoints versus other endpoint measures. *Behav Brain Res*, 73:209–214.

Noll R (2006). The blood of the insane. *Hist Psychiatry*, 17(68 Pt 4):395-418.

Nordstrom AL, Farde L (1998). Plasma prolactin and central D2 receptor occupancy in antipsychotic drug-treated patients. *J Clin Psychopharmacol*, 18:305–310

Patchev VK, Shoaib M, Holsboer F, Almeida OF (1994). The neurosteroid tetrahydroprogesterone counteracts corticotropin-releasing hormoneinduced anxiety and alters the release and gene expression of corticotropin-releasing hormone in the rat hypothalamus. *Neuroscience*, 62 (1), 265–271.

Pellock JM (1999). Managing pediatric epilepsy syndromes with new antiepileptic drugs. Pediatrics, 104 (5 Pt 1): 1106–16.

Perez-Urizar J, Granados-Soto V, Flores-Murrieta FJ, and Castaneda-Hernandez G (2000). Pharmacokinetic-pharmacodynamic modeling: why?. *Arch Med Res*, 31:539-545.

Powers ME, Yarrow JF, McCoy SC, Borst SE (2008). Growth hormone isoform responses to GABA ingestion at rest and after exercise. Med Sci Sports Exerc, 40(1):104-10

Ragueneau I, Laveille C, Jochemsen R, Resplandy G, Funck-Brentano C, and Jaillon P (1998). Pharmacokinetic-pharmacodynamic modeling of the effects of ivabradine, a direct sinus node inhibitor, on heart rate in healthy volunteers. *Clin Pharmacol Ther*, 64:192-203.

Ramsay RE, Pellock JM, Garnett WR, et al. (1991). Pharmacokinetics and safety of lamotrigine (Lamictal) in patients with epilepsy. *Epilepsy Res*, 10 (2-3): 191–200.

Riggs BL, Hodgson SF, O'Fallon WM, Chao EYS, Wahner HW, Muhs JM et al (1990). Effect of fluoride treatment on the fracture rate in postmenopausal women with osteoporosis. *N Engl J Med*, 322:802–809.

Rogawski MA, Löscher W (2004). The neurobiology of antiepileptic drugs. *Nat Rev Neurosci* , 5 (7): 553–564.

Rowland M, Tozer TN (1995). *Clinical pharmacokinetics: concepts and applications*, Williams & Wilkins eds, Baltimore.

Russell K (2004) .Biomarkers and Surrogate Markers: An FDA Perspectiva. NeuroRx_: *The Journal of the American Society for Experimental NeuroTherapeutics*, Vol. 1, 189–195.

Sasayama D, Hori H, Iijima Y, Teraishi T, Hattori K, Ota M, Fujii T, Higuchi T, Amano N and Kunugi H (2011). Modulation of cortisol responses to the DEX/CRH test by polymorphisms of the interleukin-1beta gene in healthy adults .*Behavioral and Brain Functions*, 7:23.

Schnider TW, Minto CF, Bruckert H, and Mandema JW (1996). Population pharmacodynamic modeling and covariate detection for central neural blockade. *Anesthesiology*, 85:502-512.

Schule C, Baghai TC, Eser D, Hafner S, Born C, Herrmann S, Rupprecht R (2009). The combined dexamethasone/CRH Test (DEX/CRH test) and prediction of acute treatment response in major depression. *PLoS One*, 4:e4324.

Seibyl JP, Krystal JH, Price LH, et al (1991). Effects of ritanserin on the behavioural, neuroendocrine, and cardiovascular responses to meta-chlorophenylpiperazine in healthy human subjects. *Psychiatry Res*,3 8:227–236.

Seletti B, Benkelfat C, Blier P, Annable L, Gilbert F, de Montigny C (1995). Serotonin 1A receptor activation by flesinoxan in humans. Body temperature and neuroendocrine responses. *Neuropsychopharmacology*, 13:93–104

Sheiner LB, Beal SL, Dunne A (1997). Analysis of non-randomly censored ordered categorical longitudinal data from analgesic trials (with discussion). *Journal of the American Statistical Association*, 92: 1235-55.

Sheiner LB, Stanski DR, Vozeh S, Miller RD, and Ham J (1979). Simultaneous modeling of pharmacokinetics and pharmacodynamics: application to d-tubocurarine. *Clin Pharmacol Ther*, 25:358-371.

Sieghart W, Sperk G (2002). Subunit composition, distribution and function of GABA(A) receptor subtypes. *Curr Top Med Chem*, 2 (8): 795–816.

Silverstone PH, Cowen PJ (1994). The 5-HT3 antagonist BRL 46470 does not attenuate m-chlorophenylpiperazine (mCPP)-induced changes in human volunteers. *Biol Psychiatry*, 36:309–316.

Snyder SM (1975). Opiate receptor in normal and drug altered brain function. *Nature*, 257: 185- 189.

Syvälahti EK, Kanto JH (1975). Serum growth hormone, serum immunoreactive insulin and blood glucose response to oral and intravenous diaz in man. Int J Clin Pharmacol Biopharm, 12(1-2):74-82.

Takeuchi A, Takeuchi N (1967). Anion permeability of the inhibitory post-synaptic membrane of the crayfish neuromuscular junction. *J Physiol*, 191 (3): 575–90.

Takeuchi A, Takeuchi N (1969). A study of the action of picrotoxin on the inhibitory neuromuscular junction of the crayfish. *J Physiol*, 205 (2): 377–91.

Takeuchi A, Onodera K (1972). Effect of bicuculline on the GABA receptor of the crayfish neuromuscular junction. *Nature New Biol*, 236 (63): 55–6.

Taylor, J.E. Evans, M. I. (1953). The Ohio Journal of Science, v 53:37-41.Tetrahydroprogesterone attenuates the endocrine response to stress and exerts glucocorticoid-like effects on vasopressin gene transcription inthe rat hypothalamus. *Neuropsychopharmacology*, 15 (6), 533–540.

Tsai YJ, Hoyme HE (2002). Pharmacogenomics: the future of drug therapy. *Clin Genet*, 62 (4): pp. 257–64.

Van der Graaf PH and Danhof M (1997). Analysis of drug-receptor interactions in vivo: a new approach in pharmacokinetic-pharmacodynamic modelling. *Int J Clin Pharmacol Ther*, 35:442-446.

Weinshilboum RM, Wang L (2006). Pharmacogenetics and pharmacogenomics: development, science, and translation. *Annu Rev Genomics Hum Genet*, 7: pp. 223-45.

Wessa P. (2008). Kernel Density Estimation (v1.0.6) in *Free Statistics Software (v1.1.23-r7)*, Office for Research Development and Education, Available from. http://www.wessa.net/rwasp_density.wasp/

WHO (2001). *The world health report 2001 - Mental Health: New Understanding*, New Hope. Geneva.

WHO (2005). *Mental health, facing the challenges, building solutions*. Report from the European ministerial conference.Kobenhavn.

Zhou SF (2009). Polymorphism of human cytochrome P450 2D6 and its clinical significance: Part I. *Clin Pharmacokine*, 48(11):689-723

Zuideveld KP, Maas HJ, Treijtel N, Graaf PH, Peletier LA, Danhof M (2001). A set-point model with oscillatory behaviour predicts the time course of (8-)-OH-DPAT induced hypothermia. *Am J Physiol*, 281: R2059-R2071

8

Genotoxicity Biomarkers: Application in Histopathology Laboratories

Carina Ladeira[1,2], Susana Viegas[1,2], Elisabete Carolino[1], Manuel Carmo Gomes[3] and Miguel Brito[1]

[1]*Escola Superior de Tecnologia da Saúde de Lisboa, Instituto Politécnico de Lisboa,*
[2]*Centro de Investigação e Estudos em Saúde Pública, Universidade Nova de Lisboa,*
[3]*Faculdade de Ciências, Universidade de Lisboa,*
Portugal

1. Introduction

Most cancers results from man-made and natural environmental exposures (such as tobacco smoke; chemical pollutants in air, water, food, drugs; radon; and infectious agents) acting in concert with both genetic and acquired characteristics. It has been estimated that without these environmental factors, cancer incidence would be dramatically reduced, by as much as 80%-90% (Perera, 1996). The modulation of environmental factors by host susceptibility was rarely evaluated. However, within the past few years, the interaction between environmental factors and host susceptibility factors has become a very active area of research (Perera, 2000). Molecular biology as a tool for use in epidemiological studies has significant potential in strengthening the identification of cancers associated with environmental exposures related to lifestyle, occupation, or ambient pollution. In molecular epidemiology, laboratory methods are employed to document the molecular basis and preclinical effects of environmental carcinogenesis (Portier & Bell, 1998).

Molecular epidemiology has become a major field of research and considerable progress has been made in validation and application of biomarkers and its greatest contribution has been the insights provided into interindividual variation in human cancer risk and the complex interactions between environmental factors and host susceptibility factors, both inherited and acquired, in the multistage process of carcinogenesis (Perera, 2000).

The possibility to use a biomarker to substitute classical endpoints, such as disease incidence or mortality is the most promising feature and one that is most likely to affect public health. The use of events that are on the direct pathways from the initiation to the occurrence of disease to surrogate the disease incidence is a very appealing approach, which is currently investigated in different fields (Bonassi & Au, 2002).

Biological monitoring of workers has three main aims: the primary is individual or collective exposure assessment, the second is health protection and the ultimate objective is occupational health risk assessment. It consists of standardized protocols aiming to the periodic detection of early, preferably reversible, biological signs which are indicative, if compared with adequate reference values, of an actual or potential condition of exposure, effect or susceptibility possibly resulting in health damage or disease. These signs are referred to as biomarkers (Manno et al., 2010).

There has been dramatic progress in the application of biomarkers to human studies of cancer causation. Progress has been made in the development and validation of biomarkers that are directly relevant to the carcinogenic process and that can be used in large-scale epidemiologic studies (Manno et al., 2010).

There are many important aspects to consider when a biomonitoring study is designed. For instance, there is needed a detail information on genotoxin exposure, e.g. type of toxin, duration of exposure, commencing date of exposure relative to sampling date of buccal cells, in order to achieve a meaningful interpretation of data. It will also helps to identify key variables affecting the observed frequency of biomarkers, like age, gender, vitamin B status, genotype and smoking status (Thomas et al., 2009).

Based on the impact on genotoxicity biomarkers in peripheral blood lymphocytes on the design of biomonitoring studies, Battershill et al. (2008) study have considered a strong/sufficient correlation between micronucleus (MN) frequency and increasing age. The effect is more pronounced in females than in males, with the increase more marked after 30 years of age. There are studies that also demonstrated a strong correlation between age and MN frequency and suggested that chromosome loss is a determining factor in this increase.

In what concern to gender, is also documented a gender difference in the background incidence of MN in peripheral blood lymphocytes (PBL), with the frequency being consistently higher in females. A study that assessed MN, chromosomal aberrations and sister chromatid exchange showed highly significant elevations in MN in lymphocytes of women (29% when adjusted for age and smoking) whereas chromosomal aberrations and sister chromatid exchange remained unchanged. This may reflect aneuploidy detected in MN assays (Battershill et al., 2008).

In respect to smoking, although the link between smoking and cancer is strong and exposure to genotoxic carcinogens present in tobacco smoke has been convincingly demonstrated, interestingly the same convincing association is less apparent when assessing biomonitoring studies of genotoxicity. HUMN project study about tobacco smoke, the majority of the laboratories showed no significant differences between smokers and non-smokers and the pooled analysis, interestingly, indicated an overall decrease for all smokers compared to controls (Battershill et al., 2008).

It was verified a weak/insufficient evidence for association with genotoxicity end points and alcohol consumption. Alcohol consumption has been causally associated with cancer at a number of sites (e.g. head and neck cancer). Alcoholic beverages have not been reported to induce mutagenic effects in rodents. The evidence regarding an effect of drinking alcoholic beverages on increased MN or substitute for chromosomal aberrations formation in PBL is inconclusive (Battershill et al., 2008).

2. Biomarkers – General definitions

Biomarkers have been defined by the National Academy of Sciences (USA) as an alteration in cellular or biochemical components, processes, structure or functions that is measurable in a biological system or sample. The traditional, generally accepted classification of biomarkers into three main categories - biomarkers of exposure, effect, and susceptibility; depending on their toxicological significance (Manno et al., 2010).

A biomarker can potentially be any substance, structure or process that could be monitored in tissues or fluids and that predicts or influences health, or assesses the incidence or biological behaviour of a disease. Identification of biomarkers that are on causal pathway, have a high probability of reflecting health or the progression to clinical disease, and have the ability to account for all or most of the variation in a physiological state or the preponderance of cases of the specified clinical outcome, have largely remained elusive (Davis et al., 2007).

A biomarker of exposure is a chemical or its metabolite or the product of an interaction between a chemical and some target molecule or macromolecule that is measured in a compartment or a fluid of an organism (Manno et al., 2010).

A biomarker of effect is a measurable biochemical, structural, functional, behavioural or any other kind of alteration in an organism that, according to its magnitude, can be associated with an established or potential health impairment or disease. A sub-class of biomarkers of effect is represented by biomarkers of early disease (Manno et al., 2010).

A biomarker of susceptibility may be defined as an indicator of an inherent or acquired ability of an organism to respond to the challenge of exposure to a chemical (Manno et al., 2010).

Although the different types of biomarkers are considered for classification purposes, as separate and alternative, in fact it is not always possible to attribute them to a single category. The allocation of a biomarker to one type or the other sometimes depends on its toxicological significance and the specific context in which the test is being used (Manno et al., 2010).

2.1 Genotoxicity biomarkers

As a subtype of biomarkers of effect there are biomarkers of genotoxicity, generally used to measure specific occupational and environmental exposures or to predict the risk of disease or to monitor the effectiveness of exposure control procedures in subjects to genotoxic chemicals (Manno et al., 2010).

Cytogenetic biomarkers are the most frequently used endpoints in human biomonitoring studies and are used extensively to assess the impact of environmental, occupational and medical factors on genomic stability (Barrett et al., 1997; Battershill et al., 2008) and lymphocytes are used as a surrogate for the actual target tissues of genotoxic carcinogens (Barrett et al., 1997). The evaluation of MN in PBL is the most commonly used technique, although cells such as buccal epithelium are also utilized (Battershill et al., 2008).

MN assay is one of the most sensitive markers for detecting DNA damage, and has been used to investigate genotoxicity of a variety of chemicals. MN testing with interphase cells is more suited as a cytogenetic marker because it is not limited to metaphases, and has the advantage of allowing rapid screening of a larger numbers of cells than in studies with sister chromatid exchanges or chromosomic aberrations (Ishikawa et al., 2003).

MN analysis, therefore, appears to be a good tool for investigating the effects of clastogens and aneuploidogens in occupational and environmental exposure in human epidemiological studies (Ishikawa et al., 2003) and are described as a promising approach with regard to assessing health risks (Battershill et al., 2008).

2.1.1 Cytokinesis-Block micronucleus assay

The scope and the application of cytokinesis-block MN assay (CBMN) in biomonitoring has also been expanded in recent years so that in addition to scoring MN in binucleate cells, there are proposals to evaluate MN in mononucleate cells (to provide a more comprehensive assessment of DNA damage), nucleoplasmic bridges (indicative of DNA misrepair, chromosome rearrangement or telomere endfusions) and nuclear buds (a measure of gene amplification or acentric fragments). Fenech (2007), has proposed that CBMN assay can be used to measure chromosomal instability, mitotic dysfunction and cell death (necrosis and apoptosis) and has suggested the term CBMN assay. Identification of the contents of MN (e.g. presence and absence of centromeres) is now considered important in the evaluation of MN in biomonitoring studies, providing insight into mechanisms underpinning the positive results reported, i.e. to differentiate between clastogens and aneugenic responses (Battershill, et al., 2008).

The CBMN assay is a comprehensive system for measuring DNA damage; cytostasis and cytotoxicity-DNA damage events are scored specifically in once-divided binucleated cells and include: micronucleus (MN), nucleoplasmic bridges (NPB) and nuclear buds (NBUDs). Cytostatic effects are measured via the proportion of mono-, bi- and multinucleated cells and cytotoxicity via necrotic and/or apoptotic cell ratios (Fenech, 2002a, 2006, 2007).

MN originate from chromosome fragments or whole chromosomes that lag behind anaphase during nuclear division. The CBMN assay is the preferred method for measuring MN in cultured human and/or mammalian cells because scoring is specifically restricted to once-divided binucleated cells, which are the cells that can express MN. In the CBMN assay, once-divided cells are recognized by their binucleated appearance after blocking cytokinesis with cytochalasin-B (Cyt-B), an inhibitor of microfilament ring assembly required for the completion of cytokinesis.

The CBMN assay allows measuring chromosome breakage, DNA misrepair, chromosome loss, non-disjunction, necrosis, apoptosis and cytostasis. Also measure NPB, a biomarker of dicentric chromosomes resulting from telomere end-fusions or DNA misrepair, and to measure NBUDs, a biomarker of gene amplification.

Because of its reliability and good reproducibility, the CBMN assay has become one of the standard cytogenetic tests for genetic toxicology testing in human and mammalian cells (Fenech, 2002b, 2007).

NPB occur when centromeres of dicentric chromosomes are pulled to opposite poles of the cell at anaphase. There are various mechanisms that could lead to NPB formation following DNA misrepair of strand breaks in DNA. Typically, a dicentric chromosome and an acentric chromosome fragment are formed that result in the formation of an NPB and an MN, respectively. Misrepair of DNA strand breaks could also lead to the formation of dicentric ring chromosomes and concatenated ring chromosomes which could also result in the formation of NPB. An alternative mechanism for dicentric chromosome and NPB formation is telomere end fusion caused by telomere shortening, loss of telomere capping proteins or defects in telomere cohesion. The importance of scoring NPB should not be underestimated because it provides direct evidence of genome damage resulting for misrepaired DNA breaks or telomere end fusions, which is otherwise not possible to deduce by scoring MN only (Fenech, 2007 ; Thomas et al., 2003).

NBUD are biomarkers of elimination of amplified DNA and/or DNA repair complexes. The nuclear budding process has been observed in cultures grown under strong selective conditions that induce gene amplification as well as under moderate folic acid deficiency. Amplified DNA may be eliminated through recombination between homologous regions within amplified sequences forming mini-circles of acentric and atelomeric DNA (double minutes), which localized to distinct regions within the nucleus, or through the excision of amplified sequences after segregation to distinct regions of the nucleus. The process of nuclear budding occurs during S phase and the NBUD are characterized by having the same morphology as an MN with the exception that they are linked to the nucleus by a narrow or wide stalk of nucleoplasmic material depending on the stage of the budding process. The duration of the nuclear budding process and the extrusion of the resulting MN from the cell remain largely unknown (Fenech, 2007; Serrano-García & Montero-Montoya, 2001; Utani et al., 2007).

Most chemical agents and different types of radiation have multiple effects at the molecular, cellular and chromosomal level, which may occur simultaneously and to varying extents depending on the dose. Interpretation of genotoxic events in the absence of data on effects in nuclear division rate and necrosis or apoptosis can be confounding because observed increases in genome damage may be due to indirect factors such as inhibition of apoptosis or defective/permissive cell-cycle checkpoints leading to shorter cell-cycle times and higher rates of chromosome malsegregation. Furthermore, determining nuclear division index (NDI) and proportion of cells undergoing necrosis and apoptosis provides important information on cytostatic and cytotoxic properties of the agent being examined that is relevant to the toxicity assessment. In human lymphocytes, the NDI also provides a measure of mitogen response, which is a useful biomarker of immune response in nutrition studies and may also be related to genotoxic exposure. The cytome approach in the CBMN cytome assay is important because it allows genotoxic (MN, NPB and NBUD in binucleated cells), cytotoxic (proportion of necrotic and apoptotic cells) and cytostatic (proportion and ratios of mono-, bi- and multinucleated cells, NDI) events to be captured within one assay (Fenech, 2005, 2007; Umegaki & Fenech, 2000).

In conclusion, the CBMN method has evolved into an efficient "cytome" assay of DNA damage and misrepair, chromosomal instability, mitotic abnormalities, cell death and cytostasis, enabling direct and/or indirect measurement of various aspects of cellular and nuclear dysfunction such as: unrepaired chromosome breaks fragments and asymmetrical chromosome rearrangement (MN or NPB accompanied by MN originating from acentric chromosomal fragments); telomere end fusions (NPB with telomere signals in the middle of the bridge and possibly without accompanying MN); malsegregation of chromosomes due to spindle or kinetochore defects or cell-cycle checkpoint malfunction (MN containing whole chromosomes or asymmetrical distribution of chromosome-specific centromere signals in the nuclei of BN cells); nuclear elimination of amplified DNA and/or DNA repair complexes (NBUD); chromosomal instability phenotype and breakage-fusion-bridge cycles (simultaneous expression of MN, NPB and NBUD); altered mitotic activity and/or cytostasis (NDI) and cell death by necrosis or apoptosis (ratios of necrotic and apoptotic cells) (Fenech, 2007).

2.1.2 Micronucleus in exfoliated buccal cells

Regeneration is dependent on the number and division rate of the proliferating (basal) cells, their genomic stability and their propensity for cell death. These events can be studied in the buccal mucosa (BM), which is an easily accessible tissue for sampling cells in a minimally invasive manner and does not cause undue stress to study subjects. This method is increasingly used in molecular epidemiology studies for investigating the impact of nutrition, lifestyle factors, genotoxin exposure and genotype on DNA damage, chromosome malsegregation and cell death (Thomas et al., 2009).

The assay has been successfully to study DNA damage as measured by MN or by the use of fluorescent probes to detect in BM is an indication of the regenerative capacity of this tissue. The BM provides a barrier to potential carcinogens that can be metabolized to generate potential reactive products. As up to 90% of all cancers appear to be epithelial in origin, the BM could be used to monitor early genotoxic events as a result of potential carcinogens entering the body through ingestion or inhalation. Exfoliated buccal cells have been used non-invasively to successfully show the genotoxic effects of lifestyle factors such as tobacco smoking, chewing of betel nuts and/or quids, medical treatments, such as radiotherapy as well as occupational exposure, exposure to potentially mutagenic and/or carcinogenic chemicals, and for studies of chemoprevention of cancer.

In this assay cells derived from the BM are harvested from the inside of a patient's mouth using a small-headed toothbrush. The cells are washed to remove the debris and bacteria, and a single-cell suspension is prepared and applied to a clean slide using a cytocentrifuge. The cells are stained with Feulgen and Light Green stain allowing both bright field and permanent fluorescent analysis that can be undertaken microscopically (Thomas et al., 2009).

The Buccal Mucosa Cytome (BMCyt) assay has been used to measure biomarkers of DNA damage (MN and/or nuclear buds), cytokinetic defects (binucleated cells) and proliferative potential (basal cell frequency) and/or cell death (condensed chromatin, karyorrhexis, pyknotic and karyolitic cells). The protocol can also make use of molecular probes for DNA adduct, aneuploidy and chromosome break measures within the nuclei of buccal cells. Furthermore, chromosome-specific centromeric probes have been used to measure aneuploidy by determining the frequency of nuclei with abnormal chromosome number. Tandem probes have been successfully applied to measure chromosome breaks in specific important regions of the genome (Thomas et al., 2009).

The methodology and concepts described in this protocol may be applied to other types of exfoliated cells such as those of the bladder, nose and cervix but the morphological characteristics, sampling and scoring methods are neither properly described nor standardized for cells from these tissues (Thomas et al., 2009).

The time of sampling is also an important variable to consider. As the buccal cells turn over every 7-21 days, it is theoretically possible to observe the genotoxic effects of an acute exposure approximately 7-21 days later.

Ideally, repeat sampling, at least once every 7 days after acute exposure, should be performed for 28 days or more so that the kinetics and extent of biomarker induction can be thoroughly investigated. In the case of chronic exposure due to habitual diet or alcohol consumption or smoking it is recommend that multiple samples are taken at least once every 3 months to take into account seasonal variation (Thomas et al., 2009).

The uniformity of sampling is one of the many aspects to consider; therefore a circular expanding motion is used with toothbrush sampling to enhance sampling over a greater area and to avoid continual erosion in a single region of the BM. This is performed on the inside of both cheeks using a different brush for sampling left and right areas of the mouth to maximize cell sampling and to eliminate any unknown biases that may be caused by sampling one cheek only. It is important to note that repeated vigorous brushing of the same area can lead to increased collection of cells from the less differentiated basal layer. About transportation, in some investigations buccal cells may have to be collected from a distant site which may cause sample deterioration. About cell fixation, there are many possible alternatives of fixatives such as methanol: glacial acetic acid (3:1), 80% methanol or ethanol: glacial acetic (3:1). The staining technique recommend is Feulgen because is a DNA-specific stain and because permanent slides can be obtained that can be viewed under both transmitted and/or fluorescent light conditions. There are many false-positive results in MN frequency as a result of using Romanowsky-type stains such as Giemsa, May-Grunwald Giemsa and/or Leishmann's which leads to inaccurate assessment of DNA damage. Romanowsky stains have been shown to increase the number of false positives as they positively stain keratin bodies that are often mistaken for MN and are therefore not appropriate for this type of analysis. For these reasons, it is advisable to avoid Romanowsky stains in favour of DNA-specific fluorescent-based stains such as propidium iodide, DAPI, Feulgen, Hoechst 33258 or Acridine Orange (Thomas et al., 2009).

The criterion of scoring is originally based in the described by Tolbert et al. that are intended for classifying buccal cells into categories that distinguish between "normal" cells and cells that are considered "abnormal" on the basis of cytological and nuclear features, which are indicative of DNA damage, cytokinetic failure or cell death. Therefore, some definitions of the cytological findings are (Thomas et al., 2009):

Normal "differentiated" cells have a uniformly stained nucleus, which is oval or round in shape. They are distinguished from basal cells by their larger size and by their smaller nucleus-to-cytoplasm ratio. No other DNA-containing structures apart from the nucleus are observed in these cells. These cells are considered to be terminally differentiated relative to basal cells, as no mitotic cells are observed in this population.

Cells with MN are characterized by the presence of both a main nucleus and one more smaller nuclear structures called MN. The MN are round or oval in shape and their diameter should range between 1/3 and 1/16 of the main nucleus. MN has the same staining intensity and texture as the main nucleus. Most cells with MN will ontain only one MN but it is possible to find cells with two or more MN. Baseline frequencies for micronucleated cells in the BM are usually within the 0.5-2.5 MN/1000 cells range. Cells with multiple MN are rare in healthy subjects but become more common in individuals exposed to radiation or other genotoxic events.

Cells with nuclear buds contain nuclei with an apparent sharp constriction at one end of the nucleus suggestive of a budding process, i.e. elimination of nuclear material by budding.

The NBUD and the nucleus are usually in very close proximity and appear to be attached to each other. The NBUD has the same morphology and staining properties as the nucleus; however, its diameter may range from a half to a quarter of that of the main nucleus. The mechanism leading to NBUD formation is not known but it may be related to the elimination of amplified DNA or DNA repair (Thomas et al., 2009).

The scoring method should include coded slides by a person not involved in the study in order to be a blind study. The best magnification to the observation is 1000X. An automated procedure of scoring, by image cytometry have to be developed and validated. The authors suggested first determine the frequency of all the various cell types in a minimum of 1000 cells, following this step, the frequency of DNA damage biomarkers (MN and NBUD) is scored in a minimum of 2000 differentiated cells (Thomas et al., 2009).

At the end the results with the BMCyt are dependent on the level of exposure and potency of genotoxic or cytotoxic agents, genetic background and the age and gender of the donor cells being tested (Thomas et al., 2009).

Is important to define the role of BMCyt in human biomonitoring as a new tool, less invasive in comparison with the CBMN assay, and with many potentialities in molecular epidemiology (Thomas et al., 2009).

Genotoxicity biomonitoring endpoints such as micronucleus, chromosome aberrations and 8-OHdG and DNA repair measured by comet assay are the most commonly used biomarkers in studies evaluating environmental or occupational risks associated with exposure to potential genotoxins. A review made by Knudsen and Hansen (2007) about the application of biomarkers of intermediate end points in environmental and occupational health concluded that MN in lymphocytes provided a promising approach with regard to assessing health risks but concluded that the use of chromosome aberrations in future studies was likely to be limited by the laborious and sensitive procedure of the test and lack of trained cytogeneticists. Methodologies like comet assay in lymphocytes, urine and tissues are increasingly being used as markers of oxidative DNA damage (Battershill et al., 2008).

Studies investigating correlations between endpoints used in genotoxicity biomonitoring studies have yielded inconsistent results, where we can find studies that correlate cytogenetic and comet and studies there do not achieve a correlation between micronucleus, chromosome aberrations and comet. The relative sensitivities of the different endpoints discussed, together with the importance of other factors which influence the persistence of the biomarkers such as DNA repair, may plausibly impact on background levels in the studies considered and would need to be considered before the relationship regarding increases in genotoxicity endpoints with exposure to environmental chemicals or endogenous factors is explored (Battershill et al., 2008).

2.2 Application of genotoxicity biomarkers in an occupational setting – Histopathology laboratories

A biomonitoring study was conducted in 7 histopathology laboratories in Portugal in order to assess the genotoxicity effects in occupational exposure to formaldehyde (FA).

FA is a reactive, flammable and colourless gas with a strong and very characteristic pungent odour that, when combined with air, can lead to explosive mixtures. FA occurs as an endogenous metabolic product of N-, O- and S-demethylation reactions in most living systems. It is used mainly in the production of resins and their applications, such as adhesives and binders in wood product, pulp and paper, synthetic vitreous fibre industries, production of plastics, coatings, textile finishing and also as an intermediate in the synthesis of other industrial chemical compounds. Common non-occupational sources of exposure to FA include vehicle emissions, particle boards and similar building materials, carpets, paints and varnishes, food and cooking, tobacco smoke and its use as a disinfectant (Conaway et al., 1996; Franks, 2005; IARC, 2006; Pala et al., 2008; Viegas & Prista, 2007).

Commercially, FA is manufactured as an aqueous solution called formalin, usually containing 37 to 40% by weight of dissolved FA (Zhang et al., 2009), which is commonly used in histopathology laboratories as a cytological fixative to preserve the integrity of cellular architecture for diagnosis.

Exogenous FA can be absorbed following inhalation, dermal or oral exposure, being the level of absorption dependent on the route of exposure. The International Agency for Research on Cancer (IARC) reclassified FA as a human carcinogen (group 1) in June 2004 based on *"sufficient epidemiological evidence that FA causes nasopharyngeal cancer in humans"* (IARC, 2006; Zhang et al., 2009). In their review, IARC also concluded that there was *"strong but not sufficient evidence for a causal association between leukaemia and occupational exposure to FA"* (Zhang et al., 2009, 2010). However, some studies have also led to mixed results and inconclusive evidence (Franks, 2005; Speit et al., 2010).

The inhalation of vapours can produce irritation to eyes, nose and the upper respiratory system. Whilst occupational exposure to high FA concentrations may result in respiratory irritation and asthmatic reactions, it may also aggravate a pre-existing asthma condition. Skin reactions, following exposure to FA are very common, because the chemical is both irritating and allergenic (Pala et al., 2008). FA induces genotoxic and cytotoxic effects in bacteria and mammals cells (Ye et al., 2005) and its genotoxicity and carcinogenicity has been proved in experimental and epidemiological studies that used proliferating cultured mammalian cell lines and human lymphocytes (Pala et al., 2008; Speit et al., 2007) by DNA-protein cross-links, chromosome aberrations, sister exchange chromatides, and MN (Zhang et al., 2009).

The goal of this study was to compare the frequency of genotoxicity biomarkers, provided by CBMN assay in peripheral lymphocytes and MN test in buccal cells between workers of histopathology laboratories exposed to FA and individuals non-exposed to FA and other environmental factors, namely tobacco and alcohol consumption.

The study population consisted of 56 workers occupationally exposed to FA from 7 hospital histopathology laboratories located in Portugal (Lisbon and Tagus Valley region), and 85 administrative staff without occupational exposure to FA. The characteristics of both groups are described in Table 1.

Ethical approval for this study was obtained from the institutional Ethical Board and Director of the participating hospitals, and all subjects gave informed consent to participate in this study. Every person filled a questionnaire aimed at identifying exclusion criteria like history of cancer, radio or chemotherapy, use of therapeutic drugs, exposure to diagnostic X-rays in the past six months, intake of vitamins or other supplements like folic acid as well as information related to working practices (such as years of employment and the use of protective measures). In this study, none of the participants were excluded.

	Control group	Exposed group
Number of subjects	85	56
Gender Females Masculine	 54 (64%) 31 (36%)	 37 (66%) 19 (34%)
Age (mean ±standard deviation, in years) Range	32.42±8.1 20-53	39.45±11.5 20-61
Years of employment (mean ± sandard deviation, in years) Range	-	14.5 1-33
Tobacco consumption Non-smokers Smokers	 60 (70,6%) 25(29, 4%)	 45 (80,4%) 11 (19,6%)
Alcohol consumption Non-drinkers Drinkers	 19 (22,4%) 66 (77,6%)	 19 (33,9%) 37 (66,1%)

Table 1. Characteristics of the studied sample.

2.2.1 Environmental monitoring of FA exposure

Exposure assessment was based on two techniques of air monitoring conducted simultaneously. First, environmental samples were obtained by air sampling with low flow pumps for 6 to 8 hours, during a typical working day. FA levels were measured by Gas Chromatography analysis and time-weighted average (TWA_{8h}) was estimated according to the National Institute of Occupational Safety and Health method NIOSH 2541 (NIOSH, 1994).

The second method was aimed at measuring ceiling values of FA using Photo Ionization Detection (PID) equipment (11.7 eV lamps) with simultaneous video recording. Instantaneous values for FA concentration were obtained on a per second basis. This method allows establishing a relation between workers activities and FA concentration values, as well to reveal the main exposure sources (McGlothlin et al., 2005; Viegas et al., 2010).

Measurements and sampling were performed in a macroscopic room, provided with fume hoods, always near workers breath.

2.2.2 Biological monitoring

Evaluation of genotoxic effects was performed by applying the CBMN assay in peripheral blood lymphocytes and exfoliated cells from the buccal mucosa.

Whole blood and exfoliated cells from the buccal mucosa were collected between 10 a.m. and 12 p.m., from every subject and were processed for testing. All samples were coded and analyzed under blind conditions. The criteria for scoring the nuclear abnormalities in lymphocytes and MN in the buccal cells were the ones described by, respectively, Fenech et al. (1999) and Tolbert et al. (1991).

Heparinized blood samples were obtained by venipuncture from all subjects and freshly collected blood was directly used for the micronucleus test. Lymphocytes were isolated using Ficoll-Paque gradient and placed in RPMI 1640 culture medium with L-glutamine and red phenol added with 10% inactivated fetal calf serum, 50 ug/ml streptomycin + 50U/mL penicillin, and 10 ug/mL phytohaemagglutinin. Duplicate cultures from each subject were incubated at 37°C in a humidified 5% CO_2 incubator for 44h, and cytochalasin-b 6 ug/mL was added to the cultures in order to prevent cytokinesis. After 28h incubation, cells were spun onto microscope slides using a cytocentrifuge. Smears were air-dried and double stained with May-Grünwald-Giemsa and mounted with Entellan®. One thousand cells were scored from each individual by two independent observers in a total of two slides. Each observer visualized 500 cells per individual. Cells from the buccal mucosa were sampled by endobrushing. Exfoliated cells were smeared onto the slides and fixed with Mercofix®. The standard protocol used was Feulgen staining technique without counterstain. Two thousand cells were scored from each individual by two independent observers in a total of two slides. Each observer visualized 1000 cells per individual. Only cells containing intact nuclei that were neither clumped nor overlapped were included in the analysis.

2.2.3 Statistical analysis

The deviation of variables from the normal distribution was evaluated by the Shapiro-Wilk goodness-of-fit test. The association between each of the genotoxicity biomarkers and occupational exposure to FA was evaluated by binary logistic regression. The biomarkers were dichotomized (absent/present) and considered the dependent variable in regression models where exposure was an independent variable. Odds ratios were computed to evaluate the risk of biomarkers presence and their significance was assessed. The non-parametric Kuskal-Wallis and Mann-Whitney U-tests, were also used to evaluate interactions involving confounding factors. All statistical analysis was performed using the SPSS package for windows, version 15.0.

2.2.4 Results

FA exposure levels

Results of FA exposure values were determined using the two methods described - the NIOSH 2541 method for average concentrations (TWA_{8h}) and the PID method for ceiling concentrations. For the first exposure metric, FA mean level of the 56 individuals studied was 0.16 ppm (0.04 - 0.51 ppm), a value that lies below the OSHA reference value of 0.75 ppm. The mean ceiling concentration found in the laboratories was 1.14 ppm (0.18 - 2.93 ppm), a value well above the reference of the American Conference of Governmental Industrial Hygienists (ACGIH) for ceiling concentrations (0.3 ppm). As for the different tasks developed in histopathology laboratories, the highest FA concentration was identified during macroscopic specimens' exam. This task involves a careful observation and grossing of the specimen preserved in FA, therefore has direct and prolonged contact with its vapors (Table 2).

Tasks	Ceiling values (ppm)
Macroscopic specimen's exam	2.93
Disposal of specimen and used solutions	0.95
Jar filling	2.51
Specimen wash	2.28
Biopsy exam	1.91

Table 2. FA ceiling values (ppm) by tasks in the macroscopy room.

Genotoxicity biomarkers

For all genotoxicity biomarkers under study, workers exposed to FA had significantly higher mean values than the controls (Table 3).

In peripheral blood lymphocytes, significant differences (Mann-Whitney test, $p<0.001$) were observed between subjects exposed and non-exposed to FA, namely in mean MN (respectively, 3.96±0.525 *vs* 0.81±0.172), NPB (3.04±0.523 *vs* 0.18±0.056), and NBUD (0.98±0.273 *vs* 0.07±0.028). In buccal mucosa cells, the MN mean was also significantly higher ($p=0.002$) in exposed subjects (0.96±0.277) than in controls (0.16±0.058).

	Mean, MN lymphocytes ±S.E. (range)	Mean, NPB±S.E. (range)	Mean, NBUD±S.E. (range)	Mean, MN buccal cells ±S.E. (range)
Controls	0.81±0.172 (0-7)	0.18±0.056 (0-3)	0.07±0.028 (0-1)	0.16±0.058 (0-2)
Exposed	3.96±0.525 (0-14)	3.04±0.523 (0-15)	0.98±0.273 (0-13)	0.96±0.277 (0-9)
p-value	<0.001	<0.001	<0.001	0.002

Table 3. Descriptive statistics of MN in lymphocytes and buccal cells, NPB and NBUD means in the studied population (mean ± mean standard error, range and p-value of Mann-Whitney test)

Discriminating by occupation, technologists group mean of MN in lymphocytes was 3.76±0.647; in NBP was 2.62±0.629; in NBUD was 1.09±0.401 and in MN in BM was 1.18±0.406. In pathologists, the means were 5.00±1.243; 3.75±1.467; 0.33±0.188 and in MN in BM was 0.58±0.434, respectively.

The odds ratios indicate an increased risk for the presence of biomarkers in those exposed to FA, compared to non-exposed (Table 4) and they were all significant ($p<0.001$).

	OR	CI 95%	p-value
MN lymphocytes	9.665	3.81-24.52	<0.001
NPB	11.97	4.59-31.20	<0.001
NBUD	9.631	3.12-29.70	<0.001
MN buccal cells	3.990	1.38-11.58	0.011

Table 4. Results of binary logistic regression concerning the association between FA and genotoxicity biomarkers, as evaluated by the odds ratio (OR).

Regarding the impact of the duration of exposure to FA, the mean values of MN in lymphocytes and in buccal cells tended to increase with years of exposure (Table 5) but the association was not statistically significant.

Group	Years of exposure	N	Mean MN lymphocytes ± S.E. (range)	Mean NPB± S.E. (range)	Mean NBUD± S.E. (range)	Mean MN buccal cells ± S.E. (range)
Exposed	> 5	8	2.75±0.940 (0-8)	5.13±1.381 (0-10)	1.38±0.498 (0-3)	0.63±0.625 (0-5)
	6-10	19	3.05±0.775 (0-12)	2.42±0.668 (0-9)	1.53±0.731 (0-13)	0.63±0.326 (0-6)
	11 - 20	12	5.50±1.317 (0-14)	3.33±1.443 (0-14)	0.33±0.188 (0-2)	0.83±0.458 (0-5)
	>21	15	5.00±1.151 (0-13)	2.33±1.036 (0-15)	0.73±0.248 (0-2)	1.20±0.8 (0-9)

Table 5. Descriptive statistics according to years of exposure to formaldehyde of MN in lymphocytes and buccal cells, NPB, and NBUD means in the two groups (mean ± mean standard error, range)

Age and gender are considered the most important demographic variables affecting the MN index. However, Table 6 shows that the mean of all the genotoxicity biomarkers did not differ between men and women within the exposed and the controls ($p > 0.05$).

Groups	Gender	N	Mean MN lymphocytes ± S.E. (range)	Mean NPB ± S.E. (range)	Mean NBUD ± S.E. (range)	Mean MN buccal cells± S.E. (range)
Exposed	Females	37	4.43±0.676 (0-14)	3.03±0.699 (0-15)	1.34±0.418 (0-13)	1.14±0.353 (0-8)
	Males	19	3.47±0.883 (0-13)	2.95±0.818 (0-14)	0.42±0.158 (0-2)	0.74±0.495 (0-9)
Controls	Females	54	0.87±0.229 (0-7)	0.22±0.078 (0-3)	0.11±0.043 (0-1)	0.11±0.057 (0-2)
	Males	31	0.71±0.255 (0-6)	0.10±0.071 (0-2)	0.00	0.26±0.122 (0-2)

Table 6. Descriptive statistics by gender of MN in lymphocytes and buccal cells, NPB, and NBUD means in the two groups (mean ± mean standard error, range)

In order to examine the effect of age, exposed and non-exposed individuals were stratified by age groups: 20-30, 31-40, and ≥ 41 years old (Table 7). There was no consistent trend regarding the variation of biomarkers with age, the only exception being the MN in lymphocytes in the exposed group (Kruskal-Wallis, $p= 0.006$), where the higher means where found in the older group. According to Mann-Whitney test, there is a statistical significant result between the elder and the older group (20–30 and > 41 years old, $p= 0.02$), however the comparison between 20-30 and 31–40 groups ($p= 0.262$) and 30–40 and > 41 groups ($p= 0.065$) did not reach statistical significance.

Groups	Age	N	Mean MN lymphocytes ± S.E. (range)	Mean NPB± S.E. (range)	Mean NBUD± S.E. (range)	Mean MN buccal cells ± S.E. (range)
Exposed	20-30	18	2.19±0.526 (0-8)	3.56±0.926 (0-10)	1.63±0.816 (0-13)	0.75±0.470 (0-6)
	31-40	11	3.00±0.775 (0-8)	1.20±0.467 (0-4)	0.50±0.224 (880-2)	0.40±0.221 (0-2)
	>41	27	5.54±0.876 (0-15)	3.00±0.879 (0-15)	0.69±0.234 (0-5)	1.46±0.503 (0-9)
Controls	20-30	36	0.47±0.157 (0-3)	0.14±0.071 (0-2)	0.08±0.047 (0-1)	0.19±0.96 (0-2)
	31-40	35	1.14±0.326 (0-7)	0.20±0.099 (0-3)	0.06±0.040 (0-1)	0.14±0.83 (0-2)
	>41	14	0.86±0.501 (0-6)	0.21±0.155 (0-2)	0.07±0.71 (0-1)	0.14±0.143 (0-2)

Table 7. Age effects on descriptive statistics of MN in lymphocytes and buccal cells, NPB and NBUD means in the studied population (mean ± mean standard error, range).

The interaction between age and gender in determining the frequencies of genotoxicity biomarkers was investigated and found to be significant only for MN in lymphocytes in exposed subjects (Kruskal-Wallis, $p=0.04$). In general the MN tended to be more frequent in the > 41 years old category in both genders; however women had the higher means.

Regarding smoking habits, a non-parametric analysis rejected the null hypothesis that biomarkers are the same for the four categories (control smokers and non-smokers, exposed smokers and non-smokers) (Kruskall-Wallis, $p<0.001$). However, the analysis of the interactions between FA exposure and tobacco smoke between exposed and controls (Mann-Whitney test) showed that FA exposure, rather than tobacco, has a preponderant effect upon the determination of biomarker frequencies. In the control group, non-smokers had slightly higher MN means in buccal cells in comparison with smokers; although the result did not reach statistical significance (Mann-Whitney, $p> 0.05$).

As for alcohol consumption, because uptake reported in enquires may differ considerably from real consumption, all consumers were gathered into a single entity, in contrast with non-consumers. Nevertheless, no one acknowledged having "heavy drink habits" in the questionnaires.

Overall, biomarkers in controls exhibited higher mean frequencies among alcohol consumers than among non-consumers. Among those exposed, however, mean frequencies were slightly lower among drinkers, suggesting that exposure was the major predominant factor in determining the high biomarker frequencies of those who are exposed. Differences between drinkers and non-drinkers were not statistically significant, to the exception of MN in lymphocytes in controls (Mann-Whitney, $p=0.011$), where drinkers have higher means. The interaction between alcohol consumption and smoking habits was statistically significant (Kruskal-Wallis, $p=0.043$), as subjects that do not smoke and do not drink tend to have lower frequencies of MN in buccal cells than those who drink and smoke, with a gradient of frequencies in between.

2.2.5 Discussion

Long exposures to FA, as those to which some workers are subjected for occupational reasons, are suspected to be associated with genotoxic effects that can be evaluated by biomarkers (Conaway et al., 1996; IARC, 2006; Viegas & Prista, 2007; Zhang et al., 2009). In this study the results suggest that workers in histopathology laboratories are exposed to FA levels that exceed recommended exposure limits. Macroscopic specimens' exam, in particular, is the task that involves higher exposure, because it requires a greater proximity to anatomical species impregnated with FA, as supported by the studies of Goyer et al. (2004) and Orsière et al. (2006).

A statistically significant association was found between FA exposure and biomarkers of genotoxicity, namely MN in lymphocytes, NPB, NBUD and MN in buccal cells. Chromosome damage and effects upon lymphocytes arise because FA escapes from sites of direct contact, such as the mouth, originating nuclear alterations in the lymphocytes of those exposed (He & Jin, 1998; IARC, 2006; Orsière et al. 2006; Ye et al., 2005). Our results thus corroborate previous reports (Ye et al., 2005) that lymphocytes can be damaged by long term FA exposure. Moreover, the changes in peripheral lymphocytes indicate that the cytogenetic effects triggered by FA can reach tissues faraway from the site of initial contact (Suruda et al., 1993). Long term exposures to high concentrations of FA indeed appear to have a potential for DNA damage; these effects were well demonstrated in experimental studies with animals, local genotoxic effects following FA exposure, namely DNA-protein cross links and chromosome damage (IARC, 2006).

In humans, FA exposure is associated with an increase in the frequency of MN in buccal epithelium cells (Burgaz et al., 2002; Speit et al., 2006, 2007b), as corroborated by the results presented here.

Suruda el al. (1993) claim that although changes in oral and nasal epithelial cells and peripheral blood cells do not indicate a direct mechanism leading to carcinogenesis, they present evidence that DNA alteration took place. It thus appears reasonable to conclude that FA is a cancer risk factor for those who are occupationally exposed in histopathology laboratories (IARC, 2006).

MN and NPB measured in lymphocytes had higher means in pathologists compared with technologists. This result can be explained by the exposure to higher concentrations of pathologists that perform macroscopic exam. Also this chemical mode of action is more related with the concentration than with time of exposure expressed by TWA results.

In epidemiological studies, it is important to evaluate the role played by common confounding factors, such as gender, age, smoking and alcohol consumption, upon the association between disease and exposure (Bonassi et al., 2001; Fenech at al., 1999). Concerning gender, studies realized by Fenech et al. (1999) and Wojda et al. (2007) reported that biomarker frequencies were greater in females than in males by a factor of 1.2 to 1.6 depending on the age group. With the exception of MN in the buccal cells of controls, the results presented here point to females having higher frequencies than males in all genotoxicity biomarkers, although the differences usually lacked statistical significance. Such trend is concordant with previous studies that reported higher MN frequency in lymphocytes in females and a slightly higher MN frequency in buccal cells in males (Holland et al., 2008) and that can be explained by preferential aneugenic events involving the X-chromosome. A possible explanation is the micronucleation of the X chromosome, which has been shown to occur in lymphocytes in females, both *in vitro* and *in vivo*, and that can be accounted for by the presence of two X chromosomes. This finding might explain the preferential micronucleation of the inactive X (Catalán et al., 1998, 2000a, 2000b).

Aging in humans appears to be associated with genomic instability. Cytogenetically, ageing is associated with a number of gross cellular changes, including altered size and morphology, genomic instability and changes in expression and proliferation (Bolognesi et al., 1999; Zietkiewicz et al., 2009). It has been shown that a higher MN frequency is directly associated with decreased efficiency of DNA repair and increased genome instability (Kirsch-Volders et al., 2006; Orsière et al., 2006). The data has shown a significant increase of MN in lymphocytes in the exposed group. This can be explained in light of genomic instability, understood as an increased amount of mutations and/or chromosomal aberrations that cytogenetically translate into a greater frequency of changes in chromosome number and/or structure and in the formation of micronuclei (Zietkiewicz et al., 2009). The involvement of micronucleation in age-related chromosome loss has been supported by several studies showing that the rate of MN formation increases with age, especially in women (Catalán et al., 1998). This study provides evidence that age and gender interact to determine the frequency of MN in the lymphocytes of exposed subjects. The higher incidence of MN in both genders is more manifest in older age groups and the effect of gender becomes more pronounced as age increases. Several reports link this observation to an elevated loss of X chromosomes (Battershill et al., 2008).

Tobacco smoke has been epidemiologically associated to a higher risk of cancer development, especially in the oral cavity, larynx, and lungs, as these are places of direct contact with the carcinogenic tobacco's compounds. In this study, smoking habits did not influence the frequency of the genotoxicity biomarkers; moreover, the frequencies of MN in buccal cells were unexpectedly higher in exposed non-smokers than in exposed smokers, though the difference was not statistically significant. In most reports, the results about the effect of tobacco upon the frequency of MN in human lymphocytes were negative as in many instances smokers had lower MN frequencies than non-smokers (Bonassi et al., 2003). In the current study, the analysis of the interaction between FA exposure and smoking habits indicates that exposure is preponderant in determining the frequency of biomarkers. Nevertheless, the effect of smoking upon biomarkers remains controversial. Some studies reported an increased frequency of MN in lymphocytes, NPB, and NBUD as a consequence of the tobacco-specific nitrosamine 4-(methylnitrosamino)-1-(3-pyridyl)-1-butanone (NNK). Still in this study no associations were observed between tobacco and nuclear abnormalities (El-Zein et al., 2006, 2008).

As for alcohol consumption, it did not appear to influence the frequency of genotoxicity biomarkers in study, to the exception of MN in lymphocytes in controls (Mann-Whitney, $p=0.011$), with drinkers having higher means. Alcohol is definitely a recognized genotoxic agent, being cited as able to potentiate the development of carcinogenic lesions (Ramirez & Saldanha, 2002). In our study, drinkers in the control group had higher mean frequencies of all biomarkers than non-drinkers, but the differences were only significant for MN in lymphocytes. Stich and Rosin (1983) study of alcoholic individuals, reported absence of significant differences concerning MN frequencies in buccal cells. That is important to corroborate our result, because of the lack of "heavy drinkers" in our study. The same study concluded that neither alcohol nor smoking, alone, increase MN frequency in buccal cells, but a combination of both resulted in a significant elevation in micronucleated cells in the buccal mucosa. However, the synergism between alcohol consumption and tobacco has not been observed to act upon all biomarkers and, in several studies of lifestyle factors, it was difficult to differentiate the effect of alcohol from that of smoking (Holland et al., 2008).

The CBMN assay is a simple, practical, low cost screening technique that can be used for clinical prevention and management of workers subjected to occupational carcinogenic risks, namely exposure to a genotoxic agent such as FA. The results obtained in this study provide unequivocal evidence of association between occupational exposure to formaldehyde in histopathology laboratory workers and the presence of nuclear changes.

Given these results, preventive actions must prioritize safety conditions for those who perform macroscopic exams. In general, exposure reduction to FA in this occupational setting may be achieved by the use of adequate local exhaust ventilation and by keeping biological specimen containers closed during the macroscopic exam.

3. Conclusion

Another important application of biological monitoring, besides exposure assessment, is the use of biomarkers, at either individual or group level, for the correct interpretation of doubtful clinical tests. These are usually performed as part of occupational health surveillance program when exposure assessment data are unavailable or are deemed unreliable. Health surveillance is the periodical assessment of the workers' health status by clinical, biochemical, imaging or instrumental testing to detect any clinically relevant, occupation-dependent change of the single worker's health. Biomarkers are usually more specific and sensitive than most clinical tests and may be more effective, therefore, for assessing a causal relationship between health impairment and chemical exposure when a change is first detected in exposed workers (Manno et al., 2010).

Experience in biological monitoring gained in the occupational setting has often been applied to assess (the effects of) human exposure to chemicals in the general environment. The use of biological fluids/tissues for the assessment of human exposure, effect or susceptibility to chemicals in the workplace represents, together with the underlying data (e.g. personal exposure and biological monitoring measurements, media-specific residue measurements, product use and time-activity information), a critical component of the occupational risk assessment process, a rapidly advancing science (Manno et al., 2010).

Au et al. (1998), advise to put more emphasis on monitoring populations which are known to be exposed to hazardous environmental contaminant and on providing reliable health risk evaluation. The information can also be used to support regulations on protection of the environment.

4. Acknowledgment

This work was supported by Autoridade Portuguesa para as Condições de Trabalho (ACT – Portuguese Authority for Work Conditions). http://www.act.gov.pt/. Project reference: 075MNA/06.

5. References

Au, W.; Cajas-Salazar, N. & Salama, S. (1998). Factors contributing to discrepancies in population monitoring studies. *Mutation Research,* 400, pp. 467 – 478.

Barrett, J.; Vainio, H.; Peakall, D. & Goldstein, B. (1997). 12th Meeting of the scientific group on methodologies for the safety evaluation of chemicals: susceptibility to environmental hazards. *Environmental Health Perspectives,* 104, Suppl 4, pp. 699 - 737.

Battershill, J.; Burnett, K. & Bull, S. (2008). Factors affecting the incidence of genotoxicity biomarkers in peripheral blood lymphocytes: impact on design of biomonitoring studies. *Mutagenesis,* 6, pp. 423-437.

Bolognesi, C., Lando, C.; Forni, A.; Landini, E.; Scarpato, R.; Migliori, L.& Bonassi, S. (1999). Chromosomal damage and ageing: effect of micronuclei frequency in peripheral blood lymphocytes. *Age and Ageing,* 28, pp. 393-397.

Bonassi, S.; Fenech, M., Lando, C., Lin, Y-P., Ceppi, M.; Chang, W.; Holland, N.; Kirsch-Volders, M.; Zeiger, E., Baan, S.; Barale, R., Bigatti, M., Bolognesi, C., Jia, C., Di Giorgio, M., Ferguson, L., Fucic, A., Lima, O., Hrelia, P., Krishnaja, A., Lee, T-K., Migliore, L., Mikhalevich, L.; Mirkova, E.; Mosesso, P., Müller, W.-U., Odagiri, Y., Scarfi, M.; Szabova, E.; Vorobtsova, I., Vral, A. & Zijno, A. (2001). Human MicroNucleus Project: International database comparison for results with cytokinesis-block micronucleus assay in human lymphocytes: I. Effect of laboratory protocol, scoring criteria, and host factor son the frequency of micronuclei. *Environmental and Molecular Mutagenesis,* 37, 31-45.

Bonassi, S.; Au, W. (2002). Biomarkers in molecular epidemiology studies for health risk prediction. *Mutation Research,* 511, pp. 73 – 86.

Bonassi, S.; Neri, M.; Lando, C.; Ceppi, M.; Lin, Y.; Chang, W.; Holland, N., Kirsch-Volders, M.; Zeiger, E. & Fenech, M. (2003). Effect of smoking habit on the frequency of micronuclei in human lymphocytes: results from the Human MicroNucleus project. *Mutation Research,* 543, pp. 155-166.

Burgaz, S.; Erdem, O.; Çakmak, G. & Karakaya, A. (2002). Cytogenetic analysis of buccal cells from shoe-workers and pathology and anatomy laboratory workers exposed to n-hexane, toluene, methyl ethyl ketone and formaldehyde. *Biomarker, 2,* pp. 151-161.

Catalán, J.; Autio, K.; Kuosma, E. & Norppa, H. (1998). Age-dependent inclusion of sex chromosomes in lymphocyte micronuclei in man. *Am. J. Hum. Genet.,* 63, pp.1464-1472.

Catalán, J.; Falck, G. & Norppa, H. (2000a). The X chromosome frequently lags behind in female lymphocyte anaphase. *American Journal of Human Genetics, 66,* pp. 687-691.

Catalán, J.; Surrallés, J.; Falck, G., Autio, K. & Norppa, H. (2000b). Segregation of sex chromosomes in human lymphocytes. *Mutagenesis,* 3, 251-255.

Conaway, C.; Whysner, J.; Verna, L. & Williams, G. (1996). Formaldehyde mechanistic data and risk assessment: endogenous protection from DNA adduct formation. *Pharmacol. Ther.* 71, pp. 29 – 55.

Davis, C.; & Milner, J. (2007). Biomarkers for diet and cancer prevention research: potentials and challenges. *Acta Pharmacol Sin,* Vol. 9, 28, pp. 1262-1273.

El-Zein, R.; Schabath, M.; Etzel, C.; Lopez, M.; Franklin, J. & Spitz M. (2006) . Cytokinesis-Blocked Micronucleus Assay as a Novel Biomarker for Lung Cancer Risk. *Cancer Reearch,* 66, pp. 6449 - 6456.

El-Zein, R.; Fenech, M.; Lopez, M., Spitz, M. & Etzel, C. (2008). Cytokinesis-Blocked Cytome Assay Biomarkes Identify Lung Cancer Cases amongst Smokers. *Cancer Epidemiol. Biomarkers Prev* 17, pp. 1111 - 1119.

Fenech, M.; Holland, N.; Chang, W.; Zeiger, E. & Bonassi, S. (1999). The Human MicroNucleus Project - An international collaborative study on the use of the micronucleus technique for measuring DNA damage in humans. *Mutation Research,* 428, pp. 271 - 283.

Fenech, M. & Crott, J. (2002a). Micronuclei, nucleoplasmic bridges and nuclear buds induced in folic acid deficient human lymphocytes - evidence for breakage-fusion-bridge cycles in the cytokinesis-block micronucleus assay. *Mutation Research,* 504, pp. 131-136.

Fenech, M. (2002b). Chromosomal biomarkers of genomic instability relevant to cancer. *Drug Discovery Today,* 22, pp. 1128-1137.

Fenech, M. (2005). The Genome Health Clinic and Genome Health Nutrigenomics concepts: diagnosis and nutritional treatment of genome and epigenome damage on an individual basis. *Mutagenesis,* 20, pp. 225 - 269.

Fenech, M. (2006). Cytokinesis-block micronucleus assay evolves into a "cytome" assay of chromosomal instability, mitotic dysfunction and cell death. *Mutation Research,* 600, pp.58-66.

Fenech, M. (2007). Cytokinesis-block micronucleus cytome assay. *Nature Protocols,* 5, pp. 1084-1104.

Franks, S. (2005). A mathematical model for the absorption and metabolism of formaldehyde vapour by humans. *Toxicology and Applied Pharmacology,* 206, pp. 309 - 320.

Goyer, N.; Beaudry, C. ; Bégin, D. ; Bouchard, M. ; Buissonet, S. ; Carrier, G. ; Gely, O. ; Gérin, M. ; Lavoué, L., Lefebvre, P. ; Noisel, N. ; Perraut, G. & Roberge, B. (2004). Impacts d'un abaissement de la values d'exposition admissible au formaldéhyde : industries de fabrication de formaldéhde et de résines à base de formaldéhyde. Móntreal : Institut de Recherche Robert-Sauvé en Santé et Securité du Travail 2004.

He, J-L. & Jin, H.-Y. (1998). Detection of cytogenetic effects in peripheral lymphocytes of students exposed to formaldehyde with cytokinesis-blocked micronucleus assay. *Biomed. Environm. Sci.,* 11, pp. 87-92.

Holland, N.; Bolognesi, C.; Kirsch-Volders, M.; Bonassi, S.; Zeiger, E., Knasmueller, S. & Fenech, M. (2008). The micronucleus assay in human buccal cells as a tool for biomonitoring DNA damage: The HUMN project perspective on current status and knowledge gaps, *Mutation Research*: doi: 10.1016/j.mrrev.2008.03.007.

IARC. (2006). *IARC Monographs on the Evaluation of Carcinogenic Risks to Human, volume 88: Formaldehyde, 2-Butoxyethanol and 1-tert-Butoxy-2-propanol.* World Health Organization, Lyon.

Ishikawa, H.; Tian, Y. & Yamauchi, T. (2003). Influence of gender, age and lifestyle factor son micronuclei frequency in healthy japanese populations. *Journal of Occupational Health,* 45, pp. 170-181.

Kirsch-Volders, M.; Mateuca, R.; Roelants, M.; Tremp, A., Zeiger, E.; Bonassi, S.; Holland, N.; Chang, W.; Aka, P.; DeBoeck, M.; Goddenis, L.; Haufroid, V.; Ishikawa, H.; Laffon, B.; Marcos, R.; Migliore, L., Norppa, H.; Teixeira, J.; Zijno, A. & Fenech, M. (2006). The effects of GSTM1 and GSTT1 polymorphisms on micronucleus frequencies in Human Lymphocytes in vivo. *Cancer Epidemiol Biomarkers Prev,* Vol. 5, 15, pp. 1038-1042.

Knudsen, L. & Hansen, A. (2007). Biomarkers of intermediate endpoints in environmental and occupational health. *International Journal of Hygiene and Environmental Health,* 210, pp. 461 – 470.

Manno, M.; Viau, C.; Cocker, J.; Colosio, C.; Lowry, L.; Mutti, A.; Nordberg, M. & Wang, S. (2010). Biomonitoring for occupational health risk assessment (BOHRA). *Toxicology Letters,* 192, pp. 3 – 16.

McGlothlin, J. & col. (2005). Occupational exposure assessment and control using video exposure monitoring in the pharmaceutical industry. In INTERNATIONAL SCIENTIFIC CONFERENCE (IOHA 2005), 6, 19-23 September 2005, Pilanesberg National Park North West Province, South Africa. Pilanesberg: IOHA – International Occupational Hygiene. MVS – Mine Ventilation of South Africa.

NIOSH – Manual of analytical methods. 4th ed. DHHS (NIOSH) Publication 94-113. August, 1994.

Orsière, T.; Sari-Minodier, I.; Iarmarcovai, G. & Botta, A. (2006). Genotoxic risk assessment of pathology and anatomy laboratory workers exposed to formaldehyde by use of personal air sampling and analysis of DNA damage in peripheral lymphocytes. *Mutation Research,* 605, pp.30 – 41.

Pala, M.; Ugolini, D.; Ceppi, M.; Rizzo, F.; Maiorana, L.; Bolognesi, C.; Schilirò, T.; Gilli, G.; Bigatti, P.; Bono, R. & Vecchio, D. (2008). Occupational exposure to formaldehyde and biological monitoring of Research Institute workers. *Cancer Detection and Prevention, 32,* pp. 121 – 126.

Perera, F. (1996). Molecular epidemiology: insights into cancer susceptibility, risk assessment, and prevention. *Journal of the National Cancer Institute,* 8, pp. 496 – 509.

Perera, F. & Weinstein, I. (2000). Molecular epidemiology: recent advances and future directions. *Carcinogenesis,* 21, pp. 517 – 524.

Portier, C. & Bell, D. (1998). Genetic susceptibility: significance in risk assessment. *Toxicology Letters* 102 – 103, pp. 185 -189.

Ramirez, A. & Saldanha, P. (2002). Micronucleus investigation of alcoholic patients with oral carcinoma. *Genetics and Molecular Research,* 1, pp. 246 – 260.

Serrano-García, L. & Montero-Montoya, R. (2001). Micronuclei and Chromatid Buds are result of related genotoxic events. *Environmental and Molecular Mutagenesis,* 38, pp. 38 – 45.

Speit, G. & Schmid, O. (2006). Local genotoxic effects of formaldehyde in humans measured by the micronucleus test with exfoliated epithelial cells. *Mutation Research,* 613, pp. 1-9.

Speit, G.; Schütz, P.; Högel, J. & Schmid, O. (2007a). Characterization of the genotoxic potencial of formaldehyde in V79 cells. *Mutagenesis, Vol.* 6, 22, pp. 387 – 394.

Speit, G.; Schmid, O.; Fröhler-Keller, M.; Lang, I. & Triebig, G. (2007b). Assessment of local genotoxic effects of formaldehyde in humans measured by de micronucleus test with exfoliated buccal mucosa cell. *Mutation Research*, 627, pp. 129-131.

Speit, G.; Gelbke H.-P.; Pallapies, D. & Morfeld, P. (2010). Occupational Exposure to formaldehyde, hematotoxicity and leukemia-specific chromosome changes in cultured myeloid progenitor cells - Letter, *Cancer, Epidemiology, Biomarkers & Prevention*, 7, 19, pp. 1882 - 1884.

Stich, H. & Rosin, M. (1983). Quantitating the synergistic effect of smoking and alcohol consumption with the micronucleus test on human buccal mucosa cells. *Int. J. Cancer* 31, pp. 305 - 308.

Suruda, A.; Schulte, P.; Boeniger, M.; Hayes, R.; Livingston, G.; Steenland, K., Stewart, P.; Herrick, R.; Douthit, D. & Fingerhut, M. (1993). Cytogenetic effects of formaldehyde exposure in students of mortuary science. *Cancer Epidemiology, Biomarkers & Prevention*, 2, 453 - 460.

Thomas, P.; Holland, N.; Bolognesi, C.; Kirsch-Volders, M.; Bonassi, S.; Zeiger, E.; Knasmueller, S. & Fenech, M. (2009). Buccal micronucleus cytome assay. *Nature Protocols*, 6, pp. 825-837.

Thomas, P.; Umegaki, K. & Fenech, M. (2003). Nucleoplasmic bridges are a sensitive measure of chromosome rearrangement in the cytokinesis-block micronucleus assay. *Mutagenesis*, 18, pp. 187- 194.

Tolbert, P.; Shy, C. & Allen, J. (1991). Micronuclei and other nuclear anomalies in buccal smears: a field test in snuff users. *American Journal of Epidemiology*, 8, pp. 840 - 850.

Umegaki, K.; & Fenech, M. (2000). Cytokinesis-block micronucleus assay in WIL2-NS cells: a sensitive system to detect chromosomal damage induced by reactive oxygen species and activated human neutrophils. *Mutagenesis, Vol.* 3, *15*, pp. 261-269.

Utani, K.; Kawamoto, J. & Shimizu, N. (2007). Micronuclei bearing extrachromosomal chromatin are transcriptionally competent and may perturb the cancer cell phenotype. *Mol. Cancer Res*, 5, pp. 695 - 704.

Viegas, S. & Prista, J. (2007). Cancro Nasofaríngeo e Exposição a Formaldeído: avaliação da história profissional em 63 casos registados, *Soc. Portuguesa de Medicina do Trabalho*, *6*, pp. 13 - 22.

Viegas, S.; Ladeira, C.; Nunes, C.; Malta-Vacas, J., Gomes, M., Brito, M.; Mendonça, P. & Prista, J. (2010). Genotoxic effects in occupational exposure to formaldehyde: a study in anatomy and pathology laboratories and formaldehyde- resins production. Journal of Occupational Medicine and Toxicology 5, 25, pp. 1 - 8.

Wojda, A.; Zietkiewicz, E. & Witt, M. (2007). Effects of age and gender on micronucleus and chromosome nondisjunction frequencies in centenarians and younger subjects. Mutagenesis Advance Access, pp. 1 - 6.

Ye, X.; Yan, W.; Xie, H.; Zhao, M. & Ying, C. (2005). Cytogenetic analysis of nasal mucosa cells and lymphocytes from high-level long-term formaldehyde exposed workers and low-level short-term exposed waiters. Mutation Research, *588*, pp. 22-27.

Zhang, L.; Steinmaus, C.; Eastmond, D.; Xin, X. & Smith, M. (2009). Formaldehyde exposure and leukemia: a new meta-analysis and potential mechanisms. *Mutation Research*, 681, pp. 150 - 168.

Zhang, L.; Tang, X. & Rothman, N. (2010). Occupational exposure to formaldehyde, hematoxicity, and leukemia-specific chromosome changes in cultured myeloid progenitor cells. *Cancer Epidemiology, Biomarkers & Prevention*, 19, pp. 80 - 88.

Zietkiewicz, E.; Wojda, A.; Witt, M. (2009). Cytogenetic perspective of ageing and longevity in men and women. *Jounal of Applied Genetics*, 50, pp. 261-273.

A Comparison of Biomarker and Fingerprint-Based Classifiers of Disease

Brian T. Luke and Jack R. Collins
SAIC-Frederick, NCI at Frederick, Frederick, USA

1. Introduction

1.1 Early detection of disease

Early detection of a disease is very important since it greatly improves the individual's chance of responding well to treatment. For example, the 5-year survival rate from prostate cancer is nearly 100% if it is detected early [http://www.toacorn.com/news/2005/1027/Health_and_Wellness/077.html]. Similarly, the 5-year survival rate for ovarian cancer is 95% if caught early, but since 75% of the cases are first observed in the later stages of the disease, the overall 5-year survival rate is less than 50% [http://www.information-about-ovarian-cancer.com/]. It would be nice if there was a single test to determine if an individual had cancer somewhere in their body, but unfortunately such a test does not exist. While all cancers have many factors in common, tissue differences and the body's response to different cancers make the test for ovarian cancer (CA125) very different from the test for prostate cancer (PSA). The lack of sufficient sensitivity and specificity has recently resulted in the recommendation that PSA no longer be used as a potential marker of prostate cancer [http://www.uspreventiveservicestaskforce.org/uspstf/uspsprca.htm].

Even within the same tissue, all cancers are not necessarily the same. It is well known that there are two major types of lung cancer, small cell lung cancer (SCLG) and non-small cell lung cancer (NSCLC). It is also known that NSCLC has three major sub-types; adeno-carcinoma (AC), squamous cell carcinoma (SCC), and large cell undifferentiated carcinoma (LCUC). Each of these has differences in the biochemical processes going on within the cancer cell and one should not expect that the detection, or necessarily the treatment, of these cancers will be the same. Of the four recognized forms of lung cancer (SCLG, AC, SCC and LCUC), the latter three are strictly differentiated by appearances of the cell under the microscope. It is possible that the underlying biochemical processes of an AC cell in one individual are significantly different than the biochemical processes in another individual with a cancer that appears similar. Therefore, each of these categories of lung cancer may be composed of one or more states. While the disease category represents the name of the disease based on some experimental observation, the disease state represents a grouping based on the underlying biochemical processes within the diseased cell. The detection of a disease and its treatment should be relative to specific disease states, not a disease category or individuals within that category.

1.2 Types of classifiers

A high-quality classifier would be a great aide in the early detection of disease. The general procedure is to obtain a biological specimen and search for one or more features that correctly classify the individual. The specimen can be blood, urine, mucous, or tissue sample, for example, and the feature can be the expression level of mRNA, a protein, or a metabolite. The construction of the classifier starts with obtaining a large number of features from individuals with known phenotypes, known as the training set, and constructing a classifier that sufficiently predicts each sample's phenotype. This classifier is then used on a second set of samples of known phenotype, called the testing set, to determine its overall accuracy. Since the number of features will be much larger than the number of samples in the training set, the construction of a classifier suffers from the "curse of dimensionality" [Bellman, 1957, 1961, 2003]. If the training set contains Nh healthy samples and Nd diseased samples, then virtually any classifier that uses the smaller of Nh and Nd features, such as their social security numbers, can correctly classify all samples in the training set. This extreme example would represent a case where the classifier is fitting the individuals in the training set and not their phenotype. The goal is to choose a relatively small number of features that correctly distinguishes the samples.

Two extremes in the total range of possible classifiers are fingerprint-based and biomarker-based classifiers. A fingerprint-based classifier uses a collection of features, which is also known as a panel of markers. If two individuals have the same pattern in this set of features (i.e. similar fingerprints), and one is known to have a particular disease, it is assumed that the other has this same disease. A biomarker-based classifier tries to find a very small number of features that distinguishes all healthy samples from all diseased samples. In other words, a biomarker-based classifier tries to cluster all samples of the same phenotype into the smallest possible number of clusters. The optimum biomarker would distinguish all healthy from all diseased samples, resulting in a single healthy cluster and a single disease cluster.

1.3 Selecting features

A major difference between fingerprint-based and biomarker-based classifiers is how the features are selected. In a fingerprint-based classifier, the actual classifier is used to determine who well a given set of features distinguishes the samples. An overriding heuristic is used to determine what set of features is tested in the classifier, and the quality of the classification can be used to determine which feature set is tried next. This is known as a *wrapper method*. In contrast, a biomarker-based classifier uses one or more procedures to determine which features successfully distinguish some or all of the samples in the training set. This set of putative biomarkers is then used in a different classifier, either individually or a small number together, to determine how well the healthy samples can be distinguished from the diseased samples. In other words, the selection of features for a biomarker-based classifier uses a *filter method*.

Many different procedures can be used in the wrapper method to find the optimal set of markers. Three major classes of procedures are forward-selection, reverse-selection, and multidimensional searches. The simplest forward-selection method is a Greedy Search. In this procedure all features are individually tested in the classifier and the one that performs the best is retained. All remaining features are then tested in combination with this best feature to find the feature-pair that performs the best. This procedure continues until either the addition of an additional feature does not improve the classification or a pre-set number of features are selected. An extension of this Greedy Search is known as Branch-and-Bound. In this latter procedure multiple classifiers are retained at each cycle and the search results in a population of classifiers that have the highest accuracy.

Reverse-selection works in the opposite direction. Initially, all features are used in the classifier and features that are not important to the classification are removed. In cases where the number of features is larger than the number of samples, special procedures need to be used to ensure that an important feature is not removed in the early steps of the reduction.

Multidimensional searches use a pre-defined number of features and try different combinations of features in the classifier. Examples of multidimensional search techniques are Simulated Annealing, Tabu Search, Gibbs Sampling, Genetic Algorithm, Evolutionary Programming, Ant Colony Optimization, and Particle Swarm Optimization. The first three techniques modify a single set of features while the latter four use a population of sets, where each feature set is changed throughout the search to find one or more optimal sets. It should be noted that in a Genetic Algorithm the number of features in the set can be reduced, so the pre-defined number should be considered a maximum number of allowed features in the final set.

The goal of each wrapper search technique is to find the optimal set of features, and therefore are approximations to an exhaustive search. If the objective is to find the best set of k features from a total set of K features, the number of unique combinations is generally given by $\binom{K}{k}$. If there are a total of 300 features and the goal is to find the best set of seven features, an exhaustive search would require examining 4.04×10^{13} unique sets of features. The situation is slightly more complicated for a decision tree. In this case the order of the features is important since this order determines if the feature acts on the entire set of samples, or a particular subset of samples. Here, the number of possible combinations is $\frac{K!}{(K-k)!}$ and an exhaustive search of 300 features to find the best seven-node decision tree would require examining 2.04×10^{17} trees. Since this is not computationally feasible, any result from a fingerprint-based classifier should be considered as a lower-bound to the accuracy of the classification algorithm.

In contrast, the search for the search for the best biomarker-based classifier is exhaustive. All features are examined by each filtering method and all combinations of putative biomarkers can be used in the final classifier.

1.4 Fingerprint-based classifiers

Informatic analysis has led to a new paradigm for classification known as fingerprinting or pattern matching. In this paradigm, individuals are classified based upon a particular pattern of intensities [Petricoin et al., 2003]. If an untested individual has the same pattern as a known individual, then these two have the same classification. The simplest fingerprint-based classifier is a decision tree (Figure 1). In all known applications of a decision tree to produce a classifier using spectral data [Ho et al., 2006; Liu et al., 2005; Yang et al., 2005; Yu et al., 2005], a single scoring metric (e.g. Gini Index, entropy gain, etc.) was used to determine the cut point at a given node so that the two daughter nodes were as homogeneous as possible for one or more categories (e.g. diseased versus healthy). Given the general structure of a decision tree in Figure 1, the root node (Node 1) would contain all training samples and an *m/z* value, or feature, and its cut point would be selected that best separates diseased and healthy individuals between Nodes 2 and 3. If there was still enough of a mixture in Node 2, for example, a second feature would be chosen based on the same metric that would separate the individuals into Nodes 4 and 5. The same process would be used for all heterogeneous nodes until there was a sufficient domination of one category over another.

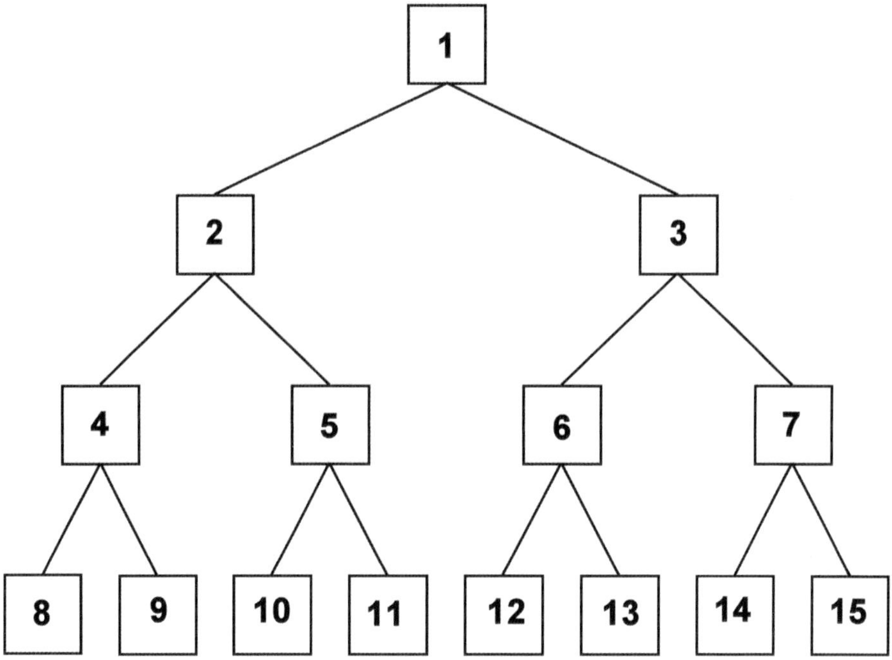

Fig. 1. Example of a 7-node decision tree.

Decision Support also uses decision trees, but an independent question is asked at each level in the tree. For example, Node 1 may be used to separate the individuals by gender, race, or other genetic difference, and then different features may be used to separate samples obtained from affected and healthy patients at a given level of stratification. Since the stratifying variables are not known ahead of time, there is no way to know the proper metric that should initially separate the training set. Therefore, the procedure used here is to construct unconstrained decision trees that best classify the training individuals.

The medoid classification algorithm is a best attempt at reproducing the algorithm used in many of the studies conducted in the laboratories of Emmanuel Petricoin and Lance Liotta [Browers et al., 2005; Conrads et al., 2004; Ornstein et al., 2004; Petricoin et al., 2004;

Srinivasan et al., 2006; Stone et al., 2005]. While these authors stated that their algorithm was quite similar to a Self-Organizing Map (SOM), their algorithm, as they described it, has virtually nothing in common with a SOM. In a SOM [Kohonen, 1988], the layout of the cells is determined *a priori*, as are the number of features, n, used in the separation. In general, the cells are placed in a rectangular or hexagonal pattern, with a maximum of four or six adjacent cells, respectively. The cells are seeded with random centroids that represent the n-dimensional coordinates of each cell. The first training sample is assigned to the cell with the closest centroid and the centroids of this and all the other cells are significantly shifted towards this sample. This procedure is repeated for all samples. Once all samples have been processed, the algorithm repetitively cycles through the list of training samples. In each subsequent cycle, the extent to which the centroid of the cell it is assigned to shifts towards that sample decreases, as does the extent to which the other centroids are affected. This shift becomes significantly smaller for cells that are further from the selected cell, as defined by the initial mapping. When finished, all samples are assigned to cells and each centroid represents an approximate average of the n features for all samples in that cell, and the distance between centroids increases as the cells become further apart in the pre-defined map.

In contrast, the algorithm used in the references cited above places the first training sample as the center of the first cell, and this cell is classified as the category of this sample. Since it is sample-centered, each cell has a medoid not a centroid. Each cell is given a constant trust radius, r. If the second sample has a distance that is larger than r from the first, it is assigned to a second cell and that cell is classified by its category; otherwise it is assigned to the first cell. This process continues until all training samples have been analyzed.

Therefore, a SOM has a fixed number of cells, each cell is described by a centroid, and the algorithm cycles through the training data many times to adjust the centroid's coordinates. The algorithm used by the groups of Petricoin and Liotta has an undefined number of cells, each described by a single sample, and the training data is only processed once.

Also grouped within the class of fingerprint-based classifiers are Support Vector Machines and Linear Discriminant Analysis. A Support Vector Machine (SVM) [Boser et al., 1992; Vapnik, 1998] is a kernel-based learning system. SVM searches for the optimal hyperplane that maximizes the margin of separation between the hyperplane and the closest data points on both sides of the hyperplane. Linear Discriminant Analysis (LDA) [Fukunaga, 1990] is a supervised learning algorithm. LDA finds the linear combination of features that maximize the between-class scatter and simultaneously minimize the within-class scatter to achieve maximum discrimination in a dataset. The within-class scatter matrix may become singular if the sample size is smaller than the dimensionality of the search space (number of features), but several techniques are available to handle this situation.

1.5 Biomarker-based classifiers

An example if a state-specific marker is shown in Figure 2. Each "+" represents, for example, the blood concentration of a particular biochemical. The individuals in the left column are in a specific disease state, while those in the right column are not and are therefore considered to be in a healthy state, at least with respect to this disease. Individuals in each state have different blood concentrations of this biochemical due to genetic and environmental differences between individuals and any experimental uncertainty in the measurement. What is clear is that the range of concentrations for individuals in the disease state is significantly higher than for those not in this state. Such a marker can be used to classify the individuals into three groups; they are in the disease state if the blood concentration is above an upper threshold, they are not in this disease state if the concentration is below a lower threshold, and they are undetermined if the blood concentration is between these thresholds.

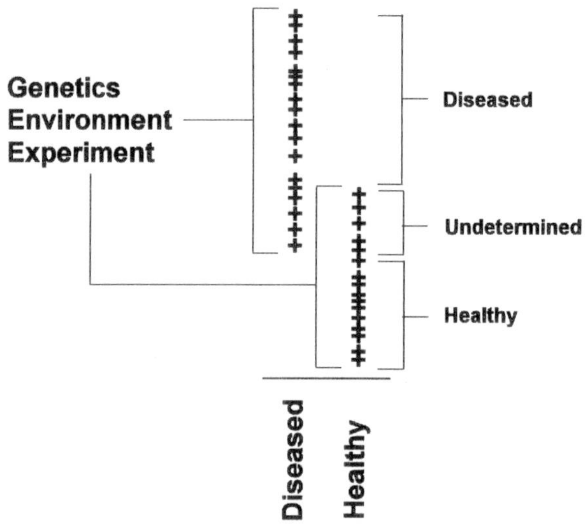

Fig. 2. Values of a state-specific marker for individuals in a disease state (left) and in a healthy state (right).

While blood concentrations of biochemicals are one possible means of examination, it is not the only one. Concentrations of biochemicals in the urine are another, but this can be extended to tears, mucous, or virtually any biofluid. Instead of directly measuring the concentration of specific compounds, mass spectra (with or without pre-fractionation) and 2D NMR of these biofluids can also be used to measure abundance. The difference with these spectral methods is that the abundance of a compound can be examined from one individual to the next without knowing the identity of this compound. Therefore, examining the intensity or area of spectral peaks is called an undirected search since a list of compounds to examine was not created before hand, while direct measurements of concentrations or intensity measurements from microarray experiments are directed searches since the search is over a set of pre-defined compounds.

In general, the set of biochemicals whose concentration is directly measured or examined by microarray analysis, as well as the set of peaks present in various spectra, are known as features. For each individual, each of these features has a corresponding value. This value can be the concentration, the logarithm of the relative fluorescence intensity, or the intensity or area of the spectral peak. The search for a putative biomarker is over the set of N available features, and each individual is represented by an array of N numbers representing the values of these features.

Since the values of many features are known for each individual, it is possible to construct classifiers using two or more features. An algorithm would search through sets of two or more features to find a set that optimally classified a given set of individuals, which is known as a training set. The goal is to maximize the number of correctly classified individuals, so if two features are used and one is that shown in Figure 2, the second feature would try to correctly resolve those in the undetermined region without upsetting the correct classification of the other individuals. Therefore, the action of this second feature in the classifier is to specifically act on those individuals in the undetermined region. The first feature (Figure 2) therefore is a state-specific marker since its intensity is largely controlled by the state of the individual, while the second feature is individual-specific since it only acts on those individuals who have an intensity of the first feature in the undetermined region.

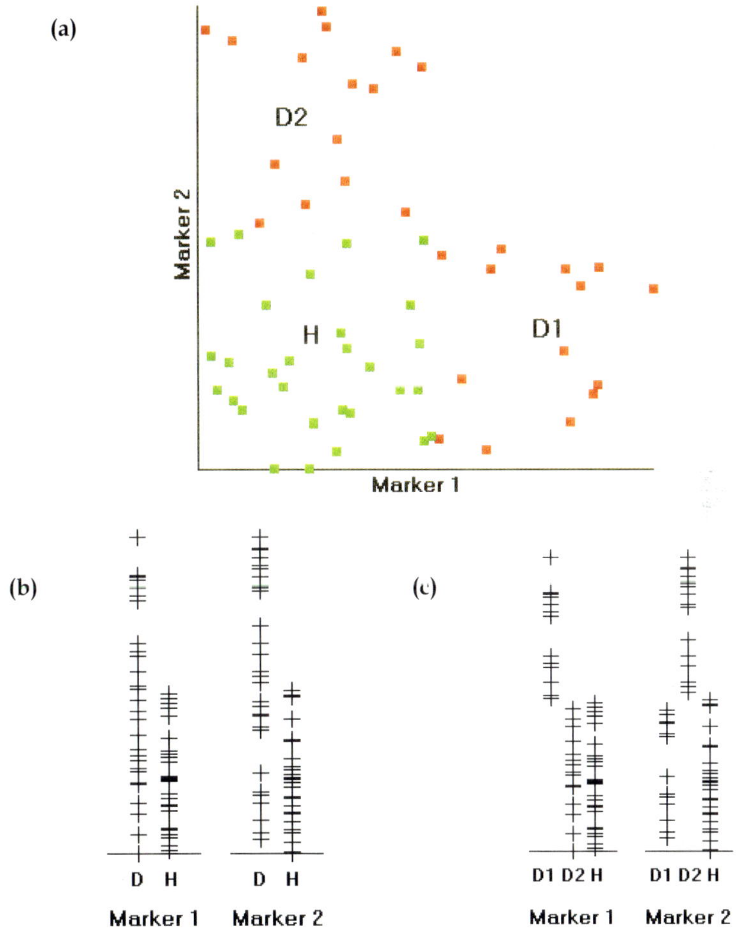

Fig. 3. (a) Scatter plot for diseased (red) and healthy (green) individuals using the values of a pair of correlated markers; (b) Values for these markers assuming one state for each category; and (c) Values for these markers assuming two disease states and one healthy state.

This argument suggests that statistical methods which find features that are significantly different in magnitude depending upon an individual's state is all that is needed to find any state-specific markers. These independent markers can be found if both the healthy and diseased categories are represented by a single state. Figure 3 displays a situation where the diseased category (shown in red) is actually composed of two states (D1 and D2). This can only be seen through the action of a concerted pair of markers, Marker 1 and Marker 2. State D1 has a high intensity in Marker 1 while State D2 has a high intensity in Marker 2, while the healthy individuals have a low intensity in both features. Figure 3 shows intensity plots for these two markers under the assumption that there is a single diseased state and a single healthy state. It is questionable whether a given statistical method would find the difference in the intensities of these features significant. Only by correctly distinguishing the state if each individual can one see that Marker 1 is a good classifier for State D1 and Marker 2 for State D2 (Figure 3).

1.6 Bias, chance and generalizability

Ransohoff [2005a, 2005b] has presented three factors that must be explored in any classification study; bias, chance and generalizability. Until now, any marker that clearly distinguishes individuals in different states, either alone or in a concerted action with another feature, is denoted as a putative biomarker. Before it can become a true biomarker one has to ensure that the marker is not due to an underlying bias. For example, if all individuals in the disease state are being given a particular drug, there is no way to determine if the change in the feature value is due to the disease or the drug. There is no way to remove this bias, and such situations should be excluded in the initial study design. As a second example, the individuals in the disease state may be significantly older than those in the healthy state. Many diseases are more prevalent in older individuals and it may be very difficult to find age-matched patients who are disease free or are not on a regular drug treatment. If a random collection of age-matched individuals without signs of the particular disease state are taken to be the healthy category, it is likely that this category will be composed of a number of states due to other diseases or drug responses. Markers separating each of these "healthy" states from the disease state would have to be found. Finding all required biomarkers would be very difficult within a single set of features. In addition, if the number of individuals in a particular healthy state was small, the significance of any biomarker may be suspect (see below). For this case, the affect of age can be examined. If there is no correlation between the feature value and the age of the individual in either the disease or healthy state, one can conclude that age is not the source of the difference in feature values.

If the available individuals in the disease and healthy states are divided into a training set and a testing set, it is theoretically possible to construct one or more classifiers using the training set that can accurately classify the individuals in the testing set without using a state-based marker. Such a classifier is a chance fit to the available data, and we have shown that accurate results can be obtained for certain classifiers without any state-specific marker being present in the set of available features. Therefore, simply constructing a good classifier is not sufficient to demonstrate the presence of a state-specific marker.

The basic assumption is that if a classifier is able to accurately classify both a training set and a testing set of data, then this classifier will be useful for all individuals in the population from which these individuals were taken. In other words, any classifier that accurately classifies a sufficient sample from a population should be generalizable to the entire population. We assert that this assumption may be true only if the classifier is strictly composed of state-specific markers. Any classifier that is a chance fit to the available data will not be generalizable to the entire population.

1.7 Coverage, uniqueness, and significance

The simplest example of fingerprinting is a straightforward decision tree, like the one shown in Figure 4. Assuming that the entire dataset is composed of 60 diseased and 60 healthy individuals, the intensity of Feature 1 splits the dataset into two groups; 40 diseased and 20 healthy individuals if the intensity of this feature is below Cut-1 and 20 diseased and 40 healthy individuals if its intensity is above Cut-1. The left branch is further divided using Feature 2 into a diseased node (D1) that contains 38 diseased and 3 healthy individuals and a healthy node (H1) that contains 2 diseased and 17 healthy individuals. The right branch is divided using Feature 3 into a healthy (H2) and a diseased (D2) terminal node.

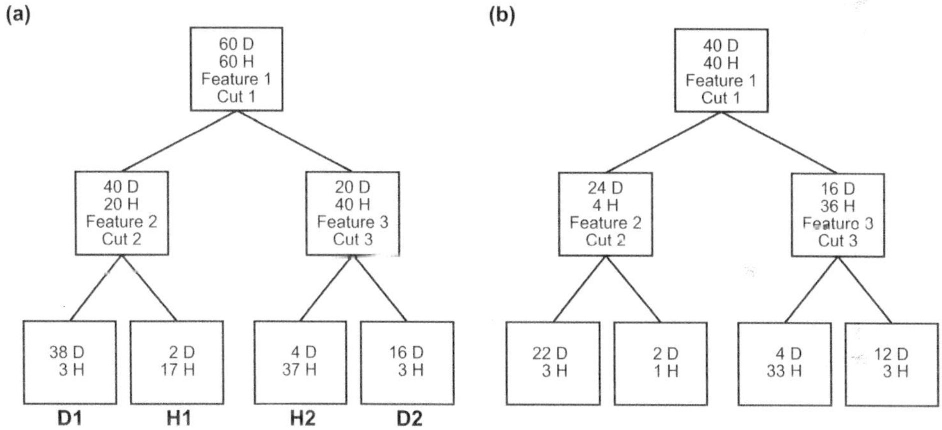

Fig. 4. (a) Hypothetical decision tree using all available data and (b) the corresponding tree when one-third of the samples are removed as testing data.

Overall this decision tree would yield a sensitivity and a specificity of 90%, but the general procedure is to divide the data into a training set and a testing set and construct the classifier using only the training data. If one-third of the data was removed to form the testing data, the situation in Figure 4b could be produced. In this example, 16 of the 20 healthy samples happened to come from H1 and 16 of 20 diseased samples from D1. This training distribution would make the use of Feature 2 unnecessary and may result in different features being used at each node. If only Features 1 and 3 were used, the training set would have a sensitivity of 90% and a specificity of 82.5%, while the testing data would have a sensitivity of 100% but a specificity of only 20%. The basic reason for this large change in sensitivity is that the fingerprint needed to describe the healthy subjects in Group H1 is no longer present in the training data.

Therefore, the first requirement of a fingerprinting method is that there must be a complete *coverage* of all required fingerprints in the training data. If a required fingerprint or proteomic pattern is missing from the training data (Figure 4), the quality of predictions for the testing data will either be greatly reduced or there will be a significant number of testing individuals that will receive an "undetermined" classification.

If a fingerprinting classifier is found that performs extremely well on classifying the training data, but classifies the testing data poorly, one can either state that the classifier is insufficient and therefore not biologically relevant, or that there was an incorrect separation of training and validation data so that effective coverage of all important fingerprints was not present in the training data. Since the discriminating fingerprints are not known, proper coverage cannot be known, and therefore proper selection of the training data cannot be known. In addition, since the quality of classifying the testing set is the metric used to determine biological relevance, the testing set is used in the process of constructing the classifier and is therefore part of the training process.

With these points in mind, an effective way to construct classifiers based on fingerprints is to include all data in the search for fingerprinting classifiers and then to selectively remove samples for the testing set in a way that preserves the coverage of the fingerprint in the training data. This statement does not suggest, in any way, that this procedure is used by other research groups who present fingerprinting classifiers, it simply states that this method is an effective way to ensure complete coverage in the training data and to effectively test for uniqueness. If Figure 4 was used as the basic classifier, all other possible three-node decision trees would have to be constructed and compared to a sensitivity and specificity of 90%. If no other three-node decision tree is found to have this overall accuracy, then the uniqueness of this classifier is established. Otherwise, each decision tree would have to be presented as a possible solution; since the important fingerprints are not known, the selection of the training set cannot be determined, and two different decision trees that imply different separations of training and validation data are therefore equally valid.

Finally, the *significance* of a fingerprinting classifier needs to be established. Permutation testing is often used to test significance, but can be used in three different ways. In the Random Forest algorithm [Breiman, 2001] the intensities of a given feature are scrambled among all data in each testing set (i.e. the out-of-bag samples) to determine the importance of that feature. The phenotypes of the samples can also be scrambled a large number of times to determine the probability that the accuracy of a given classifier occurred by chance. In this application, the phenotypes will be scrambled amongst all data to determine if a new classifier of the same form (e.g. a three-node decision tree) can be constructed with comparable accuracy. The probability that random phenotypes can be classified to a given accuracy determines the significance of a given model.

1.8 Proposed study

To test the classification ability of different algorithms, this study will attempt to build classifiers from sets of 300 possible features. In each case, the intensities of the features will be determined using a random number generator. In other words, each classifier will attempt to distinguish healthy samples from diseased ones using data that contains no information. Results using DT and MCA classifiers have been previously presented [Luke &

Collins, 2008], but these will be included here to compare to SVM, LDA, and biomarker-based classifiers. Exhaustive searches using DT, MCA, SVM and LDA are not computationally feasible, so the results presented here represent a lower bound to the accuracy that can be obtained from these methods with data that contains no information. It should also be stressed that 300 features is a very small number by current methods of analysis of biological samples, and the accuracy of all methods will not decrease as the number of features increases.

2. Methods

2.1 Decision tree

For the symmetric, 7-node decision tree shown in Figure 1, a modified Evolutionary Programming (mEP) procedure is used. Each putative decision tree classifier is represented by two 7-element arrays; the first contains the feature used at each node and the second contains the cut values. Both arrays assumed the node ordering listed in Figure 1. The only caveats are that all seven features must be different and that this ordered septet of features cannot be the same as any other putative solution in either the parent or offspring populations. When a new putative decision tree is formed, a local search is used to find optimum cut points for this septet of features.

The mEP procedure starts by randomly generating 2000 unique decision trees. Each decision tree has one or two of the features removed and unique features are selected, again requiring that the final septet is unique. The local search first tries to find optimum cut points for the new features that were added and then the search is over all seven cut points. The best set of cut points is combined with the septet of features to represent an offspring classifier. The score is the sum of the sensitivity and specificity for the training individuals over the eight terminal nodes. When the entire set of initial, or parent, decision trees have generated unique offspring, all 4000 scores are compared and the 2000 decision trees with the best score become parents for the next generation. This process is repeated for a total of 4000 generations and the best classifiers in the final population are examined.

2.2 Mediod classification algorithm

While the algorithm described by Petricoin and Liotta [Browers et al., 2005; Conrads et al., 2004; Ornstein et al., 2004; Petricoin et al., 2004; Srinivasan et al., 2006; Stone et al., 2005] used a genetic algorithm driver to search for an optimum set of features, allowing for different putative solutions to use different numbers of features (5-20 features), our algorithm uses a mEP feature selection algorithm and all putative solutions have the same number of features *n*. For a given value of *n*, *n* features were selected and the intensities of these features were rescaled for each individual using the following formula [Browers et al., 2005; Conrads et al., 2004; Ornstein et al., 2004; Petricoin et al., 2004; Srinivasan et al., 2006; Stone et al., 2005]:

$$I' = (I - Imin) / (Imax - Imin) \quad (1)$$

In this equation, I is a feature's original intensity, I' is it's scaled intensity, and Imin and Imax are the minimum and maximum intensities found for the individual among the *n* selected features, respectively. If Imin and Imax were from the same features in all samples, a baseline intensity would be subtracted and the remaining values scaled so that the largest intensity was 1.0. Each individual would then be represented as a point in an (*n*-2)-dimensional unit cube. As designed, and as found in practice, Imin and Imax do not represent the same features from one individual to the next, so this interpretation does not hold. Therefore, each individual represents a point in an *n*-dimensional unit cube.

As stated in the Background, the first training sample becomes the medoid of the first cell, with this cell being classified as the category of this sample. Each cell has a constant trust radius *r*, which is set to 0.1 $(n)^{1/2}$, or ten percent of the maximum theoretical separation in this unit hypercube. If the second sample is within *r* of the first, it is placed in the first cell; otherwise it becomes the medoid of the second cell and that cell is characterized by the second sample's category. This iteration continues until all training samples are processed. Each cell is then examined and the categories of all samples in the cell are compared to the cell's classification. This calculation allows a sensitivity and specificity to be determined for the training data, and their sum represents the score for this set of *n* features.

The mEP algorithm initially selects 2000 sets of *n* randomly selected features. The only caveat is that each set of *n* features must be different from all previously selected sets. The medoid classification algorithm then determines the score for each set of features. Again, each parent set of features generates an offspring set of features by randomly removing one or two of the features and replacing them with randomly selected features, requiring that this set be different from all feature sets in the parent population and in all offspring generated so far. The score of this feature set is determined and the score and feature set is stored in the offspring population. After all 2000 offspring have been generated the parent and offspring populations are combined. The 2000 feature sets with the best score are retained and become the parents for the next generation.

It should be noted that for a set of *n* features, the number of unique cells that can be generated is on the order of 10^n. Since no training set is ever this large (*n* is 5 or more), only a small fraction of the possible cells will be populated and classified. As will be shown in the next section, this limitation causes a significant number of the testing samples to be placed in an unclassified cell, though none of the publications that used this method [Browers et al., 2005; Conrads et al., 2004; Ornstein et al., 2004; Petricoin et al., 2004; Srinivasan et al., 2006; Stone et al., 2005] reported an undetermined classification for any of the testing samples. Instead of searching through a large number of solutions that classified the training samples to a significant extent and find those that minimized the number of unclassified testing samples, we decided to use all samples and limit the number of cells. All samples were placed in the training set and the algorithm was run with the added requirement that any set of *n* features that produced more than a selected number of cells was given a score of zero. If the number of healthy and disease medoids are sufficiently small, all other samples could then be divided to place the required number in the testing set and the remainder would be part of the training.

2.3 Support Vector Machine

A support Vector Machine (SVM) [Boser et al., 1992; Vapnik, 1998] is a kernel-based learning system. SVM searches for the optimal hyperplane that maximizes the margin of separation between the hyperplane and the closest data points on both sides of the hyperplane.

Many features in a genomic or proteomic data are irrelevant or redundant that may likely hinder the performance of a classifier. It is essential to select informative features to build a classifier. A new selection criterion is presented with a performance found to be better than or comparable to the other criteria and is applied to LDA and linear SVM as a classification method.

Support Vector Machines (SVM) [Boser, 1992; Vapnik, 1998], are becoming increasingly popular in biological problems [Noble, 2004]. SVM finds the optimal hyperplane that maximizes the margin of separation between the hyperplane and the closest data points on both sides of the hyperplane. Instead of error-risk minimization, the parameters of SVMs are determined on the basis of structural risk minimization. Thus, they have the tendency to overcome the overfitting problem. SVMs have been successful with a recursive procedure in selecting important features for cancer prediction [Guyon et al., 2002; Tang et al., 2007].

The decision functions (used to determine the class of a sample) of SVM and LDA can be expressed as a linear combination of features. They differ with regard to how the weights are determined. The weights (coefficients in the decision function) of features, which reflect the significance of the features for classification, can be served as a feature ranking criterion. This criterion corresponds to removing a feature whose elimination changes the objective function least [LeCun et al., 1990]. The criterion has been used with a recursive feature elimination scheme [Guyon et al., 2002], as described before.

Instead of judging a feature by its contribution to the classification on the full dataset, this study uses a leave-one-out cross-validation to evaluate a feature's contribution to the ensemble of classifiers. In other words, a classifier is re-trained on a new dataset formed by removing a sample from original dataset to obtain a weight for every feature. If a feature is important in differentiating samples, it should remain so when any sample is removed from a dataset. This can be indicated by the coefficient of variation of the weight value for each feature. The coefficient of variation is defined as the ratio of the standard deviation to the mean. A small coefficient of variation indicates smaller variation and a more consistent contribution of a feature to the sample classification. There are two ways to incorporate this criterion into the recursive selection process. One is to pre-select the number of iterations and the number of features at each iteration. This can be implemented by determining the coefficient of variation for each feature in current feature set and selecting k features with smallest coefficient of variation, where k is the predefined number of features for this iteration. In the second implementation, the number of iterations and the number of features at each iteration are determined during the selection process. It starts with all the features and can be described as follow:

Step 1. Compute the coefficient of variation for each feature in current feature set. In every selection cycle, the procedure initially eliminates at least certain number of features. In this study, 10% of the current features, or 1 whichever is larger, with largest coefficient of variation are eliminated.

Step 2. Let c_{min} denote the minimum coefficient of variation and c_{max} denote the maximum coefficient of variation among the remaining features.

Step 3. Select k coefficient of variation, $c_1, c_2, \ldots, c_k$, such that $c_{min} < c_1 < c_2 < \ldots < c_k = c_{max}$ and $c_1, c_2, \ldots, c_k$ divided the interval $[c_{min}, c_{max}]$ into k subintervals of equal lengths except possibly the interval $[c_{k-1}, c_{max}]$. In this study, we choose $k=8$.

Step 4. Estimate, for each c_i, $i=1,2,\ldots,k$, the performance of a classifier, which uses all the features whose coefficient of variation is less than or equal to c_i, from a cross-validation, such as, leave-one-out cross-validation.

Step 5. Find the smallest c_i from $c_1, c_2, \ldots, c_k$ which gives the best performance in Step 3.

Step 6. Choose all the features from current feature set whose coefficient of variation are less than or equal to c_i as the feature subset for this selection cycle.

The selection process is repeated until only one feature remains.

2.4 Linear Discriminate Analysis

Linear Discriminant Analysis (LDA) [Fukunaga, 1990] is a supervised learning algorithm that finds the linear combination of features that maximize the between-class scatter and simultaneously minimize the within-class scatter to achieve maximum discrimination in a dataset. The within-class scatter matrix may become singular if the sample size is smaller than the dimensionality of the search space (number of features). To overcome the singularity problem, the pseudo-inverse [Golub & Van Loan, 1983] of the within-class scatter matrix is computed in this study.

The computation of a pseudo-inverse in LDA may be demanding if the dimension of within-class scatter matrix is too large. In this study diagonal LDA is used, which is the same as LDA except that the covariance matrices are assumed to be diagonal. The diagonal LDA has been reported to be performed remarkably well compared to more sophisticated methods [Dudoit et al., 2002]. A leave-one-out procedure is again used to determine the coefficient of variation for all remaining features, and procedure outlined above is used to reduce the feature set.

2.5 Biomarker Discovery Kit

The BioMarker Discovery Kit (BMDK) represents a suite of programs with the eventual goal of constructing one or more biomarker-based classifiers. Each biomarker represents a particular feature that is associated with a particular disease state represented by a subset of the available individuals. BMDK uses 10 different methods of analysis to identify putative biomarkers. These methods determine how well each feature distinguishes some or all of the individuals in a given histology. Descriptions of each filtering method are given elsewhere [http://isp.ncifcrf.gov/abcc/abcc-groups/simulation-and-modeling/biomarker-discovery-kit/].The union of all features that have one of the top five scores for each of the 10 methods produces the set of putative biomarkers.

A single biocompound may produce more than one putative biomarker if the features are obtained from a mass spectroscopic investigation. For example, separate peaks for the +1 and +2 ion or the biocompound alone and complexed with another compound are possible. Therefore, the Pearson's correlation coefficient between all pairs of putative biomarkers across all samples is used to combine the putative biomarkers into groups. All other features in the dataset are then compared to the putative biomarkers within each group and are selected for examination if the correlation coefficient is 0.70 or higher. Each group is then represented by the single feature with the largest maximum value; all other features are discarded.

The final classifier is based on a distance-dependent K-nearest neighbor (DD-KNN) algorithm. In this classifier the un-normalized probability that an unknown sample belongs to the same group as a neighbor is given by the inverse of their distance. To account for the situation where an unknown sample has no nearest neighbors, the classifier also contains a probability that its group is unknown. This probability linearly increases from 0.0 to 0.01 as the probability of being in a neighbors group decreases from 1.0 to 0.8. For smaller probabilities of belonging to the neighbor's group, the probability of being unknown stays constant at 0.1. These probabilities are summed over all neighbors and scaled to a total probability of 1.0. Therefore, each unknown sample is described by a probability of belonging to Group-1 (e.g. healthy), Group-2 (e.g. diseased), and Undetermined. The final classification is given by a probability of membership of at least 0.5, or Undetermined if the probabilities of belonging to either group is less than 0.5.

All of the putative biomarkers are individually used to find the best 1-feature DD-KNN algorithm, and this is followed by an exhaustive search over all sets of two and three putative biomarkers. In practice, six nearest neighbors are generally used but this number can be increased if there are a large number of samples; the number of neighbors should not decrease below six. The quality of the classifier is determined using a leave-one-out procedure since this method preserves the coverage (range of intensities) for the samples to the greatest extent. Each time an optimum classifier is found, the distribution of samples in feature-space is plotted to determine the number of disease state present for each category.

3. Results

Since the datasets examined in this investigation are produced using a random number generator, the goal is to simply determine a lower-bound to the accuracy that can be obtained for 300 features for different numbers of Cases and Controls. Since these labels really have no meaning, the accuracy of a classifier will be given by the sum of the sensitivity and specificity. These are lower bounds since only five different datasets are examined for each Case/Control combination, and for all methods but BMDK only a small fraction of all possible feature-combinations are explored.

3.1 DT and MCA classifiers

For the DT and MCA classifiers, it is assumed that the dataset is divided such that two-thirds of the samples in each group are used in the training set and one-third is used in the testing set. The accuracy of the classifier is the sum of the sensitivity and specificity of the testing set.

For the DT algorithm, all samples are used in the construction of the decision tree. After the best decision tree is constructed from the evolutionary programming search over ordered sets of seven features, one-third of the samples are removed to build the testing set. This is done in a way that does not change the description of each terminal node (i.e. it stays as either a healthy or diseased node) and the sensitivity and specificity of the training and testing sets are approximately equal. This may appear to be cheating, but the goal of this investigation is to determine the minimum accuracy that could be obtained from data that contains no information.

The best quality from the five datasets for each number of Cases and Controls is given in Table 1. For 30 Cases and 30 Controls, a 7-node decision tree was able to correctly classify all 60 samples. In other words, all eight terminal nodes only contained samples from a single group. For 60 Cases and 60 Controls, a decision tree correctly classifies over 89% of the testing samples, and for 90 Cases and Controls, over 83% of the testing samples were correctly classified. It is only when the number of samples is as large or larger than the number of features that the DT classifier drops below 80% accuracy for the testing data.

Cases and Controls	**DT**	**MCA**		
		5-Feat	6-Feat	7-Feat
30	200.0	200.0	200.0	200.0
42	190.5	197.6	197.6	197.6
60	178.3	193.3	193.3	195.0
90	166.7	187.8	188.9	191.1
150	155.3	183.3	185.3	187.3
300	138.3	170.3	179.0	180.3

Table 1. Highest quality obtained using absolute differences in un-scaled peak intensities, from a decision tree (EPDT) and the medoid classifier algorithm (MCA). *Note:* Taken from [Luke & Collins, 2008] where the quality is the sum of the sensitivity and specificity.

The classifier constructed by the MCA is order dependent in that the first training sample automatically becomes the medoid of the first region. Therefore, this analysis uses all samples to construct a classifier with the requirement that the samples used as medoids cannot exceed two-thirds of either the Cases or Controls. One-third of the samples from each group are then selected as testing samples and are chosen such that the accuracy of the training set is at least as high as the testing set.

The results in Table 1 show that an MCA classifier performs excellently using datasets that contain no information. If only seven of the 300 features are used, one can find a classifier with an average sensitivity and specificity of over 90% even when there are 300 Cases and 300 Controls (200 of each in the training set and 100 of each in the testing set). If the number of features is reduced to five or six, the accuracy stays above 90% for all but the largest datasets.

3.2 SVM and LDA classifiers

The results for the SVM and LDA classifiers are shown in Table 2. As described above, all samples are used to determine which features will be used in the classifier, but the accuracy of the final classification uses the sum of the sensitivity and specificity of the testing set for 10-fold cross-validation, averaged over 100 runs where the order of the samples are scrambled before each run. SVM has an average classification accuracy over 97% when there are 90 or fewer Cases and Controls in the dataset. For LDA, the average accuracy stays above 99.7%.

For the larger datasets, the accuracy decreases significantly. When there are 150 Cases and 150 Controls, the SVM and LDA classifiers have an average accuracy of about 87 and 84%, respectively. This is better than a 7-node decision tree, but not as good as any of the MCA classifiers examined. Datasets that contain 300 Cases, 300 Controls, and only 300 features have SVM and LDA accuracies of 61.3 and 63.7% respectively, which is below the accuracy of the DT and MCA classifiers.

Cases and Controls		SVM		LDA
30		198.50		199.06
42		199.88		199.84
60		199.02		199.68
90		194.82		199.52
150		174.38		167.90
300		132.66		135.44

Table 2. Highest quality obtained using normalized feature values from support vector machine (SVM) and linear discriminate analysis (LDA) classifiers. *Note:* The quality is the sum of the sensitivity and specificity for the testing set averaged over 100 runs of 10-fold cross-validation.

3.3 BMDK Classifier

The accuracy of the BMDK classifier is shown in Table 3. This accuracy is determined from a leave-one-out cross-validation, a procedure that is known to exaggerate the accuracy of a classifier. After each sample is classified, the overall accuracy is the sum of the sensitivity and specificity minus the percentage of samples that were classified as unknown. For the smallest dataset (30 Cases and 30 Controls) a 3-feature DD-KNN classifier correctly classified 78.9% of the samples. In general, the accuracy decreased as the number of samples increased.

Cases and Controls		BMDK		
		1-Feat	2-Feat	3-Feat
30		147.4	153.3	157.8
42		142.9	136.4	137.3
60		151.7	140.0	140.1
90		123.3	137.9	137.3
150		118.0	127.3	125.3
300		115.7	121.7	122.1

Table 3. Highest quality obtained from the BioMarker Development Kit (BMDK) using absolute differences in un-scaled peak intensities. *Note:* The quality is the sum of the sensitivity and specificity minus the percent of samples undetermined using a leave-one-out cross-validation of the entire set of data.

The only exception was for one dataset with 60 Cases and 60 Controls. This increased accuracy was due to an unusual pattern in one of the randomly generated features. The intensities for this feature are shown in Figure 5, where the "+" marks in the left column are the intensities of the 60 samples in Group-1 and the marks in the right column are for the 60 samples in Group-2. While there is no overall difference between these columns, a closer examination shown a clumping of intensities in one group at values that have gaps in the other group.

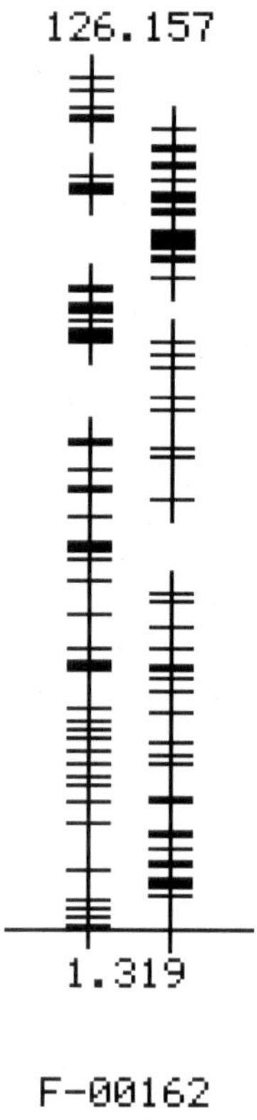

Fig. 5. Intensities for the 60 cases (left column) and 60 controls (right column) for the peak that yielded a quality score of 151.7 (sensitivity=78.3%, specificity=73.3%, undetermined=0.0%) in the dataset of random peak intensities.

In many cases the accuracy of a 3-feature classifier is not significantly better than a 2-feature classifier. This is due to the fact that as the dimensionality of the classification space increases, the separation between the samples becomes larger. This causes more samples to be classified as Undetermined. For this reason, no 4-feature classifier did better than the 3-feature classifier in any of the 30 datasets.

4. Discussion

The results presented in the tables above show that very good results can be obtained from DT, MCA, SVM and LDA classifiers for datasets that contain no information. It can be argued that the procedures used here are selected to obtain the maximum possible accuracy, and that is exactly the point. If a 7-node decision tree used 40 Cases and 40 Controls in the training set and 20 Cases and 20 Controls in the testing set and obtained an accuracy of 87.5% for the testing samples, one could propose that the set of seven features denotes a fingerprint that accurately classifies the samples. The results in Table 1 show that this accuracy can be obtained from a dataset with only 300 randomly generated feature values for each sample. A 7-feature MCA classifier is able to achieve an average accuracy of over 90% when the dataset contains 300 Cases, 300 Controls, and only 300 non-informative features. This should draw into question the results of any study that uses this classification method.

SVM and LDA classifiers have testing set accuracies above 97.4 and 99.7%, respectively, for all but the largest datasets. It is only when the number of samples is at least as large as the number of features that these methods break down. Current methods for obtaining information from biological samples generate many more features that the 300 used here.

The BMDK classifier did not achieve an average accuracy above 80% for even the smallest dataset. This result is not unexpected. Since the datasets do not contain any information, there are no biomarkers and a biomarker-based classifier should not perform well. Fortuitous results can be obtained and a closer examination of the putative biomarkers should be performed (Figure 5).

For the DT and MCA methods there is some selection of which samples should be placed in the training and testing sets, but this is basically what is required because of the coverage problem. If a given terminal node in a DT classifier contains 7 Cases and 4 Controls, and 4 of the Cases were moved to the testing set, this terminal node would change from a Case-node to a Control-node and the classification accuracy of the testing data would be decreased. The MCA classifier is based on the premise of a fingerprint that associates a sample in the testing set with a sample in the training set. If that sample were removed from the training set, the association could not be made and the accuracy of the classifier would be decreased.

5. Conclusions

The results presented here show that very good classification results can be obtained from DT, MCA, SVM, and LDA classifiers, even if the dataset contains no information. Studies using any of these methods should carefully examine whether the results are due to some underlying biology or are just fortuitous. Performing comparable examinations on randomly generated feature values, or performing analysis of the same data after the group labels of the samples has been scrambled, should be a necessary part of these investigations.

In contract, a biomarker-based classifier such as BMDK should perform poorly if the dataset contains no biological information. Even when reasonably good results are obtained, the putative biomarkers used in the classifier should be carefully examined to ensure that they really distinguish samples in one group from the other.

6. Acknowledgement

The authors would like to thank Dr. Jih-H Chen who constructed the recursive SVM and LDA programs and generated their results. This work was funded in whole with federal funds from the National Cancer Institute, National Institutes of Health, under Contract No. HHSN261200800001E and the Center for Biomedical Informatics and Information Technology (CBIIT)/Cancer Biomedical Informatics Grid (caBIG) ISRCE yellow task #09-260 to NCI-Frederick. The content of this publication does not necessarily reflect the views or policies of the Department of Health and Human Services, nor does mention of trade names, commercial products, or organizations imply endorsement by the United States Government.

7. References

Bellman, R.E. & Rand Corporation (1957). *Dynamic Programming,* Princeton University Press

Bellman, R.E. (1961). *Adaptive Control Processes: A Guided Tour,* Princeton University Press

Bellman, R.E. (2003). *Dynamic Programming,* Courier Dover Publications

Boser. B., Guyon, I. &Vapnik, V. (1992). A Training Algorithm For Optimal Margin Classifiers, In: *Proceedings of the 5th Annual Workshop on Computational Learning Theory,* pp. 114-152, New York, NY, USA

Breiman, L. (2001). Random Forests. *Machine Learning,* Vol. 45, pp. 5-32

Browers, F.M., Petricoin, E.F. 3rd, Ksinantova, L., Breza, J., Rajapakse, V., Ross, S., et al. (2005). Low Molecular Weight Proteomic Information Distinguishes Metastatic From Benign Pheochromocytoma. *Endocrine-Related Cancer* Vol. 12, pp. 263-72

Conrads, T.P., Fusaro, V.A., Ross, S., Johann, D., Rajapakse, V., Hitt, B.A., et al. (2004). High-Resolution Serum Proteomic Features For Ovarian Cancer Detection. *Endocrine-Related Cancer,* Vol. 11, pp. 163-78

Dudoit, S., Fridlyand, J., & Speed, T.P. (2002). Comparison of Discrimination Methods For Classification of Tumors Using Gene Expression Data. *Journal of the American Statistical Association,* Vol. 97, No. 457, pp. 77-87

Fukunaga, K. (1990). *Introduction to Statistical Pattern Recognition,* Academic Press, 2nd Edition, Boston, Mass, USA

Golub, G. & Van Loan, C. (1983). *Matrix Computations.* The John Hopkins University Press, Baltimore, USA

Guyon, I., Weston, J., & Barnill, S. (2002) Gene Selection for Cancer Classification Using Support Vector Machines. *Machine Learning*, Vol. 46, No. 1, pp. 389-422

Ho, D.W., Yang, Z.F., Wong, B.Y., Kwong, D.L., Sham, J.S., Wei, W.I., et al. (2006). Surface-Enhanced Laser Desorption/Ionization Time-of-Flight Mass Spectrometry Serum Protein Profiling to Identify Nasopharyngeal Carcinoma. *Cancer,* Vol. 107, pp. 99-107

Kohonen, T. (1988). Self-Organizing and Associative Memory, 2nd ed., New York, Springer-Verlag

LeCun, Y., Denker. J., & Solla, S. (1990). Optimal Brain Damage, In *Advances In Neural Information Processing System II*, Morgan Kaufmann, San Mateo, CA, USA

Liu, W., Guan, M., Wu, D., Zhang, Y., Wu, Z., Xu, M., & Lu, Y. (2005). Using Tree Analysis Pattern and SELDI-TOF-MS to Discriminate Transitional Cell Carcinoma of the Bladder Cancer From Noncancer Patients. *European Urology,* Vol. 47, pp. 456-62

Luke, B.T., & Collins, J.R. (2008). *Examining the Significance of Fingerprint-based Classifiers.* BMC Bioinformatics, Vol. 9, No. 1, (December 17), p. 545

Noble, W. (2004). Support Vector Machine Applications in Computational Biology, In: *Kernel Methods in Computational Biology*, pp. 71-92, MIT Press, Cambridge, Mass, USA

Ornstein, D.K., Rayford, W., Fusaro, V.A., Conrads, T.P., Ross, S.J., Hitt, B.A., et al. (2004). Serum Proteomic Profiling Can Discriminate Prostate Cancer From Benign Prostates In Men With Total Prostate Specific Antigen Levels Between 2.5 and 15.0 ng/ml. *Journal of Urology*, Vol. 172, pp. 1302-1305

Petricoin, E.F., Fishman, D.A., Conrads, T.P., Veenstra, T.D., & Liotta, L.A. (2003). Proteomic Pattern Diagnostics: Producers and Consumers in the era of correlative science. *BMC Bioinformatics,* Vol. 4, p. 24/comments

Petricoin, E.F., Rajapaske, V., Herman, E.H., Arekani, A.M., Ross, S., Johann, D., et al. (2004). Toxicoproteomics: Serum Proteomic Pattern Diagnostics For Early Detection of Drug Induced Cardiac Toxicities and Cardioprotection. *Toxicologic Pathology,* Vol. 32, Suppl. 1, pp. 122-30

Ransohoff, D.F. (2005a). Lessons From Controversy: Ovarian Cancer Screening and Serum Proteomics. *Journal of the National Cancer Institute,* Vol. 97, pp. 315-319

Ransohoff, D.F. (2005b). Bias as a Threat to the Validity of Cancer Molecular-marker Research. *Nature Reviews Cancer*, Vol. 5, pp. 142-149

Srinivasan, R., Daniels, J., Fusaro, V., Lundqvist, A., Killian, J.K., Geho, D., et al. (2006). Accurate Diagnosis of Acute Graft-versus-host Disease Using Serum Proteomic Pattern Analysis. *Experimental Hematology,* Vol. 34, pp. 796-801

Stone, J.H., Rajapakse, V.N., Hoffman, G.S., Specks, U., Merkel, P.A., Spiera, R.F., et al. (2005). A serum proteomic approach to gauging the state of remission in Wegener's granulomatosis. *Arthritis & Rheumatism,* Vol. 52, pp. 902-10

Tang, Z., Han, L., Lin, H., et al. (2007). Derivation of Stable Microarray Cancer Differentiating Signatures Using Consensus Scoring of Multiple Random Sampling and Gene-ranking Consistency Evaluation. *Cancer Research,* Vol. 67, No., 20, pp. 9996-10003

Vapnik, V.N. (1998). *Statistical Learning Theory*, John Wiley & Sons, New York, NY, USA

Yang, S.Y., Xiao, X.Y., Zhang, W.G., Zhang, L.J., Zhang, W., Zhou, B., et al. (2005). Application of Serum SELDI Proteomic Patterns in Diagnosis of Lung Cancer. *BMC Cancer,* Vol. 5, p. 83

Yu, Y., Chen, S., Wang, L.S., Chen, W.L., Guo, W.J., Yan, H., et al. (2005). Prediction of Pancreatic Cancer by Serum Biomarkers Using Surface-enhanced Laser Desorption/Ionization-based Decision Tree Classification. *Oncology,* Vol. 68, pp. 79-86

10

Profiling of Endogenous Peptides by Multidimensional Liquid Chromatography

Egle Machtejeviene[1] and Egidijus Machtejevas[2]
[1]Lithuanian University of Health Sciences,
[2]Merck KGaA,
[1]Lithuania
[2]Germany

1. Introduction

The state of the organism is reflected to the key process in the living body - protein metabolism. Proteomics is the large-scale study of gene expression at the protein level, which will ultimately provide direct measurement of protein expression levels and insight into the activity state of all relevant proteins (Pandey & Mann, 2000). The proteome analysis usually includes the following strategies: native protein pre-separation, then digestion followed by separation and identification, or alternatively straight digestion, separation and identification by mass spectrometry. Therefore, starting with one protein, after digestion we will end up with approximately 30 to 70 short peptide fragments. Identification of only very few of them will provide sufficient information which protein was present in the sample. The subproject of proteomics, namely the study of all peptides expressed by a certain cell, organ or organism, is termed peptidomics. The term was introduced in 2001 (Clynen et al., 2003). Peptides often have very specific functions as mediators and indicators of biological processes. They play important roles as messengers, *e.g.*, as hormones, growth factors, and cytokines, and thus have a high impact on health and disease. Peptidomics comprises not only peptides, originally synthesized by an organism to perform a certain task, but also degradation products of proteins (degradome). Therefore, proteolytic cleavage of proteins leads to peptides as indicators of protease activity, degradation, and degeneration therefore it is also reflects the organism state. The sensitivity of proteomics and peptidomics suffers from the lack of an amplification method, analogous to the polymerase chain reaction, to reveal and quantify the presence of low-abundance proteinaceous constituents therefore the display level is difficult. These challenges motivate the researches to develop reliable analytical platforms. Shortcomings in throughput are due to the absence of technologies that can deliver fast and parallel quantitative analysis of complex peptide distributions in an automated fashion. In the future, when peptidomics will be more analyzed and understood, and biomarkers identified straight capture step of biomarkers from complex bio-sample might be used. Peptidomics especially challenges the need for robust, automated, and sensitive high-throughput technologies. Most single-dimension separations lack sufficient resolution capability to resolve complex biological matrixes. For example, in human blood serum, 90 % of the protein content of serum is composed of 10 basic proteins. The remaining 10 % of serum consists of trace amounts of millions of different proteins. Thus, partial purification of proteins is necessary so that proteins in trace amounts can be identified and their exact structural analysis can be performed. Chromatographic separation techniques are well suited for the analysis of complex multi-components samples. To overcome the limited peak capacity and concentration diversities of the analytes utilizing chromatographic separation systems, multidimensional chromatography (MD-LC) has been realized by analyte transfer between different separation modes through automated valve switching (Link, 2002). Another important prerequisite for the suitability of separation systems for proteomic analysis is the ability to handle very big and very small amounts of biological material (Machtejevas et al., 2006). However, the application of several orthogonal LC separation systems also bears the danger of severe sample losses due to adsorption on the separation and capture column and sample transfer. The mass loadability of LC columns is much higher than for 2D-gelelectrophoresis systems and can be tuned to the requirements of a MD system. LC modes can be implemented into the sample clean-up which in return becomes more selective, robust and reproducible, thus enhancing the quality of the final data. The most important feature is however, that MD-LC can be automated with a high degree of robustness and reproducibility.

Most sample-preparation procedures are performed manually and are thus time-consuming and laborious. On-line sample clean-up and on-column concentrations avoid this disadvantage. There are a number of important features that is gained by having the liquid phase separation system to be operated on-line. Direct injection techniques are generally preferable, since problems involved in off-line sample pretreatments, such as time consuming procedures, errors and risk for low recoveries can be readily avoided. Introduction of the Restricted Access Materials (RAM) offers a unique and intelligent solution. It designates a support family that allows direct injection of biological fluids by limiting the accessibility of interaction sites within the pores to small molecules only. The term restricted access material is a general term for a packing material having a hydrophobic interior covered by a hydrophilic barrier. The hydrophilic barrier allows passage of small molecules to the hydrophobic part of the stationary phase, while sterically preventing large molecules, such as proteins, from interacting with this part of the stationary phase. Macromolecules are excluded and may interact only with the outer surface of the particle support coated with hydrophilic groups, which minimizes the adsorption of matrix proteins.

In a search for new stationary-phase configurations the concept of monolithic silica stationary phases was explored and investigated in depth (Unger et al., 2011). A monolith consists of a continuous rod, of a rigid, porous polymer, that has no interstitial volume but only internal porosity consisting of micro-and macropores. All of the mobile phase is forced to flow through the channels of the porous separation medium, resulting in enhanced mass transport also improved chromatographic efficiency (Meyers & Liapis, 1999) and simultaneous extension of column life time.

2. Multidimensional LC/MS approaches in proteomics and peptidomics

Two-dimensional gel electrophoresis (2D-PAGE) and mass spectrometry are well-established and the most employed techniques in proteomics today. 2D-PAGE, however, provides limited information of the total amount of proteins. Low abundant proteins and small peptides are not detected (Issaq, 2001). Additional methodologies and techniques in sample preparation, selective enrichment, high resolution separation, and detection need to be developed which would allow one to achieve even higher resolution than 2D-PAGE. Acceptable sensitivity to detect the low-abundant proteins is also still an issue. LC can address some of the above-mentioned problems. In comparison with gel-based separation methods, sample handling and preparation are simplified and automated. MD-LC has a number of advantages, such as a higher sensitivity, faster analysis time, variable sample size (preconcentration of the target substances is possible), possesses a large number of separating mechanisms, and, what is most important, and it is amenable to automation. However, because of the wide dynamic range, no single chromatographic or electrophoretic procedure is likely to resolve a complex mixture of cell or tissue proteins and peptides. Liquid chromatographic techniques are fast, quantitative, easy to automate, and can be coupled more readily to mass spectrometry than two-dimensional gel electrophoresis (Premstaller et al., 2001). The drawback of LC is the limited peak capacity of a single column. Thus, multidimensional LC is the choice, fractionating the eluent and transfer the fractions between different columns through automated valve switching (Cortes, 1990). Mass spectrometry has limitations with respect to sensitivity, therefore, a certain number of analyte molecules should be injected in order to be identified. Thus, higher amounts of the sample should be applied. Knowing the target analyte concentration in the sample provides the answer to the question: how much we should inject? In other words, the mass loadability of columns in the multidimensional column train plays a significant role, otherwise displacement phenomena and unwanted protein-protein-interactions will take place, which may change the down-stream composition of the individual fractions in an irreproducible way (Willemsen et al., 2004). Another important prerequisite for the suitability of a separation system for proteomic analysis is the ability to handle very small amounts of biological material (Premstaller et al. 2001). These methods allow one to detect low concentrations of peptides from complex mixtures with a high degree of automation.

Multidimensional (multistage, multicolumn) chromatography had been discovered early as a powerful tool to separate complex mixtures. Two of the protagonists were J.C. Giddings (Giddings, 1984, 1995) and J.F.K. Huber (Huber & Lamprecht, 1995). MD-LC is based on coupling columns in an on-line or off-line mode, which are operated in an orthogonal mode, i.e. separate the sample mixture by different separation mechanisms. The sample separated on the first column (first dimension) is separated into fractions which can then be further treated independently of each other. The practical consequence is an enormous gain in peak capacity (number of peaks resolved at a given resolution) and the potential of independent optimization of the separation conditions for each fraction. Simultaneously, there is the option of relative enrichment/depletion and peak compression by fractionation.

Multidimensional LC separation typically relies on utilizing two or more independent physical properties of the peptides to fractionate the mixture into individual components. Physical properties commonly exploited include are size, shape, charge, hydrophobicity and biomimetic or affinity interactions. These processes are the underlying phenomena for peptide/protein separations using different chromatographic modes, such as size exclusion, reversed phase, cation/anion exchange and hydrophobic interaction columns.

Biological, individual, and variations between individuals (such as gender, age and nutrition) affect peptidomes and require careful consideration in order to find valid biomarkers. A few, equally important factors for successful proteomic biomarker research are high sample quality, high sensitivity, and reproducibility which depend on proper selection of the high quality samples.

While MD-LC MS has found widespread use in the analysis of peptides from natural sources or generated by proteolytic digestion of larger proteins, the method is not suitable for analyzing proteins directly. First, proteins tend to denature under reversed-phase conditions either by stationary phase or mobile phase induced effects (strongly hydrophobic surfaces, low pH and high organic solvent concentrations) making their quantitative elution rather difficult. Observed recoveries are also often low and life time of the columns is compromised. Also, measuring the molecular mass of a protein by MS is not sufficient for its unambiguous identification. To circumvent these obstacles the proteins are digested and the separation is performed at the peptide level. One can distinguish two approaches (i) proteins are separated and then digested ("top-down" proteomics (Wolters et al., 2001)); (ii) in "shotgun" proteomics a complex protein mixture is first digested (see Figure 1, a) and peptides are then chromatographically resolved ("bottom-up" proteomics (see Figure 1, b) (Regnier et al., 2001)). In both cases, separation technologies play a critical role in protein identification and analysis.

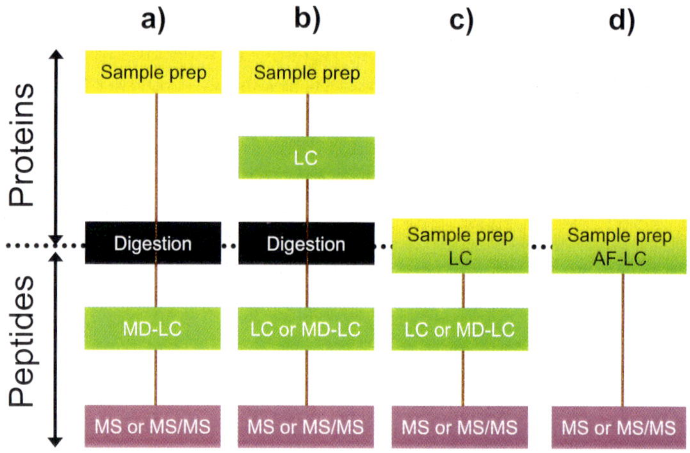

Fig. 1. Liquid chromatography workflow strategy options in proteomics. A - "bottom-up" approach, b - "top-down approach", c - selective sample clean-up directly combined with chromatographic separation ("digestion free" strategy), d - direct capture of target substances.

Even though in the "shotgun approach" sample complexity is vastly increased, there are an increasing number of reports on the comprehensive analysis of human proteomes using this strategy. Prior digestion gives access to the higher molecular weight proteins, however, at the expense of rendering the mixture much more complex. Assuming that a given biofluid contains 1,000 proteins and that each protein will generate approximately 50 proteolytic fragments, we are talking about 50,000 and more peptides to be resolved. This task can only be approached by MD protein identification technologies (Gevaert et al., 2002, Griffin et al., 2002, Walters et al., 2001, Pang et al., 2002). The disadvantage of this approach is that one ends up with an extremely large number of peptides, which need to be resolved. However such an approach could be compared to the efforts of virtually to restore the forest look after it has been completely milled to the sawdust. No one would ague that this would require a lot of guessing and speculations, multiple details might be lost or misinterpreted.

Another attractive approach is to separate proteins first by ion exchange chromatography (see Figure 1 b) according to charge and charge distribution under "soft" (biocompatible) conditions and collecting fractions. The fractions are subjected to digestion and consecutive re-injection on to a RP column is performed, whereby the separation is based on the hydrophobicity. This is particularly favorable since the mobile phase in the second dimension (RP) is compatible with the solvent requirements of mass spectrometry. The restrictions associated with this method lie in the limited size of proteins that can be investigated (MW < 20,000 Daltons) and the insolubility or incomplete separation of very hydrophobic peptides. All peptide-containing fractions are then investigated by mass spectrometry to generate a peptide map (Schulz-Knappe et al., 2001). This approach has already been found to be sufficient to deal with smaller subsets of the proteome (i.e. several hundred proteins) (Hille et al., 2001). These studies also clearly demonstrate that this methodology is not yet suitable for the analysis of a whole proteome due to its enormous complexity. Therefore, pre-selection of the protein from a given tissue or a pre-separation seems mandatory. For example, for the analysis of human urine solid-phase extraction (C-18 packings) to trap peptides, followed by IEX chromatography in the first dimension collecting 30 fractions and analysis of the collected fractions by RP LC (C-18) in the second dimension (Heine et al., 1997) was successfully employed. A similar procedure was used for the separation of proteins and peptides in human plasma filtrate and plasma (Richter et al., 1999).

It is easy to be misguided by vast amount of publications usually dealing with standard protein digests. Separation of a few digested proteins peptides are shown in Figure 2a. Easy to recognize small differences in dynamic range, and even peak distribution, therefore the conclusion could be drawn, that all what we need for successful proteomics analysis is high peak capacity separation and one dimension then would be sufficient. However, using the same chromatographic conditions and column, also injecting eight times more of a real bio-sample (amniotic fluid) we are not observing nice and even separation any longer (Figure 2b). This is a common situation with all real bio-samples.

Direct analysis of biofluids (Figure 1c and d) without prior digestion is a definitive option in biomarker discovery peptidomics. Those routes could be accomplished by employing restricted access materials. RAM columns possess a dual function: firstly, they operate as size-exclusion columns to remove high molecular weight proteins and other undesired constituents. The size characteristics of proteins in pure SEC are known to be highly dependant on eluent composition such as pH, ionic strength (I) of the buffer (which includes salt type and concentration) and on the flow-rate (Quaglia et al., 2006). Ionic strength and pH, however, can vary significantly among biofluids such as plasma and urine. The consequence will be that the sample cleanup procedures have to be adjusted individually with respect to each type of biological sample and standardised protocols have to be worked out. Secondly, the RAM column serves as trap or capture column to selectively enrich target

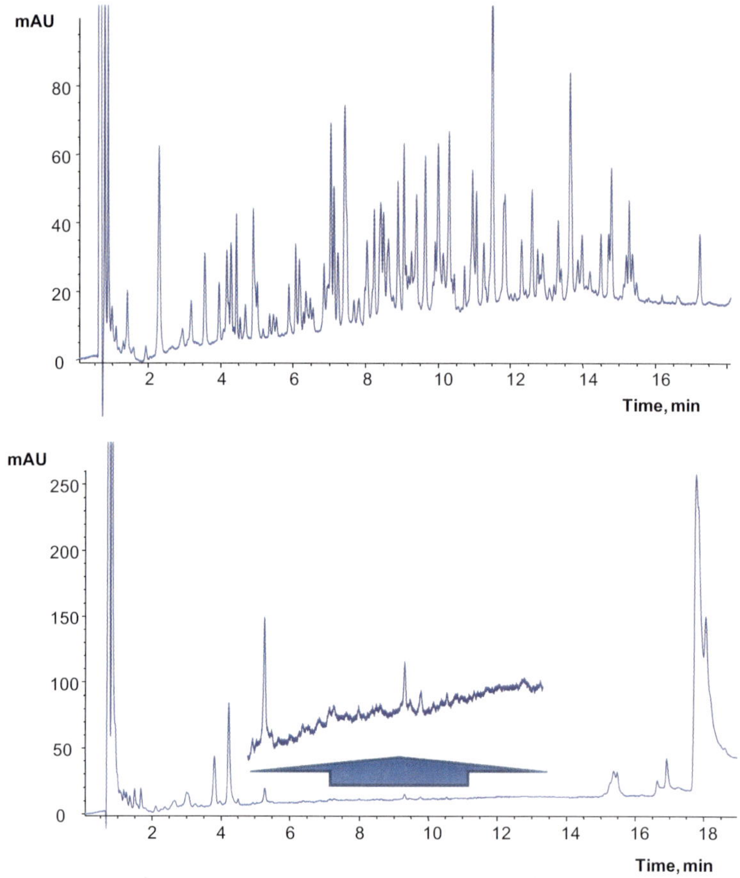

Fig. 2. Separation of standard protein digest and real biological sample analysis: upper chromatogram - 1 µl BSA digest (1mg/ml), lower chromatogram 8 µl of filtered amniotic fluid. Conditions: column - Chromolith Performance RP-18e 100 mm x 2 mm I.D.; eluents - A: 95% H_2O/5% ACN/0.1% TFA (v/v/v), B: 5% H_2O/95% ACN/0.085% TFA (v/v/v); gradient - from 5% B to 50% B in 20 min; flow rate - 0.3 ml/min, detection - UV 214 nm.

compounds in a reversed phase mode or in an ion-exchange mode. By regulating the pore size of the particles, the molecular weight exclusion can be varied as well as the molecular weight fractionation range, which allows certain analytes to be trapped at the internal surface. In this case, only proteins and peptides below a certain molecular shape and size have access to the inner pore surface of the RAM, are thus retained while the larger proteins encounter only the hydrophilic, non-adsorptive outer surface, and will be flushed out in the following washing step. Of the RAM, the strong cation exchanger with sulphonic ligands (RAM-SCX) was preferably employed in the sample clean up of proteins, which proved to show an acceptable capacity towards positively charged peptides and proteins. The features described above, when elegantly combined with column switching, become a powerful tool for direct analysis in the profiling of endogeneous peptides in a fully automated, multidimensional LC platform.

2.1 Designing a MD-LC system

The primary criteria for the choice of a separation phase system are selectivity and orthogonality, mass loadability, and biocompatibility (in case of quantitation). As a rule of thumb, the first dimension should possess a high mass loadability combined with sufficient selectivity and maintenance of bioactivity. Ion exchange chromatography (IEC) therefore is the method of choice offering charge selectivity. In principle, there are two options in IEC, either to employ a cation or anion exchanger, which in return influences the pH working range. Note that either cationic or anionic species are resolved, i.e. only a limited number of species from the whole spectrum. The IEC columns are operated via salt gradients with increasing ionic strength. Consequently, the salt load must be removed before the fractions are transferred to the second dimension column.

It is most common to use reversed phase chromatography as the second dimension. The term RP stands for a number of columns with different degrees of hydrophobicity. The most commonly applied phases are n-octadecyl bonded silicas (RP-18 columns). An intrinsic feature of RP columns is their desalting property. Salts are eluted at the front of the chromatogram, when running a gradient elution with an acidic buffer/acetonitrile mobile phase with increasing acetonitrile content. The hydrophobic surface of the RP packing and the hydrophobic eluent are not favorable with respect to providing a biocompatible environment for proteins: they may change their conformation or denature which may be seen by the appearance of broad peaks, splitting of peaks etc. RP columns possess a much lower mass loadability than IEC columns (10 mg of protein per gram of packing as compared to 100 mg in IEC). An advantage of RP is the fact that the eluents are compatible to MS, provided volatile buffers such as ammonium acetate are employed.

In case of an on-line MD-LC system, the speed of analysis in the second dimension should be as high as possible (Wagner et al., 2002). This, however, conflicts with the requirement of high resolution or high peak capacity. The highest peak capacity in gradient elution RPC is obtained with a shallow gradient at relatively low flow-rate. Thus, a compromise between the desired peak capacity and the gradient time is inevitable. Often gradient times of several hours are applied for the analysis of peptides from protein digests.

A question often arising is: How many dimensions do we need in MD-LC? It becomes obvious that as the number of dimensions increases, the peak capacity will increase. In an ideal case the total peak capacity of the MD-LC system is equal to the product of the individual orthogonal dimensions. At the same time, above two dimensions an on-line MD-LC system becomes very sophisticated in its instrumental setup and may be difficult to control. The major goal in proteomics for the common user is to design a highly efficient, error minimizing and easy-to-handle system. Reduction of the system complexity is the major demand. It is essential to select a minimum number of dimensions to handle complex separations which also should preferably include on-line sample clean-up steps.

2.2 Advantages of on-line sample clean-up approaches

Most sample-preparation procedures are performed manually and are thus time-consuming and laborious. On-line sample clean-up and on-column concentrations avoid this disadvantage. There are a number of important features that is gained by having the liquid phase separation system to be operated on-line. The overall yield in most cases is improved compared to off-line approaches and methodologies. Exposed surfaces are kept to a minimum that usually is the main cause of sample losses. Overall precision can also be controlled by having yields above 50 %. It is possible to handle yields that are lower; however, it generally is a real analytical challenge to obtain operational stability within such analytical processes. Direct injection of samples onto HPLC columns is substantially advantageous in the clinical laboratories in terms of its time- and labor-saving capabilities, in addition to other advantages given below. General direct injection methods have been devised which deal with the problem of many different proteins being present in the sample. The methods include the pre-column technique, restricted access materials, and chromatography in mobile phases containing surfactant. High performance affinity chromatography is also a direct injection technique will demonstrate its power in near feature (Figure 1 d). The characteristic and performance of each direct injection technique are comprehensively discussed below for the analysis of biological samples.

The pre-column technique is the direct injection technique that is mostly reported. The pre-column technique utilizes two columns in series (pre-column and analytical) connected by a switching valve. The most common pre-column technique employs a reversed phase pre-column and a reversed-phase analytical column: the sample is injected into an aqueous mobile phase flowing through a pre-column (1-4 cm in length, 3 - 4.6 mm I.D.) which retains lipophilic compounds, passing non-retained hydrophilic compounds to waste. The switch in valve is then changed and components retained on the pre-column are eluted onto the analytical column by increasing the solvent strength of the mobile phase. This technique serves the dual function of concentration of analyte and removal of hydrophilic substances. There are many advantages of the pre-column injection technique in comparison to traditional sample preparation techniques: time saving in comparison to the labor-intensive liquid-liquid extraction and precipitation techniques, high reproducibility and high, also a superior detection limit capabilities due to its allowance for injection of large sample volumes.

Several types of column-switching designs have been applied. The back flush design is most often used because it reduces band broadening (Yamashita et al., 1992). However some prefer the forward-flush mode to protect the analytical column from possible impurities at the head of the column. Use of an on-line ~0.5μm filter is recommended, which needs periodic replacement. A design that incorporates a second pre-column parallel to the first has been employed which increases sample throughput, by alternating injection on one pre-column and back flushing of retained compounds on the other pre-column.

Most biofluids contain large amounts of well-known proteins such as albumin and IgGs, which overwhelm the separation system and make the detection of the low abundant proteins and peptides very difficult. It is thus advantageous to remove these proteins prior to digestion or direct separation. There are alternative ways of reducing the overall protein load by specific adsorption of albumin and IgG to affinity matrices (Nakamura et al., 2002, Wang et al., 2003, Govorukhina et al., 2003). While usually an affinity matrix is generally highly specific, in high content samples the affinity ligand is limited to exhibit its specificity. There are degrees of specificity between highly selective immunoaffinity matrices and less selective but more robust affinity supports using synthetic ligands. In an effort to reduce the amount of albumin from human serum, a number of affinity matrices has been evaluated based on antibodies or dye ligands. Antibody-mediated albumin removal was efficient and selective. Dye ligand chromatography, a technique that is extensively used in protein chromatography was surprisingly effective (Andrecht et al., 2004) in particular with regard to high binding capacities and a long column lifetime, however, at the expense of selectivity.

2.3 Restricted access material columns

The direct injection of biological samples onto the chromatographic column without any sample preparation is in most cases highly problematic and may lead to an irreversible contamination of the separation columns, which deteriorate selectivity and column performance. A powerful asset to circumvent all the named problems is the implementation of restricted access material for sample preparation. Special Solid Phase Extraction (SPE) supports possessing restricted access properties have been developed (Hagestam and Pinkerton, 1985, Yu et al., 1997, Boos and Rudolphi, 1997). In 1991, Desilets et al. (Desilets, et al., 1991) introduced the restricted access term. Silica based Restricted Access Materials have been developed for the clean-up in bioanalysis; first for low molecular weight compounds in biofluids (Rbeida, et al. 2005) and subsequently for biopolymers such as peptides (Wagner et al. 2001). Those supports were able to withstand several hundred plasma or serum injections (total volume of 5–7 ml) without losing performance. The concept and the methodology were successfully used for the sample clean-up of peptides and proteins out of biofluids by extending the range of available materials employing cation and anion-exchanger RAM (Machtejevas et al., 2004)). Specific non-silica based RAM were also developed for the investigation of the food (Bovanova & Brandsteterova 2000) and environmental matrices (Hogendoorn et al., 1999). Vijayalakshmi and co-workers (Pitiot et al., 2004) have presented a new RAM called a bi-dimensional chromatographic support operating on a size exclusion mode and an affinity or pseudoaffinty mode. A survey on the current state-of-art of RAM-columns in sample pre-treatment is given Souverain et. al. (Souverain et al., 2004). A RAM support developed by Boos and Grimm (Boos & Grimm, 1999) is based on SCX-diol modification to improve performances in terms of efficiency, retention and reproducibility. Račaitytė et al. (Račaitytė et al. 2000) have shown that this type of RAMs is highly suitable for the on-line extraction and analysis of neuropeptides in plasma. Machtejevas et al. (Machtejevas et al. 2006) analyzed the pore structural parameters and size exclusion properties of LiChrospher strong cation-exchange and reverse phase restricted access materials. For peptide analysis out of the biofluids, the strong cation-exchange functionality seems to be particularly suitable mainly because of the high loadability of the strong cation-exchange restricted access material (SCX-RAM) and the fact that one can work under non-denaturing conditions to perform effective chromatographic separations. The proper column operating conditions leads to the total effective working time of the RAM column to be equal to approximately 500 injections (depending on the type of sample).

The principle of the restricted access support is based upon the presence of two chemically different surface properties of porous silica particles (Figure 3). The outer surface of the particles (25 – 40 mm O.D.) is highly biocompatible: it possesses diol modification and hence is hydrophilic, while the pore surface chemistry is tailored as a hydrophobic dispersion phase with C-18 functionality or as a strong cation exchanger with SO3 functionality. An advantage of these adsorbents relies on the simultaneous occurrence of two chromatographic separation mechanisms: selective reversed-phase interaction or ion exchange chromatography of lower molecular mass analytes and size exclusion chromatography for the macromolecular sample constituents. By regulating the pore size of the particles, a physical restriction barrier is adjusted to regulate the interval of molecules that may penetrate and, in the case of penetration, may be trapped in the functionalized pore structure. A pore size of 6 nm allows access to the pores only for analytes with a molecular mass below 15 kDa. The proteins (>15 kDa) can thus be eluted with the void volume directly into the waste. Smaller analytes, however, such as drugs and metabolites from body fluids, pesticides or hormone residues from milk or animal tissue samples, may enter the pores and interact with the n-alkyl chains or ion-exchange groups bound to the inside of the pores. When dealing with complex samples i.e. human bio-fluids, the sample clean-up and fractionation of the sample into matrix and target analytes can be achieved. Depending on the ligands present in the pores, small molecules with hydrophobic or ionic properties are selectively enriched.

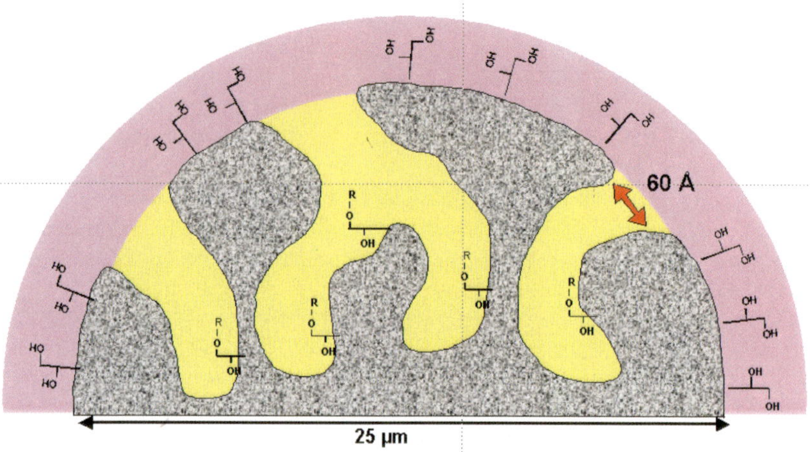

Fig. 3. Artistic representation of a SCX-RAM silica particle (LiChrospher 60 XDS (SO_3/Diol), Merck KGaA, Germany). The external surface is coated with hydrophilic, electroneutral diol-groups for the exclusion of high molecular weight components (>15 kDa); the internal surface is functionalized with ion-exchange groups accessible for low molecular weight components which may be trapped by electrostatic interaction.

The diffusion barrier can be accomplished in two ways: (i) the porous adsorbent particles have a topochemically different surface functionalization between the outer particle surface and the internal surface. The diffusion barrier is then determined by an entropy controlled size exclusion mechanism of the particle depending on the pore size of adsorbent (Pinkerton 1991); (ii) the diffusion barrier is accomplished by a dense hydrophilic polymer layer with a given network size over the essentially functionalized surface. In other words, the diffusion barrier is moved as a layer to the interfacial layer inside the adsorbent particles, the exclusion properties are controlled by the size of the polymeric network protecting the internal surface and is no longer dependant on the average pore diameter of the adsorbent (Mazsaroff & Regnier, 1988).

The SEC process is entropically driven; i.e proteins with decreasing shape and size penetrate an increasing volume of the porous particles. The SEC of proteins is commonly carried out with buffer solution containing a high salt concentration, e.g. 0.1 M, at pH 5 to 7. The high salt concentration is needed to suppress electrostatic interactions between the solute and the charged surface. In the sample clean up of the RAM-SCX column the concentration of salt is much lower e.g smaller than 20 mM and the pH is kept at approximately 3. Under these conditions, electrostatic attraction forces are dominant between the positively charged peptides and proteins whereas the negatively charged species are excluded from the pores of the RAM-SCX column through electrostatic repulsion forces (Figure 4 a).

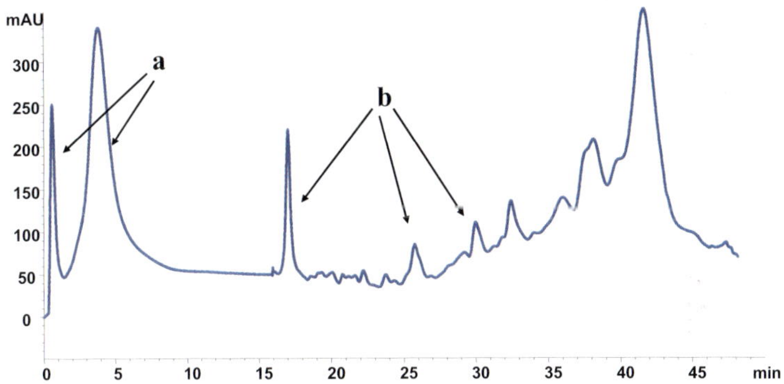

Fig. 4. Typical SCX-RAM column separation profile: peaks (a) represent physical exclusion by pore size. Trapped retained bio-molecules are separated by a gradient in the second step (b). Conditions: column - LiChrospher 60 XDS (SO_3/Diol), 25 x 4 mm I.D., flow rate - 0.5 ml/min, gradient from 0 to 1 M NaCl in 20 mM KH_2PO_4 pH 2.5, containing 5 % ACN in 30 min. Sample: 100 µl Human Hemofiltrate (3.7 mg/ml), UV detection at 214 nm.

After loading the RAM-SCX column the washing step elutes at isocratic conditions all the excluded compounds between the start and 15 minutes. After 15 minutes switching occurs and the trapped analytes are eluted from the RAM-SCX column with a strong eluent under gradient condition in the period between 15 and 45 minutes (Figure 4 b). Thus it is a charge and charge distribution selective process combined with SEC. Use of RAM-SCX allows one the direct application of biofluids onto the column. Small peptides are selectively trapped in the pores by cationic functional groups while large molecular weight biopolymers are directed to waste. This strategy performs the sample clean up and selective peptide enrichment in one simultaneous step (Figure 1 c).

Mass loadability of SPE and RAM columns play a key role in executing the sample clean-up. It is advisable to work below the overload regime of the column. Otherwise, displacement effects and other phenomena such as secondary interaction by adsorbed species might take place, which will lead to non-reproducible results (Wilemsen et al., 2004). Last statement is particularly important when the task is to monitor medium to low abundant proteins, therefore, usually large sample volumes in the millilitre range are applied. As the column lifetime is known to be limited a control measure has to be applied to check the condition of the RAM-SCX column and, if necessary, replace it by a new one. In our experience the column endured about 200 injections of urine.

Although compatibility of these stationary phases with direct biological sample injection is high, one still has to keep in mind that samples have to be filtrated or centrifuged prior to injection to remove the solid contaminants and precipitations. Even so, some components tend to agglomerate/precipitate with the time while samples queue up in autosampler. Therefore, an additional in-line filter is highly recommended. One should keep in mind that the operational flow rate has enormous impact on the molecular size distribution when employing a RAM column. Higher flow rates can shift the molecular range of the trapped molecules to lower values as smaller molecules need less time to penetrate the pores. Also higher flow rates could alter the hydrodynamic volume of the biomolecules. Higher molecular mass molecules will be enriched operating at lower flow rates. Column temperature affects the viscosity of the mobile phase and, consequently, the diffusion ratio and influences the speed of mass transfer. Carefully performed optimizations of the chromatographic parameters ensure the success of the analysis.

2.4 Monolithic silica columns

Special features of monolithic silica columns circumstanced the successful application in proteomics. In contrast to conventional particle-packed columns, monolithic silica columns are made of a continuous piece of porous silica, utilizing a sol-gel process leading to rod columns, which possess a defined bimodal pore structure with macro and meso pores in the micro- and nanometer range (see Figure 5).

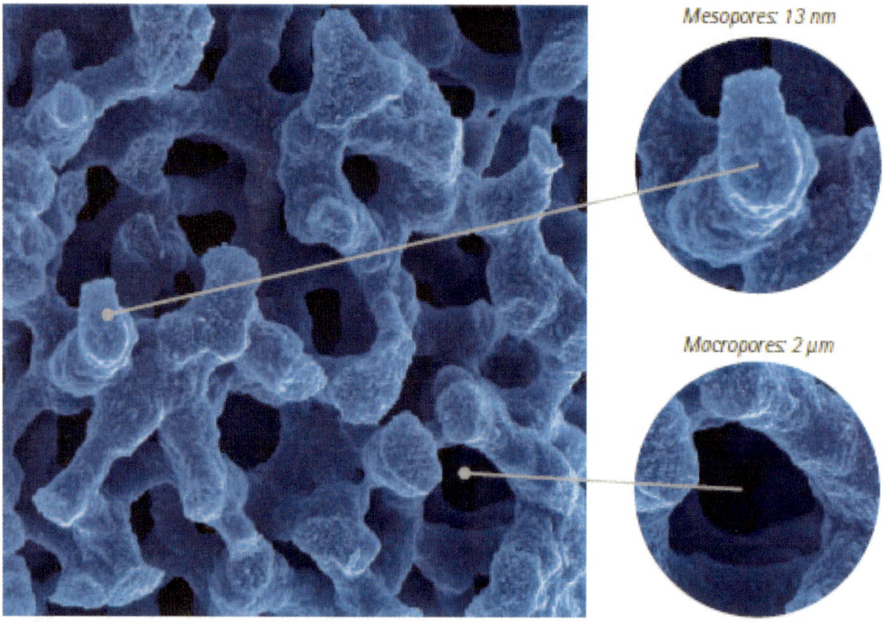

Fig. 5. SEM picture of a cross section from a silica monolith. Total porosity > 80%. The mesopores form the fine porous structure (average pore size 13 nm) and create the large uniform surface area on which adsorption takes place, thereby enabling high performance chromatographic separation. The macropores allow rapid flow of the mobile phase at low pressure. Their average size is 2 µm.

One of the major of those special features is low column backpressure. Low backpressure is not only nice to have, but a must, as setting up multidimensional separation platform for proteomics it allows one to select a desired flow-rate from a broader range (see Figure 6).

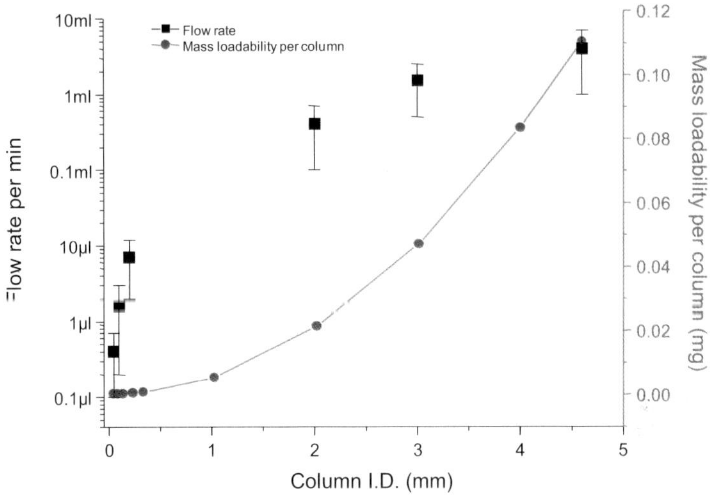

Fig. 6. Estimation of monolithic silica columns flow rates and mass loadability per column. Columns 2, 3 and 4.6 mm I.D. are 10 cm long; columns 50 µm, 100 µm and 200 µm are 15 cm long.

Prof. Regnier group, demonstrated the advantage of flow rate variation possibility for 4.6 mm I.D. Chromolith Performance column. It was concluded that silica monolith reversed-phase chromatography columns show little loss in the resolution of peptides ranging up to several thousand in molecular weight as mobile phase velocity is elevated from the conventional 2.5–25 mm/s (Xiong et al., 2004). Moreover, at 25 mm/s with a 100 mm length column, operating pressure did not exceed 150 bar. This is well within the pressure limit of most commercial LC instruments. The separation of a tryptic digest of cytochrome C in 6 and 60 min seemed almost identical. Resolution at 25 mm/s linear velocity was 77% of that at 2.5 mm/s. It was conluded that the fact that peptide separations could be achieved 10 times faster than with a conventional packed column with moderate loss in resolution could have a major impact on analytical throughput in proteomics.

Combination of different sizes fulfils the injection volume requirement for various samples. The possibility of being able to vary the flow-rate over a large area up to very high linear flow velocities combined with the robustness of the monoliths also reduce considerably the "down times" during washing and re-equilibration of the column (Rieuxet al., 2005).

Important to notice, that comparing a particulate and a silica monolithic guard column showed that the particulate column was clogging much faster than the monolithic column (Machtejevas et al., 2007). 120 injections of plasma (50 µl each injection) led to an increase of approximately 6 bar at the particulate column back pressure, while at the monolithic column the back pressure rise was only approximately 1 bar. The life time of the short silica monolithic columns used as a trap column or as a guard column heavily depends on a type and a volume of the bio-fluid injected. After injecting plasma column performance dropped drastically when the volume of half column volume was injected. For urine the column stability was at least 20 times higher. This is definitely related to the sample complexity. Comparing the life time of the same dimension of monolithic silica columns and particle packed columns under same conditions; monolithic silica column life time was at least double compared with particulate packed column of the similar dimension. This is not a surprise, as any particle packed column contains particles and frits to maintain particles in the column. The flow through between particles is much smaller that the particle size itself, for example, if the column packed with 2 µm particles the space between particles is about 0.5 µm. Monolithic silica column made as one single spongy rod, does not contains frits, and flow through pores (macropores) are about 2 µm diameter.

Capillary separations, although delivering much improved sensitivity, especially when combined with mass spectrometry, often have the drawback of reduced robustness. This is partially due to the limited stability of packed capillary columns and the risk of clogging (same aspect as discussed above). Monolithic capillary columns made of polymeric (Svec et al., 2003) or silica-based materials promise to overcome some of the limitations mentioned above, namely that of packing stability. An interesting study was performed by the Guryca et. al. to provide a side-by-side comparison of monolithic nano-LC columns used in reversed-phase chromatography of proteins tryptic digests (Guryča et al., 2008). They compared PepMap (LC Packings, Amsterdam, The Netherlands, 3 µm 100Å, ID 75 µm, 15 cm), Chromolith CapRod (Merck KGaA, Darmstadt, Germany; silica monolith-C18, ID 100 µm, 15 cm) and PS-DVB (LC Packings; polystyrene monolith, ID 100 µm, 5 cm) columns (all C18 modification), in terms of the number of peptides identified and also with respect to their chromatographic characteristics. In terms of performance the peak shapes obtained on Chromolith CapRod and PepMap columns appeared to be very similar, and the peak widths for both columns were in the range 0.3–0.4 min. The PS-DVB column exhibited somewhat disappointing performance which could be attributed, to the mobile phase composition used. However, it was concluded, that generally the performance of both silica based columns was superior to that of monolithic PS-DVB (Guryča et al., 2008). Also a similar finding was observed comparing peptide identification power. Comparing column throughput Chromolith CapRod column was superior with 5.0 µl/min in contrast to flow rates of up to 0.8 µl/min for PS-DVB column and to 0.5 µl/min for the particulate (PepMap) column. Moreover, it was found that, for short gradients, the number of identifications is not affected by the flow rate (3–10 mm/s). The results shown demonstrate the greater potential of monolithic compared to particle-based columns, as higher flows can be utilized, enabling the number of identifications per unit of time to be significantly increased. Furthermore, due to their higher porosity they have fewer tendencies to get clogged. Usually, micro columns for LC are fabricated by packing beads with a controlled range of diameters and pore sizes. To obtain a better efficiency, columns have been packed with particles of ever smaller diameters (Szabolcs et al., 2009) bringing about another practical limitation: the increase of the back pressure. To circumvent this problem, alternative chromatographic modalities such as ultrahigh-pressure liquid chromatography, open tubular chromatography, and capillary electro-chromatography have been investigated. All this has led to the use of particle sizes in the range of 3 to 5 μm as a good compromise between column efficiency and pressure drop. Moreover, it was demonstrated that the recently developed monolithic-type HPLC columns could be operated at high flow rates while maintaining a high efficiency. In this context,

(Kele & Guiochon, 2002) investigated the reproducibility of the preparation of the first columns getting reproducibilities higher than with particle based columns. Because of their capacity to perform fast separations they can be used for fast screening methods and applications in multidimensional chromatography systems. Conditioning and regeneration of these monolithic columns can be done in a short time when compared with the corresponding capillary packed columns, thus making more effective use of costly LC-MS equipment. They can be easily integrated in fully automated systems to perform unattended runs. These columns are flexible and they show a good performance at both low (1.5 µl/min) and high (4.5 µl/min) flow rates. Such flow rate range is highly compatible with MALDI plate spotting strategy. Fraction could be spotted directly, then the flow of 4 µl/min allows to spot up to 8 fractions. If the flow rate is set to 3 µl/min, and an equal flow of MALDI matrix solution is added post-column (7 mg/ml re-crystallized α-cyanohydroxycinnamic acid, 2 mg/ml ammonium phosphate, 0.1% trifluoroacetic acid, 80% acetonitrile) and the combined eluant is automatically spotted onto a stainless steel MALDI target plate every 6 s (0.6 µl/spot), a total of 370 spots obtained per original SCX fraction (Fort et al., 2009). Haffey demonstrated similar approach and obtained 3828 MALDI-TOF spots from the 12 SCX fractions (Haffey et al., 2009). Such a separation strategy offers enormous discrimination power and imposing peak capacity.

3. Application example: The case study

The analysis concept is based on an on-line sample preparation and a two-dimensional LC (see Figure 7) system: pre-separating the majority of the matrix components from the analytes which are retained on a RAM-SCX (LiChrospher 60 XDS (SO_3/Diol), two 25 x 4mm

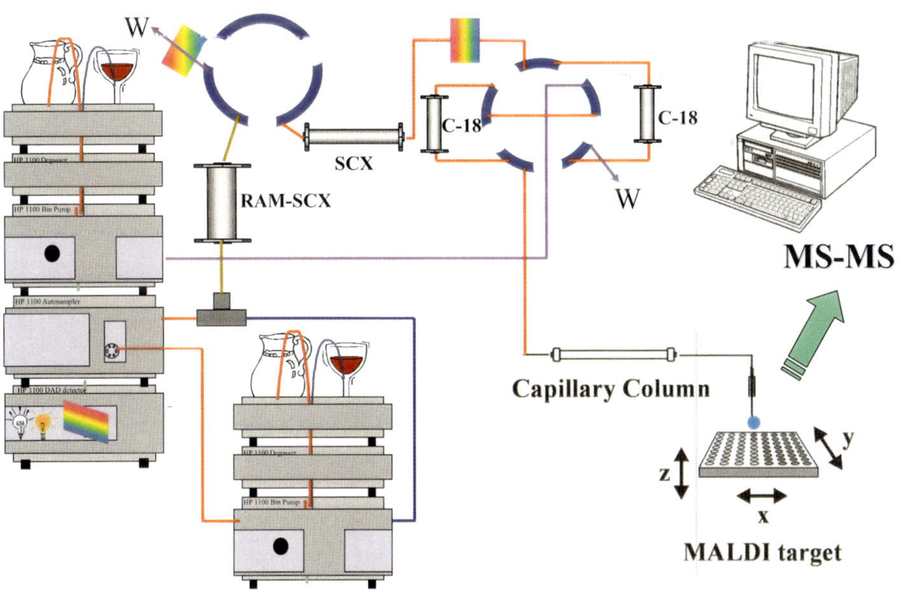

Fig. 7. Multidimensional chromatographic separation platform with integrated on-line sample clean-up.

id) column followed by a solvent switch and transfer of the trapped peptides using five salt steps by mixing 20 mM phosphate buffer (pH 2.5) (eluent A1) and 20 mM phosphate buffer with 1.5 M sodium chloride (eluent B1) at following proportions: 85/15; 70/30; 65/45; 45/55; 0/100 at the constant 0.1 ml/min flow rate was performed after the switching for the second dimensional strong cation exchange analytical separation and trapped onto the RP column by means of column switching in a way to perform two-dimensional orthogonal separations.

Desorption of the adsorbed species from the RAM-SCX column could be accomplished by employing an eluent with a higher solvent strength or pH than the eluent at the loading. We preferred the salt steps as the pH needed double time for re-equilibration. The desorption step was repeated several times to eliminate memory effects. In order to avoid sample to sample cross contamination, two blank gradients were typically applied (with specific analytes or higher loadings it could reach up to five blank gradients). The further steps of the analysis e.g. the transfer from the RAM-SCX column to the next (analytical cation exchange column) is heavily dependant on the way this transfer is performed. Three different modes could be chosen to elute the trapped sample from the RAM-SCX column: isocratic, one step elution with a strong solvent, elution with a linear gradient and elution with pulsed gradient.

A desalting and preconcentration of the fractions containing proteinaceous components were performed on two identical trap columns Zorbax 300 SB-C18, 5 µm particles, 5 x 0.3 mm I.D. obtained from Agilent (Agilent, Waldbronn, Germany). As a final column a monolithic fused silica RP-18 endcapped capillary column of dimensions 150 x 0.1 mm I.D. (Chromolith CapRod, Merck KGaA, Darmstadt, Germany) was used. We preferred the monolithic type of column over particulate capillary column for the following reasons: (a) monolithic silica columns offers high variability of flow rates adjustments, which is particularly useful in the set up of multidimensional LC MS system to adjust for different column sizes; (b) the monolithic silica columns implemented in the multidimensional LC MS system meets the requirement of high reproducibility as with particulate columns; (c) in terms of column robustness and usage flexibility monolithic silica columns are superior that packed particulate columns eg.: one could cut the top end column when damaged, furthermore, there is no change in the permeability as a result of pressure fluctuation; the end of the capillary directly connected to the MS; no frits are required etc. Standard acetonitrile gradient with 0.1 % formic acid at constant 2 µl/min flow rate separated trapped peptides in 40 min. The end of reverse phase capillary column directly inserted in an in house made robotic spotting apparatus so that the droplets are accumulated above MALDI plate and directed consequently from spot to spot with 2 minute intervals filling 100 spot MALDI plate per sample (5 fractions from the RAM-SCX column (salt steps), 20 fractions from the monolithic capillary RP 18e column, 5x20=100). After all plate positions were filled and dried out properly matrix material, consisting of α-cyano-4-hydroxycinamonic acid in 50 % acetonitrile / 4 % formic acid / water (v/v/v) of a volume of 0.5 µl was spotted on the top. The MALDI plate was kept in dark place and analysed within the 12 hours.

As already mentioned the system performs an on-line directly injected human plasma, cerebrospinal fluid and urine sample separation in a fully automated way, by a scale down strategy, gaining in sensitivity. In all peptide displays (Figure 8), between 1,000 and 4,000 mass spectrometric signals appeared, which correspond to 500 – 2,000 individual peptides.

This usually reflects redundancy (peptides that elute in more than one fraction), peptide species with and without oxidative states, and a small number of mass spectrometric derivatives, such as fragment ions.

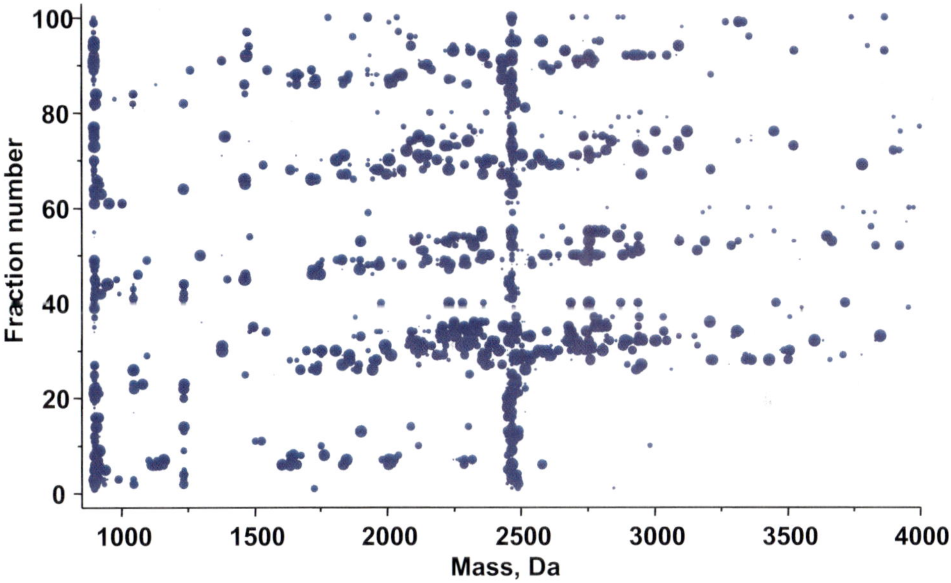

Fig. 8. Example of a human plasma peptide map. Injection volume is 48μl.

The fully automated 2D-LC system performing an effective fractionation combined with off-line MALDI TOF MS offers an enormous potential for human peptidomics screening on a daily basis. The system offers a high flexibility to be optimized for effective analysis of other biofluids such as amniotic fluid, sputum, urine, etc. The systems are completely automated and perform a high number of analysis cycles with low cost per analysis. Fast and comprehensive mapping of bio peptides and protein fragments will open possibilities to recognize novel and specific biomarkers that will help to diagnose disease and possibly provide valuable information for new drug development.

4. Conclusion

Novel restricted access materials have shown high efficiency in sample clean-up after direct on-line biofluid injections. Benefits of monolithic silica columns such as: super eminent low backpressure compared to particulate packed columns, therefore high variability of flow rates adjustments is possible; superior long term stability and data reproducibility analyzing various proteinaceous samples; much higher flow rates allows speeding up the overall analysis: fast separation, washing and re-equilibration. When those two novel developments are combined in a elegant multidimensional and fully automated way proteomic analysis could be accentuated.

In the future, proteomics will play the major role in drug discovery, accelerating the various steps involved - target identification, target validation, drug discovery (efficacy, selectivity and mode of action). Operated on a routine basis, MD-LC may provide with the desired data, and after interconnection with the biology outcome could be found.

5. References

Andrecht, S., Anders, J., Hendriks, R., Machtejevas, E., Unger, K. (2004). Effiziente Probenvorbereitung fűr die Proteomanalyse von Kőrperflűssigkeiten. *Laborwelt*, 5/2, 4–7

Boos, K.S. and Rudolphi, A. (1997). The use of restricted-access media in HPLC, Part I - Classification and review. *LC-GC Int.*, 15, 602-611

Boos, K.S. and Grimm, C.H. (1999). High-performance liquid chromatography integrated solid-phase exctraction in bioanalysis using restricted access precolumn packings. *Trends Anal. Chem.*, 18, 175-180

Bovanova, L., Brandsteterova, E., (2000). Direct analysis of food samples by high-performance liquid chromatography. *J. Chromatogr. A*, 880 149-168

Clynen, E., De Loof, A. and Schoofs, L. (2003). The use of peptidomics in endocrine research. *Gen. Comp. Endocr.*, 132, 1-9

Cortes, H.J. (1990). *Multidimensional Chromatography. Techniques and Applications*, Marcel Dekker, New York

Desilets, C.P., Rounds, M.A., Regnier, F.E. (1991). Semipermeable-surface reversed-phase media for high-performance liquid chromatography. *J. Chromatogr.*, 544, 25-39.

Fort, P.E., Freeman, W.M., Losiewicz, M.K., Sigh, R.S.J., Gardner, T.W. (2009). The Retinal Proteome in Experimental Diabetic Retinopathy: Up-regulation of Crystallins and Reversal by Systemic and Periocular Insulin. *Molecular & Cellular Proteomics*, 8, 767-779

Giddings, J.C. (1984). Two-dimensional separations: concept and promise. *Anal. Chem.*, 56, 1258–1270

Giddings, J. C. (1995). Sample dimensionality: a predictor of order-disorder in component peak distribution in multidimensional separation. *J. Chromatogr. A*, 703, 3–15

Gevaert, K., Van Damme, J., Goethals, M., Thomas, G.R., Hoorelbeke, B., Demol, H., Martens, L., Puype, M., Staes, A. and Vandekerckhove, J. (2002). Chromatographic isolation of methionine-containing peptides for gel-free proteome analysis. *Mol. Cell. Proteomics*, 1, 896-903

Govorukhina, N.I., Keizer-Gunnink, A., van der Zee, A.G.J., de Jong, S., de Bruijn, H.W.A., Bischoff, R. (2003). Sample preparation of human serum for the analysis of tumor markers. Comparison of different approaches for albumin and γ-globulin depletion. *J. Chromatogr. A*, 1009, 171-178

Guryča, V., Kieffer-Jaquinod, S., Garin, J., Masselon, C.D. (2008). Prospects for monolithic nano-LC columns in shotgun proteomics. *Anal. Bioanal. Chem.*, 392, 1291-1297.

Griffin, T.J., Gygi, S.P., Ideker, T., Rist, B., Eng, J., Hood, L. and Aebersold, R. (2002). Complementary profiling of gene expression at the transcriptome and proteome levels in Saccharomyces cerevisiae. *Mol. Cell. Proteomics*, 1, 323-333

Hagestam, I.H., Pinkerton, T.C. (1985). Internal surface reversed-phase silica supports for liquid chromatography. *Anal. Chem.*, 57 1757-1763

Haffey, W.D., Mikhaylova, O., Meller, J., Yi, Y., Greis, K.D., and Czyzyk-Krzeska M.F. (2009). iTRAQ Proteomic identification of pVHL-dependent and -independent targets of Egln1 prolyl hydroxylase knockdown in renal carcinoma cells. *Adv Enzyme Regul.*, 49(1), 121–132

Heine, G., Raida, M. and Forssmann, W.-G. (1997). Mapping of peptides and protein fragments in human urine using liquid chromatography – mass spectrometry. *J. Chromatogr. A*, 776, 117–124

Hille, J.M., Freed, A.L. and Wätzig, H. (2001). Possibilities to improve automation, speed and precision of proteome analysis: A comparison of two-dimensional electrophoresis and alternatives. *Electrophoresis*, 22, 4035–4052

Hogendoorn, E.A., Dijkman, E., Baumann, B., Hidalgo, C., Sancho, J.-V., Hernandez, F. (1999). Strategies in using analytical restricted access media columns for the removal of humic acid interferences in the trace analysis of acidic herbicides in water samples by coupled column liquid chromatography with UV detection. *Anal. Chem.*, 71 1111-1118

Huber, J.F.K. and Lamprecht, G. (1995). Assay of neopterin in serum by means of two-dimensional high-performance liquid chromatography with automated column switching using three retention mechanisms. *J. Chromatogr. B*, 666, 223–232

Issaq, H.J. (2001). The role of separation science in proteomics research. *Electrophoresis*, 22, 3629-3638

Issaq, H.J., Chan, K.C., Janini, G.M., Conrads, T.P. and Veenstra, T.D. (2005). Multidimensional separation of peptides for effective proteomic analysis. *J. Chromatogr. B*, 817, 35–47

Kele, M., Guiochon, G. (2002). Repeatability and reproducibility of retention data and band profiles on six batches of monolithic columns. *J. Chromatogr. A*, 960, 19-49.

Link, A.J. (2002) Multidimensional peptide separations in proteomics. *Trends Biotechnol.* 20(12S), 8-13

Machtejevas, E., John, H., Wagner, K., Standker, L., Marko-Varga, G., Forssmann, W-G., Bischoff, R., Unger, K.K. (2004). Automated multidimensional HPLC: sample preparation and identification of peptides from human blood filtrate. *J. Chromatography B*, 803 121-130

Machtejevas, E., Unger, K.K., Ditz, R. (2006). Multidimensional Column Liquid Chromatography (LC) in Proteomics – Where Are We Now? in *Proteomics in Drug Research*, ed. M. Hamacher, K. Marcus, K. Stühler, A. van Hall, B. Warscheid, H.E. Meyer, 89-111, Wiley-VCH, Weinheim, Germany

Machtejevas, E., Denoyel, R., Meneses, J.M., Kudirkaitė, V., Grimes, B.A., Lubda, D., Unger, K.K. (2006). Sulphonic acid strong cation-exchange restricted access columns in sample cleanup for profiling of endogeneous peptides in multidimensional liquid chromatography Structure and function of strong cation-exchange restricted access materials. *J. Chromatogr. A*, 1123, 38–46

Machtejevas, E., Andrecht, S., Lubda, D., Unger, K.K. (2007). Monolithic silica columns of various formats in automated sample clean-up/multidimensional liquid chromatography/mass spectrometry for peptidomics. *J. Chromatogr. A*, 1144 97-101

Machtejevas, E., Unger K.K. (2008). Proteomics Sample Preparation, in: Jörg von Hagen (Editor), *Sample preparation for HPLC – based proteome analysis*. 245-264, Wiley-VCH, Weinheim, Germany

Machtejevas, E., Unger, K.K. (2008). Multidimensional Liquid Chromatography: Theory and Applications in Industrial Chemistry and the Life Sciences. Steven A. Cohen and Mark R. Schure (Editors), *Peptidomics*. 207-220. John Wiley & Sons Inc., Hoboken, New Jersey, USA

Machtejevas, E., Marko-Varga. G., Lindberg, C., Lubda, D., Hendriks, R., Unger, K.K. (2009). Profiling of Endogenous Peptides by Multidimensional Liquid Chromatography: On-line Automated Sample Cleanup Procedures for Biomarker Discovery in Human Urine. *J. Sep. Sci.* 32, 2223 - 2232

Mazsaroff, I., Regnier, F.E. (1988). Phase ratio determination in an ion-exchange column having pores partially accessible to proteins. *J. Chromatogr.*, 442: 15-28

Meyers, J.J., Liapis, A.I. (1999). Network modeling of the convective flow and diffusion of molecules adsorbing in monoliths and in porous particles packed in a chromatographic column. *J. Chromatogr. A*, 852, 3-23

Nakamura, K., Suzuki, T., Kamichika, T., Hasegawa, M., Kato, Y., Sasaki, H., Inouye, K. (2002). Evaluation and applications of a new dye affinity adsorbent. *J. Chromatogr. A*, 972, 21-25

Pandey, A. and Mann, M. (2000). Proteomics to study genes and genomes. *Nature*, 405, 837-846

Pang, J.X., Ginnanni, N., Donge, A.R., Hefta, S.A. and Opiteck, G.J. (2002). Biomarker discovery in urine by proteomics. *J. Proteome Res.*, 1, 161-169

Pinkerton, T.C. (1991). High-performance liquid chromatography packing materials for the analysis of small molecules in biological matrices by direct injection. *J. Chromatogr.*, 544: 13-23

Pitiot, O., Poraht, J., Guzmann, R., Vijayalakshmi, M.A. (2004). 9th International Symposium on Biochromatography, 5–7 May, Bordeaux, France, Programme & Abstracts, p. 34

Premstaller, A., Oberacher, H., Walcher, W., Timperio, A.M., Zolla, L., Chervet, J-P., Cavusoglu, N., van Dorsselaer, A., Huber, Ch.G. (2001). High-Performance Liquid Chromatography-Electrospray Ionization Mass Spectrometry Using Monolithic Capillary Columns for Proteomic Studies. *Anal. Chem.*, 73: 2390-2396

Quaglia, M., Machtejevas, E., Hennessy, T. and Unger, K.K. (2006). Size Exclusion Chromatography (SEC) of biopolymers) Optimization strategies and trouble shouting. S. Kromidas (Editor), *HPLC Made to Measure – A Practical Handbook for Optimization*,- Wiley-VCH, Weinheim, Germany, 383-403

Račaitytė, K., Lutz, E.S.M., Unger, K.K., Lubda, D., Boos, K.S. (2000). Analysis of neuropeptide Y and its metabolites by high-performance liquid chromatography–electrospray ionization mass spectrometry and integrated sample clean-up with a novel restricted-access sulphonic acid cation exchanger. *J. Chromatogr. A*, 890: 135-144

Rbeida, O., Christiaens, B., Hubert, Ph., Lubda, D., Boos, K.-S., Crommen, J. and Chiap, P. (2005). Integrated on-line sample clean-up using cation exchange restricted access sorbent for the LC determination of atropine in human plasma coupled to UV detection. *J. Pharm. and Biomed. Anal.*, 36/5: 947-954

Regnier, F., Amini, A., Chakraborty, A., Geng, M., Ji, J., Riggs, L., Sioma, C., Wang, S. and Zhang, X. (2001). Multidimensional chromatography and the signature peptide approach to proteomics. *LC-GC*, 19, 200–213

Richter, R., Schulz-Knappe, P., Schrader, M., Standker, L., Jurgens, M., Tammen, H. and Forssmann, W.-G. (1999). Composition of the peptide fraction in human blood plasma: database of circulating human peptides. *J. Chromatogr. B*, 726, 25–35

Rieux, L., Niederlander, H., Verpoorte, E., Bischoff, R. (2005), Silica monolithic columns: Synthesis, characterisation and applications to the analysis of biological molecules. *J. Sep. Sci.*, 28, 1628–1641

Schulz-Knappe, P., Zucht, H-D., Heine, G., Jürgens, M., Hess, R. and Schrader, M. (2001). Peptidomics: the comprehensive analysis of peptides in complex biological mixtures. *Combinatorial Chemistry & High Throughput Screening*, 4, 207–217

Souverain, S., Rudaz, S., Veuthey, J.-L., (2004), Restricted access materials and large particle supports for on-line sample preparation: an attractive approach for biological fluids analysis. *J. Chromatogr. B*, 801, 141-156

Svec, F., Tennikova, T., Deyl, Z. (editors) (2003). *Monolithic materials: preparation, properties and applications*. Elsevier Amsterdam, The Netherlands, P. 800.

Szabolcs, F., Jeno, F., Katalin, G. (2009). Characterisation of new types of stationary phases for fast liquid chromatographic applications. *J. Pharm. Biomed. Anal.*, 50(5), 703-712

Unger, K.K., Machtejevas, E. (2007). Mehr als nur eine Säule – die Möglichkeiten der mehrdimensionalen LC. *Nachrichten aus der Chemie*, 6 661-664

Unger, K.K., Machtejevas, E. (2009). Peptid-Profilanalyse aus Körperflüssigkeiten. *ChromChat*, 4 44 -47

Unger K.K., Tanaka, N. and Machtejevas, E. (2011). *Monolithic silicas in separation science: Concepts, syntheses, characterization, modeling and applications*. Wiley-VCH, Weinheim, Germany, P. 374

Wagner, K., Miliotis, T., Marko-Varga, G., Bischoff, R. and Unger, K.K. (2002). An automated on-line multidimensional HPLC system for protein and peptide mapping with integrated sample preparation. *Anal. Chem.*, 74, 809–820

Wang Y.Y., Cheng, P., Chan, D.W. (2003). A simple affinity spin tube filter method for removing high-abundant common proteins or enriching low-adundant biomarkers for serum proteomic analysis. *Proteomics*, 3, 243-248

Westermeier, R., Naven, T., and Hēpker, H.-R. (2008). *Proteomics in Practice. A Guide to Successful Experimental Design* 2nd Ed. WILEY-VCH Verlag GmbH & Co. KGaA, Weinheim, Germany, P. 482

Willemsen, O., Machtejevas, E., Unger, K.K. (2004). Enrichment of proteinaceous materials on a strong cation-exchange diol silica restricted access material (RAM): protein-protein displacement and interaction effects. *J. Chromatography A*, 1025, 209-216.

Wolters, D.A., Washburn, M.P. and Yates III, J.R. (2001). An automated multidimensional protein identification technology for shotgun proteomics. *Anal. Chem.*, 73, 5683-5690

Xiong, L., Zhang, R., Regnier F.E. (2004). Potential of silica monolithic columns in peptide separations. *J. Chromatogr. A*, 1030, 187–194

Yamashita, K,, Motohashi, M., Yashiki, T. (1992). Automated high-perfomance liquid chromatographic method for the simultaneous determination of cefotiam and delta 3-cefotiam in human plasma using column switching. *J. Chromatogr.*, 577, 174-179

Yu, Z., Westerlund, D. and Boos, K.S. (1997). Determination of methotrexate and its metabolite 7-hydroxymethotrexate by direct injection of human plasma into a column-switching liquid chromatographic system using post-column photochemical reaction with fluorimetric detection. *J. Chromatogr. B*, 689, 379-386

11

Salivary Hormones, Immunes and Other Secretory Substances as Possible Stress Biomarker

Shusaku Nomura
Nagaoka University of Technology, Japan

1. Introduction

In the modern society, the issues on mental health have always been pressing and global problem, and unfortunately it remains today unsolved. It does not apply only to a personal matter, but also having a huge impact on economics as it has estimated a decade ago of that the social cost concerning mental health problem in European Union was 3 to 4% of GNP (Gabriel, 2000). However generally speaking, the mental stress is quite difficult to be aware of personally. It is hard for anyone to manage mental stress by on his/her own. Therefore it is an urgent task to figure out a "practical" methodology to evaluate, manage and control the mental stresses.

On the other hand, recent developments of the molecular analysis techniques has been revealed that particular hormones and immune substances secreted within human body change its level in responding to human mental state. For an instance, salivary Immunoglobulin-A shows a transient increase against short-term psychological stressors such as mental arithmetic task, stroop task, academic presentation (Valdimarsdottir, 1994). "All illnesses come from the mind" is no longer a folk story. These particular hormones and immune substances can potentially be a practical biomarker for human mental stress. Number of hormones and other substances in our body has been studied as a possible stress biomarker (Izawa, 2004; Wakida, 2004), and the number of academic research has been increasing as well, as shown in Figure 1. Currently it forms an interdisciplinary research field called psychoneuroendocrinology (PNE) and/or psychoneuroimmunology (PNI) (Ader, 2001) (hereafter, we use the term psychoneuroendocrine-immunology (PNEI) to indicate both PNE and PNI).

PNEI must be a contributory research field which should possibly establish "practical" criteria for objectively evaluating human mental state. However it is a relatively new field of study still developing, there are a lot of stuffs to be investigated, e.g. the precise stress response of these biomarkers in the time series, the sensitivity of the response against other than acute stressors, physiological mechanism dynamically regulating the release of these biomarkers in responding to stress.

In this chapter, PNEI research of its background, method, experiments, and mathematical modelling approach are introduced.

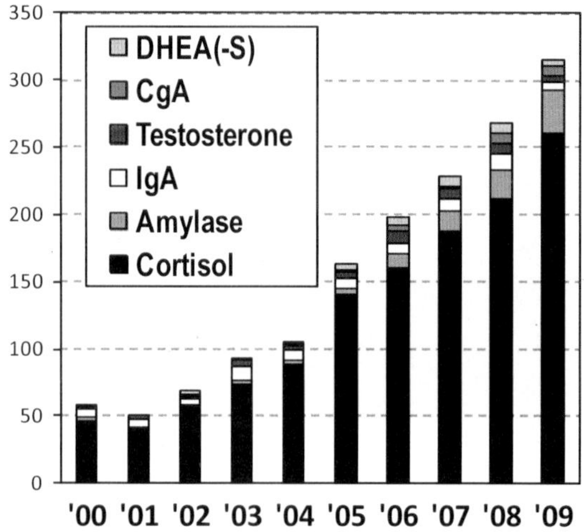

Fig. 1. Number of salivary biomarker researches: Retrieved by "PubMed" with queries "saliva", "stress" and "X (one of each substance)"

2. Stress response in our body: SAM and HPA system, and possible biomarkers

In the long history of stress research on human or animals, it has been revealed the existence of two internal stress reaction physiological pathways namely: (1) hypothalamus-pituitary-adrenal (HPA) and (2) sympatho-adrenal-medullary (SAM) system (Kirschbaum, 1994) as shown in Figure 2. When one perceives a stressful situation subjectively, one of or both SAM and HPA system is activated resulting a sort of cascade chain-reaction of a variety of bio-chemical substances inside our body along with SAM and HPA axes. During such a cascade chain-reaction, wide variety of bio-chemical substances, such as hormones, proteins, and peptides, were released into blood stream or other secretory fluid, such as saliva, urine, breast milk, sweat, etc. Therefore by monitoring such stress-related substances, the activation of SAM and/or HPA system, or nature of perceived stressor is expected to estimate to some extent. This is the background idea.

In the current PNEI studies, mainly seven biomarkers falling under the categories of hormones, immune substances, proteins and enzymes; Immunoglobulin A (IgA), cortisol, human Chromogranin A (CgA), alpha-amylase, Dehydroepiandrosterone (DHEA), Dehydroepiandrosterone sulfate (DHEA-S), and testosterone (TE), has been frequently employed (Deguchi, 2006; Bosch, 2002; Michael, 2000; Nakane, 1999; Kirschbaum, 1994). IgA, CgA, and amylase are considered to reflect SAM activation, and cortisol, DHEA, DHEA-S, and TE are considered to reflect HPA activation. The goal of PNEI study is to investigate the activations of these two systems under various stressful situations using secretory hormones and immune substances, and to demonstrate the congruity of these substances as an objective measurement of human mental stress. In the following contents, these biomarkers are described with reviewing past PNEI studies.

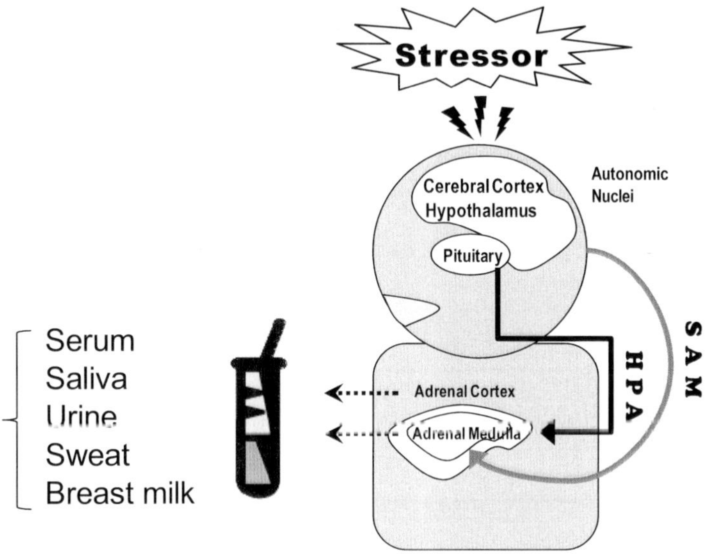

Fig. 2. Stress reaction physiological pathways: HPA and SAM system

2.1 Salivary Immunoglobulin A (IgA)

An antibody, Immunoglobulin A (IgA), is one of the most important substances in human immune system (Tsujita, 1999). It is present in almost all human secretory fluids, such as saliva, serum, urine, breast milk etc. IgA works non-specifically and therefore plays a very important role on our health, e.g. preventing bacteria from forming colonies, neutralizing toxins and enzymes produced by bacteria, and inhibiting pathogenic viruses from penetrating into the epithelial cell. Especially the salivary IgA called as "the first line of defense" since it functions in the mouse to prevent from contracting influenza or other respiratory tract infection (URTI) illnesses. In fact, clinical studies have suggested the negative correlation between the level of salivary IgA and the incidence of an acute URTI (Jemmott III, 1989). It was also reported the relevance between the level of salivary IgA and caries or periodontitis (Gregory, 1992).

On the other hand, it has been reported that salivary IgA changes its level in response to various psychological factors (Bosh, 2002), such as desirable or undesirable daily events (Stone, 1994), daily hassles (Martin, 1988), negative or positive moods (Martin, 1993), academic stresses such as examination (Jemmott III, 1983) and presentation (Evans, 1994), a short-term stressful cognitive task (Jemmott III, 1989), and relaxation (Green, 1987; Knight, 2001). These stress responses of IgA can be classified into two types: 1) a transient increase of IgA secretion immediately after an exposure of short-term laboratory stressor and subsequent recovering to the basal lever after the removal of the stressor, and 2) decline of basal IgA level several days after or during a long-term stressful situation or under chronic stress. The transient increase of IgA is considered to be regulated by autonomous nervous system (Valdimarsdottir, 1997). Thus it can be taken as a biomarker for SAM system activitiy. The decline of basal IgA level over longer period of time, by contrast, is considered to indicate chronic wear and tear of production capability. Thus it is assumed to represents some sort of long-term or chronic mental stress state while it is not necessary to consider in relation to HPA system modulation.

Although the transient increase of IgA by laboratory stressors has been consistently observed in the past PNEI studies, the decline of basal IgA over longer period of time according to chronic stress has not been always observed. A review paper on IgA studies pointed out that studies targeting on chronic stress had methodological defects such as less control of subjects' physical conditions e.g. sleep and diet, variety of saliva sampling methods, and introducing non-standardized psychological questionnaires (Bosh, 2002). Moreover the transient increase of IgA would easily mask the change in the basal IgA level over long period of time: if a subject got nervous at the moment of saliva sampling, the observed IgA level would no longer a "basal" level of the IgA of the sampling day.

There are also IgA studies focusing on the effects of various relaxing factors. These studies also reported a transient increase of IgA as the same as studies focusing on laboratory stressors. However few attempts have been made to investigate the effects of such relaxing factors with/under stressful situation (Valdimarsdottir, 1997), so it is not clear whether such a transient increase of IgA induced by relaxing factor would be derived from the same physiological mechanism as the response against laboratory stressors.

Other IgA studies have revealed that the higher cognitive process could mediate the IgA secretion. Psycho-social support alleviated the IgA secretion under long-term (Jemmott III, 1988) and short-term (Ohira, 2004) stressors. Subjects categorized in Type A trait, who are typically represented as short tempered and strong hostile, showed higher baseline of IgA and lower reactivity of IgA against an acute stressor (Ohira, 1999). Controllability of a given stressor unconsciously determined the salivary IgA (Ohira, 2001). These studies suggest that the higher cognitive process could mediate the IgA secretion. However the number of studies targeting on these potential mediators remains small.

Altogether IgA can be a useful stress biomarker, especially for laboratory stressors, representing SAM system activation, while the change in the basal IgA level over long period of time is still be a matter in discussion.

2.2 Salivary cortisol

Cortisol is the most potent glucocorticoid produced and secreted from adrenal cortex playing a quite important role for maintain our body, e.g., keeping blood glucose level adequately. Cortisol levels can be measured in serum, urine, and saliva. Cortisol is considered to be released into blood stream via activation of HPA system. In addition significant positive correlation has been obtained between salivary and blood cortisol. Therefore salivary cortisol is assumed as a possible stress biomarker representing HPA system activity.

In the past cortisol studies, a transient increase of salivary cortisol was observed by short-term laboratory stressors, such as mental arithmetic task, stroop task, and oral presentation (Dickerson, 2004; Kirschbaum, 1994). With regard to a long-term or chronic stress, higher level of cortisol secretion has been revealed to associate with chronic stress state, such as job stress (Steptoe, 2000), job loss (Ockenfels, 1995), and divorce (Powell, 2002). By contrast positive affect was found to associate with lower total cortisol secretion during daytime

(Steptoe, 2005). Cortisol has a large diurnal variation of which it starts increase at the just after awakening in the morning, reaches at the peak of the day around 30 minutes after awakening, keeps decreasing through the daytime, and then reaches a minimum level at the night. Especially the individual drastic change, increasing to the peak of the day at the morning is called "cortisol awakening response (CAR)" and it has reported that CAR is associated with chronic stress (Izawa, 2007; Clow, 2004; Schulz 1998; Pruessner, 1997). Altogether salivary cortisol can be a possible short-term and long-term stress marker.

However cortisol has been consistently reported to increase against such stressors accompanying with strong tension and threat, or psycho-social evaluation, it showed inconsistent results against relatively mild stressors such as simple arithmetic task and cognitive task (Dickerson, 2004). Some methodological defeats have been discussed on this discrepancy such as variety of biochemical analysis, saliva collection method, and subject control. Among that, the variety of the timing of saliva sampling has been frequently indicated, including the past PNEI studies with other biomarkers (Hansen, 2008; Dickerson, 2004; Bosch, 2002; Valdimarsdottir, 1997; Kirschbaum, 1994). Also it should be noted that because the stress reaction of HPA system is truly complicated and potentially mediated by variety of physiological factors, the salivary cortisol cannot be taken as a direct measure of HPA system itself but as rather an "indirect" measure (Hellhammer, 2009).

2.3 Salivary CgA

Chromogranin A (CgA), a major member of the granin family of acidic secretory glycoproteins, is known to be released from the adrenal medulla into the blood with catecholamine(Kim, 2005). Therefore it is considered to be a possible biomarker of SAM system (Nakane, 1999; Winkler, 1992). CgA has been reported to transiently increase in response to short-term laboratory stressors such as a calculation test (Nakane, 1999), white noise (Miyakawa, 2006), and a cognitive task (Kanamaru, 2006). On the other hand there are studies failed to observe increase or rather decrease against a laboratory stressors (e.g., Yamakoshi, 2009) and observed a transient increase in subjects who declared the positive affection after watching a comic video (Toda, 2007).

CgA is expected as a possible stress marker representing SAM system activity as just described. However, the number of studies on salivary CgA is still small comparing with that on Cortisol and IgA. Moreover commercial available assay protocol for CgA is limited as just one product (Human Chromogranin A EIA Kit › Yanaihara Institute Inc.). So is necessary to accumulate more studies for further discussion.

2.4 Salivary DHEA

Dehydroepiandrosterone (DHEA) and Dehydroepiandrosterone sulfate (DHEA-S) is a steroid adrenal cortex hormone like cortisol. It is thus expected as a possible stress marker representing HPA system activity. It is considered to function antagonistically with cortisol on the central nervous system and immune system (Wolf, 1999). DHEA and DHEA-S was reported to associate with superior stress tolerance (Morgan, 2009). On the contrary lowered DHEA was observed in subjects with partially or completely remitted depression (Michael, 2000). Therefore higher DHEA can be considered in relation with positive state in the context of chronic stress.

It was also reported to show a transient increase against short-term laboratory stressors like as other possible biomarkers (Shirtcliff, 2007; Sugaya, 2007; Izawa, 2008). However these studies introduced a strong and socially evaluated laboratory stressor, as typified by "Trier Social Stress Test (TSST) (Kirschbaum, 1993)," responses against relatively mild stressors such as simple arithmetic task and cognitive task is unknown.

Although DHEA in many respects paralleled cortisol secretory activity there was some dissociation in the response in the time series (Sugaya, 2007) and diurnal secretion (Hucklebridge, 2005). DHEA studies are also still small in number as depicted in Fig.1. Further studies are necessary to discuss more.

2.5 Other salivary possible biomarkers

Salivary alpha-amylase (sAA) has been reported to show a transient increase against short-term laboratory stressors along with the activation of sympathetic nervous system mediated via beta-receptor (van Stegeren, 2006; Deguchi, 2006; Yamaguchi, 2004;). Therefore it is also considered to be a possible biomarker representing SAM system activity (Bosch, 2002). However it is suggested that the activation of parasympathetic nervous system also results in a transient increase of sAA mediated via increment of saliva flow rate (Bosch, 2002).

Regarding with chronic stress sAA was reported to have no remarkable association with depression, anxiety, work stress and burnout but a small negative correlation between "social difficulties" measured with a chronic stress scale in a population of nurses (Wingenfeld, 2010). Recently alpha-amylase is used to highlight the difference in the activity of SAM system and HPA system which is measured by salivary cortisol (Strahler, 2010), and a study reported that the salivary alpha-amylase over cortisol ratio, named as AOCg, can be a better indication of stress system dysregulation than sAA or cortisol alone (Ali, 2011).

Free-3-mehoxy-4-hydroxyphenylglycol (free-MHPG) (Okamura, 2010; Buchsbaum, 1981) and testosterone was reported to show transient increase by short-term laboratory stressors, while the number of studies assessing these substances are very small and frequently showed inconsistent results (e.g. Schoofs, 2011).

2.6 Summary of possible biomarkers

In the current PNEI studies, it is suggested that the salivary biomarkers can be taken as a possible objective stress measurement. All abovementioned substances show a transient increase against short-term laboratory stressor representing the activation of human physiological stress reaction pathways, HPA and SAM systems. Cortisol is the most promising biomarker for a long-term or chronic stress, and IgA is the one for short-term laboratory stressors. However, since PNEI is relatively a new interdisciplinary study, basic problems remain unsolved such as sensitivity of these biomarkers against variety of stressful and relaxing factors, precise change in the secretion of biomarkers in the time series, the effects of long-term stress or chronic stress which might affect the change in the production speed of these biomarkers rather than a temporal change in the secretion.

A recent PNEI research for assessing all different types of biomarkers in blood, such as active natural killer (NK) cell level, varieties of T lymphocyte, dopamine, norepinephrine, and epinephrine, shows a rapid change in the composition of those substances (e.g., Kimura,

2005; Isowa, 2004). It provides quite important information for the better understanding of the human psycho-physiological stress reaction. However such a multi-assessing study is still at its infancy. Far more research needs to be conducted for more discussion.

3. Methods of PNEI Studies using saliva samples

In this chapter, the methodology of PNEI studies, i.e. experimental designs, subjects' control, preparation of stressors, analysis of biomarkers etc., is described since the variety of methodology has frequently been pointed out as one of a major confounder.

3.1 Saliva sampling method

Saliva samples have been collected frequently by "*Salivette*", which is made of dense plain cotton of a cylindrical shape about 1 cm wide and 3.5 cm long. *Salivette* is designed for one-time saliva sampling and mostly introduced in diagnosis uses. In other words, it is not suitable for repetitive saliva collection. It has high absorbability and thus deprives far more amount of saliva, about 2 mL per one sampling for 3 minute, for that of necessary to quantitative determination of biomarkers, at most 50 μL of saliva for one biomarker. Excessive saliva collection brings forth the lack of saliva and, as a result, disturbs normal saliva flow. A past study demonstrated that repetitive saliva collection in every 5 minutes resulted in the decrease of saliva volume and also the concentration of salivary IgA by sampling time as depicted in Fig.3 (Nomura, 2006). Therefore the use of *Salivette* in case of repetitive sampling is not recommended.

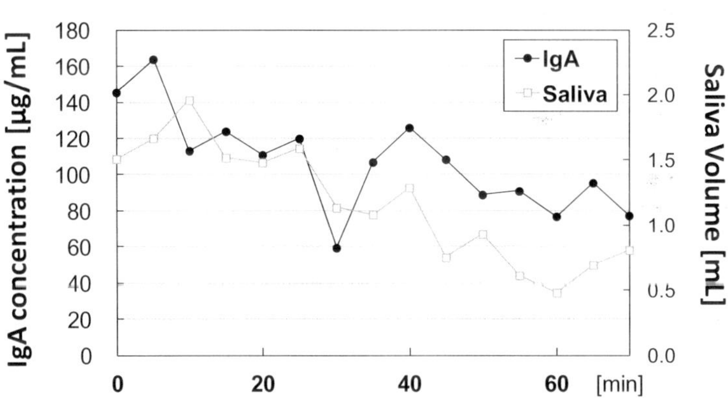

Fig. 3. The change in IgA concentration and saliva volume with repetitive saliva collection by *Salivette*

The passive drawing or the use of small cotton is recommended in case of repetitive sampling. Considering the absorption of biochemical substances by the cotton, the passive drawing is technically ideal method for saliva sampling. However it requires training for subjects to get used to dropping saliva into small cup or container. Besides it might be uncomfortable for some subjects to take saliva in this way. Taking saliva by small cotton is easiest method. Although a certain amount of biomarkers would be absorbed, it might be excluded when one focuses on the relative change in the level of biomarkers. It is important to prepare the same size and volume of cotton for the repetitive sampling otherwise the volume of saliva collection would become as an unintended confounder. The small cotton should be placed under the subjects' tongue so as to collect the fresh saliva.

Experimenter should pay attention in handling the sample saliva to avoid contingent infection of virus or other possible diseases. All experimenters should ware disposable gloves and glasses. The saliva samples should be kept in the freezer below -20 Celsius by the day of the quantitative determination of biomarkers.

3.2 Possible confounders

The natural secretion of abovementioned biomarkers has a diurnal change: the highest level is in the morning and gradually decreases afterwards to the lowest level in the night time (it should be noted that only alpha-amylase act controversy; Strahler, 2010). Therefore saliva sampling should be conducted depending on the objective of a study: (1) it should be corrected in the afternoon where the secretion of biomarkers is expected to be stable in the case of laboratory stressor studies by which a level of transient increase of these biomarkers are focused, and (2) in the morning or just after awakening in the case of chronic stress study since basal secretion level is expected to show a remarkable difference among subjects in the morning (e.g. Steptoe, 2005). Because of its remarkable diurnal change, repetitive sampling by a distinct time point of a day is recommended even in a chronic stress study.

Postprandial effects on the secretion of biomarkers are considerable. In addition pH of saliva could affect the quantitative determination of biomarkers. Subjects should not take any food or drink except for water at least an hour prior to the experiment. Hard exercise should be avoided prior to the experiment since it could make biomarkers temporary elevate. Moreover it is strongly recommended to take 5 to 10 minutes of an initial rest period before conducting experiment. If subjects were not familiar with or nervous to an experiment, most of biomarkers would increase by such a negative feeling or strain. Subjects who take any medications, especially oral contraceptive, suffer from any disease, are pregnant, or other cases in which physiological states were considered to be unusual should be excluded. Age and gender should be balanced in groups of between-subjects study since it is known to be confounders, especially for the study assessing hormones.

Subjects must be well informed about the objective and method of the study. Any experimental design targeting on human mental or physical stress should be approved by a local ethics committee or equivalent organization.

3.3 Quantitative determination of salivary biomarkers

The concentrations of salivary biomarkers have frequently been determined by enzyme-linked immunosorbent assay (ELISA). ELISA is nowadays one of major molecular determination techniques. It is much easier in treatment and cheaper in running cost than other molecular determination techniques, such as radioimmunoassay (RIA), fluorescent immunoassay (FIA), and the high performance liquid chromatography (HPLC). Several products which are designed for determination of "salivary" biomarkers, not for serum and urine, are placing on the market (e.g., Salivary Secretory IgA Indirect Enzyme Immunoassay Kit, Salimetrics, LLC., USA). By using such an ELISA kit in which all specimens and materials are included, experimenter can easily assay various biomarkers with a minimum knowledge of biochemical analysis.

The principle of ELISA is based on the antigen-antibody reaction which is for capturing a target substance and the enzyme reaction which is for detecting the mass of a target substance via optical density of reaction produced color. The brief description of ELISA (competitive method) is as follows: (1) Thaw saliva samples kept in a biological freezer by moving them into a biological refrigerator (4 Celsius). (2) Centrifuge each saliva samples for 10 minutes at 1500 rpm to precipitate mucins or other solid contents. (3) Add each saliva sample (or known samples for references) into antibody-coated 96-well micro-plate. (4) Add a constant amount of "enzyme conjugate" which is the target biomarker (antigen) combined with horseradish peroxidase (HRP) into the micro-plate and incubate for an hour. In this step, antigen-antibody reaction is occurred competitively between original target in the saliva sample and that in the enzyme conjugate. (5) Wash the micro-plate to flush unbind target. (6) Add tetramethylbenzidine (TMB) solution to induce enzyme reaction with enzyme conjugate which is captured by antigen coated on the bottom of each well of the micro-plate in the step (4). The amount of the bind enzyme conjugate, which is there as a result of competitive reaction process, can be detected as the strength of optimal color (450nm) cased by enzyme reaction. Therefore this optimal density is inversely proportional to the concentration of target containing in the original saliva sample. (7) Finally, the target concentration in each sample is determined by referencing the optimal density of the reference samples. All analysis procedures take roughly about 3 to 5 hours for one micro-plate. Correct handling of samples and specimens with well calibrated micropipette is critical for all steps.

4. Sensitivity in the response of biomarkers against laboratory stressors

In this section, the transient response of HPA and SAM above-mentioned stress biomarkers against a shot-term laboratory stressor is described with reviewing our past research (Nomura, 2006, 2009, 2010a, 2010b) and also additionally presenting some new experimental results. Especially, the transient response in the time series, i.e. the changing in the level of biomarkers in a short period of time through the onset or the end of an acute laboratory stressor, is featured. It can be highlighting the time constant of the physiological stress response of these biomarkers, or more simply the "temporal sensitivity" against the stressor.

As already described variety of salivary secretory substances are considered to be possible biomarkers as representing the activation of HPA and SAM system. Moreover there seems to be a difference in the "temporal sensitivity" among there biomarkers. Some studies demonstrated the difference in the time course response of these biomarkers against laboratory stressors. Izawa et al. (2008) demonstrated that the stress-induced transient DHEA increase took place ahead of that of cortisol in the TSST experimental session. Ali et al. (2011) also demonstrated in the same TSST session that alpha-amylase also precede cortisol response.

On the other hand whether there would be a difference in the "sensitivity of the intensity" among these biomarkers is still in the matter of discussion. A review article on cortisol described that the salivary cortisol increases against stronger and socially evaluated laboratory stressor, as typified by TSST, but have shown inconsistent results against relatively mild stressors such as simple arithmetic task and cognitive task by which IgA should always increase (Dickerson, 2004). Actually the idea of "sensitivity of the intensity" cannot stand separately from the "temporal sensitivity." The response of these biomarkers against laboratory stressors always takes place in a transient manner in a certain period of time: it gradually increases, reaches a peak, and after the removal of the stressor, it gradually decreases to the basal level. In fact, if such a transient stress-induced increase of a biomarker took place with a different time delay with respect to each biomarker, it would appear as the difference in the sensitivity of the intensity depending on the time point. Moreover in the case of that saliva sample were not taken frequently enough in the time series, it would result in the inconsistency of obtained experimental results and interpretations among the studies.

With an eye on this point, we designed an experiment to clarify the difference in the sensitivity of biomarkers against a relatively mild laboratory stressor with frequent saliva collection in the time series, as described in the next.

4.1 Experiment targeting on the difference in the sensitivity among HPA and SAM biomarkers against a mild stressor

The precise changing in the level of salivary four stress biomarkers, which were IgA, cortisol, CgA, and DHEA, were assessed continuously in the time series during which a simple calculation task was given to subjects as a mild stressor. The difference in the sensitivity of these biomarkers as a stress biomarker was expected to be illustrated. Moreover the better understanding for the dynamics of physiological stress response was expected as well since these four biomarkers represent HPA (cortisol and DHEA) and SAM (IgA and CgA) system activities respectively.

4.1.1 A stressor

Subjects, ten university male students, were instructed to conduct a simple calculation task as a mild stressor. It was a simple addition of two double-digit integers repeatedly presented on a laptop monitor every 3.0 seconds with changing the figures. It is quite similar to so-called Kraepelin psychodiagnostic test, which is typified as simple, monotonous, and boring arithmetic task, and thus frequently introduced for studies on mental work load or mental fatigue. Subjects were instructed to perform this calculation task as correct and fast as possible.

4.1.2 Procedure

Two types of experimental design of task/break schedule were prepared for this study as depicted in Figure 4. The experimental session A consists of two sets of 18 minutes of the calculation task and subsequent 9 minutes of the break. The experimental session B consists of six sets of 6 minutes of the task and subsequent 3 minutes of the break. It should be noted that the total duration of the task and break is exactly the same in both sessions: 36 minutes of the calculation task and 18 minutes of the break. After each session A and B, 20 minutes of recovering period was added during which subjects were sitting calmly on the chair.

Saliva samples were taken by a piece of cotton every three minutes during the session. Saliva was also taken at 3, 10, and 20 minutes after the last set of the task/break to observe a

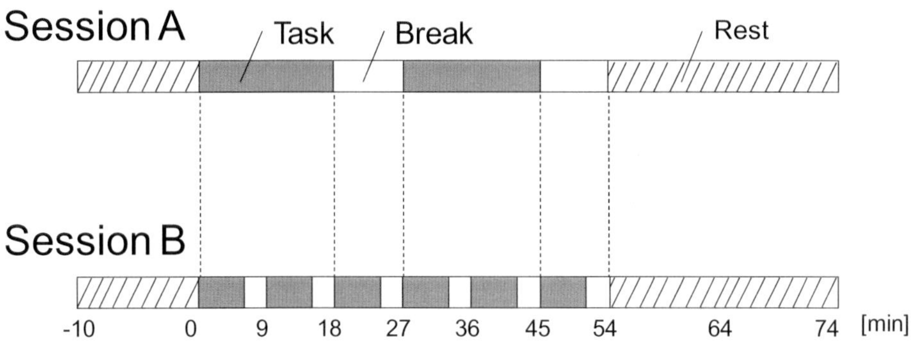

Fig. 4. Task/break schedule in session A and B

recovering process of the elevated biomarkers to a basal level. Subjects were instructed to place the cotton under his tongue for three minutes. These cottons were centrifuged at 1500 rpm for 10 minutes to remove mucin. This filtrated saliva samples were stored separately in a small polypropylene tube in freezing chamber at -20 Celsius by the day on the quantitative analysis. Four above-mentioned biomarkers, which are IgA, cortisol, CgA, and DHEA, were assessed by ELISA.

This experiment was conducted as with-in subjects design: every subject went through both sessions A and B in a randomized order. All sessions were conducted in a dark and soundproof room, one by one, and in the afternoon so as to avoid a disturbance by the large diurnal change of biomarkers in the morning.

4.1.3 Other physiological and psychological measures

Electrocardiogram (ECG) was recorded through all sessions and subsequent 20 minutes of recovering period by a multipurpose bio-signal amplifier at the rate of 500 Hz (BMS-3201, Nihon-Kohden Co.). Frequency analysis was conducted afterward to estimate the high frequency power of the ECG data in the range of 0.15 to 0.40 Hz (hereafter denoted as HF power), which has been frequently used for the index of parasympathetic nervous system activity.

Regarding with the psychological scale, "Profile of Mood State (POMS) (Japanese version)" (Yokoyama, 1993) were given to the subjects to fill up before and after the sessions. POMS is one of the most commonly used questionnaires frequently used various psychological and cognitive science studies (MacNair, 2003). It consists of 65 items concerning subjects' mood state with 5 point scale: not at all, a little, moderately, quite a lot, and extremely. These items are designed to classify into six identified mood factors: tension-anxiety (defined as T-A), depression-dejection (D), anger-hostility (A-H), fatigue-inertia (F), vigour-activity (V), and confusion-bewilderment (C). The score of each mood factors can be found by adding up the scores of corresponding items.

4.2 Results of the experiment: The difference in the sensitivity among HPA and SAM biomarkers

4.2.1 Behavior and POMS

The task performance did not show any change by repetition of the task during sessions or between the session A and B. In fact the task, which is the addition of two double-digit integers at every 3.0 seconds, is too easy for the subjects, who were university students, to find any difference in their performance.

Regarding with POMS, only the factor V (vigour-activity) out of six mood factors showed significant decrease after the calculation task ($p<.05$, t-test). Other factors did not show any significant change in the scores while the factor F (fatigue) showed a trend of decrease ($p<.1$). In other words, the calculation task introduced in our study was not an intensive stressor which gives subjects negative mood such as tension, threat, or hostility just like TSST but rather a mild stressor as we intended.

4.2.2 Profile of autonomous nervous system activities (HR, HF power of ECG)

Figure 5 shows the profile of changing in the heat rate (HR) during task/break period in the time series in the session A (Fig. 5(a)) and B (Fig. 5(b)). It should be noted each values were found by averaging every three minutes so that it makes easier to illustrate the difference in the profile with that of biomarkers as depicted later. There was no any significant change in the time series regardless of task, break, or recovering period in both session A and B, while it has a tendency to decrease in the task period. It is known through the past experimental psychological researches that the heart rate frequently decreased rather than increased under a certain type of laboratory stressors by which subjects need to concentrate on or just keep silence in perceiving the situation, such as vigilance task, noise exposure, mental arithmetic task, etc (Williams, 1986). At any rate this results again ensure the nature of the calculation task as a mild stressor as we intended.

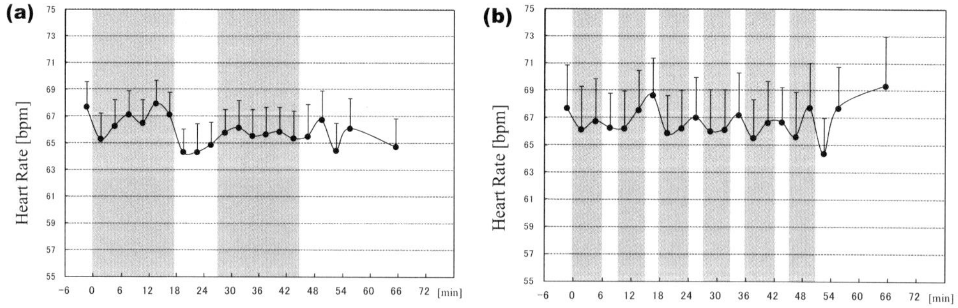

Fig. 5. Profile of heart rate in session A and B. Error bar represent standard error of the mean (S.E.M). Gray background represents a calculation task period.

Figure 6 shows the profile of changing in the high frequency power of ECG signal (HF power) during task/break period in the time series in the session A (Fig. 6(a)) and B (Fig. 6(b)). As these figures shows, HF power remarkably decreased during the task and recovered to the basal level in the subsequent break period. HF power changes according to respiratory regulated heart beat-to-beat interval modulation, which is so-called Respiratory Sinus Arrhythmia (RSA) (Andreassi, 2007). RSA is dominantly subject to the parasympathetic nervous system, so HF power is considered as an index of the parasympathetic nervous system activities. When one look at the results of our study, it is quite understandable since HF power decreased during the task and recovered in the rest period. Moreover it should be emphasized that such switch-over of the HF power took place rapidly according to the task/break schedule, and well reproduced over time regardless of the repetition of the task/break as seen the session B in particular. Therefore with regard to the "sensitivity" of HF power against a mild stressor, HF power can be compared with a binary switch as it turn on during the task and off in the break without any cumulative effect over time.

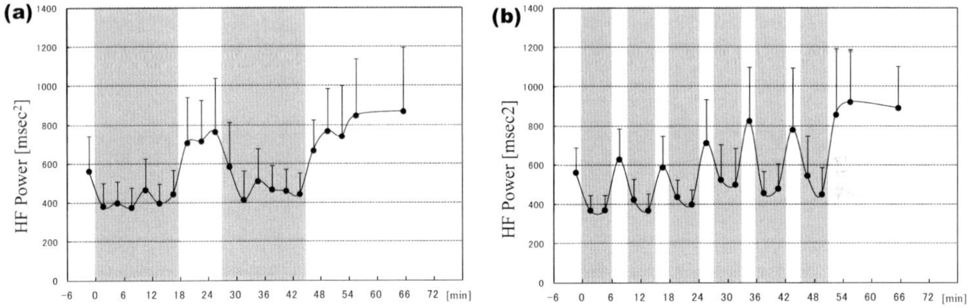

Fig. 6. Profile of HF power of ECG in session A and B. Error bar represent standard error of the mean (S.E.M). Gray background represents a calculation task period.

4.2.3 Profile of IgA

Figure 7 shows the profile of changing in the concentration of salivary secreted IgA during task/break period in the time series in the session A (Fig. 7(a)) and B (Fig. 7(b)). It increased during the task, decreased during the break, and recovered to the initial (basal) level. This simple fact demonstrates the congruity of IgA as a stress biomarker of a mild stressor.

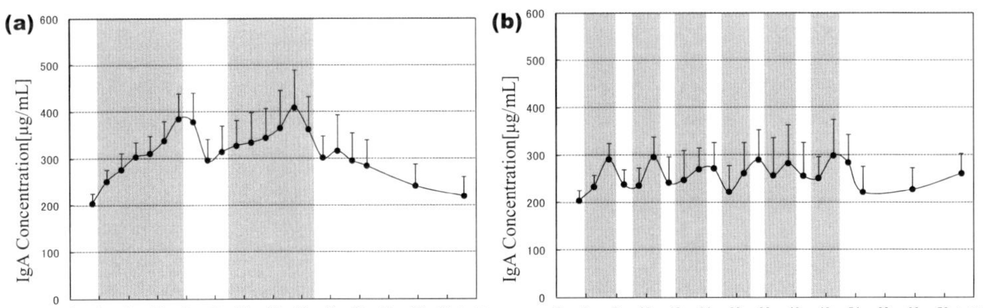

Fig. 7. Profile of IgA in session A and B. Error bar represent standard error of the mean (S.E.M). Gray background represents a calculation task period.

On the other hand IgA showed a remarkable difference in the profile over time comparing with that of HF power. In session A, IgA started to increase gradually after the onset of the first calculation task. Following the end of the first task, IgA started to decreased but because of certain latency in recovering, it did not recover to the basal level. These latencies over time in IgA increasing induced by the onset of a stressor and decreasing in the recovering resulted in cumulative profile of IgA as depicted in Fig. 7(a): where the average concentration of IgA during the first task period was significantly higher than that of the second task ($p<.01$, t-test), and it took around 30 minutes for the elevated IgA to return to the basal level. Moreover there was no significant correlation between IgA concentration and saliva flow rate. Therefore the cumulative effect observed in session A was not merely as a result of the change in saliva flow, which is thought to be mediated by the change in autonomous nervous system activity.

Comparing with the results in session A and B, there was no such remarkable cumulative effect in session B: there was no any difference in the initial (basal) level, but regarding with the total IgA secreted during all through the sessions, it was significantly higher in session A than that of B ($p<.01$). This difference in the IgA secretion profile in the session A and B is rather intriguing, because the total task/break period, and moreover the task/break ratio (2:1) were the exactly same for both session A and B. It could happen by a nonlinear feature of the IgA secretion depending on the duration of the task: IgA secretion rate might increase depending on the duration of the task. The change in the secretion rate would result in greater elevation of IgA concentration even taking an account of the difference in the duration of task period in session A, i.e. 18 minutes, and session B, 6 minutes. Subsequent recovering period was not enough in session A but appropriate in session B even it was equivalent in terms of task/break ratio. As such IgA secretion profile in the time series might reflect both the duration and repetition (or schedule) of the task/break. The idea just described was introduced into the kinetic mathematical model we proposed later (see section 5 for more detail).

With regard to the "sensitivity" against a mild stressor, IgA is not such sensitive to the onset or the end of a mild stressor as depicted in HF power profile (Fig. 6). However seen from another point, IgA secretion has cumulative feature, in other words it can represent a sort of hysteresis of a given stressor. Therefore IgA is not so sensitive against the temporal change in the situation, but it is still sensitive even for a mild stressor persisting certain time duration. In the field of dynamics, e.g. control engineering, it can be understood as the characteristic in the "time constant" or "relaxation time": in this case HF power possess small time constant against a mild stressor, and by contrast IgA possess relatively greater one. All together IgA can be a useful biomarker for a mild and long-lasting stressor.

4.2.4 Profile of cortisol

The cumulative secretion profile was more remarkable in the cortisol as depicted in Figure 8. As these figure shows salivary cortisol concentration showed a cumulative increase all through the task/break period in both session A and B. Moreover the elevated cortisol level did not recovered to the basal level despite of 20 minutes of recovering period after the sessions. HF power and saliva flow rate had no significant correlation with cortisol. It is understandable to think of that the secretion of cortisol reflects HPA system activity as already mentioned.

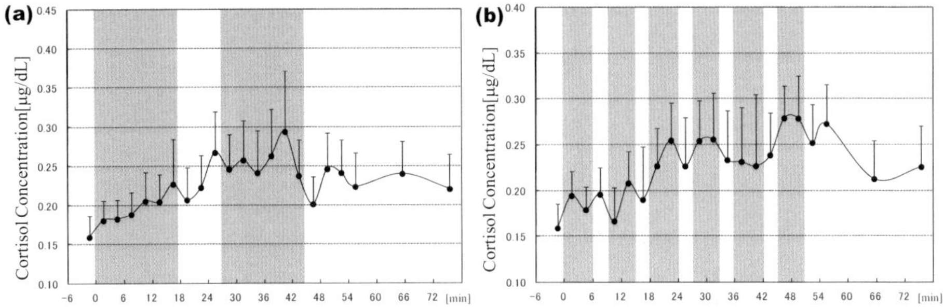

Fig. 8. Profile of cortisol in session A and B. Error bar represent standard error of the mean (S.E.M). Gray background represents a calculation task period.

With regard to the "sensitivity" against a mild stressor, it can be assumed by our experimental results that cortisol would possess greater time constant than that of IgA, then greater than HF power of course. Comparing with the profile of IgA in the session B, cortisol still showed a cumulative effect in such a short-period of but repetition of the simple calculation task. In this sense, cortisol should be much sensitive than IgA against a mild stressor.

In the past cortisol studies, the stress response of cortisol against "mild" stressors, which are typified by the cognitive tasks without any threat or performance pressure such as passive stroop task and mental arithmetic task, showed inconsistent results, while that against acute and strong stressors such as academic oral defense with psychosocial evaluation always resulted in the increase of cortisol. Then a review article concluded that cortisol can be a useful stress biomarker for an acute and stronger stressor with psychosocial evaluation rather than a mild stressor (Dickerson, 2004). However looking into the result of our experiment in which the precise changing in the level of salivary cortisol were assessed every 3 minutes, a significant stress response can be observed even by a mild stressor if only salivary cortisol was assessed by an appropriate timing and duration corresponding to a particular targets.

4.2.5 Profile of CgA

Figure 9 shows the profile of changing in the concentration of salivary secreted CgA during task/break period in the time series in the session A (Fig. 9(a)) and B (Fig. 9(b)). It increased in the task period and decreased in the break. Moreover both salivary flow rate and HF power, which represent parasympathetic nervous activities, have no significant correlation between CgA. So CgA can also be taken as a plausible biomarker for a mild stressor.

The transient increase of CgA against laboratory stressors were also observed in the past CgA studies (Miyakawa, 2006; Kanamaru, 2006; Kanamaru, 2005). However some studies showed inconsistent results (e.g., Yamakoshi, 2009). It might attributes to the nature of high "temporal sensitivity" of CgA against a mild stressor illustrated in our study. As Fig. 9(a) shows CgA seems to possess a certain time constant, however it might be smaller than that of IgA even a little greater than that HF power. This means the slight difference in the saliva sampling time and duration might result in a big difference in the level of CgA in some cases.

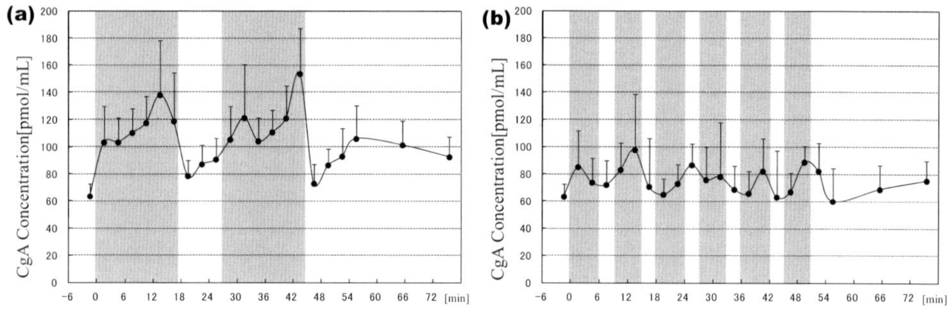

Fig. 9. Profile of CgA in session A and B. Error bar represent standard error of the mean (S.E.M). Gray background represents a calculation task period.

CgA possesses high "temporal sensitivity" as just described. On the other hand there could not find any cumulative effects like as HF power. Then it can be assumed that CgA possesses relatively small time constant. Since CgA is considered to represent sympathetic nervous system activity and thus to be a possible biomarker for SAM system activity as described in the subsection 2.3, this small time constant of CgA illustrated in our experiment is reasonable. So CgA can be a useful biomarker for detecting the change in the situation, i.e. the onset or the end of a given stressors but not suitable for estimating cumulative effect over time.

4.2.6 Profile of DHEA

The stress-induced secretion of salivary DHEA in session A and B seem to be cumulative as shown Figure 10(a) and 10(b). Moreover elevated DHEA during the both sessions did not return to the basal level during 20 minutes of recovering period, while total secretion of DHEA was larger in session A than B. Parasympathetic nervous activities indexed as HF power and saliva flow rate does not have significant correlation. There were some studies demonstrated that stress-induced DHEA secretion had reached its peak around 20 minutes after the onset of a strong stressor, TSST (Izawa, 2008; Sugaya, 2007). On the other hand looking at the result of our experiment assessing precise chaining of DHEA secretion in the time series, there might have a peak in DHEA in the last half of the second task period or much later in session A. Considering the difference in the nature of TSST and the calculation task, it can be assumed that the level of DHEA might represents the intensity of a given stressor, as the same as cortisol.

Comparing the profile of DHEA and other biomarkers, DHEA might possess relatively greater time constant: which should be ranked between that of IgA and cortisol. Therefore regarding the sensitivity of DHEA as a stress biomarker, it is not so sensitive to the onset or the end of the stressor, however it can still be a useful biomarker for long-lasting and a mild stressor like as cortisol. Since DHEA is a biomarker representing HPA system activity, it is understandable for that the stress response of DHEA was similar with cortisol. However there seems to be still a slight difference of response over time. It should be a matter in discussion in future.

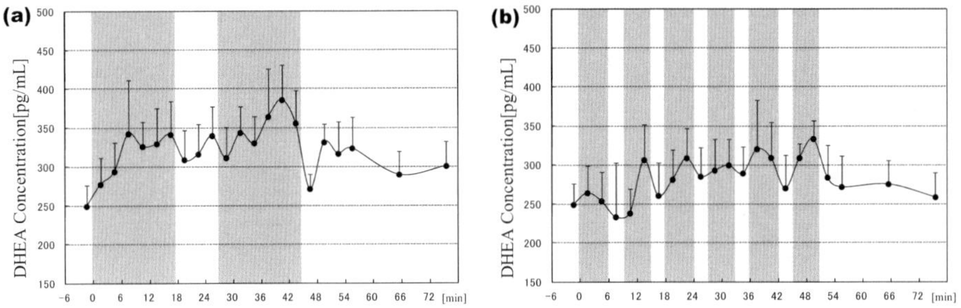

Fig. 10. Profile of DHEA in session A and B. Error bar represent standard error of the mean (S.E.M). Gray background represents a calculation task period.

4.3 Discussion of the experiment: "Sensitivity" of the biomarkers as interpreted by the time constant; SAM comes first and HPA in the later

To our knowledge our experiment was the first one to simultaneously illustrate the precise changing in the level of four stress biomarkers, which are IgA, cortisol, CgA, and DHEA, against a mild stressor. The results of our experiment plausibly demonstrate the possible candidacy of these substances as a biomarker for a mild laboratory stressor. Moreover the differences in the "sensitivity" among them as interpreted by the time constant were successfully demonstrated. The substances represents SAM system which are CgA and IgA sensitively increase and decrease by the onset and the end of the stressor, whereas those represents HPA system which are DHEA and cortisol showed cumulative effect over time. So our results might represent a part of complex dynamics of two major physiological stress reaction pathways, which are SAM and HPA. Moreover there also seems to be a difference in the time constant among SAM and HPA biomarker as CgA has the smallest, IgA places in the next, DHEA comes after IgA, and cortisol is the one which has the greatest time constant. It should represent further mechanism underlying the complexity of these systems and might be as a result of adaptive response in the sense of long evolutionary history: since cortisol possess a great impact on human physiology such as controlling blood pressure, it must be inefficient in term of energy consumption if it were as "sensitive" as CgA. In other word, it is of no use in responding a mild laboratory stressor but it should work in more critical situation in our life.

5. Kinetic model of biomarkers in the response to a mild laboratory stressor: A preliminary description

The difference in the sensitivity of stress biomarkers observed in our experiment can be restate as the difference in the time constant as described above. Here a mathematical model of the response of biomarkers is suggested to describe the experimental result as the difference in the time constant: from on/off binary response to cumulative one.

5.1 Constitution of the kinetic model

Basic assumptions for the model are introduced according to our experimental fact, and are quite simple as follows:

1. Continuity: biomarker changes continuously in the time series,
2. Homeostasis: biomarker secretion has its upper and lower limits, and
3. Stress response: biomarker increases against stressor, and its rate is linearly depend on the duration of the stressor, which means non-linear increase of IgA
4. Recovering: biomarker decrease to the basal level after the removal of the stressor.

As the most simple and well-consistent with these assumptions, the logistic function is adopted as the basis of this model. The logistic function is a nonlinear ordinary differential equation consisting of the first order of exponential increasing term and the second order of nonlinear decreasing term, as in

$$dx/dt = (a-bx)x \tag{1}$$

where x, t, a, and b are all positive values representing the concentration of biomarker, time, and increasing and decreasing coefficient respectively. This formula is called a logistic function or growth curve, and it has been applied to describe the exponential growth in the number of bacteria and its decaying, caused by environmental deterioration accompanying

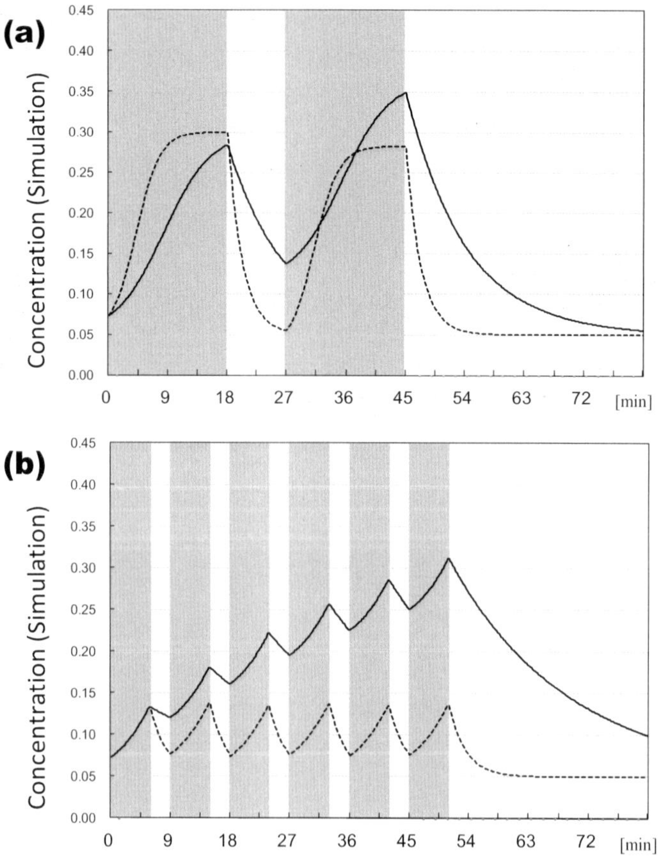

Fig. 11. Simulated biomarker secretion in session A and B.

with an increase of individual density. Moreover, it is the simplest model possessing the homeostatic property. With regard to the recovering process, a simple exponential decreasing function is introduced, as in

$$dx/dt = -cx \tag{2}$$

where *c* is a positive values representing decreasing coefficient. The stress-induced response of biomarkers, increase by a short-term laboratory stressor and decrease by its removal, was simulated with task/break schedule as the same as in the session A and B in our experiment.

5.2 Result and discussion of the numerical simulation

Figure 11(a) and 11(b) shows the results of the simulation. As expected the model successfully illustrated on/off or cumulative changing profile of biomarkers depending on the parameters. By solely changing the increasing and decreasing parameters, *a*, *b*, and *c*, the degree of such cumulative effects was able to controlled. Therefore this simple non-linear kinetic model proposed here can be assumed as a basis for the stress induced physiological response in our body. By elaborating this model though a series of experiments targeting on the variety of stressors with different schedule on various biomarkers, the dynamics of human stress reaction pathways, HPA and SAM systems, would be better understood.

6. Conclusion

In this chapter, the salivary biomarker researches as a new metric for human mental stress, its background, methods, experiments, and kinetic model approaches were introduced. Although there are numbers of technical limitation and problems to be solved, biomarkers introduced in this manuscript can be useful and unique measures for human mental states. Stress estimation by salivary biomarkers has a great methodological advantage, because saliva can be collected less-stressfully and in a noninvasive manner unlike blood and urine. Moreover it is the one and the only secretory fluid that can be collected at anytime and by anyone including children and patients in need of nursing care.

On the other hand, mathematical model approach lead us an idea of the estimation of optimal work/break schedule in the limited time avoiding excessive secretion of biochemical substances: for an instance, when one has to take a long-distance drive and reach at a destination within a limited period of time, one could estimate the optimal timing of the stop for the rest. It might be useful for a stress management in the working place as well, such as VDT workload and monitoring work. The molecular analysis techniques are advancing day by day, real-time monitoring of such a tiny amount of biomarkers might be available in the near future. Remember the difficulty of self-management of stress and the necessity of introducing objective criteria. Biomarkers introduced in this manuscript can be a possible solution, even though it still remains in the initial step.

7. Acknowledgment

This study was supported in part by "Program to Disseminate Tenure Tracking System", Promoting Science and Technology of the Ministry of Education, Culture, Sports, Science and Technology, Japan.

8. References

Ader, R.; Felten, L. & Cohen, N. (Ed(s.). (2001) *Psychoneruoimmunology* (3rd ed.), Academic Press, Waltham, Massachusetts, USA

Ali, N. & Pruessner, J.C.. (2011). The Salivary Alpha-amylase Over Cortisol Ratio as a Marker to Assess Dysregulations of the Stress Systems. *Physiology & Behavior*, [Epub ahead of print]

Andreassi, J.L. (2007). *Psychophysiology: Human Behavior & Physiological Response* (5th ed.), Psychology Press, London, England

Bosch, J.A.; Ring, C.; de Geus, E.J.; Veerman, E.C. & Amerongen, A.V. (2002). Stress and secretory immunity. *International Review of Neurobiology*, Vol.52, No.1, pp.213-253

Buchsbaum, M.S.; Muscettola, G. & Goodwin, F.K. (1981). Urinary MHPG, stress response, personality factors and patients with major affective disorders. *Neuropsychology*,Vol.7, pp.212-224

Clow, A.; Thorn, L.; Evans, P. & Hucklebridge, F. (2004). The awakening cortisol response: methodological issues and significance. *Stress*, Vol.7, No.1, pp.29-37

Deguchi, M.; Wakasugi, J.; Ikegami, T.; Nanba, S. & Yamgaguchi, M. (2006). Evaluation of driver stress using motor-vehicle driving simulator. *IEEJ Trans. Sensors and Micromachines*, Vol.126, No.8, pp.438-444

Dickerson, S.S. & Kemeny, M.E. (2004). Acute stressors and cortisol responses: A theoretical integration and synthesis of laboratory research. *Psychological Bulletin*, Vol.130, No.3, pp.335-391

Evans, P.; Bristow, M.; Hucklebridge, F.; Clow, A. & Pang, F.Y. (1994). Stress, arousal, cortisol and secretory Immunoglobulin A in students undergoing assessment. *The British journal of clinical psychology*, Vol.33, pp.575-576

Gabriel, P. & Liimatainen, M.R. (2000). *Mental health in the workplace*. International Labor Organization. 10.11.2011, Available from http://ilo.org

Green, R.G. & Green, M.L. (1987). Relaxation increases salivary Immunoglobulin A. *Psychological Reports*, Vol.61, pp.623-629

Gregory, R.L.; Kim, D.E.; Kindle, J.C.; Hobbs, L.C. & Lloyd, D.R. (1992). Immunoglobulin-degrading enzymes in localized juvenile periodontitis. *Journal of periodontal research*, Vol.27 No.3, pp.176-183

Hansen, A.M.; Garde, A.H. & Persson, R. (2008). Source of biological and methodological variation in salivary cortisol and their impact on measurement among healthy adults: A review. *The Scandinavian Journal of Clinical & Laboratory Investigation*, Vol.68, No.6, pp.448-458

Hellhammer, D.H.; Wüst, S. & Kudielka, B.M. (2009). Salivary cortisol as a biomarker in stress research. *Psychoneuroendocrinology*, Vol.34, No.2, pp.163-171

Hucklebridge, F.; Hussain, T.; Evans, P. & Clow, A. (2005). The diurnal patterns of the adrenal steroids cortisol and dehydroepiandrosterone (DHEA) in relation to awakening; *Psychoneuroendocrinology*, Vol.30, No.1, pp.51-57

Isowa, T.; Ohira, H. &d Murashima, S. (2004). Reactivity of immune, endocrine and cardiovascular parameters to active and passive acute stress. *Biological Psychology*, Vol.65, pp.101-120

Izawa, S.; Sugaya, N.; Shirotsuki, K.; Yamada, K.C.; Ogawa, N.; Ouchi, Y.; Nagano, Y.; Suzuki, K. & Nomura, S. (2008). Salivary Dehydroepiandrosterone secretion in response to acute psychosocial stress and its correlations with biological and psychological changes. *Biological Psychology*, Vol.79, No.3, pp.294-298

Izawa, S.; Sugaya, N.; Ogawa, N.; Nagano, Y.; Nakano, M.; Nakase, E.; Shirotsuki, K.; Yamada, K. C.; Machida, K.; Kodama, M. & Nomura, S. (2007). Episodic stress associated with writing a graduation thesis and free cortisol secretion after awakening. *International Journal of Psychophysiology*, Vol.64, No.2, pp.141-145

Izawa, S.; Shirotsuki, K.; Sugaya, N.; Ogawa, N.; Suzuki, K. & Nomura, S. (2004). The application of saliva to an assessment of stress: procedures for collecting and analyzing saliva and characteristics of salivary substances. *Japanese Journal of Complementary and Alternative Medicine*, Vol.4, No.3, pp.91-101

Jemmott III, J.B.; Borysenko, J.Z.; Borysenko, M.; McClelland, D.C.; Chapman, R.; Meyer, D. & Benson, H. (1983). Academic stress, power motivation, and decrease in secretion rate of salivary secretory Immunoglobulin A. *Lancet*, Vol.321, No.8339, pp.1400-1402

Jemmott III, J.B. & Magloire, K. (1988). Academic stress, social support, and secretory Immunoglobulin A. *Journal of Personality and Social Psychology*, Vol.55, No.5, pp.803-810

Jemmott III, J.B. & McClelland, D.C. (1989). Secretory IgA as a measure of resistance to infectious disease: comments on Stone, Cox, Valdimarsdottir, and Neale. *Behavioral Medicine*, Vol.15, pp.63- 71

Kanamaru, Y.; Kikukawa, A. & Shimamura, K. (2006). Salivary chromogranin-A as a marker of psychological stress during a cognitive test battery in humans. *Stress*,. Vol.9, No.3, pp.127-131

Kim, Y. & Loh, Y.P. (2005). Chromogranin A: a surprising link between granule biogenesis and hypertension. *J Clin Invest*. Vol.115, No.7, pp.1711-1713

Kimura, K.; Isowa, T.; Ohira, H. & Murashima, S. (2005). Temporal variation of acute stress responses in sympathetic nervous and immune systesm. *Biological Psychology*, Vol.70, pp.131-139

Kirschbaum, C.; Pirke, K.M. & Hellhammer, D.H. (1993). The 'Trier Social Stress Test' -a tool for investigating psychobiological stress responses in a laboratory setting. *Neuropsychobiology*. Vol.28, No.1-2, pp.76-81

Kirschbaum, C. & Hellhammer, D.H. (1994). Salivary cortisol in psychoneuroendocrine research: recent developments and applications. *Psychoneuroendocrinology*, Vol.19, No.1, pp.313-333

Knight, W.E. & Rickard, N.S. (2001). Relaxing music prevents stress-induced increase in subjective anxiety, systolic blood Pressure, and heart rate in healthy males and females. *Journal of Music Therapy*,Vol.38, pp.254-272

Martin, R.A. & Dobbin, J.P. (1988). Sense of humor, hassles, and Immunoglobulin A: evidence for a stress-moderating effect of humor. *International journal of psychiatry in medicine*, Vol.18, pp.93-105

Martin, R.B.; Guthrie, C.A. & Pitts, C.G. (1993). Emotional crying, depressed mood, and secretory Immunoglobulin A. *Behavioral Medicine*, Vol.19, No.3, pp.111-114

McNair, M.; Heuchert, P. & Shilony, E. (2003). *Profile of mood states Bibliography 1964-2002*. Multi-Health-Systems Inc, North Tonawanda, NewYork

Michael, A.; Jenaway, A.; Paykel, E.S. & Herbert, J. (2000). Altered salivary Dehydroepiandrosterone levels in major depression in adults. *Biological Psychiatry*, Vol.48, No.10, pp.989-995

Miyakawa, M.; Matsui, T.; Kishikawa, H.; Murayama, R.; Uchiyama, I.; Itoh, T. & Yoshida, T. (2006). Salivary Chromogranin A as a measure of stress response to noise. *Noise Health*. Vol.8, No.32, pp.108-113

Morgan, C.A. 3rd.; Rasmusson, A.; Pietrzak, R.H.; Coric, V. & Southwick, S.M. (2009). Relationships among plasma dehydroepiandrosterone and dehydroepiandrosterone sulfate, cortisol, symptoms of dissociation, and objective performance in humans exposed to underwater navigation stress; *Biological Psychiatry.*, Vol.66, No.4, pp.334-340

Nakane, H. (1999). Salivary Chromogranin A as index of psychosomatic stress response. *R&D Review of Toyota CRDL.*, Vol.34, No.3, pp.17-22

Nomura, S.; Tanaka, H. & Moriyama, T. (2006). Pilot Study of SIgA as a Stress Maker with Repetitive Saliva Collection, *Proceedings of the 5th International Conference of the Cognitive Science*, pp.169-170, Vancouver, Canada, July 26-29, 2006

Nomura, S.; Mizuno, T.; Nozawa, A.; Asano, H. & Ide, H. (2009). Salivary cortisol as a possible physiological biomarker for mild mental workload. *Biofeedback Research*, Vo.36, No.1, pp.23-32

Nomura, S.; Mizuno, T.; Nozawa, A.; Asano, H. & Ide, H. (2010a). Characteristics of Salivary Chromogranin A as a Short-term Mental Stress Biomarker. *Journal of Biomedical Engineering*, Vol.48, No.2, pp.207-212

Nomura, S.; Mizuno, T.; Nozawa, A.; Asano, H. & Ide, H. (2010b). Salivary DHEA as a Possible Stress-biomarker for a Mild Mental Workload. *Transactions of Human Interface Society*, Vol.12, No.3, pp.33-40

Noto, Y.; Sato, T.; Kudo, M.; Kurata, K. & Hirota, K. (2005). The relationship between salivary biomarkers and State-Trait Anxiety Inventory score under mental arithmetic stress: a pilot study. *Anesth Analg.*, Vol.101, pp.1873-1876

Ockenfels, M.C.; Porter, L.; Smyth, J.; Kirschbaum, C.; Hellhammer, D.H. & Stone, A.A. (1995). Effect of chronic stress associated with unemployment on salivary cortisol: overall cortisol levels, diurnal rhythm, and acute stress reactivity. *Psychosomatic Medicine*, Vol.57, No.5, pp.460-467

Ohira, H. (2004). Social support and salivary secretory Immunoglobulin A response in women to stress of making a public speech. *Perceptual and Motor Skills*, Vol.98, pp.1241-1250

Ohira, H. (2001). Controllability of aversive stimuli unconsciously determines volume of secretory Immunoglobulin A in saliva. *Japanese Journal of Behavioral Medicine*, Vol.6, pp.16-28

Ohira, H.; Watanabe, Y.; Kobayashi, K. & M. Kawai. (1999). The Type A behavior pattern and immune reactivity to brief stress: change of volume of secretory Immunoglobulin A in saliva. *Perceptual and Motor Skills*, Vol.89, pp.423-430

Okamura, H.; Tsuda, A.; Yajima, J.; Mark, H.; Horiuchi, S.; Toyoshima, N. & Matsuishi, T. (2010). Short Sleeping Time and Psychobiological Responses to Acute Stress. International Journal of Psychophysiology, Vol.78, No.3, pp.209-214

Powell, L.H.; Lovallo, W.R.; Matthews, K.A.; Meyer, P.; Midgley, A.R.; Baum, A.; Stone, A.A.; Underwood, L.; McCann, J.J.; Janikula Herro, K. & Ory, M.G. (2002).

Physiologic markers of chronic stress in premenopausal, middle-aged women. *Psychosomatic Medicine*, Vol.64, No.3, pp.502-509

Pruessner, J.C.; Wolf, O.T.; Hellhammer, D.H.; Buske-Kirschbaum, A.; von Auer. K.; Jobst. S.; Kaspers. F. & Kirschbaum, C. (1997). Free cortisol levels after awakening: a reliable biological marker for the assessment of adrenocortical activity. *Life Sci.* Vol.61, pp.2539-2549

Schoofs, D. & Wolfa, O.T. (2011) Are Salivary Gonadal Steroid Concentrations Influenced by Acute Psychosocial Stress? A Study Using the Trier Social Stress Test (TSST). *International Journal of Psychophysiology*, Vol.80, No.1, pp.36-43

Schulz, P.; Kirschbaum, C.; Prüßner, J. & Hellhammer, D. (1998). Increased free cortisol secretion after awakening in chronically stressed individuals due to work overload. *Stress Med.* Vol.14, No.2, pp.91–97

Shirtcliff, E.; Zahn-Waxler, C.; Klimes-Dougan, B. & Slattery, M. (2007). Salivary dehydroepiandrosterone responsiveness to social challenge in adolescents with internalizing problems. *J Child Psychol Psychiatry.*, Vol.48, No.6, pp. 580-591

Steptoe. A.; Cropley. M.; Griffith. J. & Kirschbaum, C. (2000). Job strain and anger expression predict early morning elevations in salivary cortisol. *Psychosomatic Medicine*, Vol.62, No.2, pp.286-292

Steptoe, A. & Wardle, J. (2005). Positive affect and biological function in everyday life. *Nuerobiology of Aging*, Vol.26, No.1, pp.108-112

Strahler, J.; Berndt, C.; Kirschbaum, C. & Rohleder, N. (2010). Aging Diurnal Rhythms and Chronic Stress: Distinct Alteration of Diurnal Rhythmicity of Salivary α-amylase and Cortisol. *Biological Psychology*, Vol.84, No.2, pp.248-256

Stone, A.A.; Neale, J.M.; Cox, D.S.; Napoli, A.; Valdimarsdottir, H. & Kennedy-Moore, E. (1994). Daily events are associated with a secretory immune response to an oral antigen in men. *Health Psychology*, Vol.13, No.5, pp.440-446

Sugaya, N.; Izawa, S.; Ouchi, Y.; Shirotsuki,K.; Yamada, K.C.; Ogawa, N.; Nagano, Y. & Nomura, S. (2007). Adrenal and Autonomic Responses to Psychosocial Stress in Individuals with Irritable Bowel Syndrome. *Japanese Journal of Psychosomatic Medicine*, Vol.47, No.12, pp.1013-1022

Toda, M.; Kusakabe, S.; Nagasawa, S.; Kitamura, K. & Morimoto, K. (2007). Effect of laughter on salivary endocrinological stress marker Chromogranin A. *Biomed Res.*, Vol.28, No.2, pp.15-18

Tsujita, S. & Morimoto, K. (1999). Secretory IgA in saliva can be a useful stress maker. *Environmental Health and Preventive Medicine*, Vol.4, pp.1-8

Valdimarsdottir, H.B. & Stone, A.A. (1997). Psychosocial factors and secretory Immunoglobulin A. *Critical Reviews in Oral Biology & Medicine*, Vol.8, No.4, pp.461-474

van Stegeren, A.; Rohleder, N.; Everaerd, W. & Wolf, O.T. (2006). Salivary alpha amylase as marker for adrenergic activity during stress: effect of betablockade. *Psychoneuroendocrinology*, Vol.31, No.1, pp.137-141

Wakida, S.; Tanaka, Y. & Nagai., H. (2004). High throughput screening for stress marker. *Bunseki*, Vol.2004, pp.309-316

Williams, R.B. (1986). *Patterns of reactivity and stress; Handbook of stress, reactivity, and cardiovascular disease*, John Wiley & Sons, Hoboken, New Jersey, USA

Wingernfeld, K.; Schulz, M.; Damkroeger, A.; Philippsen, C.; Rose, M. & Driessen, M. (2010). The Dirunal Course of Salivary Alpha-amylase in Nurses: An Investigation of Potential Confounders and Associations with Stress. *Biological Psychology*, Vol.85, No.1, pp.179-181

Winkler, H. & Fischer-Colbrie, R. (1992). The chromogranins A and B: the first 25 years and future perspectives. *Neuroscience*, Vol.49, No.3, pp.497-528

Wolf, O.T. & Kirschbaum, C. (1999). Actions of Dehydroepiandrosterone and its sulfate in the central nervous system: Effects on cognition and emotion in animals and humans. *Brain Res Rev.*, Vol.30, No.3, pp.264-288

Yamaguchi, M., Kanemori, T., Knemaru, M., Takai, N., Yasufumi, M. & Yoshida, H. (2004). Performance evaluation of salivary amylase activity monitor. *Biosens.Bioelectron.*, Vol.20, pp.491-497

Yamakoshi, T.; Park, S.B.; Jang, W.C.; Kim, K.; Yamakoshi, Y. & Hirose, H. (2009). Relationship between salivary chromogranin-A and stress induced by simulated monotonous driving. *Med Biol Eng Comput.*, Vol.47, pp.449-456.

Yokoyama, K. & Araki, S. (1993). *Nihongo ban POMS tebiki* (the guide of profile of mood states Japanese version, 5th ed.), Kaneko Shobo, Tokyo, Japan

12

8-Nitroguanine, a Potential Biomarker to Evaluate the Risk of Inflammation-Related Carcinogenesis

Ning Ma[1], Mariko Murata[3],
Shiho Ohnishi[2], Raynoo Thanan[2],
Yusuke Hiraku[3] and Shosuke Kawanishi[2]
[1]*Faculty of Health Science,*
Suzuka University of Medical Science, Suzuka, Mie,
[2]*Faculty of Pharmaceutical Sciences,*
Suzuka University of Medical Science, Suzuka, Mie,
[3]*Department of Environmental and Molecular Medicine,*
Mie University Graduate School of Medicine, Tsu, Mie,
Japan

1. Introduction

Recently, chronic inflammation induced by infection has been postulated to be an important risk factor of various cancers (Schetter et al., 2010; Aggarwal & Sung, 2011; Kamp et al., 2011; Rook & Dalgleish, 2011; Trinchieri, 2011). Many malignancies arise from areas of infection and inflammation (Balkwill & Mantovani, 2001; Coussens & Werb, 2002). Epidemiological and experimental studies have provided evidence showing that chronic infection and inflammation contribute to a substantial part of environmental carcinogenesis (Coussens & Werb, 2002; IARC, 2003). It has been estimated that chronic inflammation accounts for approximately 25 % of human cancers (Hussain S. P. & Harris, 2007). International Agency for Research on Cancer (IARC) has estimated that infectious diseases account for approximately 18 % of cancer cases worldwide (IARC, 2003). During inflammation, nitric oxide (NO) and reactive oxygen species (ROS) are generated from inflammatory cells and considered to play the key role in carcinogenes (Hofseth et al., 2003a; Hofseth et al., 2003b; Hussain S. P. et al., 2003; Ohshima et al., 2003). Inducible nitric oxide synthase (iNOS) catalyzes the production of NO particularly during inflammation, leading to generation of various reactive nitrogen species (RNS), such as NOx and peroxynitrite ($ONOO^-$). RNS generated during infection with influenza viruses can mediate the formation of 8-nitroguanine, a nitrative lesion of nucleic acids, via $ONOO^-$ formation (Maeda H. & Akaike, 1998; Akaike et al., 2003). 8-Nitroguanine formed in DNA is chemically unstable, and thus can be spontaneously released, resulting in the formation of an apurinic site (Yermilov et al., 1995a). The apurinic site can form a pair with adenine during DNA synthesis, leading to G:C-to-T:A transversions (Kawanishi & Hiraku, 2006) (Fig. 1). Thus, 8-nitroguanine is a potentially mutagenic DNA lesion, which can participate in initiation and promotion in the infection-related carcinogenesis (Loeb & Preston, 1986; Kawanishi et al., 2006). Our studies have demonstrated that 8-nitroguanine is formed at the sites of carcinogenesis in humans and experimental animals (Ma et al., 2004; Pinlaor et al., 2004b; Ding et al., 2005; Horiike et al., 2005; Ma et al., 2006; Hoki et al., 2007a; Hoki et al., 2007b; Fujita et al., 2008; Ma et al., 2008; Tanaka et al., 2008; Ma et al., 2009; Ma et al., 2010). Moreover, our studies have demonstrated that 8-nitroguanine was formed in Oct3/4-positve stem cells in *S. haematobium*-associated cystitis and cancer tissues. Inflammation by *S. haematobium* infection may increase the number of mutant stem cells, in which iNOS-dependent DNA damage occures via NF-κB activation leading to tumor development (Ma et al., 2011).

We describe the procedures of these experiments including the 8-nitroguanine antibody produce method, and employed this rabbit anti-8-nitroguanine polyclonal antibody to examine the formation and localization of 8-nitroguanine in patients and animals with inflammation related carcinogenesis by the immunohistochemical method in our laboratory. These protocols provide a detailed description of methodologies successfully used to define the pattern of 8-nitroguanine expression in pathological samples. Visualization of nuclear 8-nitroguanine expression aids in assessment of potential sites of nitrative DNA damage within inflammation-related carcinogenesis. On the basis of our results, we propose that 8-nitroguanine is a promising biomarker to evaluate the potential risk of inflammation-mediated carcinogenesis.

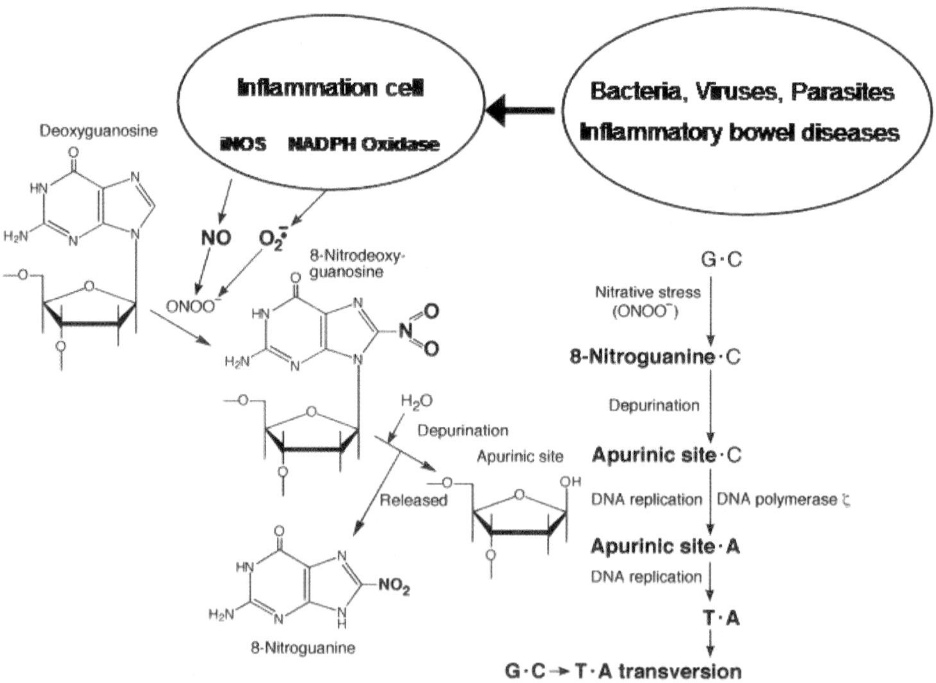

Fig. 1. Formation of 8-nitroguanine during chronic inflammation and proposed mechanism of mutation.

2. Immunohistochemical identification of 8-nitroguanine

2.1 Production of anti-8-nitroguanine antibody

Anti-8-nitroguanine polyclonal antibody was produced by a modified method (Akaike et al., 2003). 8-Nitroguanosine was incubated with sodium metaperiodate for 20 min at room temperature and then conjugated with rabbit serum albumin (RSA) for 1 h followed by incubation with sodium borohydride for 1 h. The conjugate was dialyzed against 150 mM NaCl overnight. 8-Nitroguanine–aldehyde–RSA conjugate mixed with Freund's complete adjuvant was injected in rabbit by intracutaneous administration. After 4 weeks of the immunization, the same antigen was given and the blood was taken two weeks later. We immobilized 8-nitroguanine in a cellulofine GCL-2000m column (Seikagaku Kogyo, Tokyo, Japan), and then purified the antibody by affinity chromatography.

2.2 Specificity of anti-8-nitroguanine antibody

Specificity of the purified antibody was examined by a dot immunobinding assay and absorption test (Pinlaor et al., 2004a). Purified antibody gave a strong immunostaining only on the spot of 8-nitroguanine conjugate (Fig. 2A). The immunoreactivity disappeared only when the antibody was pre-incubated with 8-nitroguanine. In contrast, immunoreactivity with 8-nitroguanine conjugate did not disappear when the antibody was preincubated with 3-nitrotyrosine, guanosine, 8-oxo-7,8-dihydro-2'-deoxyguanosine (8-oxodG), deoxyguanosine, 8-bromoguanosine, and xanthosine (Fig. 2B).

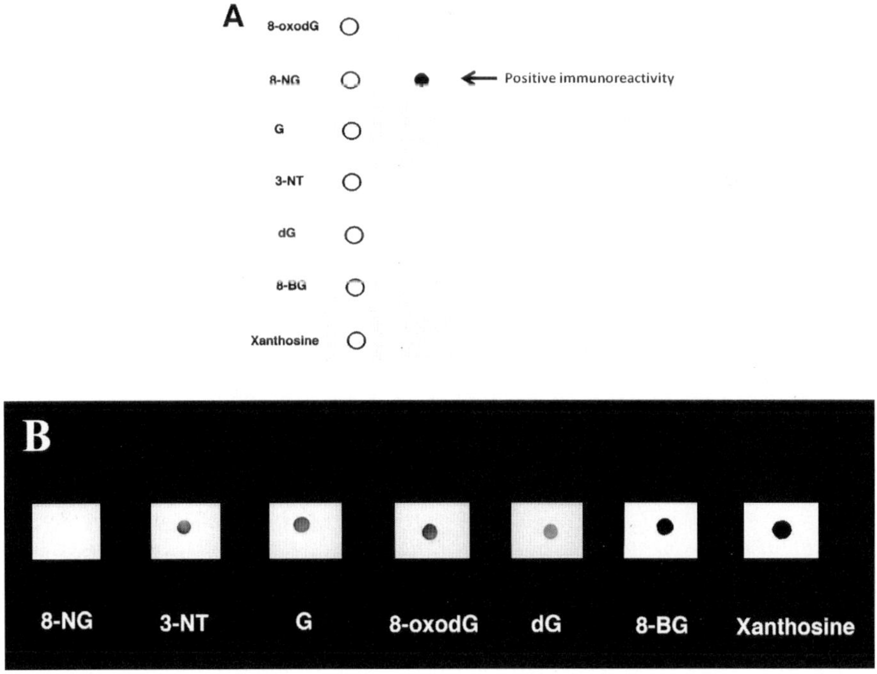

Fig. 2. Dot immunobinding assay and absorption test of anti-8-nitroguanine antibody.

Antigen–antibody reactions were visualized by the peroxidase-anti-peroxidase method. Purified antibody gave a strong immunostaining only on the spot of 8-nitroguanine conjugate (A). 8-Nitroguanine, 3-nitrotyrosine, guanosine, 8-oxodG and deoxyguanosine were incubated with the antibody at the concentration of 0.7 μg/ml, and were applied to 8-nitroguanine conjugate. Immunoreactivity disappeared only when the antibody was pretreated with 8-nitroguanine (B). 8-NG, 8-nitroguanine; 3-NT, 3-nitrotyrosine; G, guanosine; dG, deoxyguanosine and 8-BromoG, 8-bromoguanosine.

2.3 Materials and animals

2.3.1 Donor tissue source

Rat, mouse, hamster, served as the donor tissue source in accordance with the guidelines Proper Care and Use of Laboratory Animals in Research. For the patient's operation samples, written informed consent was obtained from each patient, and the study protocol followed the ethical guidelines of the Declaration of Helsinki.

2.3.2 Chemicals and reagents for immunohistochemistry (IHC) and special equipment

Silanized slides (Dako, Japan)

Dapi-Fluoromount-G™ Mounting Medium (Southern Biotech, Birmingham, USA)

Malinol mounting medium (Muto Pure Chemicals Co. Tokyo,Japan)

3,3′-Diaminobenzidine tetrahydrochloride dehydrate (DAB) (Dojindo, Kumamoto, Japan)

Goat anti-rabbit γ-globulin-HRP (Medical Laboratories, Nagoya, Japan)

Normal goat serum (Medical Laboratories, Nagoya, Japan)

Difco™ Skim milk (Becton, Dickinson and Company, Sparks, USA)

Rabbit anti-8-nitroguanine antibody (Made by Ma N. et al, Suzuka University of Medical Science, Japan)

Anti-8-hydorxy-2′-deoxyguanosine monoclonal antibody (Japan Institute for the Control of Aging, Shizuoka, Japan)

Rabbit peroxidase-anti-peroxidase (PAP) (ab28054, abcam, Tokyo, Japan)

Alexa 488-labeled goat antibody against mouse IgG (Molecular Probes Inc., Eugene, Oregon, USA)

Alexa 594-labeled goat antibody against rabbit IgG (Molecular Probes Inc., Eugene, Oregon, USA)

Other antibodies from abcam or Santa Cruz Biotechnology, Inc. USA.

Tris-HCl (Sigma, St. Louis, MO, USA)

Sodium chloride (Nacalai, Kyoto, Japan)

Sodium pentobarbital (Nacalai, Kyoto, Japan)

Ethanol (Nacalai, Kyoto, Japan)

Xylene (Nacalai, Kyoto, Japan)

Paraformaldehyde (Nacalai, Kyoto, Japan)

Monobasic and dibasic salts of sodium and potassium phosphate (Nacalai, Kyoto, Japan)

Confocal laser scanning microscopy (FV-1000D, Olympus, Tokyo, Japan)

Fluorescent light microscope (BX53, Olympus, Tokyo, Japan)

Sliding microtome (RM2265, Leica, Germany)

2.4 Detailed procedure for IHC

2.4.1 Time required for immunohistochemistry of 8-nitroguanine

Average time for immunohistochemical (IHC) localization of 8-nitroguanine is 2-3 days, not including preparation and mounting of tissues. Albeit, time varies with duration of antibody incubation of second antibody in double fluorescent immunohistochemistry.

2.4.2 Preparation of animal tissues for IHC

1. Animal is weighed and anesthetized by intraperitoneal injection of 50 mg/kg sodium pentobarbital.
2. After the animal has fallen asleep, firmly pinch the foot with a pair of tweezers. If there is no response, then proceed with the surgery.
3. Position the animal on its back. Open the abdominal cavity with a midline incision to the sternum. Make a diagonal cut to each side of the sternum through the rib cage extending to either side of the neck. Care should be taken not to sever any vessels or puncture the heart. The sternum may now be clamped back with hemostatic forceps to give access to the heart.
4. Cut the connective tissue surrounding the diaphragm and make a lateral cut on each side of the animal to allow proper drainage of perfusate.
5. Lift the lungs to expose the descending aorta and occlude the vessel using hemostatic forceps.
6. Make a small incision in the right atrium.
7. Insert an i.v. catheter into the left ventricle. Remove the needle from the catheter. Position so that the tip of the catheter resides within the aortic arch. The optimal size of the catheter for transcardial perfusion is 18 and 22 gauge for rat and mouse, respectively.
8. Connect the catheter to the perfusion apparatus and begin the flow of 0.9% NaCl into the animal. For an adult rat 80 ml 0.9% saline should be infused over 3 min. For a mouse 20 ml saline should be infused over 2 min. Progress of the perfusion may be monitored by assessment of the eyes and gums which should be blanched toward the end of this step.
9. Switch perfusion to 0.1 M phosphate buffer (PB) containing 4% paraformaldehyde. It is common to see turgor and twitching of the upper extremities at the initial flow of fixative into the animal. Perfuse an adult rat, 300 ml of fixative over 10 min should be

used. For a mouse approximately 80 ml over 5 min of fixative should be infused. After completion of the procedure, the arms and tip of the nose should be stiff.

10. Disconnect the rat or mouse from the perfusion apparatus and carefully remove the organ to avoid damage to the tissue. After carefully removing organ from the body, continue fixation of adult tissue at room temperature for 3 h.
11. Following incubation, tissue for IHC should be paraffin-embedded and then sectioned at 5μm thickness onto silanized glass slides. Slides may be stored at ambient temperature in slide cases until use.

2.4.3 Detailed procedure for IHC staining

Step A. Immunofluorescent staining procedure

1. Paraffin sections of human or animal tissues are deparaffinized in xylene for 3 min with frequent shaking in a glass box. Then, the sections are treated in xylene in another glass box for 3 min, followed by the treatment with 100, 90, 80, 70, and 50% (v/v) ethanol for 30–60 sec. To insure complete removal of paraffin, soak sections in PBS for 30 min.
2. To retrieve the antigens, the sections are heated in 5% (w/v) urea for 5 min in a microwave oven, and then left sections on the 5% urea until the temperature reducing to room temperature.
3. Rinse sections in PBS at room temperature, 3 times for 5 min each.
4. Block sections by 30 min incubation in PBS containing 5% (v/v) normal goat serum antibody buffer, or 5% (w/v) skim milk.
5. The sections are incubated with the primary antibody, rabbit polyclonal anti-8-nitroguanine antibody (1–2μg/ml), overnight at room temperature. When double immunofluorescence labeling study is performed, mouse monoclonal antibody is mixed with anti-8-nitroguanine antibody and the sections are treated with this mixture. Note: the final concentration of antibody depends on the specific antibody preparation being used and may need to be empirically determined.
6. The sections are washed with PBS at room temperature, 3 times for 5 min each.
7. The sections are incubated with the secondary antibody, Alexa 594-labeled goat antibody against rabbit IgG (1:400) for 3 h at room temperature. When double immunofluorescence labeling study is performed, Alexa 488-labeled goat antibody against mouse IgG (1:400) is mixed with Alexa 594-labeled goat antibody against rabbit IgG and the sections are treated with this mixture. Note: if primary serum is derived from a source other than rabbit, then the choice of secondary antibody should be adjusted accordingly for specificity.
8. Wash sections with PBS 3 times over 30 min.
9. Pipet Dapi-Fluoromount-G™ Mounting Medium onto the section and then cover with a cover glass. Dry overnight covered at 4°C on a refrigerator.
10. The stained sections are examined under a fluorescent microscope.

Step B. Peroxidase anti-peroxidase immunohistochemical method

1. Deparaffinize as Step A (1)
2. To retrieve the antigens as Step A (2).
3. Rinse sections in PBS at room temperature, 3 times for 5 min each.

4. The sections are incubated with 3% H_2O_2 for 30 min, and rinse sections in PBS for 10 min at room temperature.
5. Block sections by 30 min incubation in PBS containing 5% (v/v) normal goat serum or 5% (w/v) skim milk.
6. The sections are incubated with the primary antibody, rabbit polyclonal anti-8-nitroguanine antibody (1–2 μg/ml), overnight at room temperature.
7. Wash sections in PBS at room temperature, 3 times for 5 min each.
8. The sections are incubated with goat anti-rabbit IgG antibody (1:200) for 3h at room temperature, fellow by wash in PBS, 3 times for 5 min each.
9. The sections are incubated with peroxidase anti-peroxidase complex (PAP, 1:200) for 2h at room temperature, fellow by wash in PBS, 3 times for 5 min each.
10. Equilibrate sections in 0.05 M Tris, pH 7.5 with two washes for 10 min each.
11. Incubate sections in DAB/Tris solution 10 mg 3,3-diaminobenzidine tetrahydrochloride dihydrate in 100 ml 0.05 M Tris, pH 7.4; filter under a hood with general usage filter paper. Incubate sections in developer for up to 15 min. Check sections frequently under a microscope for the degree of development, and reaction product is brown.
12. Terminate reaction by washing sections 3 times for 10 min each in 0.05 M Tris, pH 7.4.
13. Wash sections 2 times for 5 min in distilled water (DW).
14. Counterstain sections with Mayer hematoxylin for 1-1.5 min if necessary.
15. Wash sections 2 times for 5 min in DW.
16. Dehydrate sections in Coplin jars containing graded ethanol 50–80%, 3 min each; twice in 95% ethanol 3 min each; and 3 times in 100% ethanol 3 min each. Tissue is cleared by incubation 3 times for 5 min each in xylene, and coverslipped using Maninol mounting medium.

Step C. Pre-absorption immunostaining

To prepare pre-absorbed 8-nitroguanine antibody place equal amounts of 8-nitroguanine antibody in 1.5 ml Eppendorf microfuge tubes. For the primary antibody to be pre-absorbed pure 8-nitroguanine is added to give a final protein concentration greater than 1 μg/ml. An equal amount of diluents without 8-nitroguanine is added to the control antiserum. Mixtures are incubated for 2 h at room temperature and then diluted to their final working concentration with antibody buffer. Pre-absorption is then continued by incubation overnight at 4°C prior to use. Control and pre-absorbed antibody are used in parallel at StepA or StepB. Proceed as StepA (1) through (10).

3. 8-Nitroguanine accumulation in inflammation-related cancer

3.1 Application of Immunochemistry employing anti-8-nitroguanine antibody

We have performed immunohistochemical analysis for 8-nitroguanine formation in various clinical specimens and animal models of inflammation-related carcinogenesis. We have firstly demonstrated that 8-nitroguanine is formed at the sites of carcinogenesis regardless of etiology, and we have proposed the possibility that 8-nitroguanine is a potential biomarker to evaluate the risk of inflammation-associated carcinogenesis (Kawanishi & Hiraku, 2006; Kawanishi et al., 2006). In clinical specimens, 8-nitroguanine was formed in the gastric grand epithelial cells of patients with gastritis caused by *Helicobacter pylori* (*H. pylori*) infection (Ma et al., 2004), hepatocytes of patients with chronic hepatitis C (Horiike et al., 2005), oral precancerous lesions oral lichen planus (OLP) (Chaiyarit et al., 2005) and oral leukoplakia (Ma et al., 2006), soft tissue sarcoma (Hoki et al., 2007a; Hoki et al., 2007b) and Epstein-Barr virus (EBV)-associated nasopharyngeal carcinoma (NPC) (Ma et al., 2008).

In animal models, 8-nitroguanine was formed in a mouse model of inflammatory bowel disease (IBD) (Ding et al., 2005). 8-Nitroguanine was formed in the bile duct epithelium of the liver of hamsters infected with the liver fluke, *Opisthorchis viverrini*, which causes cancer of intrahepatic bile duct (Pinlaor et al., 2003; Pinlaor et al., 2004a). The treatment with praziquantel, an antiparasitic drug, reduced 8-nitroguanine formation (Pinlaor et al., 2006).

3.1.1 *H.pylori* gastritis and eradication treatment

H. pylori infection, which is the major cause of atrophic gastritis, is a high risk factor for gastric carcinoma (Peek & Blaser, 2002). Lipopolysacharide (LPS), a component of Gram-negative bacteria such as *H. pylori*, is a TLR4 ligand that induces inflammatory responses via NF-κB expression (Maeda S. et al., 2001). NF-κB, which is involved in the regulation of iNOS, had been reported to function as a tumor promoter in inflammation-associated cancer (Surh et al., 2001; Pikarsky et al., 2004). In patients with *H.pyroli*-induced gastritis or gastric ulcers, iNOS is expressed in the infiltrating inflammatory cells (Mannick et al., 1996). ROS and RNS generated by inflammatory cells may contribute to carcinogenesis through the formation of DNA base lesions, such as 8-oxodG, which can lead to a G:C-to-T:A transversion (Shibutani et al., 1991; Kawanishi & Murata, 2006). 8-oxodG, a marker of oxidative DNA damage, is found at a significantly increased level in the gastric epithelium of *H. pylori*-infected patients (Baik et al., 1996; Pignatelli et al., 2001). Therefore, in addition to 8-oxodG formation, the accumulation of 8-nitroguanine may play a key role in the initiation and/or promotion of inflammation-mediated carcinogenesis. To evaluate whether nitrative DNA damage plays a role early in the carcinogenic process triggered by *H. pylori* and the affection of *H. pylori* eradication treatment on 8-nitroguanine formation, we used a double-immunofluorescence staining procedure to compare the formation of both 8-nitroguanine and 8-oxodG in the gastric epithelium of gastritis patients with and without *H. pylori* infection, and before and after *H. pylori* eradication treatment patients.

The formation of 8-nitroguanine and 8-oxodG in gastric epithelium in gastritis patients with *H. pylori* infection is shown in Fig. 3. Notably, intense immunoreactivity of both lesions was observed to co-localize in gastric gland epithelial cells in patients with *H. pylori* infection (Fig. 3, HP(+)). On the other hand, in gastritis patients without *H. pylori* infection, little or no immunoreactivity was observed in gastric gland epithelial cells (Fig. 3, HP(-)). 8-Nitroguanine formation was observed in both the nuclei and the cytoplasm of the labeled epithelial cells, suggesting that it can form in both DNA and RNA. The 8-oxodG immunoreactivity was coincident with that of 8-nitroguanine within the nuclei of gastric gland cells and surface epithelial cells in *H. pylori*-infected patients (Fig. 3, merged labeling in yellow). Regardless of the *H. pylori* infection status, immunoreactivity of 8-nitroguanine and 8-oxodG was observed in inflammatory cells.

Moreover, we found that 8-nitroguanine formation in patients with *H. pylori* infection was dramatically decreased by eradication. After eradication, reduction of 8-nitroguanine and 8-oxodG formation in the epithelia was observed in 58% and 53% patients, respectively (Fig.

4A, B). Despite the complete eradication of *H. pylori*, reduced 8-nitroguanine and 8-oxodG production by infiltrating inflammatory cells were found only in 26% and 36% patients, respectively. Mean 8-nitroguanine and 8-oxodG immunoreactivities in inflammatory cells was not significantly decreased after the eradication treatment.

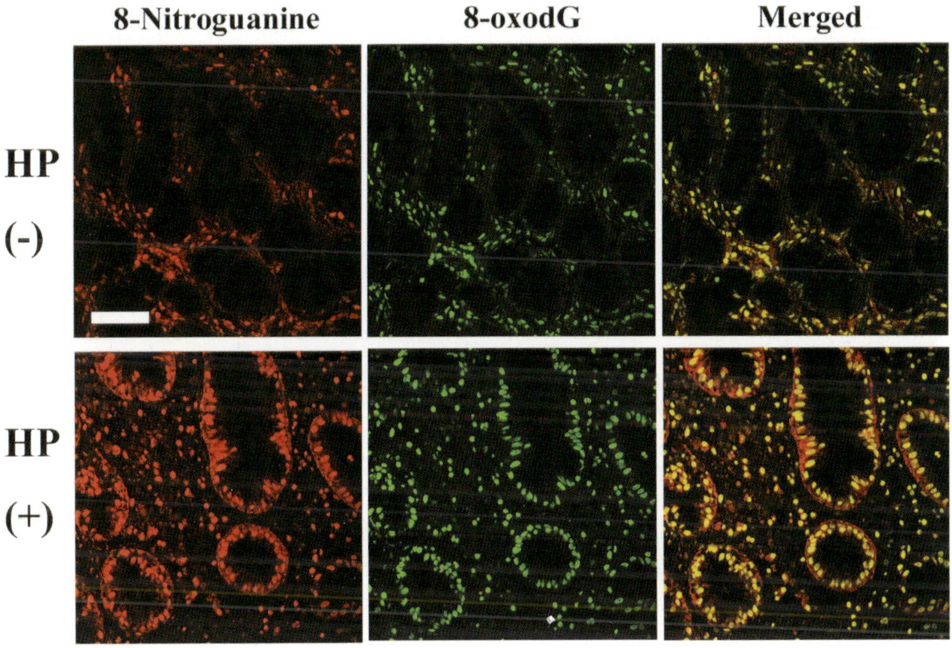

Fig. 3. 8-Nitroguanine and 8-oxodG formation in gastritis patients with and without *H. pylori* infection. Double immunofluorescence staining of paraffin sections shows the localization of 8-oxodG and 8-nitroguanine in the gastric epithelium. In *H. pylori*-infected patients (HP(+)), the immunoreactivity of 8-nitroguanine and 8-oxodG co-localizes primarily in the nuclei of gastric gland epithelial cells and in some inflammatory cells in the corpus (Merged). In chronic gastritis patients without *H. pylori*-infection (HP(-)), the immunoreactivity of 8-nitroguanine and 8-oxodG is observed mainly in the inflammatory cells, while the gastric gland epithelial cells displayed little or no immunoreactivity. Scale bar represents 50 μm.

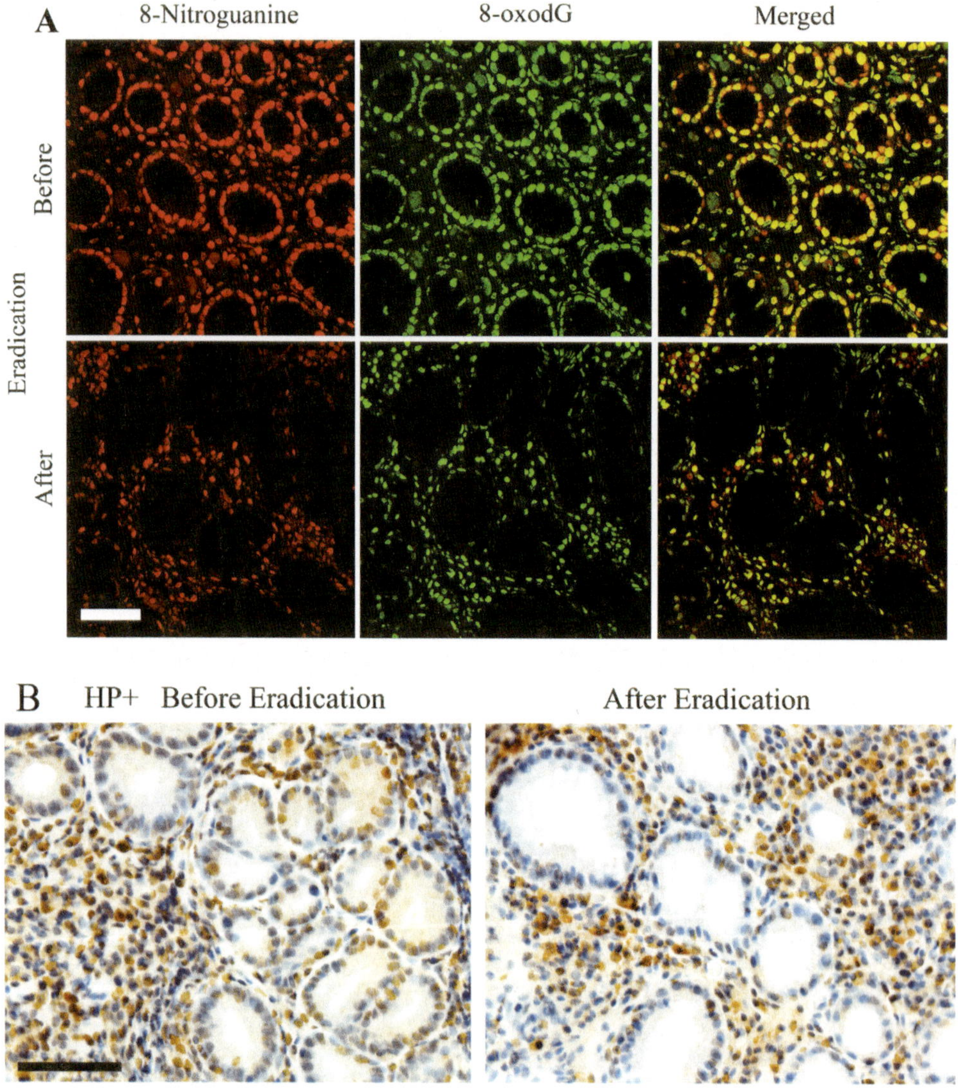

Fig. 4. Detective 8-nitroguanine and 8-oxodG formation in the *H. pylori* eradication patients by double immunofluorescent method (A) and peroxidase anti-peroxidase immunohistochemical method (B). Positive immunoreactivity for 8-nitroguanine was predominantly localized in the nuclei and cytosol of foveolar cells, neutrophils and lymphocytes. The immunoreactivity of 8-nitroguanine and 8-oxodG on the nuclei of foveolar cells was greater reduced after successful *H. pylori* eradication. Conversely, reduced 8-nitroguanine and 8-oxodG formation in infiltrating inflammatory cells did not significantly decrease after the treatment. Scale bar represents 50 μm.

The mechanisms by which *H. pylori* infection causes gastric cancer have been investigated. LPS, a component of Gram-negative bacteria, including *H. pylori*, is a ligand of TLR4. TLR4 is involved in activation of the transcription factor NF-κB (Maeda H. & Akaike, 1998), which mediates expression of iNOS and various inflammatory cytokines. Alternatively, the Cag-positive *H.pylori* strain induces an intense inflammatory response, including interleukin-8 (IL-8) production by epithelial cells and subsequent production of tumor necrosis factor (TNF-α) by inflammatory cells (Peek & Blaser, 2002). The host immune response to *H. pylori* mediated by cytokines, resulting in iNOS expression, may lead to an increase in the accumulation of 8-nitroguanine and 8-oxodG in gastric epithelium.

3.1.2 Leukoplakia, oral lichen planus and oral cancer

More than 300,000 new cases are being diagnosed with oral squamous cell carcinoma annually in the world (Sudbo & Reith, 2005). Oral leukoplakia is a precancerous lesion characterized by white plaque and hyperkeratosis (Neville & Day, 2002; Reibel, 2003). Five to 15% of leukoplakia is histologically classified as dysplasia (Suarez et al., 1998; Sudbo & Reith, 2005). The presence of epithelial dysplasia may be important in predicting malignant development. A substantial part of dysplasia is reported to develop into oral carcinoma (Lumerman et al., 1995; Sudbo & Reith, 2005). Oral lichen planus (OLP) is a chronic inflammatory mucosal disease (Scully et al., 1998). Several pathological features indicate that OLP is an immunologically mediated inflammatory response, including an intense, band-like infiltrate of predominantly T-lymphocytes subjacent to epithelium. Basal epithelial cells are the target for immune destruction by cytotoxic T-lymphocytes (Tyldesley & Appleton, 1973; Dekker et al., 1997). The most important complication of OLP is development of oral squamous cell carcinoma (OSCC) (Rajentheran et al., 1999; Mignogna et al., 2004).

Antioxidants have induced regression of precancerous oral lesions including leukoplakia (Enwonwu & Meeks, 1995), suggesting that ROS are involved in the pathogenesis of precancerous lesions. ROS are considered to participate in carcinogenesis by forming oxidative DNA lesions, such as 8-oxodG (Kawanishi et al., 2001; Kawanishi et al., 2002).

A chronic inflammatory infiltration was generally present in oral tissues of leukoplakia patients (Rodriguez-Perez & Banoczy, 1982). Expression of COX-2, an inflammatory mediator, was increased in oral mucosa with various lesions of leukoplakia, including hyperplasia and dysplasia (Renkonen et al., 2002; Altorki et al., 2004). These reports implicate that inflammation may mediate the development of oral cancer from leukoplakia. Therefore, we examined whether nitrative stress contributes to the development of oral carcinogenesis from leukoplakia through DNA damage.

We demonstrated that accumulation of 8-nitroguanine and 8-oxodG was observed in oral epithelium of biopsy specimens from patients with OLP and OSCC, whereas no immunoreactivity was observed in normal oral mucosa (Chaiyarit et al., 2005). 8-Nitroguanine and 8-oxodG were also observed in oral epithelium of patients with leukoplakia (Ma et al., 2006). Co-localization of 8-nitroguanine and iNOS was found in oral epithelium of patients with OLP, OSCC and leukoplakia. Immunoreactivity of 3-nitrotyrosine, which is formed by protein tyrosine nitration and considered to be a biochemical marker for inflammation, was also observed in oral epithelial cells. Accumulation of p53 was observed in oral epithelium in OLP and leukoplakia, and more prominent expression of this protein was observed in OSCC patients. Our findings demonstrate that iNOS-dependent DNA damage may lead to p53 accumulation not only in OLP and leukoplakia, but also in OSCC. It is concluded that the formation of 8-nitroguanine and 8-oxodG may contribute to the development of oral cancer from OLP and leukoplakia.

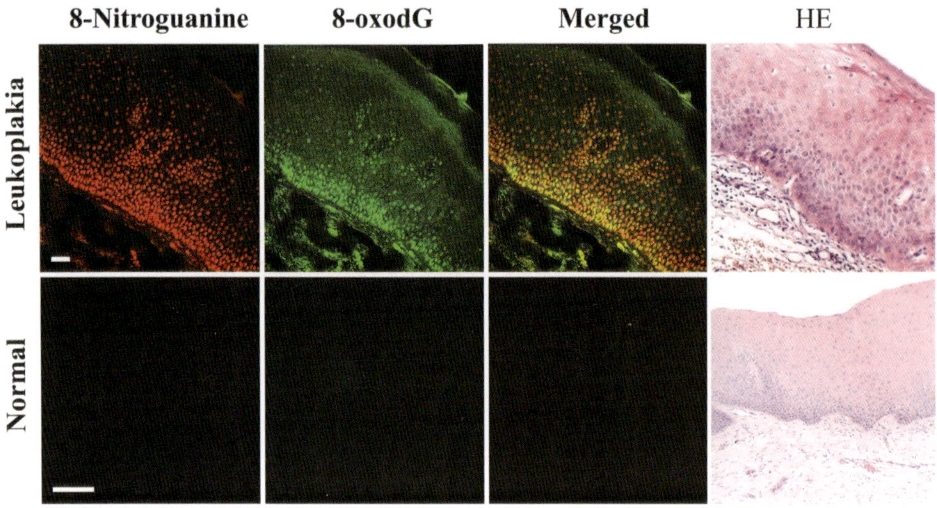

Fig. 5. Localization of 8-nitroguanine and 8-oxodG and histopathological changes in oral tissues of leukoplakia patients. Paraffin sections were immunostained with anti-8-nitroguanine antibody and anti-8-oxodG antibody using double immunofluorescence technique as described in immunofluorescent staining procedure procedures. Strong 8-nitroguanine and 8-oxodG immunoreactivities are observed in the nucleus of the same epithelial cells in supra-basal and basal layers and epithelial-connective tissue interface area of leukoplakia patients. The distribution of 8-nitroguanine- and 8-oxodG-positive cells is similar to that of dysplastic epithelial cells. Little or no immunoreactivity of 8-nitroguanine and 8-oxodG was observed in normal mucosa. Scale bar represents 50 μm.

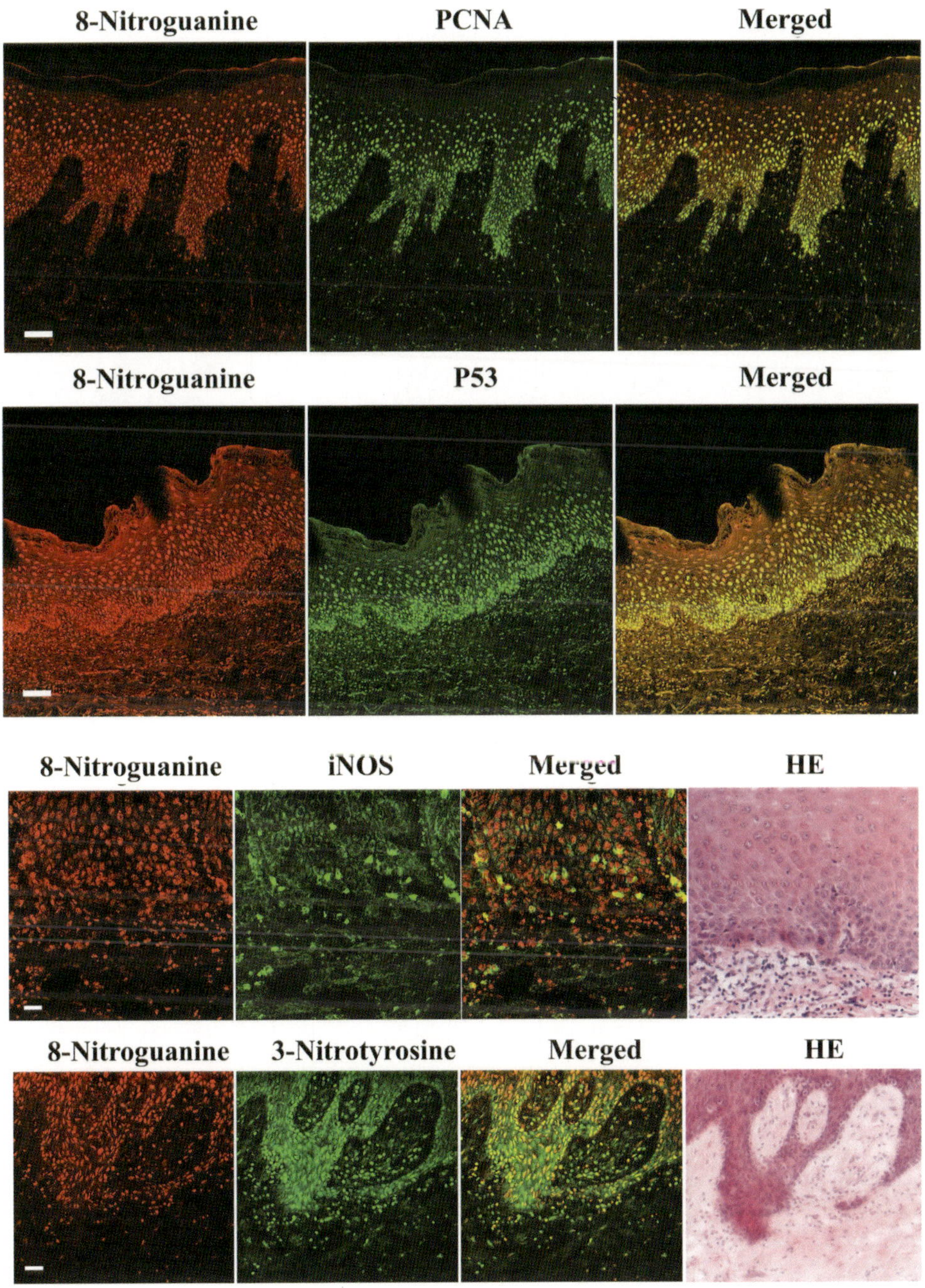

Fig. 6. Localization of 8-nitroguanine, PCNA, p53, iNOS and 3-nitrotyrosine in oral tissues of leukoplakia patients. Paraffin sections were immunostained with anti-8-nitroguanine

antibody and anti-PCNA or anti-3-nitrotyrosine or anti-iNOS, p53 antibody using double immunofluorescence technique. 8-Nitroguanine formation is observed mainly in the nucleus of oral epithelial cells. Strong expression of PCNA and p53 was observed in the nucleus of 8-nitroguanine-positive cells in the basal layer. iNOS expression is strongly observed in inflammatory cells and weakly in the cytoplasm of epithelial cells. Moreover, strong 8-nitroguanine and 3-nitrotyrosine immunoreactivities are observed in the nucleus of the same epithelial cells. Scale bar represents 50 μm.

3.1.3 Epstein-Barr virus and nasopharyngeal carcinoma

NPC is a human epithelial tumor with a high prevalence in the southern Chinese population. In southern China, the incidence rate is about 25–50 per 100,000 person-year and 100-fold higher than that in the Western world. In contrast to other head cancer and epithelial malignancy in general, a unique feature of NPC is its strong association with Epstein-Barr virus (EBV) (McDermott et al., 2001). Various transcription factors are known to participate in iNOS expression including signal transducers and activators of transcription (STATs), such as STAT1α and STAT3 (Tedeschi et al., 2003; Lo et al., 2005). Epidermal growth factor receptor (EGFR) physically interacts with STAT3 in the nucleus, leading to transcriptional activation of iNOS (Lo et al., 2005). STAT3 is repeatedly activated through phosphorylation via the expression of latent membrane protein 1 (LMP1) as well as EGFR (Chen et al., 2003; Tao et al., 2005), and interleukin-6 (IL-6) is required for LMP1-mediated STAT3 activation (Chen et al., 2003). In addition, LMP1-mediated iNOS expression was reported in EBV-infected epithelium cell lines, which play a role in colonization independent of anchorage and tumorigenicity in nude mice (Yu et al., 2002). We performed double immunofluorescent staining method to examine the formation of DNA lesions, 8-nitroguanine and 8-oxodG in surgical and biopsy specimens of nasopharyngeal tissues from NPC patients and chronic nasopharyngitis patients. We also examined the expression of iNOS, STAT3, EGFR and IL-6 in these specimens to examine contribution of these molecules to iNOS expression for 8-nitroguanine formation.

Using biopsy and surgical specimens of nasopharyngeal tissues from NPC patients in southern China, we performed double immunofluorescent staining to examine the formation of 8-nitroguanine and 8-oxodG (Ma et al., 2008; Huang et al., 2011). Intensive immunoreactivity of iNOS was detected in the cytoplasm of 8-nitroguanine-positive cancer cells. DNA lesions and iNOS expression were also observed in epithelial cells of EBV-positive patients with chronic nasopharyngitis but weaker than those in NPC patients (Fig. 7.). No or few DNA lesions were observed in EBV-negative subjects. EGFR and phosphorylated STAT3 were strongly expressed in cancer cells of NPC patients, suggesting that the STAT3-dependent mechanism is important to the carcinogenesis (Ma et al., 2008). IL-6 was expressed mainly in inflammatory cells of nasopharyngeal tissues of EBV-infected patients. We also found that serum levels of 8-oxodG were significantly higher in NPC patients than control subjects (Huang et al., 2011). Collectively, these findings indicate that the nuclear accumulation of EGFR and activation of STAT3 by IL-6 play a key role in iNOS expression and resultant DNA damage, leading to EBV-related NPC.

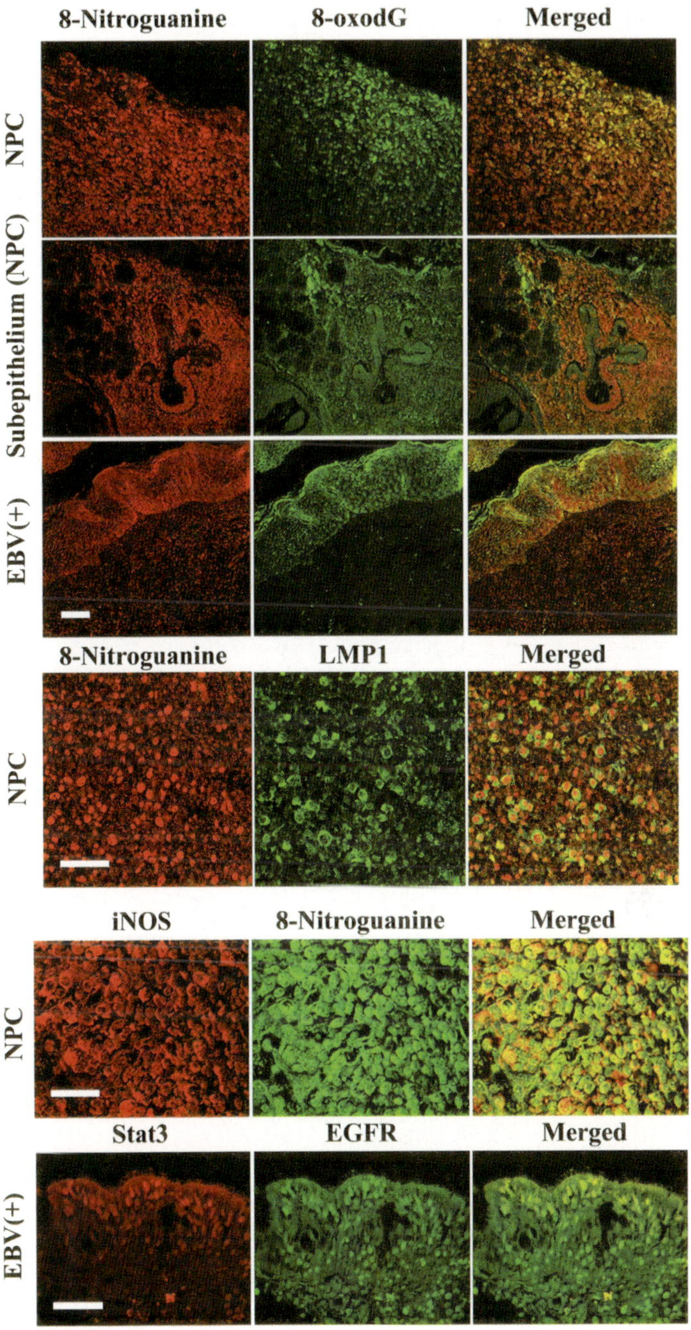

Fig. 7. Formation of 8-nitroguanine and 8-oxodG and expression of LMP, iNOS, STAT3 and EGFR in the nasopharyngeal tissues of NPC and chronic nasopharyngitis patients.

8-Nitroguanine and 8-oxodG are co-localized in cancer cells. These DNA lesions are formed mainly in the nucleus and weakly in the cytoplasm. The formation of these DNA lesions was also observed in inflammatory cells in stroma in NPC patients and the epithelium in patients with chronic nasopharyngitis. Immunoreactivity of LMP1 is clearly observed along cell membrane and the cytoplasm of cancer cells. iNOS and 8-nitroguanine are colocalized in cancer cells of NPC patients. Expression of EGFR and STAT3 are colocalized in nasopharyngeal epithelical cells of EBV-positive chronic nasopharyngitis patients. Scale bar represents 50 μm.

3.1.4 Inflammatory bowel diseases and colon cancer

Ulcerative colitis and Crohn's disease are well known as chronic inflammatory diseases in the lower bowel, and share many clinical and pathological characteristics. These diseases are referred to as inflammatory bowel disease (IBD), which leads to long-term impairment of intestinal structure and function (Podolsky, 2002). A large number of immunological abnormalities have been noted in patients with IBD (Bouma & Strober, 2003). It is well established that an increased cancer risk occurs in tissues undergoing chronic inflammation. Epidemiological studies have suggested that the incidence of colorectal cancer in IBD is greater than the expected incidence in the general population (Ekbom et al., 1990; Langholz et al., 1992; Choi & Zelig, 1994; Pikarsky et al., 2004). The histological and molecular signatures suggest an inflammation-driven carcinogenesis process in IBD patients. To evaluate whether nitrative DNA damage plays a role in the carcinogenic process triggered by IBD, we prepared a mouse model of IBD induced by transfer of $CD45RB^{high}CD4^{+}$ T cells lacking regulatory T cells to SCID mice (Powrie et al., 1993; Philippe et al., 2003), since mouse models of IBD can result from either excessive effector T cell function or deficient regulatory T cell function (Bouma & Strober, 2003). We performed a double immunofluorescent staining procedure to examine the formation of 8-nitroguanine and 8-oxodG in the colon tissues. We also examined the expression of iNOS by immunohistochemistry. To evaluate the proliferating activity of colonic epithelial cells and their response to DNA damage, we also examined the expression of p53 in the colon tissues.

In the$CD45RB^{high}CD4^{+}$Tcell-transferred mouse, significant 8-nitroguanine accumulation was induced in the nuclei and the cytoplasm of epithelial cells, and was also present in infiltrated cells supposed to be inflammatory cells in lamina propria. 8-Nitroguanine was formed in most of 8-oxodG-immunoreactive nuclei of epithelial cells and infiltrated cells (Fig. 8). When the sections were pretreated with RNase, 8-nitroguanine immunoreactivity was more clearly observed in the nuclei of epithelial cells (Ding et al., 2005). This result suggests that 8-nitroguanine was formed in genomic DNA. iNOS was expressed in the cytoplasm of epithelial cells and infiltrated cells in the lamina propria of the IBD mouse model (Fig. 8). iNOS was expressed mainly in 8-nitroguanine immunoreactive epithelial cells (Fig. 8). However, no or little 8-nitroguanine, 8-oxodG and iNOS were observed in non-treated control mice. In the IBD mouse model, significant p53 was accumulated in the nuclei of regenerated epithelial cells. P53 was also expressed in some infiltrated cells. P53 expression was overlapped with 8-nitroguanine (Fig. 8). The mice of IBD model that we used by transfer of $CD45RB^{high}CD4^{+}$ T cells showed the similar results of histopathological analysis and immunohistochemical staining. No or little expression of p53 was observed in non-treated control mice.

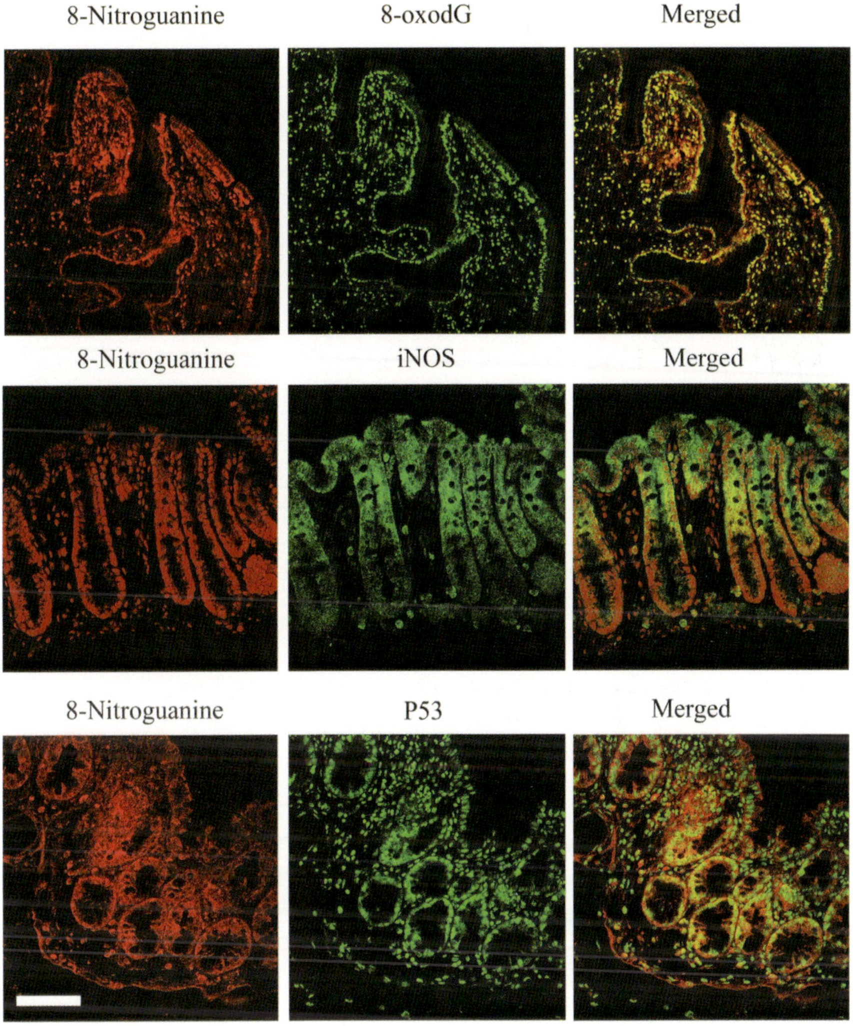

Fig. 8. Formation of 8-nitroguanine, 8-oxodG, iNOS and p53 in the mouse model of inflammatory bowel disease. 8-Nitroguanine is accumulated in the nuclei and the cytoplasm of epithelial cells. 8-Nitroguanine is also present in infiltrated cells. 8-oxodG formation is observed in the nuclei of epithelial cells and the infiltrated cells in lamina propria, 8-oxodG and 8-nitroguanine co-localized in the nuclei of most epithelial cells and infiltrated cells, iNOS is expressed in the cytoplasm of epithelial cells and infiltrated cells in lamina propria, and iNOS and 8-nitroguanine colocalized in the cytoplasm of many epithelial cells and some infiltrated cells. Double immunostaining for 8-nitroguanine and p53, significant p53 expression is observed in the nuclei of regenerated epithelial cells and some infiltrated cells. P53 is also induced in the cytoplasm of many epithelial cells in lower portions of the gland. P53 is expressed in most of 8-nitroguanine-immunoreactive epithelial cells. Scale bar represents 50 μm.

4. Concluding

We have investigated the mechanisms of oxidative and nitrative DNA damage induced by various inflammatory conditions. In relation to inflammation-related carcinogenesis, we examined the formation of 8-nitroguanine and 8-oxodG in human samples and animals. It is noteworthy that DNA damage was specifically induced at sites of carcinogenesis under various inflammatory conditions. In human samples, 8-nitroguanine formation was observed in gastric gland epithelial cells of patients with *H. pylori* infection (Ma et al., 2004) and in hepatocytes of patients with chronic hepatitis C (Horiike et al., 2005). 8-Nitroguanine was also formed in oral epithelium of OLP and OSCC patients (Chaiyarit et al., 2005; Ma et al., 2006). Moreover, in hamsters infected with the liver fluke *Opisthorchis viverrini* causing cholangiocarcinoma, 8-nitroguanine formation was induced in bile duct epithelium (Pinlaor et al., 2004b). 8-Nitroguanine formation was also found in colonic gland epithelial cells of mouse model of IBD (Ding et al., 2005). Therefore, 8-nitroguanine could be used as a potential biomarker to evaluate the risk of inflammation-related carcinogenesis. Recently, 8-nitroguanosine has been reported to be a highly redox-active molecule that strongly stimulates O_2•-generation from NADPH-dependent reductases (Sawa et al., 2003). 8-Nitroguaninemay be a cofactor for redox reaction and cell signaling implicated in diverse physiological and pathological events (Zaki et al., 2005). More importantly, experimental evidence has suggested that 8-nitroguanine is a mutagenic DNA lesion, which preferentially leads to G:C-to-T:A transversions (Yermilov et al., 1995b; Suzuki et al., 2005), in addition to 8-oxodG (Shibutani et al., 1991; Bruner et al., 2000). Indeed, G:C-to-T:A transversions have been observed *in vivo* in the *ras* gene (Bos, 1988) and the *p53* tumor suppressor gene in lung and liver cancer (Takahashi et al., 1989; Prahalad et al., 1999). We also investigated the role of DNA damage in carcinogenesis initiated by *K-ras* mutation, using conditional transgenic mice. Immunohistochemical analysis revealed that mutagenic 8-nitroguanine and 8-oxodG were apparently formed in adenocarcinoma caused by mutated *K-ras*. 8-Nitroguanine was co-localized with iNOS, NF-κB, IKK, MAPK, MEK, and mutated *K-ras*, suggesting that oncogenic *K-ras* causes additional DNA damage via signaling pathway involving these molecules. It is noteworthy that *K-ras* mutation mediates not only cell over-proliferation but also the accumulation of mutagenic DNA lesions, leading to carcinogenesis (Ohnishi et al., 2011). These findings imply that DNA damage mediated by ROS and RNS may participate in carcinogenesis via activation of protooncogenes and inactivation of tumor suppressor genes. In conclusion, oxidative and nitrative DNA damage could be promising biomarkers to evaluate the risk of carcinogenesis induced by a wide variety of chemicals and inflammatory conditions.

5. Acknowledgments and funding

This work was supported by a Grant-in-Aid from the Ministry of Education, Culture, Sports, Science and Technology of Japan and Otsuka Pharmaceutical Co., Ltd. Japan.

6. References

Aggarwal, B. B. and Sung B. (2011). The relationship between inflammation and cancer is analogous to that between fuel and fire. *Oncology (Williston Park)*, Vol.25, No.5 (Apr 30), pp. (414-418), 0890-9091 (Print)

Akaike, T., Okamoto S., Sawa T., Yoshitake J., Tamura F., Ichimori K., Miyazaki K., Sasamoto K. and Maeda H. (2003). 8-Nitroguanosine formation in viral pneumonia and its implication for pathogenesis. *Proc Natl Acad Sci U S A,* Vol.100, No.2 (Jan 21), pp. (685-690), 0027-8424 (Print)

Altorki, N. K., Subbaramaiah K. and Dannenberg A. J. (2004). COX-2 inhibition in upper aerodigestive tract tumors. *Semin Oncol,* Vol.31, No.2 Suppl 7 (Apr), pp. (30-36), 0093-7754 (Print)

Baik, S. C., Youn H. S., Chung M. H., Lee W. K., Cho M. J., Ko G. H., Park C. K., Kasai H. and Rhee K. H. (1996). Increased oxidative DNA damage in Helicobacter pylori-infected human gastric mucosa. *Cancer Res,* Vol.56, No.6 (Mar 15), pp. (1279-1282), 0008-5472 (Print)

Balkwill, F. and Mantovani A. (2001). Inflammation and cancer: back to Virchow? *Lancet,* Vol.357, No.9255 (Feb 17), pp. (539-545).

Bos, J. L. (1988). Ras oncogenes in hematopoietic malignancies. *Hematol Pathol,* Vol.2, No.2 pp. (55-63), 0886-0238 (Print)

Bouma, G. and Strober W. (2003). The immunological and genetic basis of inflammatory bowel disease. *Nat Rev Immunol,* Vol.3, No.7 (Jul), pp. (521-533), 1474-1733 (Print)

Bruner, S. D., Norman D. P. and Verdine G. L. (2000). Structural basis for recognition and repair of the endogenous mutagen 8-oxoguanine in DNA. *Nature,* Vol.403, No.6772 (Feb 24), pp. (859-866), 0028-0836 (Print)

Chaiyarit, P., Ma N., Hiraku Y., Pinlaor S., Yongvanit P., Jintakanon D., Murata M., Oikawa S. and Kawanishi S. (2005). Nitrative and oxidative DNA damage in oral lichen planus in relation to human oral carcinogenesis. *Cancer Sci,* Vol.96, No.9 (Sep), pp. (553-559), 1347-9032 (Print)

Chen, H., Hutt-Fletcher L., Cao L. and Hayward S. D. (2003). A positive autoregulatory loop of LMP1 expression and STAT activation in epithelial cells latently infected with Epstein-Barr virus. *J Virol,* Vol.77, No.7 (Apr), pp. (4139-4148), 0022-538X (Print)

Choi, P. M. and Zelig M. P. (1994). Similarity of colorectal cancer in Crohn's disease and ulcerative colitis: implications for carcinogenesis and prevention. *Gut,* Vol.35, No.7 (Jul), pp. (950-954), 0017-5749 (Print)

Coussens, L. M. and Werb Z. (2002). Inflammation and cancer. *Nature,* Vol.420, No.6917 (Dec 19-26), pp. (860-867).

Dekker, N. P., Lozada-Nur F., Lagenaur L. A., MacPhail L. A., Bloom C. Y. and Regezi J. A. (1997). Apoptosis-associated markers in oral lichen planus. *J Oral Pathol Med,* Vol.26, No.4 (Apr), pp. (170-175), 0904-2512 (Print)

Ding, X., Hiraku Y., Ma N., Kato T., Saito K., Nagahama M., Semba R., Kuribayashi K. and Kawanishi S. (2005). Inducible nitric oxide synthase-dependent DNA damage in mouse model of inflammatory bowel disease. *Cancer Sci,* Vol.96, No.3 (Mar), pp. (157-163), 1347-9032 (Print)

Ekbom, A., Helmick C., Zack M. and Adami H. O. (1990). Increased risk of large-bowel cancer in Crohn's disease with colonic involvement. *Lancet,* Vol.336, No.8711 (Aug 11), pp. (357-359), 0140-6736 (Print)

Enwonwu, C. O. and Meeks V. I. (1995). Bionutrition and oral cancer in humans. *Crit Rev Oral Biol Med,* Vol.6, No.1 pp. (5-17), 1045-4411 (Print)

Fujita, N., Sugimoto R., Ma N., Tanaka H., Iwasa M., Kobayashi Y., Kawanishi S., Watanabe S., Kaito M. and Takei Y. (2008). Comparison of hepatic oxidative DNA damage in patients with chronic hepatitis B and C. *J Viral Hepat,* Vol.15, No.7 (Jul), pp. (498-507), 1365-2893 (Electronic)

Hofseth, L. J., Khan M. A., Ambrose M., Nikolayeva O., Xu-Welliver M., Kartalou M., Hussain S. P., Roth R. B., Zhou X., Mechanic L. E., Zurer I., Rotter V., Samson L. D. and Harris C. C. (2003a). The adaptive imbalance in base excision-repair enzymes generates microsatellite instability in chronic inflammation. *J Clin Invest,* Vol.112, No.12 (Dec), pp. (1887-1894), 0021-9738 (Print)

Hofseth, L. J., Saito S., Hussain S. P., Espey M. G., Miranda K. M., Araki Y., Jhappan C., Higashimoto Y., He P., Linke S. P., Quezado M. M., Zurer I., Rotter V., Wink D. A., Appella E. and Harris C. C. (2003b). Nitric oxide-induced cellular stress and p53 activation in chronic inflammation. *Proc Natl Acad Sci U S A,* Vol.100, No.1 (Jan 7), pp. (143-148), 0027-8424 (Print)

Hoki, Y., Hiraku Y., Ma N., Murata M., Matsumine A., Nagahama M., Shintani K., Uchida A. and Kawanishi S. (2007a). iNOS-dependent DNA damage in patients with malignant fibrous histiocytoma in relation to prognosis. *Cancer Sci,* Vol.98, No.2 (Feb), pp. (163-168), 1347-9032 (Print)

Hoki, Y., Murata M., Hiraku Y., Ma N., Matsumine A., Uchida A. and Kawanishi S. (2007b). 8-Nitroguanine as a potential biomarker for progression of malignant fibrous histiocytoma, a model of inflammation-related cancer. *Oncol Rep,* Vol.18, No.5 (Nov), pp. (1165-1169), 1021-335X (Print)

Horiike, S., Kawanishi S., Kaito M., Ma N., Tanaka H., Fujita N., Iwasa M., Kobayashi Y., Hiraku Y., Oikawa S., Murata M., Wang J., Semba R., Watanabe S. and Adachi Y. (2005). Accumulation of 8-nitroguanine in the liver of patients with chronic hepatitis C. *J Hepatol,* Vol.43, No.3 (Sep), pp. (403-410), 0168-8278 (Print)

Huang, Y. J., Zhang B. B., Ma N., Murata M., Tang A. Z. and Huang G. W. (2011). Nitrative and oxidative DNA damage as potential survival biomarkers for nasopharyngeal carcinoma. *Med Oncol,* Vol.28, No.1 (Mar), pp. (377-384), 1559-131X (Electronic)

Hussain, S. P. and Harris C. C. (2007). Inflammation and cancer: an ancient link with novel potentials. *Int. J. Cancer,* Vol.121, No.11 (Dec 1), pp. (2373-2380),

Hussain, S. P., Hofseth L. J. and Harris C. C. (2003). Radical causes of cancer. *Nat Rev Cancer,* Vol.3, No.4 (Apr), pp. (276-285), 1474-175X (Print)

Kamp, D. W., Shacter E. and Weitzman S. A. (2011). Chronic inflammation and cancer: the role of the mitochondria. *Oncology (Williston Park),* Vol.25, No.5 (Apr 30), pp. (400-410, 413), 0890-9091 (Print)

Kawanishi, S. and Hiraku Y. (2006). Oxidative and nitrative DNA damage as biomarker for carcinogenesis with special reference to inflammation. *Antioxid Redox Signal,* Vol.8, No.5-6 (May-Jun), pp. (1047-1058), 1523-0864 (Print)

Kawanishi, S., Hiraku Y., Murata M. and Oikawa S. (2002). The role of metals in site-specific DNA damage with reference to carcinogenesis. *Free Radic Biol Med,* Vol.32, No.9 (May 1), pp. (822-832), 0891-5849 (Print)

Kawanishi, S., Hiraku Y. and Oikawa S. (2001). Mechanism of guanine-specific DNA damage by oxidative stress and its role in carcinogenesis and aging. *Mutat Res,* Vol.488, No.1 (Mar), pp. (65-76), 0027-5107 (Print)

Kawanishi, S., Hiraku Y., Pinlaor S. and Ma N. (2006). Oxidative and nitrative DNA damage in animals and patients with inflammatory diseases in relation to inflammation-related carcinogenesis. *Biol Chem,* Vol.387, No.4 (Apr), pp. (365-372), 1431-6730 (Print)

Kawanishi, S. and Murata M. (2006). Mechanism of DNA damage induced by bromate differs from general types of oxidative stress. *Toxicology,* Vol.221, No.2-3 (Apr 17), pp. (172-178), 0300-483X (Print)

Langholz, E., Munkholm P., Davidsen M. and Binder V. (1992). Colorectal cancer risk and mortality in patients with ulcerative colitis. *Gastroenterology,* Vol.103, No.5 (Nov), pp. (1444-1451), 0016-5085 (Print)

Lo, H. W., Hsu S. C., Ali-Seyed M., Gunduz M., Xia W., Wei Y., Bartholomeusz G., Shih J. Y. and Hung M. C. (2005). Nuclear interaction of EGFR and STAT3 in the activation of the iNOS/NO pathway. *Cancer Cell,* Vol.7, No.6 (Jun), pp. (575-589), 1535-6108 (Print)

Loeb, L. A. and Preston B. D. (1986). Mutagenesis by apurinic/apyrimidinic sites. *Annu Rev Genet,* Vol.20, pp. (201-230), 0066-4197 (Print)

Lumerman, H., Freedman P. and Kerpel S. (1995). Oral epithelial dysplasia and the development of invasive squamous cell carcinoma. *Oral Surg Oral Med Oral Pathol Oral Radiol Endod,* Vol.79, No.3 (Mar), pp. (321-329), 1079-2104 (Print)

Ma, N., Adachi Y., Hiraku Y., Horiki N., Horiike S., Imoto I., Pinlaor S., Murata M., Semba R. and Kawanishi S. (2004). Accumulation of 8-nitroguanine in human gastric epithelium induced by Helicobacter pylori infection. *Biochem Biophys Res Commun,* Vol.319, No.2 (Jun 25), pp. (506-510), 0006-291X (Print)

Ma, N., Kawanishi M., Hiraku Y., Murata M., Huang G. W., Huang Y., Luo D. Z., Mo W. G., Fukui Y. and Kawanishi S. (2008). Reactive nitrogen species-dependent DNA damage in EBV-associated nasopharyngeal carcinoma: the relation to STAT3 activation and EGFR expression. *Int J Cancer,* Vol.122, No.11 (Jun 1), pp. (2517-2525), 1097-0215 (Electronic)

Ma, N., Sasaki T., Sakata-Haga H., Ohta K., Gao M., Kawanishi S. and Fukui Y. (2009). Protective effect of taurine against nitrosative stress in the stomach of rat with water immersion restraint stress. *Adv Exp Med Biol,* Vol.643, pp. (273-283), 0065-2598 (Print)

Ma, N., Sasoh M., Kawanishi S., Sugiura H. and Piao F. (2010). Protection effect of taurine on nitrosative stress in the mice brain with chronic exposure to arsenic. *J Biomed Sci,* Vol.17 Suppl 1, pp. (S7), 1423-0127 (Electronic)

Ma, N., Tagawa T., Hiraku Y., Murata M., Ding X. and Kawanishi S. (2006). 8-Nitroguanine formation in oral leukoplakia, a premalignant lesion. *Nitric Oxide,* Vol.14, No.2 (Mar), pp. (137-143), 1089-8603 (Print)

Ma, N., Thanan R., Kobayashi H., Hammam O., Wishahi M., Leithy T. E., Hiraku Y., Amro E. K., Oikawa S., Ohnishi S., Murata M. and Kawanishi S. (2011). Nitrative DNA damage and Oct3/4 expression in urinary bladder cancer with Schistosomahaematobium infection. *Biochem Biophys Res Commun,* (Sep 17), pp. 1090-2104 (Electronic)

Maeda, H. and Akaike T. (1998). Nitric oxide and oxygen radicals in infection, inflammation, and cancer. *Biochemistry (Mosc),* Vol.63, No.7 (Jul), pp. (854-865), 0006-2979 (Print)

Maeda, S., Akanuma M., Mitsuno Y., Hirata Y., Ogura K., Yoshida H., Shiratori Y. and Omata M. (2001). Distinct mechanism of Helicobacter pylori-mediated NF-kappa B activation between gastric cancer cells and monocytic cells. *J Biol Chem,* Vol.276, No.48 (Nov 30), pp. (44856-44864), 0021-9258 (Print)

Mannick, E. E., Bravo L. E., Zarama G., Realpe J. L., Zhang X. J., Ruiz B., Fontham E. T., Mera R., Miller M. J. and Correa P. (1996). Inducible nitric oxide synthase, nitrotyrosine, and apoptosis in Helicobacter pylori gastritis: effect of antibiotics and antioxidants. *Cancer Res,* Vol.56, No.14 (Jul 15), pp. (3238-3243), 0008-5472 (Print)

McDermott, A. L., Dutt S. N. and Watkinson J. C. (2001). The aetiology of nasopharyngeal carcinoma. *Clin Otolaryngol Allied Sci,* Vol.26, No.2 (Apr), pp. (82-92), 0307-7772 (Print)

Mignogna, M. D., Fedele S., Lo Russo L., Lo Muzio L. and Bucci E. (2004). Immune activation and chronic inflammation as the cause of malignancy in oral lichen planus: is there any evidence ? *Oral Oncol,* Vol.40, No.2 (Feb), pp. (120-130), 1368-8375 (Print)

Neville, B. W. and Day T. A. (2002). Oral cancer and precancerous lesions. *CA Cancer J Clin,* Vol.52, No.4 (Jul-Aug), pp. (195-215), 0007-9235 (Print)

Ohnishi, S., Saito H., Suzuki N., Ma N., Hiraku Y., Murata M. and Kawanishi S. (2011). Nitrative and oxidative DNA damage caused by K-ras mutation in mice. *Biochem Biophys Res Commun,* Vol.413, No.2 (Sep 23), pp. (236-240), 1090-2104 (Electronic)

Ohshima, H., Tatemichi M. and Sawa T. (2003). Chemical basis of inflammation-induced carcinogenesis. *Arch Biochem Biophys,* Vol.417, No.1 (Sep 1), pp. (3-11), 0003-9861 (Print) 0003-9861 (Linking)

Peek, R. M., Jr. and Blaser M. J. (2002). Helicobacter pylori and gastrointestinal tract adenocarcinomas. *Nat Rev Cancer,* Vol.2, No.1 (Jan), pp. (28-37), 1474-175X (Print)

Philippe, D., Dubuquoy L., Groux H., Brun V., Chuoi-Mariot M. T., Gaveriaux-Ruff C., Colombel J. F., Kieffer B. L. and Desreumaux P. (2003). Anti-inflammatory properties of the mu opioid receptor support its use in the treatment of colon inflammation. *J Clin Invest,* Vol.111, No.9 (May), pp. (1329-1338), 0021-9738 (Print)

Pignatelli, B., Bancel B., Plummer M., Toyokuni S., Patricot L. M. and Ohshima H. (2001). Helicobacter pylori eradication attenuates oxidative stress in human gastric mucosa. *Am J Gastroenterol,* Vol.96, No.6 (Jun), pp. (1758-1766), 0002-9270 (Print)

Pikarsky, E., Porat R. M., Stein I., Abramovitch R., Amit S., Kasem S., Gutkovich-Pyest E., Urieli-Shoval S., Galun E. and Ben-Neriah Y. (2004). NF-kappaB functions as a tumour promoter in inflammation-associated cancer. *Nature,* Vol.431, No.7007 (Sep 23), pp. (461-466), 1476-4687 (Electronic)

Pinlaor, S., Hiraku Y., Ma N., Yongvanit P., Semba R., Oikawa S., Murata M., Sripa B., Sithithaworn P. and Kawanishi S. (2004a). Mechanism of NO-mediated oxidative and nitrative DNA damage in hamsters infected with Opisthorchis viverrini: a model of inflammation-mediated carcinogenesis. *Nitric Oxide,* Vol.11, No.2 (Sep), pp. (175-183), 1089-8603 (Print)

Pinlaor, S., Hiraku Y., Yongvanit P., Tada-Oikawa S., Ma N., Pinlaor P., Sithithaworn P., Sripa B., Murata M., Oikawa S. and Kawanishi S. (2006). iNOS-dependent DNA damage via NF-kappaB expression in hamsters infected with Opisthorchis viverrini and its suppression by the antihelminthic drug praziquantel. *Int J Cancer,* Vol.119, No.5 (Sep 1), pp. (1067-1072), 0020-7136 (Print)

Pinlaor, S., Ma N., Hiraku Y., Yongvanit P., Semba R., Oikawa S., Murata M., Sripa B., Sithithaworn P. and Kawanishi S. (2004b). Repeated infection with Opisthorchis viverrini induces accumulation of 8-nitroguanine and 8-oxo-7,8-dihydro-2'-deoxyguanine in the bile duct of hamsters via inducible nitric oxide synthase. *Carcinogenesis,* Vol.25, No.8 (Aug), pp. (1535-1542), 0143-3334 (Print)

Pinlaor, S., Yongvanit P., Hiraku Y., Ma N., Semba R., Oikawa S., Murata M., Sripa B., Sithithaworn P. and Kawanishi S. (2003). 8-Nitroguanine formation in the liver of

hamsters infected with Opisthorchis viverrini. *Biochem Biophys Res Commun,* Vol.309, No.3 (Sep 26), pp. (567-571), 0006-291X (Print)
Podolsky, D. K. (2002). Inflammatory bowel disease. *N Engl J Med,* Vol.347, No.6 (Aug 8), pp. (417-429), 1533-4406 (Electronic)
Powrie, F., Leach M. W., Mauze S., Caddle L. B. and Coffman R. L. (1993). Phenotypically distinct subsets of CD4+ T cells induce or protect from chronic intestinal inflammation in C. B-17 scid mice. *Int Immunol,* Vol.5, No.11 (Nov), pp. (1461-1471), 0953-8178 (Print)
Prahalad, A. K., Manchester D. K., Hsu I. C., Inmon J. and Gallagher J. E. (1999). Human placental microsomal activation and DNA adduction by air pollutants. *Bull Environ Contam Toxicol,* Vol.62, No.1 (Jan), pp. (93-100), 0007-4861 (Print)
Rajentheran, R., McLean N. R., Kelly C. G., Reed M. F. and Nolan A. (1999). Malignant transformation of oral lichen planus. *Eur J Surg Oncol,* Vol.25, No.5 (Oct), pp. (520-523), 0748-7983 (Print)
Reibel, J. (2003). Prognosis of oral pre-malignant lesions: significance of clinical, histopathological, and molecular biological characteristics. *Crit Rev Oral Biol Med,* Vol.14, No.1 pp. (47-62), 1544-1113 (Electronic)
Renkonen, J., Wolff H. and Paavonen T. (2002). Expression of cyclo-oxygenase-2 in human tongue carcinoma and its precursor lesions. *Virchows Arch,* Vol.440, No.6 (Jun), pp. (594-597), 0945-6317 (Print)
Rodriguez-Perez, I. and Banoczy J. (1982). Oral leukoplakia. A histopathological study. *Acta Morphol Acad Sci Hung,* Vol.30, No.3-4 pp. (289-298), 0001-6217 (Print)
Rook, G. A. and Dalgleish A. (2011). Infection, immunoregulation, and cancer. *Immunol Rev,* Vol.240, No.1 (Mar), pp. (141-159), 1600-065X (Electronic)
Sawa, T., Akaike T., Ichimori K., Akuta T., Kaneko K., Nakayama H., Stuehr D. J. and Maeda H. (2003). Superoxide generation mediated by 8-nitroguanosine, a highly redox-active nucleic acid derivative. *Biochem Biophys Res Commun,* Vol.311, No.2 (Nov 14), pp. (300-306), 0006-291X (Print)
Schetter, A. J., Heegaard N. H. and Harris C. C. (2010). Inflammation and cancer: interweaving microRNA, free radical, cytokine and p53 pathways. *Carcinogenesis,* Vol.31, No.1 (Jan), pp. (37-49), 1460-2180 (Electronic)
Scully, C., Beyli M., Ferreiro M. C., Ficarra G., Gill Y., Griffiths M., Holmstrup P., Mutlu S., Porter S. and Wray D. (1998). Update on oral lichen planus: etiopathogenesis and management. *Crit Rev Oral Biol Med,* Vol.9, No.1 pp. (86-122), 1045-4411 (Print)
Shibutani, S., Takeshita M. and Grollman A. P. (1991). Insertion of specific bases during DNA synthesis past the oxidation-damaged base 8-oxodG. *Nature,* Vol.349, No.6308 (Jan 31), pp. (431-434), 0028-0836 (Print)
Suarez, P., Batsakis J. G. and el-Naggar A. K. (1998). Leukoplakia: still a gallimaufry or is progress being made?--A review. *Adv Anat Pathol,* Vol.5, No.3 (May), pp. (137-155), 1072-4109 (Print) 1072-4109 (Linking)
Sudbo, J. and Reith A. (2005). The evolution of predictive oncology and molecular-based therapy for oral cancer prevention. *Int J Cancer,* Vol.115, No.3 (Jun 20), pp. (339-345), 0020-7136 (Print)
Surh, Y. J., Chun K. S., Cha H. H., Han S. S., Keum Y. S., Park K. K. and Lee S. S. (2001). Molecular mechanisms underlying chemopreventive activities of anti-inflammatory phytochemicals: down-regulation of COX-2 and iNOS through

suppression of NF-kappa B activation. *Mutat Res,* Vol.480-481, (Sep 1), pp. (243-268), 0027-5107 (Print)

Suzuki, N., Yasui M., Geacintov N. E., Shafirovich V. and Shibutani S. (2005). Miscoding events during DNA synthesis past the nitration-damaged base 8-nitroguanine. *Biochemistry,* Vol.44, No.25 (Jun 28), pp. (9238-9245), 0006-2960 (Print)

Takahashi, T., Nau M. M., Chiba I., Birrer M. J., Rosenberg R. K., Vinocour M., Levitt M., Pass H., Gazdar A. F. and Minna J. D. (1989). p53: a frequent target for genetic abnormalities in lung cancer. *Science,* Vol.246, No.4929 (Oct 27), pp. (491-494), 0036-8075 (Print)

Tanaka, H., Fujita N., Sugimoto R., Urawa N., Horiike S., Kobayashi Y., Iwasa M., Ma N., Kawanishi S., Watanabe S., Kaito M. and Takei Y. (2008). Hepatic oxidative DNA damage is associated with increased risk for hepatocellular carcinoma in chronic hepatitis C. *Br J Cancer,* Vol.98, No.3 (Feb 12), pp. (580-586), 0007-0920 (Print)

Tao, Y., Song X., Deng X., Xie D., Lee L. M., Liu Y., Li W., Li L., Deng L., Wu Q., Gong J. and Cao Y. (2005). Nuclear accumulation of epidermal growth factor receptor and acceleration of G1/S stage by Epstein-Barr-encoded oncoprotein latent membrane protein 1. *Exp Cell Res,* Vol.303, No.2 (Feb 15), pp. (240-251), 0014-4827 (Print)

Tedeschi, E., Menegazzi M., Margotto D., Suzuki H., Forstermann U. and Kleinert H. (2003). Anti-inflammatory actions of St. John's wort: inhibition of human inducible nitric-oxide synthase expression by down-regulating signal transducer and activator of transcription-1alpha (STAT-1alpha) activation. *J Pharmacol Exp Ther,* Vol.307, No.1 (Oct), pp. (254-261), 0022-3565 (Print)

Trinchieri, G. (2011). Inflammation in cancer: a therapeutic target? *Oncology (Williston Park),* Vol.25, No.5 (Apr 30), pp. (418-420), 0890-9091 (Print)

Tyldesley, W. R. and Appleton J. (1973). Observations on the ultrastructure of the epithelium in oral lichen planus. *J Oral Pathol,* Vol.2, No.1 pp. (46-57), 0300-9777 (Print)

Yermilov, V., Rubio J., Becchi M., Friesen M. D., Pignatelli B. and Ohshima H. (1995a). Formation of 8-nitroguanine by the reaction of guanine with peroxynitrite in vitro. *Carcinogenesis,* Vol.16, No.9 (Sep), pp. (2045-2050), 0143-3334 (Print)

Yermilov, V., Rubio J. and Ohshima H. (1995b). Formation of 8-nitroguanine in DNA treated with peroxynitrite in vitro and its rapid removal from DNA by depurination. *FEBS Lett,* Vol.376, No.3 (Dec 4), pp. (207-210), 0014-5793 (Print)

Yu, J. S., Tsai H. C., Wu C. C., Weng L. P., Li H. P., Chung P. J. and Chang Y. S. (2002). Induction of inducible nitric oxide synthase by Epstein-Barr virus B95-8-derived LMP1 in Balb/3T3 cells promotes stress-induced cell death and impairs LMP1-mediated transformation. *Oncogene,* Vol.21, No.52 (Nov 14), pp. (8047-8061), 0950-9232 (Print)

Zaki, M. H., Akuta T. and Akaike T. (2005). Nitric oxide-induced nitrative stress involved in microbial pathogenesis. *J Pharmacol Sci,* Vol.98, No.2 (Jun), pp. (117-129), 1347-8613 (Print)

13

Novel Tissue Types for the Development of Genomic Biomarkers

Zinaida Sergueeva, Heather Collins, Sally Dow, Mollie McWhorter and Mark L. Parrish
Covance Genomics Laboratory, Seattle, Washington, USA

1. Introduction

Imagine a simple clinical test that can not only diagnose a disease, but that can also identify the exact, personal therapeutic regime to cure it. Not only that, imagine tests that can accurately predict the potential of developing a disease and provide an individualized roadmap on how it will progress. Now imagine that all you had to do was to spit in a vial, or have a few hairs plucked for the analysis. While the promise of "personalized medicine" is technologically a reality, it relies on the development of disease and progression biomarkers.

The ideal biomarker should have a number of characteristics, including: having an analyte that is accessible using noninvasive protocols, inexpensive to quantify, specific to the disease of interest, translatable from model systems to humans, and the ability to provide a reliable early indication of disease before clinical symptoms appear. Biomarkers that can be used to stratify disease and assess response to therapeutics are also medically valuable.

Although most current biomarkers utilize protein or metabolic analytes, it can be difficult to develop new protein-based biomarkers. This is due to the inherent complexity of the protein composition of biological samples, the assorted posttranslational modifications of proteins, and the low abundance of many proteins of interest in most biological samples (especially blood). Similarly, the detection of metabolic analytes is difficult due to the complex biological matrix from which they are measured.

Detecting specific nucleic acids, while not trivial, is generally much easier. Synthetic complimentary oligonucleotides can deliver sufficient detection specificity in most cases, and PCR or other DNA amplification methods can be used to improve the detection limit. There are numerous examples of genomic biomarkers that have become powerful tools for molecular diagnostics and outcome prediction (Cronin et al., 2007; Guttmacher & Collins, 2002; Hamburg & Collins, 2010; Klein et al., 2009; Tainsky, 2009; L. J. van 't Veer et al., 2002). RNA and DNA biomarkers are used routinely for screening patients to diagnose and subtype disease, as well as to monitor therapy and predict progression. Discovery of microRNAs, and lately lncRNAs (long non-coding RNAs), further increased their importance and broadened their clinical application (Gibb, Brown, & Lam, 2011; Laterza et al., 2009). Low complexity, no known post-processing modifications, simple detection and amplification methods, tissue-specific expression profiles, and sequence conservation between humans and model organisms make extracellular miRNAs ideal candidates for genomic biomarkers to reflect and study various physiopathological conditions of the body.

Ideally, the most clinically powerful information would come directly from the tissue of interest. To understand cancer, one must look at malignant cells, much as one must analyze brain tissue to understand the complexities of neuroscience. However, many of these tissues are difficult to access or impossible to reach without potential injury to the patient. Alternative, or "surrogate", tissues can provide a means of assessing the genomic changes in the tissue of interest, without fear of harming the donor. For example, surrogate tissues may contact the tissue of interest and retain sloughed cells, secreted molecules or the contents of dying cells. While these molecular signals may not exactly mirror the tissue of origin, in many cases they are reproducible and can clearly point to underlying biology. Clinical material suitable for biomarker testing can be divided into 2 different types. The first are those that require minimally invasive procedures to obtain. This type includes blood, cerebrospinal fluid, tissue biopsies and so on. Type 2 tissues are those that can be obtained without any invasive means: hair, saliva, tears, epidermal cells, urine, etc. In some cases, acquisition of the material may not be passive. Examples of Type 1 and Type 2 samples are listed in Table 1.

Type 1 Samples	**Type 2 Samples**
Whole Blood	Hair
Serum	Tears
Plasma	Breast Milk
Cerebral Spinal Fluid	Vaginal Secretions
Nasal Scrape	Semen
Sputum (Lavage)	Saliva
Bone Marrow	Urine
Skin Punch	Feces
Buccal Swab	Sweat
Ductal Lavage	Nipple Aspirate Fluid
Dental Plaque	
Vascular Plaque	

Table 1. Example sample types for the development of genomic biomarkers.

The easier it is to provide a sample for biomarker testing, the greater will be the utilization and utility. There is emerging data that many tissues and fluids that have been largely ignored, hold numerous important analytes that can be exploited for biomarker development. Relative ease of acquisition and rich genomic information, make these surrogate tissues ideally suited for the development of new biomarkers. By casting a wider net over the potential sources of biomarkers, we can increase the odds of finding clinically important ones that will make predictive, personalized healthcare a reality (Hood & Friend, 2011). In this review we will provide examples of various surrogate tissues that are being utilized for the development of genomic biomarkers, and highlight important concepts for successful collection and handling of them.

2. Clinically important tissues

2.1 Blood

2.1.1 Whole blood

Peripheral blood remains the most commonly studied tissue due to the minimally invasive nature of sample collection and the vascularization of most tissues. Peripheral whole blood is a rich source of validated and potential biomarkers, whether they are protein, genomic, or metabolic in nature. While the methods for extraction and profiling of blood DNA are well established, the isolation of RNA and microRNA from whole blood, and studies on their transcript abundance (commonly called gene expression studies), still pose many technical challenges. These include transcriptomic changes induced by *ex vivo* handling and the interference of highly abundant globin mRNA.

Pre-analytical variables such as the degradation of RNA by endogenous RNases and unintentional expression of individual genes after drawing blood could lead to false assessment of potential markers. The introduction of blood collection systems containing stabilizing additives has significantly improved the RNA quantity and quality of blood samples (Rainen et al., 2002; Thach, 2003). RNA stabilization systems have the advantage of storing the collected samples at more accessible temperatures before shipment to the laboratory for analysis, resulting in reduced pre-analytical variability. A well-described method for RNA stabilization in human blood is the PAXgene™ system (Chai et al., 2005; Rainen et al., 2002). The Tempus™ Whole Blood RNA isolation system offers an alternative approach to peripheral blood RNA isolation suitable for gene expression profiling as well (Asare et al., 2008). Recently RNAlater™, a common stabilization reagent for RNA in cells and tissues, has been successfully used for RNA stabilization in human peripheral blood (Weber et al., 2010). The downside of the latter method is that pre-filled RNAlater™ blood collection tubes are not currently available commercially.

All the described methods are able to stabilize transcription and isolate total RNA with good quality and in appropriate quantities. However, RNA stabilization/isolation methods can critically impact differential expression results. For example, the failure of PAXgene™ to stabilize specific transcripts was reported in several studies (Asare et al., 2008; Kågedal et al., 2005). Until more broad studies are done, it is recommended that a researcher should pre-validate the whole blood stabilization/isolation conditions with the transcripts of interest. We find that strict adherence to the manufacturer's protocol for collection and storage, including how the reagent is mixed with the blood at the time of collection, is critical to successful expression profiling.

The discovery of microRNAs has opened new opportunities for markers in the diagnosis of cancer (Wang et al., 2009). MicroRNAs are small (typically ~22 nt in size) regulatory RNA molecules that function to modulate the activity of specific mRNA targets and play important roles in a wide range of physiologic and pathologic processes (Mattick & Makunin, 2005). MicroRNAs are an ideal class of blood-based biomarkers for disease detection because: (i) miRNA expression is frequently dysregulated in disease, (ii) expression patterns of miRNAs are tissue-specific, and (iii) miRNAs have unusually high stability in most tissues and can be recovered from formalin-fixed, paraffin embedded samples.

Several studies have reported optimized isolation protocols to enhance the recovery of microRNAs in the stabilized samples. For example it was shown that microRNAs could be isolated from PAXgene-stabilized blood of sufficient quantity and quality that is suitable for downstream applications (Kruhøffer et al., 2007).

Another problem hampering the analysis of microarray gene expression data in whole blood is the presence of globin. Globin mRNA in red blood cells accounts for over 70% of all mRNA in whole blood and interferes with the accurate assessment of other genes (Field et al., 2007; Wright et al., 2008). Several approaches have been developed to mitigate this effect and tested in microarray experiments (Liu et al., 2006; Vartanian et al., 2009; Wright et al., 2008). Globin reduction techniques based on biotinylated DNA capture oligos (Ambion GLOBINclear processing protocol) produced sensitive results but was least reproducible among all the methods tested (Vartanian et al., 2009). An alternative protocol with globin PNAs (peptide nucleic acid inhibitory oligos) proved to be the best in sensitivity and reproducibility, but was the most time-consuming and required the highest amount of total RNA input (Liu et al., 2006; Vartanian et al., 2009). An alternative approach was suggested by Eklund and colleagues (Eklund et al., 2006). NuGEN's Ovation WB sample preparation protocol, based on single primer isothermal amplification (SPIA), generates cDNA target. The hybridization kinetics of the cDNA target are less affected than cRNA targets by the abundant globin RNA present in whole blood extract. The high specificity and sensitivity of cDNA targets, and the highly reproducible SPIA protocol have been shown to be as good or better for mitigating the interference of globin transcripts compared to other protocols (Fricano et al., 2011; Li et al., 2008; Parrish et al., 2010). The strong performance of this technique, and the relatively low input requirements (50ng of total RNA) have made the NuGEN Ovation WB protocol the method of choice for gene expression profiling in the microarray community.

2.1.2 Serum and plasma

Both plasma and serum are widely used specimen types for molecular diagnostics. Nucleic acids that can be found in small amounts in cell-free preparations of whole blood are frequently called "circulating nucleic acids". To date, a number of studies show that plasma and serum nucleic acids can serve as both tumor- and fetal-specific markers for cancer detection and prenatal diagnosis, respectively. For example, several studies reported increased concentrations of DNA in the plasma or serum of cancer patients sharing some characteristics with DNA of tumor cells (Leon et al., 1977; Stroun et al., 1989). Interestingly, DNA levels decreased by up to 90% after radiotherapy, while persistently high or increasing DNA concentrations were associated with a lack of response to treatment (Anker et al., 2001). RNA has also been found circulating in the plasma or serum of normal subjects and cancer patients (Feng et al., 2008; Tsui et al., 2002, 2006). The recent discovery that serum and plasma contain a large amount of stable miRNAs derived from various tissues/organs has lead to multiple studies on circulating miRNA expression as well (Mitchell et al., 2008; Chen et al., 2008; Zhu et al., 2009).

Analysis of circulating nucleic acids, however, requires modified extraction methods to utilize plasma or serum as the source material. First, plasma and serum are biospecimens that have a very high concentration of protein that can interfere with sample preparation and detection techniques. Second, the yield of circulating nucleic acids from small volume plasma or serum samples (< 1 mL) usually falls below the limit of accurate quantification by spectrometry and calls for an alternative way to assess the efficiency of nucleic acids recovery. Several serum/plasma extraction kits are now available commercially through Qiagen, Norgen and other companies. These kits successfully address the problems mentioned above, employing column-based purification methods and various carriers. We suggest the use of carefully selected extraction spike-ins to allow researchers to evaluate the efficiency of the circulating nucleic acids isolation.

2.1.3 Circulating tumor cells

Circulating tumor cells (CTCs) are cells that have been sloughed off of primary tumors and circulate in the bloodstream. Their numbers can be very small (1-10 cells per mL of whole blood) and these cells are not easily detected. Even though CTCs were first observed by Thomas Ashworth back in 1869, the technology with the requisite sensitivity and reproducibility to detect CTC in patients with metastatic disease was developed only recently (Sleijfer et al., 2007). While the presence of circulating tumor cells themselves can serve as a marker of poor clinical outcome, there is an opportunity to develop new biomarkers by studying the gene or protein expression in these cells. Changes in the phenotype of tumor cells can occur after the original diagnosis and resistance to a treatment can only be inferred after the treatment has failed. CTCs offer a tool to understand the complex biology of tumor cells, without the need of invasive biopsies.

Recently, CTCs have been the target of multiple molecular profiling studies (Bosma et al., 2002; Punnoose et al., 2010; Smirnov et al., 2005; Tewes et al., 2009). mRNA expression and DNA mutations can be measured from captured CTCs. RT-PCR using a multi-marker panel of cancer-associated genes was found to be the most sensitive technique for the detection of CTC in blood of breast cancer patients (Bosma et al., 2002; Tewes et al., 2009). Another approach involves the analysis of CTC-enriched samples by microarray gene expression profiling, where numerous genes like S100A14 and S100A16 have been detected (Smirnov et al., 2005).

2.1.4 Dried blood spots

The method of collecting capillary blood on filter paper was introduced in Scotland by Robert Guthrie in 1963 and since then has become a mainstream approach for blood sample collection from newborns in more than 20 countries (Consultant Paediatricians and Medical Officers of Health of the SE Scotland Hospital Region, 1968; Scriver, 1998). These samples were found invaluable for screening for congenital metabolic disorders. Dried blood spots (DBS) are easily acquired through a simple needle stick and transfer to paper cards that are stored and handled at room temperature in ambient atmospheric conditions. This approach eliminates many costly, time-consuming, and unpleasant aspects of sample collection, and can also significantly reduce the cost for shipping samples. The collection of DBS samples requires very little infrastructure and can be done in resource-limiting locations. Vidal-Taboada and colleagues even showed that both patients and investigators prefer this as a method of DNA collection and storage (Vidal-Taboada et al., 2006).

The limitation of small sample volume has restricted the usage of dried blood spots for the development of molecular diagnostics until recently. Advances in technology have overcome many of the problems with reduced sensitivity and specificity. For example, the development of whole genome amplification (WGA) protocols allow researchers to perform reliable genome-wide scans using archived residual blood samples from newborn screening programs, which are standard practice in several countries (Hollegaard et al., 2009). Several studies have shown that despite being considered too vulnerable to degradation by ribonucleases, RNA could be recovered from DBS samples that had been stored for 15-20 years, and be successfully amplified by reverse transcription-PCR (Karlsson et al., 2003; Zubakov et al., 2008). Also, dried blood spots recently become the sample type of choice for HIV screening in low-resource settings (Sherman et al., 2005; Uttayamakul et al., 2005).

2.2 Cerebrospinal fluid

Cerebrospinal fluid (CSF) is a cell-free, colorless liquid that occupies the subarachnoid space and the ventricular system around and inside the brain and spinal cord. It is usually obtained through lumbar puncture. CSF has been rediscovered in the post-genomic era, as a great source of potential protein biomarkers for various diseases as it bathes the brain and other neurological tissues. Analysis of CSF allows rapid screening, low sample consumption, and accurate protein identification by proteomic technology (Guerreiro et al., 2006; Zheng et al., 2003). Brain proteins in CSF are also important for diagnosis of non-inflammatory CNS diseases. Examples of conditions in which these proteins are diagnostically relevant include degenerative diseases (Otto et al., 1997; Ranganathan et al., 2005), tumors (Zheng et al., 2003), hypoxias and brain infarction (Schaarschmidt et al., 1994).

Advancements in nucleic acid (NA) amplification techniques have transformed the diagnosis of bacterial and viral infections of the central nervous system. Because of their enhanced sensitivity, these methods enable detection of very low amounts of pathogenic genomes in cerebrospinal fluid. Diagnosis of several viral CNS infections, such as herpes encephalitis, enterovirus meningitis and other viral infections occurring in human immunodeficiency virus-infected persons are currently performed using cerebrospinal fluid (Cinque, Bossolasco, & Lundkvist, 2003). MicroRNAs are also becoming an important analyte in CSF for the identification of neurological disease (Baraniskin et al., 2011; Cogswell et al., 2008; De Smaele et al., 2010). For example, miRNAs isolated from the frozen cerebrospinal fluid of Alzheimer disease-affected (AD) and non-affected patients showed distinctly different expression profiles (Cogswell et al., 2008). Notably miRNAs linked to immune cell functions including innate immunity and T cell activation and differentiation were up-regulated in AD.

Combining mRNA studies with protein expression analysis may provide a more global picture of the biological processes associated with CNS disorders. Information gathered could lead to the development of select biological indices (biomarkers) for guiding CNS diagnosis and therapy.

2.3 Saliva

Saliva is an easily obtainable tissue that has been used in forensics for decades (Sweet et al., 1997). However, new molecular profiling kits for voluntary saliva collection have made saliva an increasingly useful clinical biomarker tissue. The collection process is non-invasive, and can even be collected at home or in isolated locations using some of the newer collection kits (Oragene or Norgen products). This ease of collection results in higher compliance by the patients. As is often the case in biological samples, the difference in yield is usually a donor dependent value (van Schie & Wilson, 1997). It is possible that saliva samples could replace blood samples for DNA studies. A study in Australia and New Zealand compared 10 matched pairs of blood and saliva, as well as nearly 2000 samples of either blood (Australia) or saliva (New Zealand; Oragene collection system) for genotyping. This study was larger than the van Schie & Wilson study, but corroborated that there is a donor dependency to DNA yield. Because of the larger sample number, they saw more sample variance. However, they also concluded that variance had more to do with collection, processing and donor variability than variance due to tissue type (Bahlo et al., 2010). The collection and processing methods can all eventually be controlled. In most cases there was enough mass from 1 ml of saliva sample to yield at least 4ug of DNA, which is enough DNA for most molecular biology assays.

2.4 Skin

2.4.1 Skin tissue

Readily-accessible and as well-tolerated as punch biopsies (Camidge et al., 2005), skin is comprised of various layers of cells, making it useful for phenotypic and histological studies. Moreover, as a constantly dividing tissue with cells at various stages of development, skin provides insight into important signaling networks such as EGF, Wnt, Notch and cell proliferation (Phillips & Sachs, 2005).

Wee1 inhibitors have been examined as a way to bypass the G2 checkpoint, sensitizing p53 negative cells to DNA-damaging agents (Wang et al., 2001). In research conducted by Mizuarai et al., p53 negative rat skin xenograft tumors, p53 positive and negative cultured cancer cells, and p53 positive rat skin tissues were subjected to gemcitabine alone or in combination with the Wee-1 inhibitor MK-1775 (Mizuarai et al., 2009). Gene expression data identified five genes as potential biomarkers present in both tumor and skin.

Because of its strong potential as a surrogate tissue, it is important to address storage and handling challenges faced when using skin. Due to its protective nature, skin is shielded by nucleases and difficult to homogenize. We have found immediate preservation in RNAlater following the manufacturer's protocol (rather than flash-freezing) and thorough pulverization are paramount to extracting sufficient quantities of high-quality nucleic acid (data not shown).

2.4.2 Skin tissue alternatives

Synthetic skin is a relatively new surrogate tissue that lends itself to investigation of a wide variety of processes while reducing the need for volunteer recruitment or laboratory animal testing (Poumay & Coquette, 2007). For extracting nucleic acids, we have found that synthetic skin is less susceptible to nucleic acid degradation and more easily homogenized than real human skin (data not shown). Synthetic skin has recently been used to study processes such as wound healing (Koria et al., 2003), epithelial development (Taylor et al., 2009), effects of cosmetics on skin (Faller et al., 2002), and even differential gene expression in skin disorders.

Yao et al. identified the overexpression of type I IFN-inducible genes in psoriatic biopsies by comparing biopsies of normal, healthy donor skin and non-lesional skin to psoriatic donor skin (Yao et al., 2008). To better understand the degree of type I IFN-inducible gene overexpression in psoriasis, blood from healthy donors and normal keratinocyctes (EpiDerm, MatTek, Inc.) were stimulated with various members of the type I IFN family. Ex vivo blood and in-vitro keratinocyte data showed overall agreement in up-regulated type I IFN-inducible genes. While only 1% of upregulated probes from the stimulation study were overexpressed in non-lesional compared to normal skin, 11.7% of the upregulated probes were overexpressed in lesional compared to non-lesional skin, suggesting type I IFNs may be a prospective target for psoriatic treatment.

2.5 Hair follicles

Hair follicles are different from skin and blood, in that they are made up of stem cells, which control the growth and cycling of hair. The stem cells are contained within the follicle and are often called the bulge. It is this fact which makes hair follicle gene expression particularly intriguing: "stem cells in the epidermis and hair follicle serve as the ultimate source of cells for both of these tissues, understanding the control of their proliferation and differentiation is key to understanding disorders related to disruption in these processes," (Cotsarelis, 2006).

Advances in hair follicle extraction, isolation, and amplification techniques along with the relative ease of collection of the tissue, and the abundance on most, hair follicle collection is being increasingly examined as a good investigatory and clinical biomarker tissue. To date most research has been in diseases involving skin conditions (Ohyama et al., 2006). However, hair follicles are also being examined for markers in to quantify exposures to pharmaceuticals (Reiter et al., 2008) or toxicology to certain drug targets (Kim et al., 2006).

Hair follicles are obtained using tweezers, grasping at the hair as near to the scalp as possible, and quickly yanking upwards. The follicle should be clearly present and immediately preserved in the appropriate preservation solution. For those with longer hair, we have found it helpful to cut the hair close to the follicle, before preservation. Although it is possible to achieve results with a single or a few (3 follicles), it is often better to acquire a larger set (15 follicles), to ensure the needed mass for evaluation will be met. The follicles for the experiment should be taken from a similar location for each extraction, as there might be slight gene expression changes with different hair locations (head, arm, and eyebrow). We recommend behind the ear for collection of the desired hairs for most applications. There are several different preservation solutions such as RNAlater (Ambion) or SD Lysis Buffer (Promega). Following preservation, follow the manufacturer guidelines on storage and extraction/isolation of the RNA.

2.6 Feces

Often overlooked, stool is an important source of potential biomarkers for a number of clinical indications. While the identification of infection and various metabolic imbalances are easily identified, feces can also yield RNA, DNA and miRNA for use in biomarker development. This is largely due to the shedding of epithelial cells in the gastrointestinal track (Osborn & Ahlquist, 2005). With the use of highly sensitive detection techniques, one can identify genetic aberrations in the genomes of these cells and understand or diagnose, non-invasively, the pathology of the patient's disease. However, the extraction and purification of nucleic acids in feces is quite challenging due to its low abundance and the high level of contaminants like humic acid. Thankfully, there are a number of commercial kits available for fecal DNA isolation, and new techniques such as synchronous coefficient of drag alteration (SCODA) show promise in further purifying and concentrating this rare DNA (Broemeling et al., 2008; Marziali et al., 2005). Interestingly, both the amount and integrity of DNA in feces have been shown to identify colorectal cancer patients (Klaassen et al., 2003; Osborn & Ahlquist, 2005). A variety of mutations found in this DNA have been identified in the stool of colorectal cancer patients. Genes identified with mutations include KRAS, TP53 and APC, among several others (Osborn & Ahlquist, 2005; Young & Bosch, 2011). The most interesting of these is the adenomatous polyposis coli gene (APC). Mutations in the APC gene have been shown to drive the growth of adenomas, and their identification in stool samples allows the early detection of early stage colorectal neoplasia (Jen et al., 1994; Traverso et al., 2002). Analysis of fecal DNA has also been used to identify pancreatic adenocarcinoma (Caldas et al., 1994).

The isolation and analysis of RNA from fecal samples has also gained a great deal of attention. While less stable than DNA, RNA provides a snapshot of the transcriptional activity of exfoliated cells; reflecting both genomic and environmental influences. Changes in gene expression may more fully reflect a target tissue's response to therapeutic agents. Alexander and Raicht demonstrated the ability to extract RNA from stool and suggested its use as a method for the early detection of colon tumors (Alexander & Raicht, 1998). One such transcript with potentially diagnostic value is cyclooxygenase 2 (COX-2) which can separate colorectal cancer patients from healthy patients (Kanaoka et al., 2004). Still others are exploiting fecal RNA to better understand infant health (Chapkin et al., 2010; Davidson et al., 1995; Kaetter et al., 2007).

2.7 Urine

Urine is an ideal source for the identification of new biomarkers as it is easily and non-invasively collected. It has long been a standard fluid for the measurement of metabolites, proteins, and infectious agents. Recent data has demonstrated that not only can these traditional analytes can be identified, but RNA, DNA miRNA can be extracted and profiled. While less stable than the other nucleic acids, mRNA can be detected in urine. Keller and colleagues have demonstrated that this stability is likely due to protection of the mRNA in protein/lipid vesicles called exosomes (Keller et al., 2011; Nilsson et al., 2009). Further, mRNA patterns from urine sediments have been suggested for the development of ovulation and fertility biomarkers (Campbell & Rockett, 2006). miRNAs have also been uniquely identified in urine (Weber et al., 2010), and their stability has also been linked to exosomes (Record et al., 2011; Valadi et al., 2007). Differential detection of miRNAs in urine is showing promise in the non-invasive detection of lupus, nephropathy, renal allograft rejection and urothelial cancer (Lorenzen et al., 2011; Wang et al., 2010; Wang et al., 2011; Yamada et al., 2011).

Urinary DNA is a complex target, with both host and non-host DNA being present and clinically relevant. Patient DNA is readily extracted from urine with methylation patterns that have been shown to have utility in the diagnosis of cancer and kidney injury (Chen et al., 2011; Kang et al., 2011). Microbial DNA is also extracted in urine. Through the expanding discipline of microbial metagenomics, we now understand that the relative distribution of microbial DNA has important clinical utility (Nelson et al., 2010; Virgin & Todd, 2011). New improvements in next generation sequencing and microarray technology are showing how the interactions between microbial communities and their host are measurable and are correlated with the health of the host. Urine, like feces, has the potential to provide an easily accessed fluid type, whose flora may provide an exquisitely sensitive measure of pathological state. For example, the microbiome of urine can be used to monitor asymptomatic sexually transmitted disease and is highly correlated to data generated from the urethra swabs (Dong et al., 2011; Nelson et al., 2010). As more work is done in this field, it is likely that more examples will be uncovered.

2.8 Nipple aspirate fluid

The breast is a complex organ whose architecture is intertwined with its biology. Even the structure of the nipple is multifaceted and not completely well understood (Love & Barsky, 2004). However, it does provide unique access to fluid that can be leveraged for biomarker development. Nipple aspirate fluid (NAF) and ductal lavage contain cells that have been used for the diagnosis and monitoring of breast cancer (Lang & Kuerer, 2007; Li et al., 2005; Mendrinos et al., 2005; Sauter et al., 1997). NAF is generally obtained either through spontaneous emission or suction, while ductal lavage requires the use of a microcatheter to enter the duct orifice to rinse and collect fluid. Although more invasive, ductal lavage yields more cells (Dooley et al., 2001; Li et al., 2005). These cells originate from the ductal epithelium and by studying them in the NAF, we can glean important information about the active biology within the ducts without the risks associated with biopsy (Dooley et al., 2001; King & Love, 2006; Miller et al., 2006). Much of this work has focused on the early identification of neoplasia using proteomic or cytological analysis of the cells isolated from this fluid (Dooley et al., 2001; Harigopal & Chhieng, 2010; King & Love, 2006; Mendrinos et al., 2005; Wrensch et al., 1992; Wrensch et al., 2001). Recent work has focused on the genomic profiling of NAF cells in order to identify early biomarkers that may predict progression, before morphological changes are evident. For example, the methylation of key tumor suppressor genes can be a highly effective means of predicting tumorgenesis. Preliminary work using NAF samples has demonstrated this as a feasible biomarker of early cancer detection (Krassenstein, 2004). However, measuring the methylation status of key genes in NAF-derived cells is generally not a sensitive enough technique on its own to diagnose disease or predict progression (Euhus et al., 2007; Fackler et al., 2006; Locke et al., 2007).

Mitochondrial sequencing has been shown to be a sensitive way of identifying neoplastic tissues (Czarnecka et al., 2006; Jakupciak et al., 2008; Jakupciak et al., 2008). Mutations in the mitochondrial genome are often found at higher rates than in normal tissues. It is likely that in many cases, these mutations are directly linked to disease pathogenesis, while in others this linkage may only be an effect of other processes. Various groups have applied different techniques to sequence mtDNA from NAF. Zhu and colleagues showed that mutations in mtDNA can be detected non-invasively from NAF using sequencing (Zhu et al., 2005). Jakupciak and colleagues used a mitochondrial resequencing microarray and were able to demonstrate the detection of mutations and a high correlation to traditional sequencing methods (Jakupciak et al., 2008). These methods show great promise for clinical use, although further work is required to validate the approaches. Interestingly, traditional methodologies for mtDNA sequencing, such as Sanger sequencing or hybridization-based resequencing, are substantially impacted by the presence of normal cells. This background of normal cells attenuates the positive mutational signals, leading to poor discrimination of bases. While Zhu and colleagues did not find this to be true in their study, it is likely that as next generation sequencing methodologies are applied to NAF profiling, we will be able to discriminate and quantify the differences between normal and tumor cells with high resolution (Zhu et al., 2005).

Genomic and mitochondrial DNA statuses are important factors in understanding the genetic context of disease. However, tumorigenesis is a dynamic process that is influenced by heredity and environment. RNA profiling is a way of linking these factors in a measurable way. Due to their low numbers, breast fluid-derived cells are difficult targets for gene expression profiling. With recent advances in mRNA amplification methodologies, there are now tools that allow these studies (Van Gelder et al., 1990). For example, Single-Primer, Isothermal Amplification (SPIA) is one of several techniques that can amplify and label mRNA for microarray or RT-qPCR analysis (Kurn et al., 2005). Various studies have shown the utility of gene expression in identifying gene expression patterns of tumors that subclassify breast cancer and help to predict outcome (Cronin et al., 2007; Ma et al., 2003; van de Vijver et al., 2002). It is conceivable that these same transcript signatures will be obtained from isolated cells from ductal fluid.

3. Factors that impact genomic sample quality and utility

3.1 Sample collection

The utility of a given sample to yield a clinically meaningful result is dependent on many factors. These include when and how samples were collected, the preservation method used to stabilize the analytes, shipping and storage effects, and the correct association of patient data with the sample. Variation in any of these areas can have a substantial impact on the usefulness of a sample.

There is conflicting data as far as the effect of time delay between sample collection and the time of extraction of RNA. Some studies report that any delay in getting the sample from the living state to a preserved state (frozen, in formalin (FFPE) or RNAlater) will decrease the quality of the sample (Hong et al., 2010). There are other studies that indicate that there is at least a 16 hour window in which the sample collection and the QC metrics of BioAnalyzer assessment do not show any degradation (Micke et al., 2006). In our experience, we have found that any interruption of sample collection state en route to preservation could lead to degradation of the RNA (unpublished observation). Lisowski and colleagues found that as FFPE sample slices aged, signal intensity by in situ hybridization (ISH) was impacted. If they sliced from the block right before extracting RNA, the signal was clearer and stronger (Lisowski et al., 2001). While some tissues are considered homogenous, studies by Irwin and Dyroff show that there are different physiological responses to different sections of liver in response to drugs (Dyroff et al., 1986; Irwin et al., 2005).

3.2 Shipping and storage

With the advent of electronic tracking by the shipping industry, as well as a societal expectation of overnight shipments, samples can safely and quickly travel from a clinical site to a separate processing facility. FedEx pioneered the idea of hub shipments and overnight travel, but others have adopted and emulated their practices. Some couriers will replenish dry ice on shipments traveling more than 24 hours (World Courier). Coupled with this is the need for the initial shipper to pack the samples in such a fashion that they will be held at the correct temperature for at least 24 hours. Written or web based guidance should be given to all collection sites with explicit details as to size of shipping containers and amount of dry ice to use to ensure safe passage of the samples.

3.3 Sample handling and logistics – Barcoding and annotation

Clinical studies need the support of large numbers of samples to confirm the efficacy and safety of a drug. With the expanded usage of biomarkers in clinical trials, even more samples and patients may be needed to fully discover the population that will best be served by a given therapy. One clinical collection set can consist of as little as one sample or up to potentially 100 samples from a single patient in one day. The number of samples needed to generate statistically significant data will number in the tens of thousands across the different stages of a clinical trial. Clinical trial involvement necessitates scrupulous tracking of many details about each sample. Historically, this was all done on paper, but with increasing computing power and usage, tracking of the samples can be more effectively done by utilizing well built database systems. Effective use of computers also increases the option of analyzing samples across multiple trials, including the option of comparing biomarkers for a more customized treatment approach. To accomplish this, companies are relying on electronic data capture such as LIMS (Laboratory Information Management system), EMR (Electronic Medical Records) or CTMS (Clinical Trial Management System) and barcodes on individual samples (Burczynski et al., 2005; B. Choi et al., 2005; Niland & Rouse, 2010).

There is more than one approach towards connecting the annotation about a sample and an identifier on the sample container. Some systems rely on human readable text on the labels to tell the person handling the container what should be in it. There is the potential for error when depending on a human to read or type (Turner et al., 2003). Sometimes these labels with text also have a barcode on them. This type of barcoding system is referred to as an intelligent barcode system, only because there is specific sample information, other than the barcode, on the label. Other systems make full use of contemporary technology to track samples (naïve barcodes). With the use of the naïve barcode system, the sample collector needs to be able to associate the sample with a related database. This can be done by the collector writing on a piece of paper, which is then entered into the database at a later time by a data entry clerk. Alternatively, technology may be fully leveraged by supplying the collection sites with barcode readers, and access to the appropriate database, to associate the barcode on the container, with the given patient ID.

There are pros and cons for each of these barcoding methods. Having an intelligent barcode (pre-association of barcode with patient ID/time point) means that the person doing the collection needs only to find the correct label for the given sample, as the time point information should already be tracked in a database. If the labels are printed in a sequential fashion, then this may be simple. The con to this system is that if for some reason the correct label cannot be found, there is not usually a means to associate a new label with the sample.

Generally, projects that use this kind of labeling do not have any computer connection from the collection sites to the database storing the sample information. Before the advent of ubiquitous computers and hand held devices, associating the sample label information to a matching piece of paper seemed an effective way to track samples.

The major drawback with the naïve barcode system (barcoded tubes that are associated at the point of collection with the sample) is that if the association of sample to barcode is not made by the collection site, then the container is just a tube of tissue, useless for further study. To effectively use the naïve barcode, sites benefit from having access to the database while collecting samples. This can be as simple as barcode scanners that allow some amount of data entry. In some instances, double barcode labels can be supplied to the sites, one is affixed to the form and one is placed on the tube, with the association in to the database to be made later.

One method of association, which is a compromise between the intelligent barcode method and the naïve barcode method, is done by associating barcoded containers into a kit at a central laboratory assembly site. Then the kits are shipped to various collection sites. As the kit leaves the facility, the internal containers are still a naïve barcoded container, however at this point, they are associated with a tube type and a destination, all of this information is tracked at a the central laboratory, not on the containers. At the collection site, the kit is associated to a patient. This reduces the amount of data entry needed. The practice of associating the kit barcode at the site of collection to the patient ID allows some flexibility, while still allowing tracking of the tubes within the kits to be organized. This method ensures the highest quality association between a given sample and the donor.

In addition, given the current increase of hand held scanners with WiFi access, immediate computer access is no longer a large barrier. Car rental agencies and store inventory systems have been using portable scanners to track inventory for decades; similarly, it isn't too difficult to adopt similar technology for use in clinical trial data collection. The New York subway system integrates data from barcoded tickets, generated from identified machines, all with customer anonymity, to track where passenger flow is most active. There are some groups who have started to study the benefits of this type of live data association in studies involving human donors or patients (Avilés et al., 2008). While it is not essential for the sites to have computer access, as the paper trail of requisition forms is still common,, instant computer contact by the collection site does make the tracking easier. Handwriting barcodes and manual association outside of the database defeats the efficiency of the naïve barcode system, although downstream sample processing can make use of the barcoding system if there is a barcode and the association is made to the patient identifier.

In addition, there is an added benefit of naïve barcodes for double blind studies. Double blind studies mask the sample identity, including patient and treatment information. This is to prevent bias in the study and to protect the identity of the study patients. In the past a double tier system of identification numbers would cryptically hide the patient information from those involved in the collection or the analysis of the study. Only a select few would have access to source information about both the patient and drug information. Unique barcodes on the container, without any study information on the label, can provide a double blind labeling system, as long as the sample is always tracked in the LIMS system.

4. Conclusion

Technology has finally caught up with science fiction. The idea of a pin prick to divine ones' future is fast becoming a reality. Science is moving medicine in a direction where patient care will be predicted and prevented, and not watched from afar. Data-rich and highly sensitive techniques like microarray profiling, quantitative PCR, and Next Generation Sequencing are the genomics tools that are helping to drive these changes. However, to extract the greatest utility, tests need to be simple to complete, cost effective and as non-invasive as possible. Clinical impact is directly related to the availability and cost of a test. Consider the case of standard tumor biopsy. Depending on the disease and tumor location, a biopsy can be minor surgery involving a team of doctors, nurses, radiologists, and specialists. Recovery from a biopsy is often brief, but in some cases can lead to a costly overnight hospital stay. In the end, the actual cost of obtaining material for a test can be in the thousands of dollars, while the test itself, may only be a couple of hundred of dollars. For many biomarkers, there is more cost associated with the acquisition of sample, than the test itself. It is for this reason it makes both clinical and financial sense to find ways to make sample acquisition more cost effective and less precarious for the patient.

By studying often overlooked sample types, we may identify a treasure trove of clinically useful biomarkers. While not every surrogate tissue will yield a disease or response-specific biomarker, there is substantial data to justify the investigation. There is undeniable value in the use of biomarkers in drug development and patient care, but this value is tempered with the cost of sample acquisition. Developing methods for the acquisition of clinically useful and easily obtainable samples is important as we move from a drug discovery process that is focused on finding the right drugs to one that focuses on finding the right patients.

5. Acknowledgements

The authors are indebted to our many colleagues at the Covance Genomics Laboratory (formally the Rosetta Gene Expression Laboratory) for years of dedication and collaboration. We also give thanks to our clients, who have continued to challenge the norm and helped us develop new and novel approaches for biomarker development.

6. References

Alexander, R. J., & Raicht, R. F. (1998). Purification of total RNA from human stool samples. *Digestive Diseases and Sciences*, *43*(12), 2652–2658.

Anker, P., Lyautey, J., Lederrey, C., & Stroun, M. (2001). Circulating nucleic acids in plasma or serum. *Clinica Chimica Acta*, *313*(1-2), 143-6.

Asare, A. L., Kolchinsky, S. A., Gao, Z., Wang, R., Raddassi, K., Bourcier, K., & Seyfert-Margolis, V. (2008). Differential gene expression profiles are dependent upon method of peripheral blood collection and RNA isolation. *BMC Genomics*, *9*, 474.

Avilés, W., Ortega, O., Kuan, G., Coloma, J., & Harris, E. (2008). Quantitative assessment of the benefits of specific information technologies applied to clinical studies in developing countries. *The American Journal of Tropical Medicine and Hygiene*, *78*(2), 311-5.

Bahlo, M., Stankovich, J., Danoy, P., Hickey, P. F., Taylor, B. V., Browning, S. R., The Australian and New Zealand Multiple Sclerosis Genetics Consortium, Brown, M.

A., & Rubio, J. P. (2010). Saliva-derived DNA performs well in large-scale, high-density single-nucleotide polymorphism microarray studies. *Cancer Epidemiology, Biomarkers & Prevention, 19*(3), 794-8.

Baraniskin, A., Kuhnhenn, J., Schlegel, U., Chan, A., Deckert, M., Gold, R., Maghnouj, A., Zöllner, H., Reinacher-Schick, A., Schmiegel, W., Hahn, S.A., Schroers, R. (2011). Identification of microRNAs in the cerebrospinal fluid as marker for primary diffuse large B-cell lymphoma of the central nervous system. *Blood, 117*(11), 3140-6.

Bosma, A. J., Weigelt, B., Lambrechts, A. C., Verhagen, O. J. H. M., Rodenhuis, S., & Veer, L. J. V. (2002). Detection of Circulating Breast Tumor Cells by Differential Expression of Marker Genes Detection of Circulating Breast Tumor Cells by Differential Expression of Marker Genes. *Clinical Cancer Research*, 1871-1877.

Broemeling, D. J., Pel, J., Gunn, D. C., Mai, L., Thompson, J. D., Poon, H., & Marziali, A. (2008). An instrument for automated purification of nucleic acids from contaminated forensic samples. *Journal of the Association for Laboratory Automation, 13*(1), 40-48.

Burczynski, M. E., Oestreicher, J. L., Cahilly, M. J., Mounts, D. P., Whitley, M. Z., Speicher, L. A., & Trepicchio, W. L. (2005). Clinical pharmacogenomics and transcriptional profiling in early phase oncology clinical trials. *Current Molecular Medicine, 5*(1), 83-102.

Caldas, C., Hahn, S. A., Hruban, R. H., Hahn, A., Redston, M. S., Yeo, J., & Kern, S. E. (1994). Detection of K-ras Mutations in the Stool of Patients with Pancreatic Adenocarcinoma and Pancreatic Ductal Hyperplasia. *Cancer*, 3568-3573.

Camidge, D. R., Pemberton, M. N., Growcott, J. W., Johnstone, D., Laud, P. J., Foster, J. R., Randall, K. J., et al. (2005). Assessing proliferation, cell-cycle arrest and apoptotic end points in human buccal punch biopsies for use as pharmacodynamic biomarkers in drug development. *British Journal of Cancer, 93*(2), 208-15.

Campbell, K. L., & Rockett, J. C. (2006). Biomarkers of ovulation, endometrial receptivity, fertilisation, implantation and early pregnancy progression. *Paediatric and Perinatal Epidemiology, 20 Suppl 1*, 13-25.

Chai, V., Vassilakos, A., Lee, Y., Wright, J. A., & Young, A. H. (2005). Optimization of the PAXgene™ blood RNA extraction system for gene expression analysis of clinical samples. *Journal of Clinical Laboratory Analysis, 19*(5), 182–188.

Chapkin, R. S., Zhao, C., Ivanov, I., Davidson, L. A., Goldsby, J. S., Lupton, J.R., Mathai, R. A., et al. (2010). Noninvasive stool-based detection of infant gastrointestinal development using gene expression profiles from exfoliated epithelial cells. *American Journal of Physiology. Gastrointestinal and Liver Physiology, 298*(5), G582-9.

Chen, P. C., Tsai, M. H., Yip, S., Jou, Y. C., Ng, C. F., Chen, Y., Wang, X., Huang, W., Tung, C. L., Chen, G. C., Huang, M. M., Tong, J. H., Song, E. J., Chang, D. C., Hsu, C. D., To, K. F., Shen, C. H., & Chan, M. W. (2011). Distinct DNA methylation epigenotypes in bladder cancer from different Chinese sub-populations and its implication in cancer detection using voided urine. *BMC Medical Genomics, 4*(1), 45.

Chen, X., Ba, Y., Ma, L., Cai, X., Yin, Y., Wang, K., Guo, J., Zhang, Y., Chen, J., Guo, X., Li, Q., Li, X., Wang, W., Zhang, Y., Wang, J., Jiang, X., Xiang, Y., Xu, C., Zheng, P., Zhang, J., Li, R., Zhang, H., Shang, X., Gong, T., Ning, G., Wang, J., Zen, K., Zhang, J., & Zhang, C. Y. (2008). Characterization of microRNAs in serum: a novel class of biomarkers for diagnosis of cancer and other diseases. *Cell Research, 18*(10), 997-1006.

Choi, B., Drozdetski, S., Hackett, M., Lu, C., Rottenberg, C., Yu, L., Hunscher, D., & Clauw, D. (2005). Usability comparison of three clinical trial management systems. *American Medical Informatics Association Symposium Proceedings,* (2005) 921.

Cinque, P., Bossolasco, S., & Lundkvist, A. (2003). Molecular analysis of cerebrospinal fluid in viral diseases of the central nervous system. *Journal of Clinical Virology, 26*(1), 1-28.

Cogswell, J. P., Ward, J., Taylor, I. A., Waters, M., Shi, Y., Cannon, B., Kelnar, K., Kemppainen, J., Brown, D., Chen, C., Prinjha, R. K., Richardson, J. C., Saunders, A. M., Roses, A. D., & Richards, C. A. (2008). Identification of miRNA changes in Alzheimer's disease brain and CSF yields putative biomarkers and insights into disease pathways. *Journal of Alzheimer's Disease, 14*(1), 27-41.

Consultant Paediatricians and Medical Officers of Health of the SE Scotland Hospital Region. (1968). Population screening by Guthrie test for phenylketonuria in South-east Scotland. Report by the consultant paediatricians and medical officers of health of the S.E. Scotland Hospital Region. *British Medical Journal, 1*(5593), 674-6.

Cotsarelis, G. (2006). Gene expression profiling gets to the root of human hair follicle stem cells. *The Journal of Clinical Investigation, 116*(1), 19-22.

Cronin, M., Sangli, C., Liu, M.-L., Pho, M., Dutta, D., Nguyen, A., Jeong, J., Wu, J., Langone, K. C., & Watson, D. (2007). Analytical validation of the Oncotype DX genomic diagnostic test for recurrence prognosis and therapeutic response prediction in node-negative, estrogen receptor-positive breast cancer. *Clinical Chemistry, 53*(6), 1084-91.

Czarnecka, A. M., Golik, P., & Bartnik, E. (2006). Mitochondrial DNA mutations in human neoplasia. *Journal of Applied Genetics, 47*(1), 67-78.

Davidson, L. A., Jiang, Y. H., Lupton, J R, & Chapkin, R. S. (1995). Noninvasive detection of putative biomarkers for colon cancer using fecal messenger RNA. *Cancer Epidemiology, Biomarkers & Prevention, 4*(6), 643-7.

De Smaele, E., Ferretti, E., & Gulino, A. (2010). MicroRNAs as biomarkers for CNS cancer and other disorders. *Brain Research, 1338*, 100-11.

Dong, Q., Nelson, D. E., Toh, E., Diao, L., Gao, X., Fortenberry, J. D., & Van der Pol, B. (2011). The microbial communities in male first catch urine are highly similar to those in paired urethral swab specimens. *PloS One, 6*(5), e19709.

Dooley, W. C., Ljung, B. M., Veronesi, U., Cazzaniga, M, Elledge, R. M., O'Shaughnessy, J. A., Kuerer, H. M., Hung, D. T., Khan, S. A., Phillips, R. F., Ganz, P. A., Euhus, D. M., Esserman, L. J., Haffty, B. G., King, B. L., Kelley, M. C., Anderson, M. M., Schmitt, P. J., Clark, R. R., Kass, F. C., Anderson, B. O., Troyan, S. L., Arias, R. D., Quiring, J. N., Love, S. M., Page, D. L., & King, E. B. (2001). Ductal lavage for detection of cellular atypia in women at high risk for breast cancer. *Journal of the National Cancer Institute, 93*(21), 1624-32.

Dyroff, M. C., Richardson, F. C., Popp, J. A., Bedell, M. A., & Swenberg, J. A. (1986). Correlation of O4-ethyldeoxythymidine accumulation, hepatic initiation and hepatocellular carcinoma induction in rats continuously administered diethylnitrosamine. *Carcinogenesis, 7*(2), 241-6.

Eklund, A. C., Turner, L. R., Chen, P., Jensen, R. V., deFeo, G., Kopf-Sill, A. R., & Szallasi, Z. (2006). Replacing cRNA targets with cDNA reduces microarray cross-hybridization. *Nature Biotechnology, 24*(9), 1071-3.

Euhus, D. M., Bu, D., Ashfaq, R., Xie, X.-J., Bian, A., Leitch, A. M., & Lewis, C. M. (2007). Atypia and DNA methylation in nipple duct lavage in relation to predicted breast cancer risk. *Cancer Epidemiology, Biomarkers & Prevention, 16*(9), 1812-21.

Fackler, M. J., Malone, K., Zhang, Z., Schilling, E., Garrett-Mayer, E., Swift-Scanlan, T., Lange, J., Nayar, R., Davidson, N. E., Khan, S. A., & Sukumar, S. (2006). Quantitative multiplex methylation-specific PCR analysis doubles detection of tumor cells in breast ductal fluid. *Clinical Cancer Research, 12*(11), 3306-10.

Faller, C., Bracher, M., Dami, N., & Roguet, R. (2002). Predictive ability of reconstructed human epidermis equivalents for the assessment of skin irritation of cosmetics. *Toxicology In Vitro, 16*(5), 557-72.

Feng, G., Li, G., Gentil-Perret, A., Tostain, J., & Genin, C. (2008). Elevated serum-circulating RNA in patients with conventional renal cell cancer. *Anticancer Research, 28*(1A), 321-6.

Field, L. A., Jordan, R. M., Hadix, J. A., Dunn, M. A., Shriver, C. D., Ellsworth, R. E., & Ellsworth, D. L. (2007). Functional identity of genes detectable in expression profiling assays following globin mRNA reduction of peripheral blood samples. *Clinical Biochemistry, 40*(7), 499-502.

Fricano, M. M., Ditewig, A. C., Jung, P. M., Liguori, M. J., Blomme, Eric A. G., & Yang, Y. (2011). Global transcriptomic profiling using small volumes of whole blood: a cost-effective method for translational genomic biomarker identification in small animals. *International Journal of Molecular Sciences, 12*(4), 2502-17.

Gibb, E. A., Brown, C. J., & Lam, W. L. (2011). The functional role of long non-coding RNA in human carcinomas. *Molecular Cancer, 10*(1), 38.

Guerreiro, N., Gomez-Mancilla, B., & Charmont, S. (2006). Optimization and evaluation of surface-enhanced laser-desorption/ionization time-of-flight mass spectrometry for protein profiling of cerebrospinal fluid. *Proteome Science, 4*, 7.

Guttmacher, A. E., & Collins, F. S. (2002). Genomic Medicine-A Primer. *New England Journal of Medicine, 347*(19), 1512–1520.

Hamburg, M., & Collins, F. S. (2010). The path to personalized medicine. *New England Journal of Medicine, 363*(4), 301–304.

Harigopal, M., & Chhieng, D. C. (2010). Breast Cytology : Current Issues and Future Directions. *Cancer*, 81-89.

Hollegaard, M. V., Grauholm, J., Børglum, A., Nyegaard, M., Nørgaard-Pedersen, B., Ørntoft, T., Mortensen, P. B., Wiuf, C., Mors, O., Didriksen, M., Thorsen, P., Hougaard, D. M. (2009). Genome-wide scans using archived neonatal dried blood spot samples. *BMC Genomics, 10*, 297.

Hong, S. H., Baek, H. A., Jang, K. Y., Chung, M. J., Moon, W. S., Kang, M. J., Lee, D. G., & Park H. S. (2010). Effects of delay in the snap freezing of colorectal cancer tissues on the quality of DNA and RNA. *Journal of the Korean Society of Coloproctology, 26*(5), 316-23.

Hood, L., & Friend, S. H. (2011). Predictive, personalized, preventive, participatory (P4) cancer medicine. *Nature Reviews. Clinical Oncology, 8*(3), 184-7.

Irwin, R. D., Parker, J. S., Lobenhofer, E. K., Burka, L. T., Blackshear, P. E., Vallant, M. K., Lebetkin, E. H., Gerken, D. F., & Boorman, G. A. (2005). Transcriptional profiling of the left and median liver lobes of male f344/n rats following exposure to acetaminophen. *Toxicologic Pathology, 33*(1), 111-7.

Jakupciak, J. P., Maggrah, A., Maragh, S., Maki, J., Reguly, B., Maki, K., Wittock, R., Robinson, K., Wagner, P. D., Thayer, R. E., Gehman, K., Gehman, T., Srivastava, S., Ngom, A., Dakubo, G. D., & Parr, R. L. (2008). Facile whole mitochondrial genome resequencing from nipple aspirate fluid using MitoChip v2.0. *BMC Cancer, 8*, 95.

Jakupciak, J. P., Maragh, S., Markowitz, M. E., Greenberg, A. K., Hoque, M. O., Maitra, A., Barker, P. E., Wagner, P. D., Rom, W. N., Srivastava, S., Sidransky, D., & O'Connell, C. D. (2008). Performance of mitochondrial DNA mutations detecting early stage cancer. *BMC Cancer, 8*, 285.

Jen, J., Powell, S. M., Papadopoulos, N., Smith, K. J., Hamilton, S. R., Vogelstein, B., & Kinzler, K. W. (1994). Molecular determinants of dysplasia in colorectal lesions. *Cancer Research, 54*(21), 5523.

Kaeffer, B., des Robert, C., Alexandre-Gouabau, M.-C., Pagniez, A., Legrand, A., Amarger, V., Küster, A., Piloquet, H., Champ, M., Le Huërou-Luron, I., & Rozé, J. C. (2007). Recovery of exfoliated cells from the gastrointestinal tract of premature infants: a new tool to perform "noninvasive biopsies?". *Pediatric Research, 62*(5), 564-9.

Kågedal, B., Lindqvist, M., Farnebäck, M., Lenner, L., & Peterson, C. (2005). Failure of the PAXgene blood RNA system to maintain mRNA stability in whole blood. *Clinical Chemical Laboratory Medicine, 43*(11), 1190–1192.

Kanaoka, S., Yoshida, K.-I., Miura, N., Sugimura, H., & Kajimura, M. (2004). Potential usefulness of detecting cyclooxygenase 2 messenger RNA in feces for colorectal cancer screening. *Gastroenterology, 127*(2), 422-427.

Kang, S. W., Shih, P., Mathew, R., Mahata, M., Biswas, N., Rao, F., Yan, L., Bouchard, J., Malhotra, R., Tolwani, A., Khandrika, S., Mehta, R. L., & O'Connor, D. T. (2011). Renal kallikrein excretion and epigenetics in human acute kidney injury: Expression, mechanisms and consequences. *BMC Nephrology, 12*(1), 27.

Karlsson, H., Guthenberg, C., von Döbeln, U., & Kristenssson, K. (2003). Extraction of RNA from dried blood on filter papers after long-term storage. *Clinical Chemistry, 49*(6), 979-81.

Keller, S., Ridinger, J., Rupp, A.-K., Janssen, J. W., & Altevogt, P. (2011). Body fluid derived exosomes as a novel template for clinical diagnostics. *Journal of Translational Medicine, 9*(1), 86.

Kim, S. J., Dix, D. J., Thompson, K. E., Murrell, R. N., Schmid, J. E., Gallagher, J. E., & Rockett, J. C. (2006). Gene expression in head hair follicles plucked from men and women. *Annals of Clinical and Laboratory Science, 36*(2), 115-26.

King, B. L., & Love, S. M. (2006). The intraductal approach to the breast: raison d'être. *Breast Cancer Research 8*(2), 206.

Klaassen, C. H. W., Jeunink, M. A. F., Prinsen, C. F. M., Ruers, T. J. M., Tan, A. C. I. T. L., Strobbe, L. J. A., & Thunnissen, F. B. J. M. (2003). Quantification of human DNA in feces as a diagnostic test for the presence of colorectal cancer. *Clinical Chemistry, 49*(7), 1185-7.

Klein, T., Altman, R., Eriksson, N., Gage, B., Kimmel, S., Lee, M., Limdi, N., et al. (2009). Estimation of the warfarin dose with clinical and pharmacogenetic data. *New England Journal of Medicine, 360*(8), 753–64.

Koria, P., Brazeau, D., Kirkwood, K., Hayden, P., Klausner, M., & Andreadis, S. T. (2003). Gene expression profile of tissue engineered skin subjected to acute barrier disruption. *The Journal of Investigative Dermatology, 121*(2), 368-82.

Krassenstein, R. (2004). Detection of breast cancer in nipple aspirate fluid by CpG island hypermethylation. *Clinical Cancer Research, 10*(1), 28-32.

Kruhøffer, M., Dyrskjøt, L., Voss, T., Lindberg, R. L. P., Wyrich, R., Thykjaer, T., & Orntoft, T. F. (2007). Isolation of microarray-grade total RNA, microRNA, and DNA from a single PAXgene blood RNA tube. *The Journal of Molecular Diagnostics, 9*(4), 452-8.

Kurn, N., Chen, P., Heath, J. D., Kopf-Sill, A., Stephens, K. M., & Wang, S. (2005). Novel isothermal, linear nucleic acid amplification systems for highly multiplexed applications. *Clinical Chemistry, 51*(10), 1973-81.

Lang, J. E., & Kuerer, H. M. (2007). Breast ductal secretions: clinical features, potential uses, and possible applications. *Cancer Control: Journal of the Moffitt Cancer Center, 14*(4), 350-9.

Laterza, O. F., Lim, L., Garrett-Engele, P. W., Vlasakova, K., Muniappa, N., Tanaka, W. K., Johnson, J. M., Sina, J. F., Fare, T. L., Sistare, F. D., & Glaab, W. E. (2009). Plasma microRNAs as sensitive and specific biomarkers of tissue injury. *Clinical Chemistry, 55*(11), 1977-83.

Leon, S. A., Shapiro, B., Sklaroff, D. M., & Yaros, M. J. (1977). Free DNA in the serum of cancer patients and the effect of therapy free DNA in the serum of cancer patients and the effect of therapy. *Cancer*, 646-650.

Li, Jinong, Zhao, J., Yu, X., Lange, J., Kuerer, H., Krishnamurthy, S., Schilling, E., et al. (2005). Identification of biomarkers for breast cancer in nipple aspiration and ductal lavage fluid. *Clinical Cancer Research 11*(23), 8312-20.

Li, L., Ying, L., Naesens, M., Xiao, W., Sigdel, T., Hsieh, S., Martin, J., et al. (2008). Interference of globin genes with biomarker discovery for allograft rejection in peripheral blood samples. *Physiological Genomics, 32*(2), 190-7.

Lisowski, A. R., English, M. L., Opsahl, A. C., Bunch, R. T., & Blomme, E. A. G. (2001). Effect of the storage period of paraffin sections on the detection of mRNAs by in situ hybridization. *Journal of Histochemistry & Cytochemistry, 49*(7), 927-928.

Liu, J., Walter, E., Stenger, D., & Thach, D. (2006). Effects of globin mRNA reduction methods on gene expression profiles from whole blood. *The Journal of Molecular Diagnostics, 8*(5), 551-558.

Locke, I., Kote-Jarai, Z., Fackler, M. J., Bancroft, E., Osin, P., Nerurkar, A., Izatt, L., et al. (2007). Gene promoter hypermethylation in ductal lavage fluid from healthy BRCA gene mutation carriers and mutation-negative controls. *Breast Cancer Research 9*(1), R20.

Lorenzen, J. M., Volkmann, I., Fiedler, J., Schmidt, M., Scheffner, I., Haller, H., Gwinner, W., et al. (2011). Urinary miR-210 as a mediator of acute T-Cell mediated rejection in renal allograft recipients. *American Journal of Transplantation 11*(10), 2221-7.

Love, S. M., & Barsky, S. H. (2004). Anatomy of the nipple and breast ducts revisited. *Cancer, 101*(9), 1947-57.

Ma, X.-J., Salunga, R., Tuggle, J. T., Gaudet, J., Enright, E., McQuary, P., Payette, T., et al. (2003). Gene expression profiles of human breast cancer progression. *Proceedings of the National Academy of Sciences of the United States of America, 100*(10), 5974-9.

Marziali, A., Pel, J., Bizzotto, D., & Whitehead, L. A. (2005). Novel electrophoresis mechanism based on synchronous alternating drag perturbation. *Electrophoresis, 26*(1), 82-90.

Mattick, J. S., & Makunin, I. V. (2005). Small regulatory RNAs in mammals. *Human Molecular Genetics, 14 Spec No*(1), R121-32.

Mendrinos, S., Nolen, J. D. L., Styblo, T., Carlson, G., Pohl, J., Lewis, M., & Ritchie, J. (2005). Cytologic findings and protein expression profiles associated with ductal carcinoma of the breast in ductal lavage specimens using surface-enhanced laser desorption and ionization-time of flight mass spectrometry. *Cancer, 105*(3), 178-83.

Micke, P., Ohshima, M., Tahmasebpoor, S., Ren, Z.-P., Ostman, A., Pontén, F., & Botling, J. (2006). Biobanking of fresh frozen tissue: RNA is stable in nonfixed surgical specimens. *Laboratory Investigation, 86*(2), 202-11.

Miller, M. J., Cazzaniga, Massimiliano, & Casadio, C. (2006). Cytologic findings of breast ductal lavage and concurrent fine needle aspiration in pleomorphic lobular carcinoma in situ: a case report. *Acta Cytologica, 52*(2), 207-10.

Mitchell, P. S., Parkin, R. K., Kroh, E. M., Fritz, B. R., Wyman, S. K., Pogosova-Agadjanyan, E. L., Peterson, A., et al. (2008). Circulating microRNAs as stable blood-based markers for cancer detection. *Proceedings of the National Academy of Sciences of the United States of America, 105*(30), 10513-8.

Mizuarai, S., Yamanaka, K., Itadani, H., Arai, T., Nishibata, T., Hirai, H., & Kotani, H. (2009). Discovery of gene expression-based pharmacodynamic biomarker for a p53 context-specific anti-tumor drug Wee1 inhibitor. *Molecular Cancer, 8*, 34.

Nelson, D., Pol, B. V. D., Dong, Q., & Revanna, K. (2010). Characteristic male urine microbiomes associate with asymptomatic sexually transmitted infection. *PLoS One, 5*(11), 1-7.

Nelson, K. E., Weinstock, G. M., Highlander, S. K., Worley, K. C., Creasy, H. H. H., Wortman, J. R. R., Rusch, D. B., et al. (2010). A catalog of reference genomes from the human microbiome. *Science, 328*(5981), 994–999.

Niland, J. C., & Rouse, L. (2010). Clinical research systems and integration with medical systems, In: *Biomedical Informatics for Cancer Research*, M. F. Ochs, J. T. Casagrande, & R. V. Davuluri, (Eds.) DOI 10.1007/978-1-4419-5714-6_2

Nilsson, J., Skog, J., Nordstrand, A., Baranov, V., Mincheva-Nilsson, L., Breakefield, X. O., & Widmark, A. (2009). Prostate cancer-derived urine exosomes: a novel approach to biomarkers for prostate cancer. *British Journal of Cancer, 100*(10), 1603-7.

Ohyama, M., Terunuma, A., Tock, C. L., Radonovich, M. F., Pise-masison, C. A., Hopping, S. B., Brady, J. N., Udey, M. C., & Vogel, J. C. (2006). Characterization and isolation of stem cell – enriched human hair follicle bulge cells. *The Journal of Clinical Investigation, 116*(1).

Osborn, N. K., & Ahlquist, D. A. (2005). Stool screening for colorectal cancer: Molecular approaches. *Gastroenterology, 128*(1), 192-206.

Otto, M., Stein, H., Szudra, A., Zerr, I., Bodemer, M., Gefeller, O., Poser, S., et al. (1997). S-100 protein concentration in the cerebrospinal fluid of patients with Creutzfeldt-Jakob disease. *Journal of Neurology, 244*(9), 566-70.

Parrish, M. L., Wright, C., Rivers, Y., Argilla, D., Collins, H., Leeson, B., Loboda, A., Nebozhyn, M., Marton, M. J., & Lejnine, S. (2010). cDNA targets improve whole blood gene expression profiling and enhance detection of pharmocodynamic biomarkers: a quantitative platform analysis. *Journal of Translational Medicine, 8*, 87.

Phillips, R. L., & Sachs, A. B. (2005). Skin biopsies for the measurement of clinical pharmacodynamic biomarkers. *Current Opinion in Biotechnology, 16*(6), 687-90.

Poumay, Y., & Coquette, A. (2007). Modelling the human epidermis in vitro: tools for basic and applied research. *Archives of Dermatological Research, 298*(8), 361-9.

Punnoose, E. A., Atwal, S. K., Spoerke, J. M., Savage, H., Pandita, A., Yeh, R.-F., Pirzkall, A., et al. (2010). Molecular biomarker analyses using circulating tumor cells. *PLoS One, 5*(9), e12517.

Rainen, L., Oelmueller, U., Jurgensen, S., Wyrich, R., Ballas, C., Schram, J., Herdman, C., et al. (2002). Stabilization of mRNA expression in whole blood samples. *Clinical Chemistry, 48*(11), 1883-90.

Ranganathan, S., Williams, E., Ganchev, P., Gopalakrishnan, V., Lacomis, D., Urbinelli, L., Newhall, K., et al. (2005). Proteomic profiling of cerebrospinal fluid identifies biomarkers for amyotrophic lateral sclerosis. *Journal of Neurochemistry, 95*(5), 1461-71.

Record, M., Subra, C., Silvente-Poirot, S., & Poirot, M. (2011). Exosomes as intercellular signalosomes and pharmacological effectors. *Biochemical Pharmacology, 81*(10), 1171-82.

Reiter, M., Pfaffl, M. W., Schönfelder, M., & Meyer, H. H. D. (2008). Gene expression in hair follicle dermal papilla cells after treatment with stanozolol. *Biomarker Insights, 4*, 1-8.

Sauter, E. R., Ross, E., Daly, M., Klein-Szanto, A., Engstrom, P. F., Sorling, A., Malick, J., et al. (1997). Nipple aspirate fluid: a promising non-invasive method to identify cellular markers of breast cancer risk. *British Journal of Cancer, 76*(4), 494-501.

Schaarschmidt, H., Prange, H. W., & Reiber, H. (1994). Neuron-specific enolase concentrations in blood as a prognostic parameter in cerebrovascular diseases. *Stroke, 25*(3), 558-65.

Scriver, C. R. (1998). A simple phenylalanine method for detecting phenylketonuria in large populations of newborn infants, by Robert Guthrie and Ada Susi, Pediatrics, 1963;32:318-343. *Pediatrics, 102*(Supplement_1), 236-237.

Sherman, G. G., Stevens, G., Jones, S. A., Horsfield, P., & Stevens, W. S. (2005). Dried blood spots improve access to HIV diagnosis and care for infants in low-resource settings. *Journal of Acquired Immune Deficiency Syndromes (1999), 38*(5), 615-7.

Sleijfer, S., Gratama, J.-W., Sieuwerts, A. M., Kraan, J., Martens, J. W. M., & Foekens, J. A. (2007). Circulating tumour cell detection on its way to routine diagnostic implementation? *European Journal of Cancer, 43*(18), 2645-50.

Smirnov, D. a, Zweitzig, D. R., Foulk, B. W., Miller, M. C., Doyle, G. V., Pienta, K. J., Meropol, N. J., et al. (2005). Global gene expression profiling of circulating tumor cells. *Cancer Research, 65*(12), 4993-7.

Stroun, M., Anker, P., Maurice, P., Lyautey, J., Lederrey, C., & Beljanski, M. (1989). Neoplastic characteristics of the DNA found in the plasma of cancer patients. *Oncology, 46*(5), 318-22.

Sweet, D., Lorente, M., Lorente, J. a, Valenzuela, a, & Villanueva, E. (1997). An improved method to recover saliva from human skin: the double swab technique. *Journal of Forensic Sciences, 42*(2), 320-2.

Tainsky, M. (2009). Genomic and proteomic biomarkers for cancer: a multitude of opportunities. *Biochim Biophysica Acta, 1796*(2), 176-193.

Taylor, J. M., Street, T. L., Hao, L., Copley, R., Taylor, M. S., Hayden, P. J., Stolper, G., et al. (2009). Dynamic and physical clustering of gene expression during epidermal barrier formation in differentiating keratinocytes. *PloS One, 4*(10), e7651.

Tewes, M., Aktas, B., Welt, A., Mueller, S., Hauch, S., Kimmig, R., & Kasimir-Bauer, S. (2009). Molecular profiling and predictive value of circulating tumor cells in patients with metastatic breast cancer: an option for monitoring response to breast cancer related therapies. *Breast Cancer Research and Treatment, 115*(3), 581-90.

Thach, D. (2003). Assessment of two methods for handling blood in collection tubes with RNA stabilizing agent for surveillance of gene expression profiles with high density microarrays. *Journal of Immunological Methods, 283*(1-2), 269-279.

Traverso, G., Shuber, A., Levin, B., Johnson, C., Olsson, L., Schoetz Jr, D. J., Hamilton, S. R., et al. (2002). Detection of APC mutations in fecal DNA from patients with colorectal tumors. *New England Journal of Medicine, 346*(5), 311–320.

Tsui, N. B. Y., Ng, E. K. O., & Lo, Y. M. D. (2002). Stability of endogenous and added RNA in blood specimens, serum, and plasma. *Clinical Chemistry, 48*(10), 1647-53.

Tsui, N. B. Y., Ng, E. K. O., & Lo, Y. M. D. (2006). Molecular analysis of circulating RNA in plasma. *Methods in Molecular Biology, 336*, 123-34.

Turner, C. L., Casbard, A. C., & Murphy, M. F. (2003). Barcode technology: its role in increasing the safety of blood transfusion. *Transfusion, 43*(September), 1200-1209.

Uttayamakul, S., Likanonsakul, S., Sunthornkachit, R., Kuntiranont, K., Louisirirotchanakul, S., Chaovavanich, A., Thiamchai, V., et al. (2005). Usage of dried blood spots for molecular diagnosis and monitoring HIV-1 infection. *Journal of Virological Methods, 128*(1-2), 128-34.

Valadi, H., Ekström, K., Bossios, A., Sjöstrand, M., Lee, J. J., & Lötvall, J. O. (2007). Exosome-mediated transfer of mRNAs and microRNAs is a novel mechanism of genetic exchange between cells. *Nature Cell Biology, 9*(6), 654-9.

van 't Veer, L. J., Dai, H., van de Vijver, M. J., He, Y. D., Hart, A. a M., Mao, M., Peterse, H. L., van der Kooy, K., Marton, M. J., Witteveen, A. T., Schreiber, G. J., Kerkhoven, R. M., Roberts, C., Linsley, P. S., Bernards, R., & Friend S. H. (2002). Gene expression profiling predicts clinical outcome of breast cancer. *Nature, 415*(6871), 530-6.

van de Vijver, M. J., He, Y. D., van't Veer, L. J., Dai, H., Hart, A. A. M., Voskuil, D. W., Schreiber, G. J., Peterse, J. L., Roberts, C., Marton, M. J., Parrish, M., Atsma, D., Witteveen, A., Glas, A., Delhaye, L. van der Velde, T., Bartelink, H., Rodenhuis, S., Rutgers, E. T., Friend, S. H., & Bernards, R. (2002). A gene-expression signature as a predictor of survival in breast cancer. *The New England Journal of Medicine, 347*(25), 1999-2009.

Van Gelder, R. N., von Zastrow, M. E., Yool, A., Dement, W. C., Barchas, J. D., & Eberwine, J. H. (1990). Amplified RNA synthesized from limited quantities of heterogeneous cDNA. *Proceedings of the National Academy of Sciences of the United States of America, 87*(5), 1663-7.

van Schie, R. C., & Wilson, M. E. (1997). Saliva: a convenient source of DNA for analysis of bi-allelic polymorphisms of Fc gamma receptor IIA (CD32) and Fc gamma receptor IIIB (CD16). *Journal of Immunological Methods, 208*(1), 91-101.

Vartanian, K., Slottke, R., Johnstone, T., Casale, A., Planck, S. R., Choi, D., Smith, J. R., Rosenbaum, J. T., & Harrington, C. A. (2009). Gene expression profiling of whole blood: comparison of target preparation methods for accurate and reproducible microarray analysis. *BMC Genomics, 10*, 2.

Vidal-Taboada, J. M., Cucala, M., Mas Herrero, S., Lafuente, A., & Cobos, A. (2006). Satisfaction survey with DNA cards method to collect genetic samples for pharmacogenetics studies. *BMC Medical Genetics, 7*, 45.

Virgin, H. W., & Todd, J. A. (2011). Metagenomics and Personalized Medicine. *Cell, 147*(1), 44-56.

Wang, G, Tam, L. S., Li, E. K. M., Kwan, B. C. H., Chow, K. M., Luk, C. C. W., Li, P. K. T., & Szeto, C.-C. (2011). Serum and urinary free microRNA level in patients with systemic lupus erythematosus. *Lupus, 20*(5), 493-500.

Wang, G., Kwan, B. C.-H., Lai, F. M.-M., Chow, K.-M., Li, P. K.-T., & Szeto, C.-C. (2011). Elevated levels of miR-146a and miR-155 in kidney biopsy and urine from patients with IgA nephropathy. *Disease Markers, 30*(4), 171-9.

Wang, G., Tam, L.-S., Li, E. K.-M., Kwan, B. C.-H., Chow, K.-M., Luk, C. C.-W., Li, P. K.-T., & Szeto, C. –C. (2010). Serum and urinary cell-free MiR-146a and MiR-155 in patients with systemic lupus erythematosus. *The Journal of Rheumatology, 37*(12), 2516-22.

Wang, Jin, Chen, Jinyun, Chang, P., LeBlanc, A., Li, D., Abbruzzesse, J. L., Frazier, M. L., Killary, A. M., & Sen, S. (2009). MicroRNAs in plasma of pancreatic ductal adenocarcinoma patients as novel blood-based biomarkers of disease. *Cancer Prevention Research, 2*(9), 807-13.

Wang, Yuli, Li, Jun, Booher, R. N., Kraker, A., Lawrence, T., Leopold, W. R., & Sun, Y. (2001). Radiosensitization of p53 mutant cells by PD0166285 , a novel G 2 checkpoint abrogator. *Cancer Research*, 8211-8217.

Weber, D. G., Casjens, S., Rozynek, P., Lehnert, M., Zilch-Schöneweis, S., Bryk, O., Taeger, D., Gomolka, M., Kreuzer, M., Otten, H., Pesch, B., Johnen, G., & Brüning, T. (2010). Assessment of mRNA and microRNA stabilization in peripheral human blood for multicenter studies and biobanks. *Biomarker Insights, 5*, 95.

Weber, J. A., Baxter, D. H., Zhang, S., Huang, D. Y., How Huang, K., Jen Lee, M., Galas, D. J., & Wang, K. (2010). The microRNA spectrum in 12 body fluids. *Clinical Chemistry, 56*(11), 1733.

Wrensch, M. R., Petrakis, N. L., King, E. B., Miike, R., Mason, L., Chew, K. L., Lee, M. M., Ernster, V. L., Hilton, J. F., Schweitzer, R., Goodson, W. H., & Hunt, T. K. (1992). Breast cancer incidence in women with abnormal cytology in nipple aspirates of breast fluid. *American Journal of Epidemiology, 135*(2), 130-41.

Wrensch, M. R., Petrakis, N. L., Miike, R., King, E. B., Chew, K., Neuhaus, J., Lee, M. M., & Rhys, M. (2001). Breast cancer risk in women with abnormal cytology in nipple aspirates of breast fluid. *Journal of the National Cancer Institute, 93*(23), 1791-1798.

Wright, C., Bergstrom, D., Dai, H., Marton, M., Morris, M., Tokiwa, G., Wang, Y., & Fare, T. (2008). Characterization of globin RNA interference in gene expression profiling of whole-blood samples. *Clinical Chemistry, 54*(2), 396-405.

Yamada, Y., Enokida, H., Kojima, S., Kawakami, K., Chiyomaru, T., Tatarano, S., Yoshino, H., et al. (2011). MiR-96 and miR-183 detection in urine serve as potential tumor markers of urothelial carcinoma: correlation with stage and grade, and comparison with urinary cytology. *Cancer Science, 102*(3), 522-9.

Yao, Y., Richman, L., Morehouse, C., de los Reyes, M., Higgs, B. W., Boutrin, A., White, B., Coyle, A., Krueger, J., Kiener, P. A., Jallal, B. (2008). Type I interferon: potential therapeutic target for psoriasis? *PLoS One, 3*(7), e2737.

Young, G. P., & Bosch, L. J. W. (2011). Fecal Tests: From Blood to Molecular Markers. *Current Colorectal Cancer Reports, 7*(1), 62-70.

Zheng, P.-P., Luider, T. M., Pieters, R., Avezaat, C. J. J., van den Bent, M. J., Sillevis Smitt, P. A. E., & Kros, J. M. (2003). Identification of tumor-related proteins by proteomic analysis of cerebrospinal fluid from patients with primary brain tumors. *Journal of Neuropathology and Experimental Neurology, 62*(8), 855-62.

Zhu, W., Qin, W., Atasoy, U., & Sauter, E. R. (2009). Circulating microRNAs in breast cancer and healthy subjects. *BMC Research Notes, 2*, 89.

Zhu, W., Qin, W., Bradley, P., Wessel, A., Puckett, C. L., & Sauter, E. R. (2005). Mitochondrial DNA mutations in breast cancer tissue and in matched nipple aspirate fluid. *Carcinogenesis, 26*(1), 145-52.

Zubakov, D., Hanekamp, E., Kokshoorn, M., van Ijcken, W., & Kayser, M. (2008). Stable RNA markers for identification of blood and saliva stains revealed from whole genome expression analysis of time-wise degraded samples. *International Journal of Legal Medicine, 122*(2), 135-42.

14

Computer Simulation Model System for Interpretation and Validation of Algorithms for Monitoring of Cancer Patients by Use of Serial Serum Concentrations of Biomarkers in the Follow-Up After Surgical Procedures and Other Treatments – A Computer Simulation Model System Based on the Breast Cancer Biomarker TPA

Flemming Lund[1], György Sölétormos[1],
Merete Frejstrup Pedersen[1] and Per Hyltoft Petersen[1,2]
[1]*Department of Clinical Biochemistry, Hillerød Hospital, University of Copenhagen,*
[2]*Norwegian Quality Improvement of Primary Care Laboratories (NOKLUS), Section for General Practice, University of Bergen, Bergen,*
[1]*Denmark*
[2]*Norway*

1. Introduction

Concentrations of biomarkers for cancers (tumour markers) in plasma vary over time, and the ideal biomarker is a component which reflects the size of the tumour. Optimal interpretation of serial data on biomarkers during monitoring of patients following treatment of malignant disease is therefore vital for early prediction of reappearance of the tumour or metastases. Consequently, an ideal tumour biomarker will signal such reappearance before being detected by other relevant methods. On the other hand any false positive signals which can lead to superfluous investigations and unnecessary anxiety for the patient must be avoided. Because the biomarkers are produced in small amounts and released to plasma during healthy conditions, and because concentrations in plasma vary over time, it is necessary to be able to distinguish between true and false signals when serial measurements after treatment are to be interpreted. Here, different algorithms are proposed in literature, and this chapter deals with validation of some of these algorithms designed for the biomarker TPA (tissue polypeptide antigen) used in follow-up in treated breast tumours.

In contrast to the common statistics used for comparing two or several groups or some distributions, the purpose with the algorithms for bio-markers is to decide at each sampling and measurement time whether there is a reappearance of the tumour and whether or not there are metastases.

Several algorithms to interpret serial measurements of these markers for monitoring have been proposed and used in clinical trials. The simplest algorithm, used by all kit manufactures and included in their inserts, as also published by Barak et al. (1990), is a cut-off which defines relapse when the marker concentration exceeds this concentration. All algorithms include a cut-off, either directly in the interpretation or indirectly as an algorithm to be used either below or above the cut-off value. Some algorithms are based on two measurements (e.g. a minimum and the latest measured value) and crossing of the cut-off limit, while others include rules for the size of a critical difference of 25 % (Tondini & Hayes, 1989) or a doubling (Söletormos et al., 1996) or significant change (Söletormos et al., 1996) according to the reference change value (RCV) concept introduced by (Harris & Yasaka, 1983). An increase of 25% either below or above the cut-off for both measured concentrations (Dinistrian et al., 1991), and also a doubling or significant change when all measurements are above the cut-off value has been proposed (Söletormos et al., 1996). Others are based on three measurements, where the last measurement is a third, confirmatory test for the increase, and these have also been recommended when crossing the cut-off (Chan et al. 1997; Molina et al., 1995; Nicolini et al., 1991; Söletormos et al., 1996), in addition to algorithms where all measurements are below the cut-off (Bonfrer, 1990) as well as for situations where all measurements are above the cut-off (Bonfrer, 1990; Mughal et al., 1983; Söletormos et al., 1996).

All these algorithms give different signals for the same monitoring data, and a comparison of outcomes in the form of true positive and false positive results based on computer simulations of relevant monitoring situations has been performed (Söletormos et al., 2000b). These illustrate for each algorithm the advantages in terms of time to detection of reappearance, and disadvantages in the form of false positive signals. The basic biological and clinical data for estimated values of within-subject biological variation of serum-TPA (CV_B) during *steady-state* are available (Söletormos et al., 2000a). The rates of exponential increases in serum TPA during tumour growth are based on monitoring data from breast cancer patients (Söletormos et al., 2000a).

It has been demonstrated by Iglesias et al. (2005) that, for monitoring, the benefit of using the RCV (Harris & Yasaka, 1983) compared to a cut-off depends on the distance between the cut-off and the first measured concentration of the difference between two consecutive measurements to be compared to the RCV. When this distance is small, the probability of crossing the cut-off by the second measurement is higher than the probability of obtaining a significant change between the two measurements. Larger distances speak in favour of the reference change value.

The purpose of this chapter is to demonstrate the influence of the distance between the cut-off and the initial (baseline) concentration for TPA in serum in a simulation study like the paper on the tumour marker CA 15-3 (Petersen et al., 2011). This is done by challenging the different algorithms, where crossing the cut-off is part of the criterion, by computer simulations of various situations of monitoring breast cancer, imitating various exponential increases corresponding to recurrent cancer and a range of values of biological variation in order to validate the algorithms.

2. Interpretation of serial TPA concentrations

2.1 Materials and methods

The materials were data and parameters for breast cancer patients obtained from the literature (Söletormos et al., 1996; Söletormos et al., 2000a).

2.1.1 Cut-off

The cut-off concentration for TPA during treatment and follow-up of women with breast cancer is 95 U/L, recommended by the manufacture of the TPA kit (AB Sangtec Medical, Bromma, Sweden).

2.1.2 *Steady-state*, biological and analytical variation

The variations during the stable period of monitoring breast cancer patients are considered as *steady-state* and expressed as within-subject biological variation (CV_B) and analytical variation (CV_A) according to Sölétormos et al. (2000a). However, the within-subject biological variation, CV_B, is not homogeneous. Therefore CV_B for 5th, 50th and 95th percentile has been used with the analytical variation CV_A as a constant.

For TPA the 50th percentile for within-subject biological variation, CV_B%, is 24.5% and analytical variation, CV_A%, is 8.4%.

For TPA the 95th percentile of within-subject biological variation, CV_B%, is 48.9% and analytical variation, CV_A%, is 8.4%

For TPA the 5th percentile of within-subject biological variation, CV_B%, is 8.5% and analytical variation, CV_A%, is 8.4% (Söletormos et al., 2000a).

2.1.3 Tumour biomarker increase

The estimated values for the rate of increase (λ) in biomarkers after relapse in women with breast cancer are available (Söletormos et al., 2000a). The increase is assumed to be exponential ($e^{\lambda t}$) and the λ-values for the 5%, 50%, and 95% percentiles are 0.0132, 0.0346, and 0.0907, respectively (Söletormos et al., 2000a).

2.1.4 Algorithms

Barak et al. {1}:

Two consecutive measurements. The first below and the second above cut-off (Barak et al., 1990).

Tondini & Hayes {2}:

At least two measurements. The last measurement is above cut-off and at least 25% higher than any previous measurement below the cut-off concentration (Tondini & Hayes, 1989).

Söletormos et al. A {3}:

At least two measurements. The last measurement is above cut-off and at least twice (doubling) of any previous measurement below the cut-off (Söletormos et al., 1996).

Chan et al. {4}:

Three consecutive measurements. The last and middle concentrations are both above the cut-off and the first is below the cut-off (Chan et al., 1997).

Söletormos et al. B {5}:

At least three measurements. The last concentration is higher than the penultimate concentration and both are above the cut-off. The penultimate concentration is significantly higher than any previous measurement below the cut-off (Söletormos et al., 1996).

Molina et al. {6}:

Three consecutive measurements. The first concentration is below twice the cut-off (doubling) and the last two are both above twice the cut-off (doubling) (Molina et al., 1995).

Nicolini et al. {7}:

Three consecutive measurements. The first measured concentration is below the cut-off. The middle concentration is above the cut-off and the last measured concentration is >30 % higher than the middle measured concentration (Nicolini et al., 1991).

2.1.5 Methods

The basic principles and methods have been presented previously (Petersen et al., 2011; Söletormos et al., 2000b), and the basic model and the additional calculations of results for the varying start concentrations of TPA between the cut-off and these initial concentrations are described in detail below.

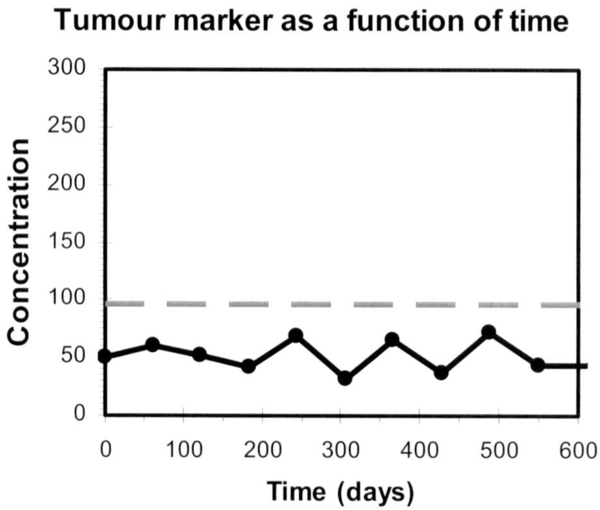

Illustration of simulated data for steady-state concentrations (-•-), with a mean concentration 50 U/L, CV_B = 24.5% and CV_A = 8.5%. Baseline (starting) concentration 50 U/L and the cut-off concentration, 95 U/L, (- - - -). Sampling frequency every two months (61 days).

Fig. 1A. *Steady-state* graph

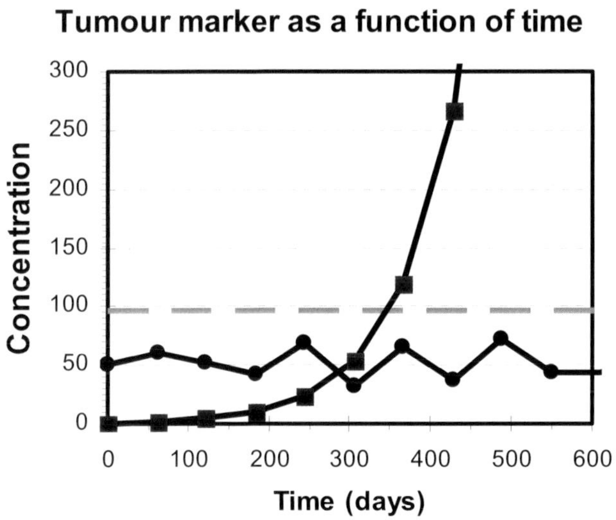

Illustration of simulated data for steady-state concentrations (-•-), with a mean concentration 50 U/L, CV_B = 24.5% and CV_A = 8.5%, and tumours with exponential growth λ = 0.0132 (-■-)), according to 0.95* $e^{\lambda^* t}$ U/L. Baseline (starting) concentration 50 U/L and the cut-off concentration, 95 U/L, (- - - -). Sampling frequency every two months (61 days).

Fig. 1B. *Steady-state* and tumour growth graphs.

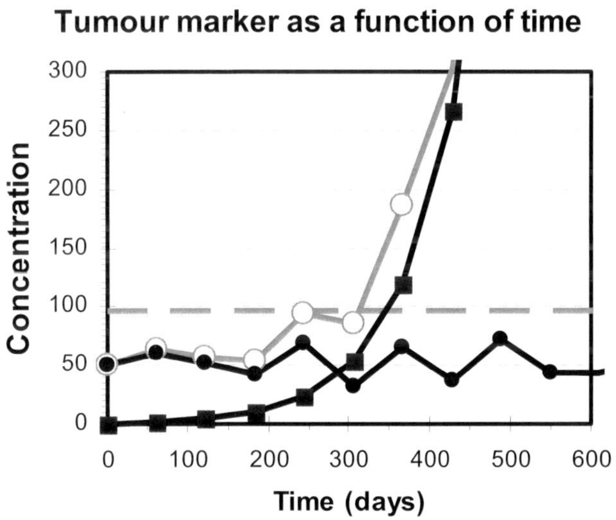

Illustration of simulated data for steady-state concentrations (-•-), with a mean concentration 50 U/L, CV_B = 24.5% and CV_A = 8.5%, and tumour with exponential growth λ = 0.0132 (-■-)),according to 0.95* $e^{\lambda^* t}$ U/L. Baseline (starting) concentration for the course is 50 U/L and the cut-off concentration, 95 U/L, (- - - -). Sampling frequency every two months (61 days). The (-○-) graph is the addition result of steady-state concentrations (-•-) plus 0.95* $e^{\lambda^* t}$ U/L.

Fig. 1C. Steady-state, tumour growth and resulting graphs.

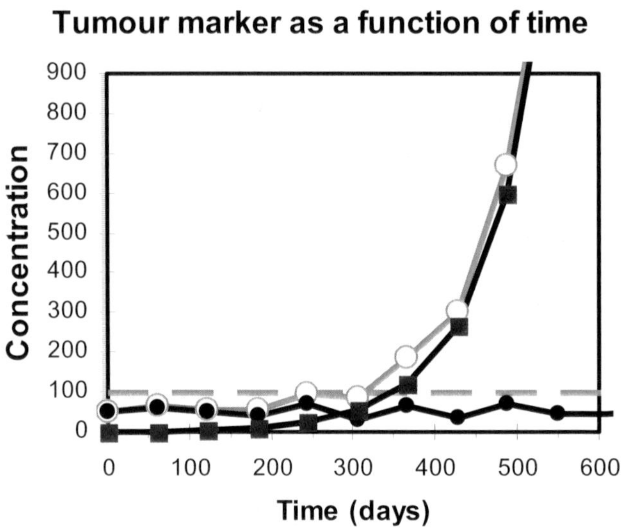

The same as fig. 1C except chanced scale of concentrations U/L. The resulting graph and the exponential graph will in time be nearly indistinguishable, here after approx. 500 days.

Fig. 1D. Steady-state, tumour growth and resulting graphs.

2.1.6 Basic simulation

Simulation of concentration data using Microsoft Excel version 2003.

2.1.7 Steady-state

For each patient, a series of "concentrations" of biomarker was calculated from simulated data as a function of time 'after treatment'. For each 'sample' during *steady-state* conditions, the resulting concentration value ($\mathbf{c}_{ij}$) is calculated from a chosen '*steady-state*' concentration ($\mathbf{c}_{s\text{-}s}$) with the addition of a random number ($random_i$) from a Gaussian distribution multiplied by 'the *steady-state* within-subject biological variation' (CV_B), plus a new random number ($random_j$) from a Gaussian distribution multiplied by the analytical variation (CV_A) according to the model (Bliss, 1967):

$$\mathbf{c}_{ij} = \mathbf{c}_{s\text{-}s} * [1 + random_i * CV_B \%/100 + random_j * CV_A \%/100]$$

This is performed for 50 samples in series, numbered from 1 to 50 and each corresponding to a specific day of monitoring when sampling is performed every two months (61 days), and further performed for each patient with new random Gaussian numbers for a total of 1000 surrogate patients. The result is a series of random concentration values with a mean close to the chosen value ($\mathbf{c}_{s\text{-}s}$). Fig. 1A illustrates a steady-state situation, where the fluctuations are based on within- subject biological variation (CV_B) plus analytical imprecision variation (CV_A).

2.1.8 Tumour growth

Based on data from Sölétormos *et al.* (1997, 2000a), increases in biomarkers are shown to be associated with progression of disease and it is found that the concentrations of biomarkers have an exponential relation with time. However, the rate of tumour growth can vary considerably. The rate of increase is expressed as λ in the exponential function as a factor in the exponent in $e^{\lambda t}$ or as $\exp(\lambda t)$. The rate of increase λ (also called slope) was calculated for TPA in patients Sölétormos *et al.* (2000a) and found as 5th percentile (λ = 0.0132), as 50th percentile (λ = 0.0346) and as 95th percentile (λ = 0.0907). Therefore, in the simulation model tumour growth is described as an exponential increase in the biomarker TPA. The start concentration (t = 0) of the biomarker originating from the tumour is arbitrarily selected as an amount corresponding to a concentration 100 times lower than the cut-off concentration (0.95 U/L). The resulting function of the TPA from the tumour is then expressed as $0.95e^{\lambda t}$ or as 0.95 $\exp(\lambda t)$. See Fig 1B as an example of an exponential tumour growth where λ = 0.0132.

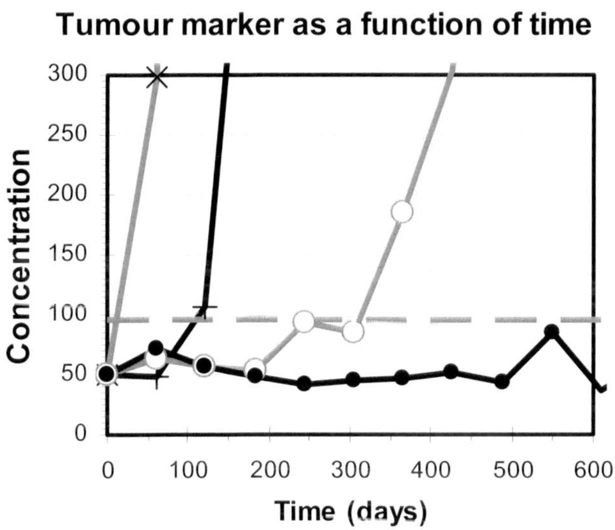

Illustration of simulated data for steady-state concentrations (-•-), with a mean concentration 50 U/L and CV_B = 24.5% and CV_A = 8.5%., and tumours with exponential growth λ = 0.0132 (-○-), λ = 0.0346(-+-) , and λ = 0.0907 (-x-) according to 0.95* $e^{\lambda * t}$ U/L. Baseline (starting) concentration for the four courses is 50 U/L and the cut-off concentration, 95 U/L, (- - - -). Sampling frequency every two months (61 days).

Fig. 2. Different rates of tumour growth increase.

As a resulting graph the tumour concentration is now added to the *steady-state* concentration (*steady-state* concentration + initial tumour (0.95 U/L)). An example is illustrated in Fig 1C. At first, the resulting graph has nearly the same concentration as the *steady-state* graph, but after some time TPA products from the tumour take over as the dominating contributor. Thereafter *steady-state* concentrations might be neglected as the resulting graph will be close to the exponential tumour graph (see Fig 1D). This process is repeated until a total of 1000 'patient pathways' are evaluated using the same parameters. In Fig 2 is illustrated an example of the resulting graphs from 3 different rates of tumour increases (slopes = λ) and a steady-state situation where λ = 0. When λ is high, the biomarker will increase fast and correspondingly the smaller slopes will show later increases.

2.1.9 Testing the algorithms by application to the simulated data

For each 'patient', the investigated algorithm is applied in sequential order and when a sample is positive according to the algorithm, it is recorded as a positive biomarker signal (POS). Summing up all the 1000 simulated 'patients', the percentage that are positive in each sample number (same days) is calculated, resulting in a growing graph in a plot of percentage biomarker positive as a function of sample number or day/months. This is illustrated in figure 3 for four different values of λ, including zero (= *steady-state*).

The slopes become steeper for increasing λ-values, which means that the detection of tumour growth is earlier for fast growing tumours, as expected. The POS signals for the *steady-state* situation (λ = 0.000) represent false positive signals (in the example in Fig. 3 it is 0% after 600 days, approximately 20 months). In *steady-state,* POS signals will be recorded as false positive because no tumour growth is simulated, and therefore the POS signals cannot be considered true positives. For the three other graphs, the POS signals are recorded as true positives because an exponential tumour growth is simulated. In validation of the different algorithms, the time for 100% POS is important, but from a theoretical point of view, the most interesting variables are the lowest □-values (0.000 and 0.0123), which are the most difficult to distinguish - and at the same time very important for follow-up of tumour-producing biomarkers after surgery, chemotherapy etc.

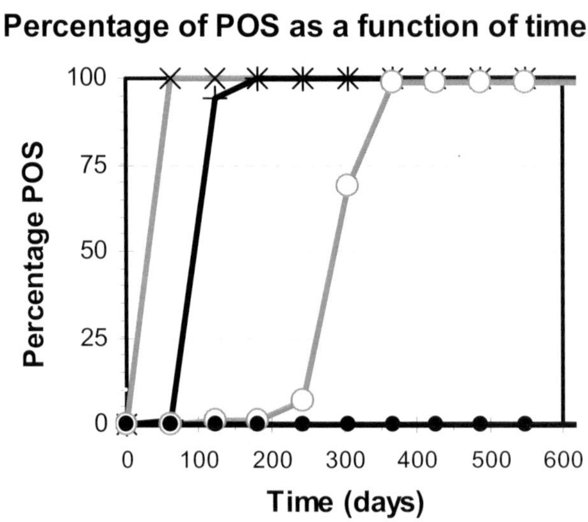

Illustration of the algorithm from Barak et al.{1} considered POS when the concentration first exceeds the cut-off (TPA = 95U/L). Percentage POS as a function of time for four different exponential increases with λ = 0.0132 (-○-), λ = 0.0346 (-+-), and λ = 0.0907 (-x-) according to 0.95* $e^{\lambda * t}$ U/L. The steady-state simulation is represented by λ = 0.0000 (-•-).

Fig. 3. Percentage positive patients (POS) as a function of time.

2.1.10 Varying *steady-state* and start (baseline) concentrations

For each algorithm, a number of steady-state and start concentrations are used (2.38, 4.75, 9.5, 14.3, 19.0, 23.8, 28.5, 38.0, 47.5, 57.0, 66.5, 76.0, 85.5, and 95.0 U/L) where the concentration in the first 'sample' is fixed at 0.1 % below the stated concentration in order to ensure that at least one sample from each 'patient' is below the cut-off threshold. The percentage of positives at a certain time/sample is illustrated as a function of the starting concentration for each algorithm (see e.g. Fig 4).

2.1.11 Biological variation of tumour growth

As defined in the tumour growth situation, the exponential function is added to the steady-state including a biological variation CV_B. This exponential function can further be varied by multiplying the concentration due to the exponential function by a random factor times 0.25, which corresponds to an extra biological variation in tumour growth of 25 %.

As previously defined, the tumour growth is expressed as an exponential function: $0.95*e^{\lambda t}$, where λ is the slope and t is the time (days or months). The 25% extra biological variation within the tumour growth is then expressed with:

$$(1 + random_k*0.25)*0.95*e^{\lambda t},$$

where $random_k$ is a new random number from a Gaussian distribution, and the start concentration of tumour growth is still expressed by the factor 0.95, when t = 0, i.e. 1% of cut-off concentration.

2.2 Results

Results for each algorithm are presented with illustrations of the characteristics for each algorithm.

2.2.1 Algorithm {1} Barak et al.

Two consecutive measurements. The first below and the second above the cut-off (Barak et al., 1990).

In Fig. 4, the fastest tumour growth (λ = 0.0907) is 100 % percentages positive (POS) after two months for all start concentrations (sample 2), whereas the remaining graphs have almost the same development, with POS increasing from 0% at approximately 57 U/L to approximately 50% POS at 95 U/L. After six months (sample 4), the next lower slope (λ = 0.0346) reaching 100% POS for all start concentrations, whereas the lowest slope (λ = 0.0132) and *steady-state* (λ = 0.0000) slowly increase to approximately 85% POS near the cut-off of 95 U/L. At ten months (sample 6), the slowest tumour growth has separated from the *steady-state* concentrations, increasing from 0 to 100% POS for starting concentrations between 30 and 70 U/L, and false positive (FP) is still zero up to approximately 57 U/L, but has increased to 97% at 95 U/L.

It is clear from Fig. 4 that true positive (TP) graphs increase with increasing starting concentrations, whereas FP graphs are zero for the low starting concentrations and increase over time for starting concentrations above 57 U/L.

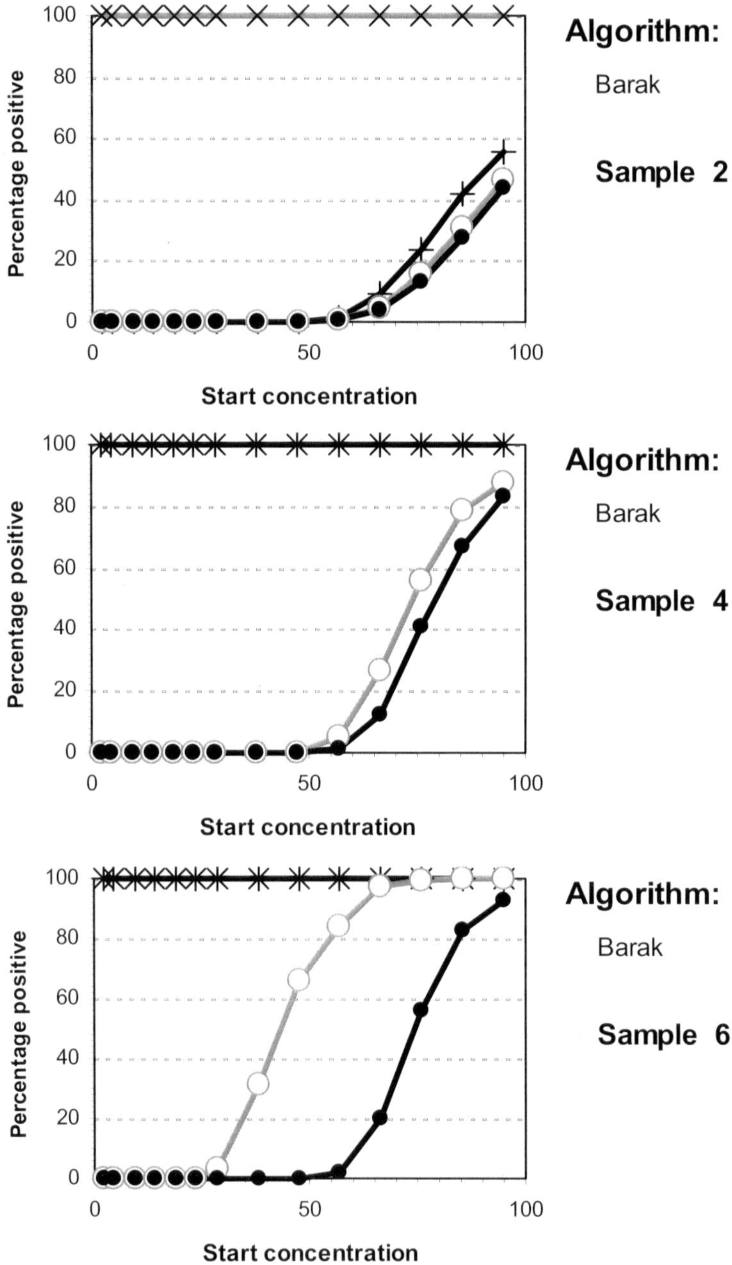

Percentage positive (POS) as a function of starting concentration (TPA U/L) for algorithm {1} Barak et al. after 2 months (sample 2), 6 months (sample 4) and 10 months (sample 6). Same slope symbols as in Fig. 2.

Fig. 4. Percentages positive signals at three different times.

With the only criterion as crossing the cut-off, the algorithm {1} from Barak et al. is very simple. In this way the time for progression detection is short – however the percentages of FP are unacceptably high - especially with start concentrations near cut-off - i.e. from approx 57 U/L to cut-off (95 U/L). After 1 year the FP is 98% near the cut-off.

In comparison with the other algorithms, which all have more restrictive criteria for recording a positive signal (POS) as in progression of tumour growth, the percentage of FP results decreases. Table 1 lists FP after one and two years, and the algorithm Barak et al. {1} has the highest FP (i.e. 98%) rate in 'patients'. However, if the start concentration is below 57 U/L, the algorithm Barak et al. {1} has only few percentages FP (i.e. 3%) and at the same time the fastest detection time for progression. Only Tondini & Hayes {2} has comparable "good" POS results for TPA.

2.2.2 Algorithm {2} Tondini & Hayes

Two consecutive measurements. The last measurement is above the cut-off and at least 25% higher than any previous concentration below the cut-off value (Tondin & Hayes, 1989).

The only difference between algorithm Barak et al. {1} and algorithm Tondini & Hayes {2} is that, in the latter algorithm, the criterion is 25% higher concentration above cut-off compared to the lowest value below cut-off. Many (simulated) patients will be recorded similarly as algorithm Barak et al. {1} - especially with low start concentration. Therefore, the performances of these two algorithms are comparable. Algorithm Tondini & Hayes {2} shows only moderately lower percentages of positives (POS) for the lower tumour growths and the steady-state situation at 6 months, i.e. also slightly lower FP between 55 and 95 U/L during the first half of the year (compare Fig. 4 and Fig. 5 at sample 4).

Although there are a few more restrictions in algorithm Tondini & Hayes {2}, the detection time for TP patients is practically the same – however, the percentage of FP is still unacceptable with start concentrations near cut-off.

2.2.3 Algorithm {3} Sölétormos et al. A

At least two measurements. The last measurement is above cut-off and at least 100% higher than any previous measurement below the cut-off (doubling) (Söletormos et al., 1996).

This algorithm is comparable to the algorithm Tondini & Hayes {2}. The only difference is that the increase is not 25% but 100% for the last concentration over cut-off. In other words the three first algorithms are very similar.

The slightly more restrictive criterion with algorithm Söletormos et al. A {3} results in much lower FP signals with start concentrations near cut-off (see Fig. 5). For example the percentages of FP signals are reduced from 98% by algorithm Barak et al. {1} to 32% by algorithm Söletormos et al. A {3} after 1 year just below 95 U/L (cut-off) (see Table 1). However, after 6 months it is not possible to distinguish between the slowest tumour growth and healthy steady-state patients (see Fig. 5). Comparison of the algorithm from Söletormos et al. A {3} with Barak et al. {1} and Tondini & Hayes {2} shows nearly the same results with low start concentrations (below 57 U/L) where all three algorithms have only few FP signals.

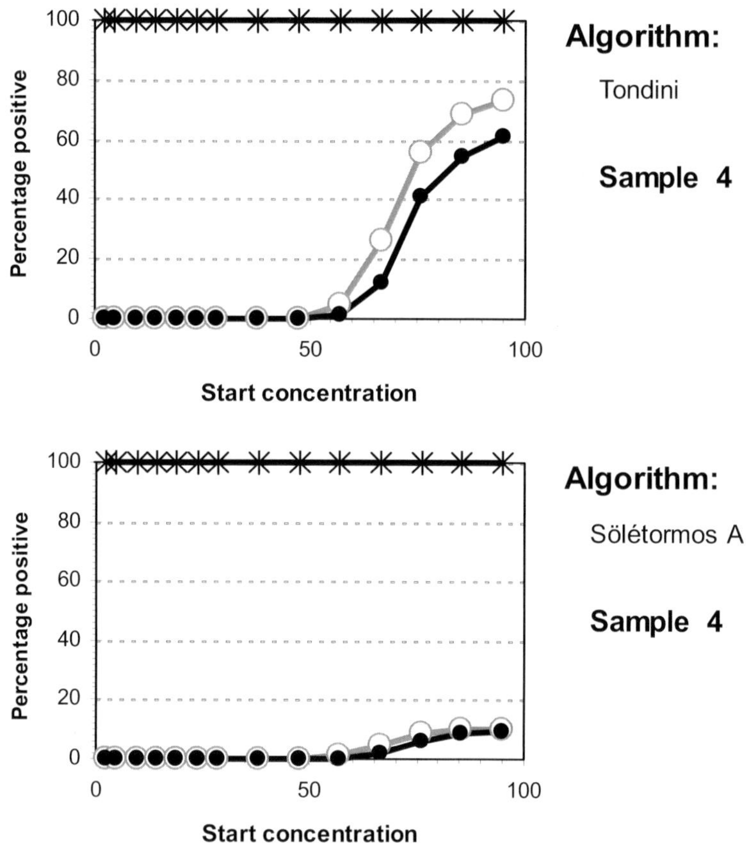

Comparison of the algorithms of algorithm {2} Tondini & Hayes, and algorithm {3} Söletormos et al. A at 6 months (sample 4). Percentage positive (POS) as a function of starting concentration as for Fig. 3. The only difference between the two algorithms is the size of increase after crossing the cut-off, i.e. 25% and 100%, respectively. For symbols see Fig. 3.

Fig. 5. Comparison of two different algorithms.

All three algorithms have also the same tumour detection time – except Söletormos et al. A {3} which has extended the time by two months for the slowest tumour growth (see Table 1).

The next four algorithms presented here - all have a characteristic in common – they all need at least three measurements. As a consequence, the earliest detection time for tumour progression is 4 months. In Table 1, these algorithms are marked with a footnote: 'Three sample points are needed'.

2.2.4 Algorithm {4} Chan et al.

Three consecutive measurements. The last and penultimate concentrations are both above the cut-off, and the first measured concentration is below cut-off (Chan et al., 1997).

The algorithm Chan et al.{4} appears similar to algorithm Barak et al. {1} with the addition of a confirmation of crossing the cut-off. When the graph is crossing the cut-off (95 U/L) - the next sample should also be above cut-off. In this way the percentage FP signals may be reduced – from 98% FP by algorithm Barak et al. {1} to 64% FP by algorithm Chan et al. {4} after 1 year below 95 U/L. As a consequence - the detection times are correspondingly 2 months later for all 3 slopes.

Algorithm	Slope 0.0907: 100% at time	Slope 0.0346: 100% at time	Slope 0.0123: 100% at time	False positive below 95 U/L at 1 year	False positive below 95 U/L at 2 years	False positive below 57 U/L at 1 year	False positive below 57 U/L at 2 years
Barak et al. {1}	2 months	6 months	12 months	98%	100%	3%	4%
Tondini and Hayes {2}	2 months	6 months	12 months	91%	100%	3%	4%
Söletormos et al. A {3}	2 months	6 months	14 months	32%	70%	2%	3%
Chan et al. {4}	[4 months][1]	8 months	14 months	64%	91%	0%	0%
Söletormos et al. B {5}	[4 months][1]	8 months	16 months	6%	24%	0%	0%
Molina et al. {6}	[4 months][1]	8 months	16 months	0%	0%	0%	0%
Nicolini et al. {7}	[4 months][1]	[8 months][2]	[14 months][3]	6%	10%	0%	0%

[1]Three sample points are needed for the algorithm. [2] Only at start concentrations below 57 U/L obtain 100%. [3]Only at start concentrations below 28 U/L obtain 100%.

Times for detection of 100 % tumour progression using the different algorithms are listed for three slopes. Percentages of false positive results after 1 and 2 years with TPA start concentrations below 95 U/L and 57 U/L for each algorithm are also listed. All results are generated from 1000 computer simulations.

Table 1. Performance results from seven algorithms.

2.2.5 Algorithm {5} Sölétormos et al. B

At least three measurements. The last measured concentration is higher than the penultimate concentration, both above the cut-off, and higher than the third to last measured concentration. The penultimate concentration is significantly higher than any previous measurements below the cut-off (Söletormos et al., 1996).

In a comparison of algorithm Chan et al. {4} with algorithm Söletormos et al. B {5}, the latter algorithm is much more restrictive in recording positive signals (POS). The last measurement demands an increase compared to the penultimate value – and this penultimate value has to have a significant increase compared to earlier measurements (see below). The more restrictive criteria are shown to give much lower FP signals – even after two years, the percentages of FP results are 24% compared to 91% at algorithm Chan et al. {4} below 95 U/L. Again more restrictive criteria have a 'cost' in regard to detection time - here at the slowest slope, which is extended by two months at algorithm Söletormos et al. B {5}. On the other hand these algorithms show only 0% FP results at low start concentrations, i.e. below 57 U/L.

The significant increase, or reference change value (RCV), was introduced by Harris and Yasaka (1983) in order to detect a significant change in consecutive measurements, and was defined as RCV = $1.96*2^{1/2}*CV_B$, where the 1.96 is the standard deviation from a Gaussian distribution corresponding to a two-tailed probability of 5 %, and $2^{1/2}$ relates to the variation of differences $CV_{Difference} = (CV_B^2 + CV_B^2)^{1/2}$ or the CV_B^2 can be substituted by the combination of biological and analytical variation. The calculation in the computer system is the test of the difference between two consecutive measurements (as a percentage) in regard to the RCV.

2.2.6 Algorithm {6} Molina et al.

Three consecutive measurements. The first is below cut-off and the next two measurements are both over double the cut-off value (Molina et al., 1995).

This algorithm Molina et al. {6} is comparable with algorithm Chan et al. {4} - a confirmation of crossing cut-off with an extra sample - but at algorithm Molina et al.{6}, there is a doubling of the cut-off (to 190 U/L).

This very restrictive criterion results in 0% FP results – even also near cut-off. This algorithm has the lowest number of FP, i.e. 0%, in comparison to all the other algorithms. And, again, strict restrictions inhibit the ability to detect early tumour progression – algorithm Molina et al. {6} has the longest detection time shared with algorithm Söletormos et al.B {5} and algorithm Nicolini et al {7}.

2.2.7 Algorithm {7} Nicolini et al.

Three consecutive measurements. The first measured concentration is below the cut-off, the middle measured concentration is above the cut-off and the last is more than 30% higher than the middle value (7).

The algorithm Nicolini et al. {7} can also be compared with algorithm Chan et al. A crossing of cut-off has to be confirmed by a new sample – but this new sample has to be 30% higher compared to the second measurement over cut-off.

This 30% higher concentration for the two last measurements is difficult to fulfil for the two slowest tumour growths for starting concentrations just below the cut-off. The exponential function simulated from tumour growth has to have some time before an increase effect is observed in the results. As a consequence, the graphs decrease with increasing starting concentrations without the possibility of giving a positive signal (POS), because when crossing the cut-off too slowly, there will never be a POS signal. This is illustrated in Fig. 6 where the graphs for sample 10 and sample 13 are almost identical.

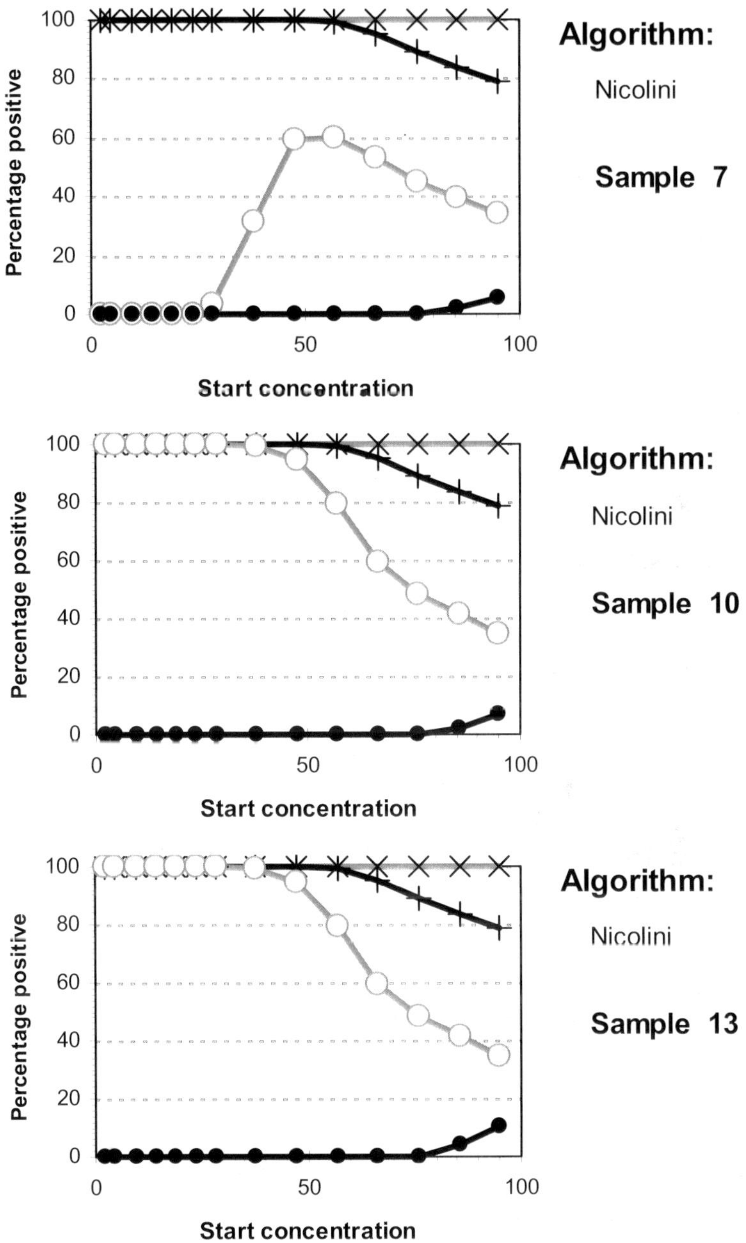

Percentage positive (POS) as a function of starting concentration for algorithm {7} Nicolini et al. after 1 year (sample 7), after 18 months (sample 10), and after two years (sample 13). After sample 8 (14 months) the figures will "freeze" and be identical for the three tumour slopes.

Fig. 6. Results from Algorithm {7} Nicolini et al. at different times

It has to be underlined that, in this way, the algorithm Nicolini et al. {7} will never achieve 100% POS with start concentrations near cut-off. The 100% POS will only be fulfilled at start concentrations below 28 U/L, for the two slowest slopes (see footnotes in Table 1)

2.2.8 Overall results

The characteristics for the seven algorithms are summarised in Table 1 with the time for 100% true positive results (TP) for each slope of tumour growth, and with percentage false positive (FP) at two years for both start concentrations of 57 U/L and 95 U/L (cut-off).

The two first algorithms (Barak et al. {1} and Tondini & Hayes {2}) in Table 1 show the fastest time to detect 100% positive signals in patients for each of the investigated three slopes. However, these algorithms also show the highest percentage of false positive (FP) signals, both after 1 and 2 years. All the other algorithms also show FP results of lower and varying percentages - except algorithm Molina et al. {6} with zero FP. The algorithm Molina et al. {6} on the other hand also needs the longest time for 100% positive results shared with algorithm Söletormos et al. B {5}. The algorithm Nicolini et al. {7} has partly the same long time, but only at start concentrations below 57 U/L and below 28 U/L for the slopes 0.0346 and 0.0132, respectively. Above these start concentrations, the algorithm Nicolini et al. {7} will never obtain 100% positive results (see also Fig 6). In other words after 14 months the two slowest slopes will "freeze" and have the same results. Only FP percentages will increase slowly.

Overall, all the algorithms are comparable when the start concentrations are below 57 U/l with only few FP results for the algorithms from Barak et al. {1}, Tondini & Hayes {2} and Söletormos et al. A {3}. The other algorithms are even better as regards the percentage of FP results. However, they need longer time for detection of tumour progression.

In the clinical situation, when the TPA start concentration is below 57 U/L, it should be recommended to use the algorithm Barak et al. {1} in order to obtain an early detection of tumour progression. However, when the TPA start concentration is above 57 U/L and up to just below 95 U/L, it should be recommended to use the algorithm Molina et al. {6}– even with a longer detection of tumour progression – in order to avoid any false positive signals.

In a clinical situation using the Nicolini et al. {7} algorithm, several patients with slow tumour growth and with high biomarker (TPA) start concentration near cut-off will never be recorded as positive tumour patients – hopefully treatment action will be taken based on high concentrations or other clinical signals.

In this investigation the performances of the algorithms have been studied using results from the biomarker TPA. The same procedure has been used on the same algorithms with results from the biomarker CA 15-3 (Petersen et al., 2011). The results from these two investigations are very similar. The properties from the algorithms on detection time of progression, the percentages of false positive patients (FP), the dependence on start concentration both near cut-off and approx half cut-off – all the overall characteristic results and figures from each algorithm were relatively identical using different biomarkers, i.e. TPA and CA 15-3.

These results indicate that the relative performance of the investigated algorithms for early detection of tumour progression and avoiding FP results - seems to be independent of the biomarker in the present model and set-up.

It must be underlined that this statement may only be valid based on general considerations. For example biomarkers with relative low *steady-state* variation combined with high rates of tumour increase may change some of the algorithm performances according to the detection time of progression and percentage of FP signals. In this situation the performance from algorithm Nicolini et al. {7} could be better, because start concentration near cut-off may achieve 100% TP signals within an acceptable timeframe compared with a never ending timeframe in this TPA investigation. Nevertheless, the relative information from the algorithms on performance will still stand. In other words - the best ability to detect tumour progression will often be obtained by using the algorithm from Barak et al. {1} and the best ability to get low FP signals will often be obtained by using the algorithm from Molina et al. {6} - and this is noteworthy: independent of the biomarker.

2.2.9 Performance of the algorithms with impact from extreme values of within-subject biological variation (CV_B)

An important assumption for calculation of within-subject biological variation as the square root of the mean of the variances from the individual coefficients of variation of reference individuals in projects on biological variation is that these variations are distributed homogeneously. If there is variance homogeneity, this pooled coefficient of variance represents all individuals of the reference group and it is correct to use this pooled CV_B in the simulations as a factor for the random Gaussian values. This assumption, however, is not fulfilled for TPA (Sölétormos et al. 2000a), where the range of coefficients of variation goes from 8.5% and 48.9% and represents individual CV_B-values, from which the extreme values used for the challenging of algorithms in the simulations are selected.

The results in Table 1 are based on CV_B = 24.5% (within-subject biological variation). This value is based on a 50th percentile from an investigation on 127 patients (Söletormos et al., 2000b). Due to the lack of variance homogeneity, we have also investigated the impact on the results from the algorithms based on a 95th percentile where CV_B = 48.9%.

The results for CV_B = 48.9% are listed in Table 2 where it can be seen that the detection times for tumour progression are practically the same as for the 50th percentile of biological variation. Only algorithm Söletormos et al. B {5} shows a 2 months later detection time for a slope of 0.0123. Nearly all algorithms show an increased percentage of false positive signals (the four first algorithms are already close to 100 % for $CV_{B,}$ = 24.5% for the highest start concentrations) with the higher biological variation CV_B. Only the algorithm Molina et al. {6} maintains 0% FP results in situations with high biological variations. It should also be noted that the algorithm results from Söletormos et al. A {3} and Söletormos et al. B {5} both markedly increase the number of FP results, when the biological variation, CV_B, is high and the start concentration is below cut-off. For Söletormos et al. B {5} this is partly due to the algorithm, where the significant change in the criterion is based on the 50th percentile of biological variation CV_B = 24.5% whereas the simulation is based on the much higher extreme CV_B = 48.9%. Consequently the use of significant change in the algorithm makes it sensitive to lack of variance homogeneity.

Algorithm	Slope 0.0907: 100% at time	Slope 0.0346: 100% at time	Slope 0.0123: 100% at time	False-positive below 95 U/L at 1 year	False positive below 95 U/L at 2 years	False positive below 57 U/L at 1 year	False positive below 57 U/L at 2 years
Barak et al. {1}	2 months (2 months)	6 months (6 months)	12 months (12 months)	98% (98%)	100% (100%)	45% (3%)	70% (4%)
Tondini and Hayes {2}	2 months (2 months)	6 months (6 months)	12 months (12 months)	95% (91%)	100% (100%)	45% (3%)	70% (4%)
Söletormos et al. A {3}	2 months (2 months)	6 months (6 months)	14 months (14 months)	76% (32%)	98% (70%)	35% (2%)	65% (3%)
Chan et al. {4}	[4 months][1] ([4months][1])	8 months (8 months)	14 months (14 months)	65% (64%)	91% (91%)	6% (0%)	13% (0%)
Söletormos et al. B {5}	[4 months][1] ([4months][1])	8 months (8 months)	18 months (16 months)	19% (6%)	47% (24%)	3% (0%)	7% (0%)
Molina et al. {6}	[4 months][1] ([4months][1])	8 months (8 months)	16 months (16 months)	0% (0%)	0% (0%)	0% (0%)	0% (0%)
Nicolini et al. {7}	[4 months][1] ([4months][1])	[8 months][2] ([8 months][2])	[14 months][4] ([14 months][3])	16% (6%)	29% (10%)	0% (0%)	0% (0%)

[1]Three sample points are needed for the algorithm. [2] Only at start concentrations below 57 U/L obtain 100%. [3]Only at start concentrations below 28 U/L obtain 100%. [4] Only at start concentration below 19 U/L. Test of robustness of the algorithms when the biological variation, CV_B, is increased from 24.5% to 48.9%. Times for detection of tumor progression using the different algorithms are listed for three slopes. Percentages false positive results (FP) after 1 and 2 years with TPA start concentrations below 95 U/L and 57 U/L for each algorithm are also listed. All results are generated from 1000 computer simulations. Results from biological variation of CV_B = 48.9% and CV_B = 24.5% just below in (brackets).

Table 2. Performance of seven algorithms with increased biological variation.

On the other hand the results indicate that the algorithm from Molina et al. {6} is most robust against increased biological variation CV_B values.

In the other extreme situation with a very low biological variation 5th percentile (CV_B = 8.5%), the performances from the algorithms are listed in Table 3.

The most striking results in the table is the impact from low biological variation CV_B on the false positive number (FP) from algorithm Söletormos et al. A {3} and algorithm Söletormos et al. B {5}. These algorithms show low percentage of FP results, when the biological variation CV_B is low – and on the other hand - a high number of FP results when the biological variation CV_B is high, as discussed above. It should also be noted that the detection time for the slowest slope is two months earlier for Söletormos et al. A {3}, who at the same time show very low percentages of FP signals. In a clinical situation with a patient, where the biological variation is known to be low, the best algorithm for interpreting monitoring biomarker results will thus be the algorithm Söletormos et al. A {3}. In this situation very early detection times are combined with very low FP signals. It is notable that the algorithms {1} Barak et al., {2} Tondini and Hayes and {4} Chan et al. for the high start concentrations have high percentages of FP after two years.

Algorithm	Slope 0.0907: 100% at time	Slope 0.0346: 100% at time	Slope 0.0123: 100% at time	False-positive below 95 U/L at 1 year	False positive below 95 U/L at 2 years	False positive below 57 U/L at 1 year	False positive below 57 U/L at 2 years
Barak et al. {1}	2 months (2 months)	6 months (6 months)	12 months (12 months)	98% (98%)	100% (100%)	0% (3%)	0% (4%)
Tondini and Hayes {2}	2 months (2 months)	6 months (6 months)	12 months (12 months)	65% (91%)	94% (100%)	0% (3%)	0% (4%)
Söletormos et al. A {3}	2 months (2 months)	6 months (6 months)	12 months (14 months)	1% (32%)	1% (70%)	0% (2%)	0% (3%)
Chan et al. {4}	[4 months][1] ([4months][1])	8 months (8 months)	14 months (14 months)	68% (64%)	92% (91%)	0% (0%)	0% (0%)
Söletormos et al. B {5}	[4 months][1] ([4months][1])	8 months (8 months)	14 months (16 months)	0% (6%)	0% (24%)	0% (0%)	0% (0%)
Molina et al. {6}	[4 months][1] ([4months][1])	8 months (8 months)	16 months (16 months)	0% (0%)	0% (0%)	0% (0%)	0% (0%)
Nicolini et al. {7}	[4 months][1] ([4months][1])	[8 months][2] ([8 months][2])	[14 months][2] ([14 months][3])	0% (6%)	0% (10%)	0% (0%)	0% (0%)

[1]Three sample points are needed for the algorithm. [2] Only at start concentrations below 57 U/L obtain 100%. [3]Only at start concentrations below 28 U/L obtain 100%.
Test of robustness of the algorithms when the biological variation is decreased from CV_B = 24.5% to CV_B = 8.5%. Times for detection of tumor progression using the different algorithms are listed for three slopes. Percentages false positive results after 1 and 2 years with TPA start concentrations below 95 U/L and 57 U/L for each algorithm are also listed. All results are generated from 1000 computer simulations. Results from biological variation of CV_B = 8.5% and CV_B = 24.5 % just below in (brackets).

Table 3. Performance of seven algorithms with decreased biological variation.

In conclusion, the most robust algorithm against biological variation is the algorithm Molina el al. {6}. And the most sensitive algorithms with influence from biological variations CV_B are the algorithms Söletormos et al. A {3} and Söletormos et al. B {5}.

2.2.10 Biological variation of tumour growth

Just as we have investigated the impact of biological variation, CV_B, on the performance in a *steady-state* situation, we have also challenged the variation in progression conditions. Thus, we have included a variation of 25% with the selected three slopes in the simulation model and compared the results with the results in Table 1.

Nearly all the results were close to the same as in Table 1 when this variation of 25% was included in the exponential function. The false positive (FP) results chanced only a few per cent for the most algorithms and maximum increases in percentages were 4% found at the algorithms Barak et al. {1} and Tondini & Hayes {2} below 57 U/L after two years.

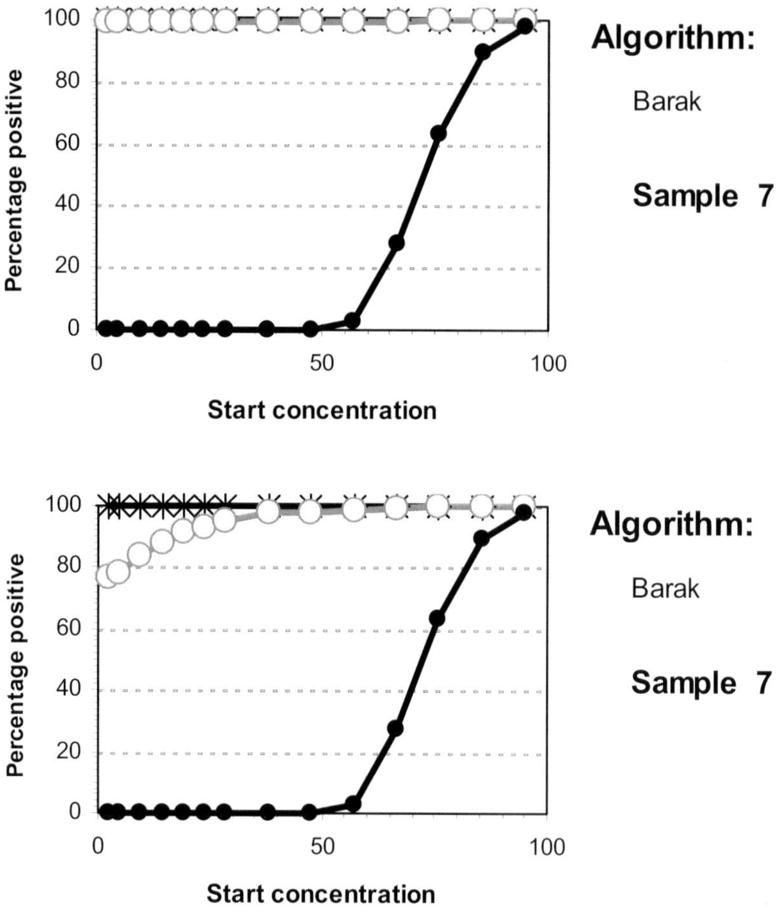

Percentage positive patients (POS) as a function of starting concentrations for algorithm Barak et al. {1} after one year. The upper figure shows results from the "normal" rate of increase. The figure below shows results from a modified rate of increase, including biological variation in the exponential function of tumour growth of 25%. For the slowest slope (λ =0.0132) (---o---), the modified slope shows a reduced number of percentage positives from start concentration 0 up to approx 57 U/L TPA with percentage positives increasing from 78% to 100%, respectively.

Fig. 7. Impact of biological variation on exponential tumour growth.

Also the detection times for progression using the three slopes with biological variation were nearly the same as the results without variation. An example of the minor changes in results including variation of tumour growth is illustrated in Fig. 7. Results from the algorithm Barak et al.{1} include a variation of exponential function of 25%; only the slowest slope for tumour growth shows a slightly reduced number of percentages of positive results compared to the "normal" slope. The most marked change was found with algorithm Söletormos et al. A {3}. This algorithm showed two months extended detection time at the middle fast slope ($\lambda = 0.0346$) – and similarly the algorithm Molina et al. {6} showed two months extended detection time at the slowest slope.

Overall, the biological variation of tumour growth has only minimal effects on the results and does not change the conclusions based on results in Table 1; it may therefore be excluded from further computer simulation investigations.

3. Conclusion

The start concentration of the biomarker TPA is a very important parameter in the examination of the performance of the algorithm, i.e. time for detection of progression and percentage of false positive results (FP). Start concentrations near cut-off will give more FP in nearly every algorithm – but the algorithms with low FP results also have longer tumour detection time. All the investigated algorithms performed comparable in FP results, when the start concentration was low, i.e. below 57 U/L.

These overall conclusions are relatively identical to the conclusion on results from the same algorithms using biomarker CA 15-3 (Petersen et al., 2011) – this indicates that the relative performance of algorithms is independent of the biomarker.

Differences in biological variation, CV_B, have an influence on the performance of nearly all the algorithms. Only the algorithm Molina et al {6} has unchanged results with the different biological variations, CV_B, – in other words this algorithm is the most robust against increasing biological variation CV_B. Some algorithms show better performance when the biological variation CV_B is low. When the biological variation CV_B is low the algorithm Söletormos et al. A {3} has the best performance as regards early progression detection and simultaneously low number of FP results.

The biological variation of the tumour growth up to 25% has only a minor influence on the performance of the algorithms and does not chance the overall conclusions.

In a clinical situation the start concentration should be the point for selecting the best algorithm. When the start concentration is near the cut-off, the algorithm Molina et al. {6} could be used to avoid too many FP results. When the start concentration is below 57 U/L, the algorithm Barak et al. {1} could be used to have a short progressive detection time with only few FP results.

3.1 Computer simulations

A summary of new important conclusions from this investigation:

a. The relative performances of algorithms are independent of the biomarker.

b. Some algorithms are more robust against increased biological variation than others.
c. Variation in tumour growth has only limit impact on the performances of the algorithms.

These conclusions are based on computer simulations. In the computer simulations, the *steady-state* variation and the rate of tumour increase (λ = slope) are based on clinical data from the literature and the simulations are based on random counts generated from a Gaussian distribution from the computer multiplied by the parameters borrowed from publications. Furthermore, the cost-price for the clinical investigations compared with computer simulation is enormous and the computer simulation is a convenient, easy and quick method to compare algorithm performances based on the same simulated data-points. Thus, computer simulation should be a tool to select the "right" algorithm before a clinical investigation regarding for example low number of false positive (FP) signals. Computer simulations are thus not a substitute for clinical investigations, but a supplementary tool in helping to interpret biomarker variations and challenge the algorithms with extreme parameters in the model.

Thus, the advantage of computer simulations is that it is relatively easy to vary the parameters in the simulation model and examine the impact on the performances of the algorithms. In this investigation we have investigated these performances under standard conditions as well as under extremes with conditions of varied CV_B in *steady-state* and varying slopes of tumour growth. In addition, we have tested the robustness of the algorithms by using extreme values for CV_B and we have tested for variation in the exponential slopes of tumour growth.

Parameters which interestingly could also be varied are sampling intervals or the starting points of the exponential tumour growth.

In this study we have chosen a sampling interval of every two months, which is a relevant time schedule for monitoring of patients with breast cancer during follow-up after treatment (Söletormos et al., 2000b). Obviously, a sampling interval of one month could give earlier detection of tumour growth progression. However, in many of the algorithms the number of FP signals will simultaneously increase, and, conversely, longer sampling intervals will reduce FP signals, but true signals will be delayed.

We have chosen arbitrarily the starting point of exponential tumour growth to be 1% of cut-off. The impact on the performances of the algorithms when varying this starting point for the contribution from the growing tumour may be comparable for all the algorithms. If, for example, a starting point of 50% of the cut-off concentration was selected - the time for crossing cut-off would be shortened, so the progression detection time would possibly be earlier, whereas the percentages of FP would be unchanged for all algorithms.

3.2 Future research

In this investigation, we have investigated and challenged the seven algorithms, but the effect of sampling interval and of the start value of the contribution of marker from the tumour has not been studied. Furthermore, this computer model for simulations can be used for evaluation of other algorithms which can be tested and compared to the existing algorithms, before they are published or introduced in the clinic.

4. References

Barak, M., Steiner, M., Finkel, B., Abrahamson, J., Antal, S., & Gruener, N. (1990). CA-15.3, TPA and MCA as markers for breast cancer, *Eur J Cancer*, 26, pp. 577-80

Bliss, CI. (1967). *Statistics in Biology*, McGraw-Hill Book Company, New York

Bonfrer, JMG. (1990). Working group on tumor marker criteria (WGTMC). *Tumor Biol*, 11, pp. 287-8

Chan, DW., Beveridge,RA., Muss, H., Fritsche, HA., Theriault, R., Kiang, D., et al.. (1997). Use of Truquantt BR radioimmunoassay for early detection of breast cancer recurrence in patients with stage II and stage III disesase. *J Clin Oncol.* 15, pp. 2322-8

Dinistrian, AM., Schwartz, MK., Greenberg, EJ., Smith, CA. & Schwartz, DC. (1991) CA 15-3 and carcinoembryonic antigen in the clinical evaluation of breast cancer. *Clin Chim Acta*, 200, pp. 81-94

Harris, EK. & Yasaka, T. (1983) On the calculation of a reference change for comparing two consecutive measurements. *Clin Chem*, 29, pp. 25-30

Iglesias, N., Hyltoft Petersen, P. & Ricos, C. (2005). Power functions of the reference change value in relation to cut-off points, reference intervals and index of individuality. *Clin Chem Lab Med*, 43, pp. 441-8

Molina, R., Zanón, G., Filella, X., Moreno, F., Jo, J., Daniels M, et al. (1995) Use of serial carcinoembryonic antigen and CA 15-3 assays in detecting relapses in breast cancer patients. *Breast Cancer Res Treat*, 36, pp. 41-8

Mughal, AW., Hortobagyi, GN., Fritsche, HA., Buzdar, AU., Yap, HY. & Blumenschein GR. (1983) Serial carcinoembryonic antigen measurements during treatment of metastatic breast cancer. *JAMA*, 249, pp.1881-6

Nicolini, A., Colombini, C., Luciani, L., Carpi, A. & Giuliani L. (1991) Evaluation of serum CA 15-3 and TPA in the post-operative follow-up of breast cancer patients. *Br J* Cancer, 64, pp.154-8

Petersen, PH., Sölétormos, G., Pedersen, MF. & Lund F. Interpretation of increments in serial tumour biomarker concentrations depends on the distance of the baseline concentration from the cut-off. *Clin Chem Lab Med*, 49 pp. 303-10

Sölétormos, G., Fogh, JM., Sehested-Hansen, B., Spang-Thomsen, M., Schiøler, V., Dombernowsky, P. & Skovgaard, T. (1997) Carcino-embryonic antigen in monitoring the growth of human colon adenocarcinoma tumour cells SK-CO-1 and HT-29 in vitro and in nude mice. *Eur J Cancer*, 33, pp.108-14

Sölétormos, G., Hyltoft Petersen, P. & Dombernowsky P. (2000a) Assessment of CA 15.3, CEA and TPA concentrations during monitoring of breast cancer. *Clin Chem Lab Med*, 38, pp. 453-63

Sölétormos, G., Hyltoft Petersen, P. & Dombernowsky P. (2000b) Progression criteria for cancer antigen 15.3 and carcinoembryonic antigen in metastatic breast cancer compared to computer simulation of marker data. *Clin Chem*, 46, pp. 939-49

Sölétormos, G., Nielsen, D., Schiøler, V., Skovsgaard, T. & Dombernowsky P. (1996) Tumor markers cancer antigen 15.3 and carcinoembryonic antigen in the clinical evaluationof breast cancer. *Clin Chem*, 42, pp. 564-75

Tondini, C. & Hayes DF. (1989) Circulating tumor markers in breast cancer. *Hematol Oncol Clin N Am*, 3, pp. 653-74

15

The Discovery of Cancer Tissue Specific Proteins in Serum: Case Studies on Prostate Cancer

Spiros D. Garbis[1,2,*] and Paul A. Townsend[1,*]
[1]*Cancer Sciences, Faculty of Medicine, University of Southampton, Southampton,*
[2]*Biomedical Research Foundation, Academy of Athens, Athens,*
[1]*UK*
[2]*Greece*

1. Introduction

Carcinogenesis remains a complex and unpredictable process that involves defects in multiple signalling pathways. Environmental determinants and lifestyle practices may contribute toward their onset by the exposure to a variety of carcinogenic agents. Since the process of carcinogenesis involves the **synergistic induction** in multiple pathways inside the cell, an effective means to investigate and understand them is to engage a global approach that identifies and considers multiple changes simultaneously at the protein level (Albini & Sporn, 2007; Alderton, 2007; Hanahan & Weinberg, 2011; Mueller & Fusenig, 2004). Such an approach can be effectively engaged with the use of discovery proteomics that allows for the large-scale analysis of protein identity and expression (Anderson, Anderson, et al., 2009; Cox & Mann, 2011; Cravatt, Simon, & Yates, 2007; Diamandis, 2004; Nilsson et al., 2010; Walther & Mann, 2010; Wright, Han, & Aebersold, 2005). There is increasing strong evidence that tumorigenesis occurs in the **tissue microenvironment** as a whole, involving the active crosstalk between epithelial, endothelial, immune and stromal cells (Albini &Sporn, 2007; Alderton, 2007; Mueller & Fusenig, 2004). Consequently, the analysis at the whole tissue level is a logical initial step in the identification of tissue-specific or tissue-prevalent proteins occurring at larger concentration levels relative to those found in the systemic circulation, wherein their secretion and shedding may occur (Hanash, Pitteri, & Faca, 2008). Provided that the expressed tissue specific and prevalent proteins found in the serum or plasma represent phenotypic cancer pathophysiological events, then these proteins may be potential cancer biomarkers and/or physiologic treatment targets (Hanash, Pitteri, & Faca, 2008).

Research involving the mass spectrometry (MS) based proteomic study of fresh-frozen whole prostate tissue biopsies, cell-culture models and blood sera originating from well-defined clinical designs are discussed. Emphasis is given to those approaches involving the hyphenation of liquid chromatography with mass spectrometry by means of electrospray

* Corresponding Authors

ionization (LC-MS) for the analysis of proteins derived from prostate cancer clinical specimens (S. D. Garbis et al., 2011; S. D. Garbis et al., 2008). One of the several challenges of the serum and plasma proteomic methods involve the removal of high abundant proteins (i.e. albumin, IgGs, etc.) for the in-depth analysis of the lower abundant proteins where potential biomarkers can be revealed (S. D. Garbis et al., 2011; Hanash et al., 2008). However, their removal typically results in the co-removal of a significant percentage of the lower abundant tissue specific proteins. At the same token, the co-analysis of both high and low abundance proteins and their endogenously occurring cleavage products (**serum degradome**) may confer greater insight on serum biochemistry and cancer biology. The principle themes to be covered in the present book chapter includes the development and application of quantitative bottom-up LC-MS proteomic methods in the analytical characterization of (i) fresh frozen cancerous breast and prostate tissue biopsy specimens to define proteins expressed by the tumour microenvironment, (ii) the discovery of tissue_ specific serum biomarkers that are secreted in the systemic circulation of clinical utility to the medical practitioner, (iii) the future perspective on the use of targeted and high-throughput LC-MS based analysis approaches for the validation of biomarker discovery findings spanning large scale specimens sets including healthy specimen cohorts], and (iv) the use of lab-on-chip formats to further enhance LC-MS analysis sensitivity, selectivity and specificity at multiple orders of magnitude lower clinical specimen amounts currently used. The analytical attributes intrinsic to these methods allow the generation of a panel of protein biomarkers with multiple molecular features as reflected on measurable analytical variables that include the chromatographic retention times indexes, the concentration level, the amino acid sequence of the proteolytic peptide, uniquely traceable or surrogate, to one particular protein, and its *in vivo* modification status. The uniqueness in molecular features encoded in a given biomaker panel is accomplished by an ensemble of analytical variables that are explicitly dependent on the collective physico-chemical properties of the proteins and their surrogate peptides that constitute this panel. The end-product from the use of such methods is the determination of tumor "signatures" at the serum or plasma level based on rationally derived protein-panels with a high degree of specificity and sensitivity that uniquely identify a particular cancer type, its stage and its applicability to personalized intervention protocols.

2. Critical elements for the study of biomarkers

Prostate cancer imposes an ever increasing healthcare burden to males worldwide due to do their higher life expectancies, the prevalence of high fat diets and sedentary lifestyles, exposure to environmental pollutants, sexual habits, etc (Albini & Sporn, 2007; De Marzo et al., 2004; DeMarzo, Nelson, Isaacs, & Epstein, 2003; Hammarsten & Hogstedt, 2002; Jemal, Siegel, Xu, & Ward, 2010; Pfeffer et al., 2002). Early detection is of vital importance in reducing mortality. However, the early detection of cancer is hampered by the lack of effective analytical methods. This lack in analytical efficiency has often resulted in the erroneous assessment and derivation of biological indicators, or biomarkers, of prostate cancer disease (Balk, Ko, & Bubley, 2003; Thompson et al., 2005). The reasons for the ineffective utility of these biomarkers are multi-fold and include the following, (i) they lack specificity and selectivity to the cancer type of interest, (ii) their reproducible detection is poor, (iii) the sensitivity of available methods, especially as they refer to biological fluids such as serum and plasma, is poor relative to the natural abundance levels of the tissue-specific secreted or shedded molecular entities of disease, and (iv) the majority of the available analytical protocols measure biomarkers at the DNA and mRNA level, which may not reflect the phenotypic aspects of disease (Adewale et al., 2008; Buchen, 2011; Lin et al., 2005; Rahbar et al., 2011; Sawyers, 2008; Turteltaub et al., 2011). In addition, the availability of more selective prognosis strategies may also help identify patient cohorts, or even single individuals, eligible for adjuvant therapy (i.e., **personalized medicine**). Hence, new biomarkers for asymptomatic prediction, diagnosis, prognosis and response to treatment at the protein level are warranted to improve clinical intervention. It is assumed that one of the critical parameters for the staging of disease and/or treatment intervention is the difference in concentration levels found for the respective biomarkers. This especially becomes true when the complexity of the derived proteomes is decoded in the form of biological pathways and their networks that allow the interrogation of novel candidate protein markers as physiologic targets. Consequent to with this notion, the family of protein markers that will encompass the molecular biology of carcinogenesis will include not only tissue specific proteins but also proteins that reflect systemic changes that predispose a seemingly healthy individual to a longer-term initiation to event of carcinogenesis (Adewale et al., 2008; Buchen, 2011; DeMarzo et al., 2004; Hanahan & Weinberg, 2011; Joyce, 2005; Rahbar et al., 2011; Sawyers, 2008; Turteltaub et al., 2011). In addition to protein markers, and in particular enzyme species, other biological indicators of disease and its pre-disposition, may include co-factors (i.e., vitamin species) and protein end-products such as 1° and 2° metabolites in the form nucleic acids, amino acids, fatty acids and xenobiotic species in their parent and biotransformed moieties. This integrated monitoring of these biomolecular entities at multiple levels may impart more accuracy and reliability in functionally capturing biochemical pathways of disease. A general example may include an *in vivo* phosphorylation at the catalytic domain of a protein substrate leading to the inhibition of the metabolism of its affiliated ligand. The absence of biotransformed ligand constitutes a proof-positive indicator in the functional annotation of the protein under consideration. A case in point is the polymorphism of the enzyme species 5-methyl-tetrahydrofolate reductase (5-MTHFR) leading to altered concentration levels of 5-methyl tetrahydrofolate (5MTHF), a metabolically active form of folic acid. The polymorphism of 5-MTHFR has been implicated as a cause to the sub-clinical deficiency of folic acid observed in the older human adult populations, despite their adequate intake of this essential nutrient. The ability, therefore, to quantitatively monitor both the polymorphic 5-MTHFR enzyme and its biotransformation product 5-MTHF can better capture this event (Antoniades et al., 2009; S. D. Garbis, Melse-Boonstra, West, & van Breemen, 2001; Melse-Boonstra et al., 2006; Yetley et al., 2011). The unique analytical versatility and adaptability of MS based methods in detecting diverse biomolecular species imparts a unique opportunity in both customizing and validating key mechanisms of disease and its etiology. From this perspective, modulating these **mechanism based biomarkers** may cause the induction or inhibition of a given carcinogenesis pathway (Kocher & Superti-Furga, 2007). Consequently, such types of biomarkers make for better candidates as treatment targets that can be modulated with medicinal agents and other clinical intervention schemes. Our working hypothesis is based on the assumption that the key difference between the early, asymptomatic disease (low disease burden) versus that of late stage, metastatic disease (high disease burden) is the concentration level found for these mechanistic biomarkers either in their native

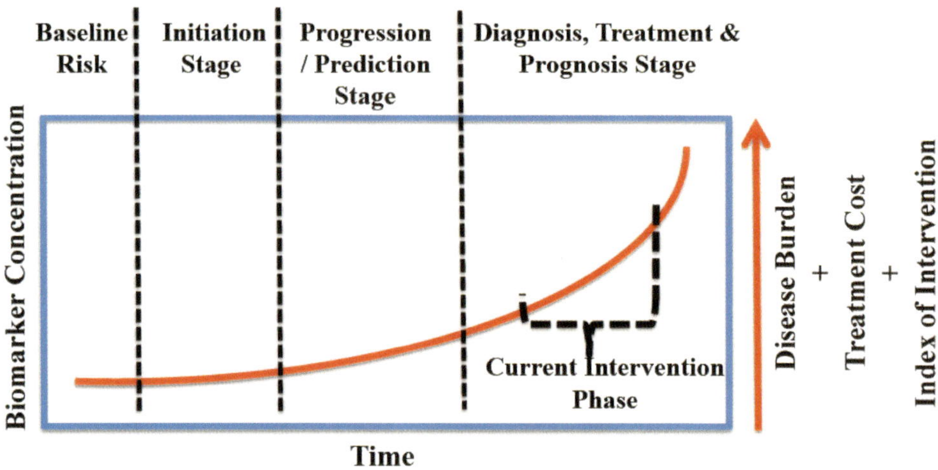

Fig. 1. A key parameter to the utility of a given biomarker is its concentration level in the assessment of disease and its treatment. The current detection methods detect biomarker levels that reflect late stage disease wherein treatment options are limited. The more sensitive and selective the analysis method the greater the effectiveness in capturing the disease progression at the initiation stage wherein its reversal is possible with cancer chemoprevention, nutritional/functional food intervention, and other low-toxicity treatment protocols.

or *in vivo* modified form (i.e., post translational modified proteins, biotransformed 1° and 2° metabolites). As such, the ability to capture very low levels of these protein markers and their surrogate end-products provides greater assurance in capturing their disease potential at the progression or even initiation stage whose effects can be reversed with less toxic intervention protocols (see Figure 1). The present discourse will focus on protein-based markers of prostate carcinogenesis.

3. Analytical chemistry background

The selection of the analytical method for the investigation of a biological specimen depends on the clinical query to be solved. However, the essential features to this selection process is for the analytical method to impart: (a) qualitative effectiveness for the identification of as many proteins as possible, (b) quantitative effectiveness to reveal absolute or relative concentrations of these proteins. The advent of mass spectrometry (MS) based techniques as compared to the other analytical techniques (i.e., molecular spectroscopy based such as fluorescence, UV-VIS, NMR; X-Ray crystallography) has allowed for the simultaneous protein identification and quantification in very small amounts of biological material, at analyte detection limits that may exceed those of fluorescence based ELISA assays as applied to clinical specimens (S. D. Garbis et al., 2011; Rubakhin, Romanova, Nemes, & Sweedler, 2011). A major milestone to the effective use of MS techniques to the analysis of a vastly larger range of biomolecules (e.g., metabolites, peptides, proteins, nucleic acids, fatty acids, steroids, etc.) was the advent of the electrospray ionization source (ESI) and its micro-

and nano- flow derivatives (Wilm, 2011). As a soft-ionization source, ESI made it possible to introduce the thermally labile biomolecular species to become introduced to the gas phase from its initial liquid phase in its charged state with an intact chemical integrity. Consequently, the ESI source allowed the interfacing of liquid phase sample introduction systems (i.e., liquid chromatography and capillary electrophoresis) with the vacuum-system encased MS platforms (i.e., quadrupolar, ion trapping, time-of-flight, or hybrids thereof, etc.). (Cox & Mann, 2011; Cravatt et al., 2007; Diamandis, 2004; Kocher & Superti-Furga, 2007; Nilsson et al., 2010; Walther & Mann, 2010). The development of novel analytical methods that are based on the combined use of liquid chromatography and tandem mass spectrometry (LC-MS) techniques for the bottom-up or top-down proteome analysis of a wide spectrum of both low and high abundant proteins in clinical tissue and sera dates back to the late nineties with the introduction of the Multi-Dimensional Protein Identification Technology (MudPIT) by John Yates (Fournier, Gilmore, Martin-Brown, & Washburn, 2007). The MuDPIT approaches constituted an alternative to the Two-Dimensional Gel Electrophoresis (2DGe) approaches in their ability to capture and identify a wider spectrum of proteins and at lower abundance levels. These in-depth LC-MS proteomic methods employ the orthogonal use of various high-performance liquid chromatographic (HPLC) chemistries, based on the principles of strong ion exchange (XIC), size-exclusion (SEC), hydrophilic interaction (HILIC), affinity capture (biological and chemical), reverse phase (RPC) and others. These separation techniques allow the isolation, separation and enrichment of proteins and surrogate peptides found in extracts derived form clinical specimens such as tissues, blood plasma and sera. Overall, the LC-MS proteomic methods incorporate the combined use of both nano-electrospray ionization (nESI) and off-line matrix-assisted laser desorption ionization (MALDI) interfaces, to ensure the broadest possible surrogate peptide coverage for a given protein. The bottom-up analysis approach, which is based on the analysis of surrogate tryptic peptides, is well suited for a robust and sensitive protein analysis strategy (taking into consideration individual protein hydrophobicity, charge, or post-translational modification). These complementary methodological approaches provide a more comprehensive and reproducible proteomics assessment of clinical tissue and sera specimens. This has become yet more evident with the use of the latest tandem MS-MS analyzer platforms that include the quadrupole time-of-flight QqTOF and Orbitrap based geometries. These MS platforms exhibit high-sensitivity (limit of detection < 10 fmol on-column allowing the use of very low signal accumulation times) and ultra-high resolution (≥ 30,000, translating to 1-3 ppm mass accuracies) at very high signal sampling speeds (≥ 30 Hz). Such performance characteristics allow the detection > 3,000 proteins at > 99% confidence derived from cell culture lysates and spanning over 4-orders of magnitude natural concentration abundance in a single LC-MS analysis run (Cox & Mann, 2011; Liu, Belov, Jaitly, Qian, & Smith, 2007; Mann & Kelleher, 2008; Ong & Mann, 2005). One of several key advantages of the non-gel LC-MS based methods is that they allow the analysis of a much wider spectrum of proteins than that typically covered with the classical gel-based approaches. This spectrum includes proteins that are membrane bound or membrane associated; proteins that exhibit alkaline (pI > 8) and acidic (pI < 5) character; proteins with low (<10 kDa) or high (>200 kDa) molecular weights; and proteins that have undergone *in vivo* modifications (i.e. phosphorylation, acetylation, methylation, glycosylation, etc.) occurring in minor molar ratios (oftentimes < 1:1000) relative to their native counterparts (S. Garbis, Lubec, & Fountoulakis, 2005; Lubec & Afjehi-Sadat, 2007; Nilsson et al., 2010; van Bentem, Mentzen, de la Fuente, & Hirt, 2008). Currently more than 150 different types of *in vivo* modifications are possible (Seymour et al., 2006; Shilov et al., 2007). The ability to detect and discriminate these post-translational modified proteins constitutes a major advancement in the more comprehensive understanding of signaling cascades at the protein level allowing for a more direct appreciation of protein-protein interaction and consequently biological pathways and their networks (Kocher & Superti-Furga, 2007; Mann & Kelleher, 2008; Ong & Mann, 2005; van Bentem et al., 2008). It is assumed that the vast majority of proteins have undergone multiple and diverse *in vivo* modifications that define their induction or silencing status. Such protein traits can only be captured with tandem MS spectra generated at high sensitivity and high resolution providing unequivocal evidence in the annotation of their *in vivo* modification at the precise amino acid location in single LC-MS experiment (Liu et al., 2007; Mann & Kelleher, 2008; Ong & Mann, 2005; Papayannopoulos, 1995). Conceptually, a vast array of *in vivo* modifications can be captured and stored for later use as means to provide a multifactorial understanding of biological pathways and their networks. The current biochemical assays such as Immunohistochemistry and Western blots fail to account for these intrinsic protein *in vivo* modification traits. It is this limitation that has often resulted in the analysis bias between the MS and biochemical assay measurements (Diamandis, 2004; Lubec & Afjehi-Sadat, 2007; Nilsson et al., 2010).

The collective LC-MS analysis characteristics constitute a major advancement toward an in-depth proteome analysis of the fresh-frozen tumor specimens.Advanced proteomics approaches can bridge the gap between the genetic and epigenetic alterations underlying cancer and cellular physiology. The precepts of multidimensional liquid chromatography hyphenated with high resolution, tandem mass spectrometry (MDLC-MS-MS) techniques in combination with the use of isobaric tags for relative and absolute quantification (iTRAQ™) of whole tissue biopsies of various types of cancer tissue (i.e., breast, prostate, cervical) has played a key role in bridging this gap. In general, a key advantage of 2DLC-MS-MS methods that utilize isobaric stable isotope based approaches (i.e., cICAT, TMT, iTRAQ, etc.) is the ability to conduct multiplex experiments, whereby specimen extracts can be analyzed concurrently under the same experimental conditions. This multiplexing advantage reduces systematic error, and improves the signal-to-noise of the precursor MS and product ion MS-MS response allowing for a greater number of proteins to be quantitatively profiled (DeSouza et al., 2005; S. D. Garbis et al., 2008; Glen et al., 2008; Pichler et al., 2011; Wu, Wang, Baek, & Shen, 2006). Advancements made to liquid chromatography and mass spectrometry stand to further potentiate the utility of these isobaric stable isotope tags (Fournier et al., 2007; Pichler et al., 2011). Other key attributes that make MS based methods the premier choice for the analysis of small amounts of clinically valuable and complex biological specimens along with reduced requirements for stable isotope reagents is driven by the increased automation and miniaturization imparted by lab-on-a-chip formats (Everley, Krijgsveld, Zetter, & Gygi, 2004; Koster & Verpoorte, 2007; Rubakhin et al., 2011; Tsougeni et al., 2011). These themes are covered within the context of case studies in the analysis of clinical whole tissue biopsies and their sera for prostate cancer.

4. Prostate cancer

4.1 The quantitative proteomic profiling of clinical whole tissue biopsies derived from benign prostate hyperplasia and prostate cancer

Prostate whole tissue biopsies exhibit extensive biological variability when accounting for the diversity in human subjects and the heterogeneity and size of the tissue specimen itself. These variables must be taken into consideration when executing its proteomic study. Factors such as tissue procurement, histopathology pre-assessment, storage, handling, and pre-analytical processing, and instrumental performance verification with standardization (chromatographic and nano-ESI ionization efficiency, MS and MS-MS sensitivity, resolution, accuracy and precision) are variables that need to be optimized for any given proteomic study. The optimization of these variables will minimize the histopathological, biological, pre-analytical and analytical variability so essential to a reproducible and information-rich proteomic output (Buchen, 2011; Cox & Mann, 2011; Diamandis, 2004; Hilario & Kalousis, 2008; Nilsson et al., 2010).

Several multiplex proteomics studies that rely on the use of cysteine-specific isotope-coded affinity tags (cICAT), stable isotope labeling with amino acids in cell culture (SILAC), difference gel electrophoresis (DIGE) and trypsin-mediated ^{18}O isotope labeling have been successful in detecting differentially expressed proteins in combined specimen samples (DeSouza et al., 2005; Everley et al., 2004; Hood et al., 2005). Despite their advantages however, intrinsic limitations exist for each of these approaches. The cICAT approach allows only the labeling of proteins containing cysteine residues on tractable peptides upon proteolysis making this approach unsuitable as a comprehensive and in-depth protein discovery tool. The cICAT approach has been used for the quantitative proteomic profiling in secondary prostate cancer cell cultures. In one such study, 524 secreted proteins were from the LNCaP neoplastic prostate epithelium of which 9% of these were found to be differentially expressed (Martin et al., 2004). In another study involving the same cell culture model in response to androgen exposure resulted in the identification of 1064 proteins of which approx. 21% of these proteins were modulated (Wright et al., 2004).

Another label-based approach for prostate biomarker discovery efforts makes use of heavy water. In such an approach, $H_2{}^{18}O$ water is used instead of regular water for the solution phase trypsinization process thus allowing the trypsin-mediated ^{18}O stable isotope incorporation (^{18}O labeling) for those proteins extracted from one specimen category (i.e. control, treated or diseased states). This process leads to the exchange of two equivalents of ^{16}O with two equivalents of the ^{18}O stable isotope at the carboxyl terminus of the resulting tryptic peptides coined as the «heavy» peptides. The heavy water approach was applied to proteins extracted from benign prostate hyperplasia (BPH) vs. prostate cancer (PCa) cells isolated from a single formalin-fixed paraffin embedded (FFPE) prostate cancer tissue specimen (Hood et al., 2005). This study resulted in the quantitative profiling of only 68 proteins. The limited proteins amounts along with their cross-linked form limit the utility of FFPE as a viable specimen source for proteomic assessment. Another confounding factor in the practical utility of the ^{18}O labeling strategy, which also applies in cICAT labeling case, is that only two samples can be analyzed per experiment.

A gel-based relative quantitative approach that has been used for prostate cancer cells is known as the differential gel-electrophoresis (DIGE). The DIGE method represents a variant of the classical 2-D gel electrophoresis (2DGE) technique whereby CyDye fluorescence probes are used as tags to covalently modify proteins without affecting their electrophoretic properties. Consequently, the resulting CyDye fluorescence labeled proteins originating from multiple biological specimens migrate to almost the same location of a 2-D gel. Using this approach, up to three different fluor labeled samples can be combined and 2DGE separated in a single experiment thus allowing better spot matching and reduction in gel-to-gel non-reproducibility. One fundamental drawback to the DIGE approach is its MS-incompatibility because of the ionization suppression effects induced by fluor labeled reagents. Consequently, all the intrinsic gel-based limitations also apply for the DIGE approach (S.Garbis et al., 2005; Garcia-Ramirez et al., 2007; Lubec & Afjehi-Sadat, 2007; Wu et al., 2006). The use of the DIGE based method was applied to the study of perturbed protein networks in LNCaP prostate cancer cells administered to both androgen and anti-androgen exposure resulting in the quantitative profiling of 107 proteins (Rowland et al., 2004).

The development and application of a quantitative proteomic method involving the use of off-line size-exclusion chromatography (SCX) followed by the on-line reverse phase (RP) chromatography hyphenated with high resolution, tandem mass spectrometry (2DLC-MS-MS) in combination with the use of isobaric tags for relative and absolute quantification (iTRAQ™) was applied to the analysis of clinical whole tissue biopsies derived from patients with benign prostate hyperplasia (BPH, n=10) and prostate cancer (PCa, n=10)(S. D. Garbis et al., 2008). Key advantages to this approach include the ability to conduct multiplex experiments, whereby up to eight samples can be analyzed concurrently under the same 2DLC-MS conditions, resulting in reduced systematic error and increased electrospray ionization efficiency leading to higher sensitivity; in addition, since protein identification and quantification is based on tandem mass spectrometric (MS-MS) evidence, increased selectivity, specificity and confirmatory power are achieved. This study resulted in the reproducible quantitative profiling of 827 proteins of which 65 were differentially expressed. The access to well defined human whole prostate tissue biopsies allowed for the investigation of the stromal vs. epithelial cell interaction in the manifestation of prostate cancer. An essential requirement to the iTRAQ 2DLC-MS-MS approach is the use effective liquid chromatographic technique to impart sufficient separation of the large number of tryptic peptides generated. This will reduce the co-eluting peptides that would otherwise result in erroneous product ion MS-MS spectra negating the accurate relative quantification efficiency and protein identification accuracy (Fournier et al., 2007). The modulated proteins identified were implicated in the inflammation response (Albini et al., 2007; Albini, Tosetti, Benelli, & Noonan, 2005; DeSouza et al., 2005; Goldstraw, Fitzpatrick, & Kirby, 2007; Nelson, DeMarzo, DeWeese, & Isaacs, 2005), the modulation of the androgen (Cheung-Flynn et al., 2005; De Leon et al., 2011; Hildenbrand et al., 2011; McKeen et al., 2011; Milad et al., 1995; Miyoshi et al., 2003; Nelson et al., 2005; M. H. Yang & Sytkowski, 1998), and prostate cancer metastasis (Ablin, Kynaston, Mason, & Jiang, 2011; Dabbous, Jefferson, Haney, & Thomas, 2011; Di Cristofano et al., 2010; Grisendi, Mecucci, Falini, & Pandolfi, 2006; Hale, Price, Sanchez, Demark-Wahnefried, & Madden, 2001; Jiang & Ablin, 2011; Khanna et al., 2004; C. J. Kim, Sakamoto, Tambe, & Inoue, 2011; Krust, El Khoury, Nondier, Soundaramourty, & Hovanessian, 2011; Moretti et al., 2011; Okuda et al., 2000; Planche et al., 2011; Sun, Song, et al., 2011; Sun, Zhao, et al., 2011; Weng, Ahlen, Astrom, Lui, & Larsson, 2005; Yu & Luo,

2006), as essential hallmark features for these prostate cancer tissue specimens. Another interesting finding that also goes toward validating the accuracy of the proteomic method is the differential expression of several prostate specific cancer markers such as the prostate-specific transglutaminase, the prostate associated gene 4 protein, the prostatic acid phosphatase, and the prostate specific membrane antigen (see Figure 2). The presence of the prostate-specific transglutaminase in PCa has been recently reported as a potential anti-tumour target (Ablin et al., 2011; Jiang & Ablin, 2011). Yet another important finding from this study were proteins reported to be implicated as potential cancer chemoprevention targets also affiliated with poor nutritional status and metabolic syndrome disease (Das et al., 2011; De Nunzio et al., 2011; DeMarzo et al., 2003; Dong, Zhang, Hawthorn, Ganther, & Ip, 2003; Gonzalez-Moreno et al., 2011; Jeronimo et al., 2004; J. Kim et al., 2005; Kuemmerle et al., 2011; Menendez & Lupu, 2007; Nelson et al., 2005; Oh et al., 2006; Sytkowski, Gao, Feldman, & Chen, 2005; Toki et al., 2010; Tsavachidou et al., 2009; Walsh, 2010; C. M. Yang, Yen, Huang, & Hu, 2011; Zeliadt & Ramsey, 2010). These proteins include the retinol binding protein I, selenium binding protein 1, fatty acid synthase, and insulin-regulated lipase and are oftentimes synergistically expressed with other proteins implicated in the inflammation response and androgen regulation.

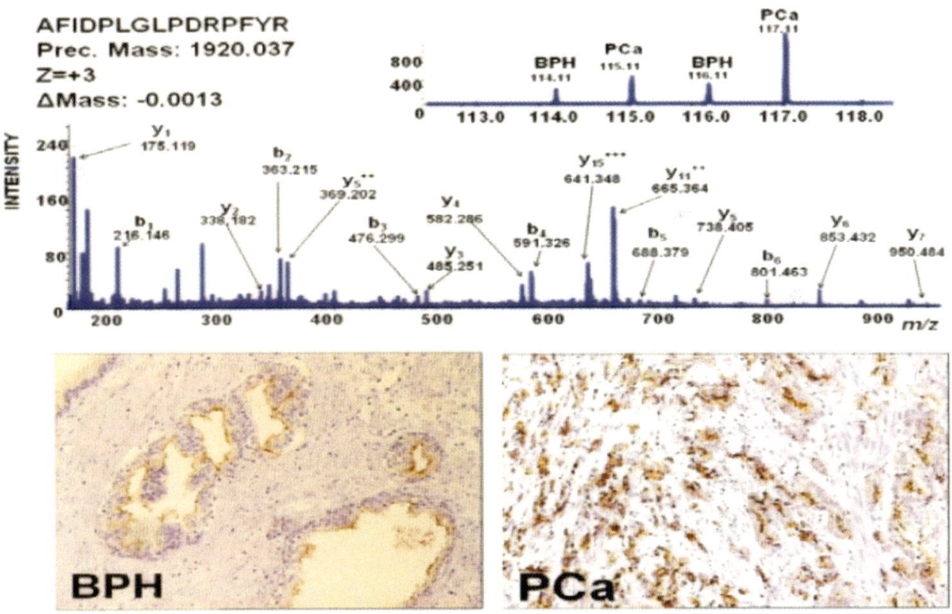

Fig. 2. A surrogate peptide sequence and its relative quantification indicating the over expression of prostate-specific membrane antigen (PSMA) in prostate cancer (PCa) vs. benign prostate hyperplasia (BPH) with corresponding immunohistochemical confirmation for these specimen categories that effectively corroborate the quantitative proteomic findings (S. D. Garbis et al., 2008).

4.2 The quantitative proteomic profiling of clinical serum samples derived from benign prostate hyperplasia

Tissue proteomics is considered a logical first step for the novel discovery of tumour-derived proteins as they exist in higher concentrations due to their more direct proximity to cancer cells (Cravatt et al., 2007; Hanash et al., 2008; Joyce, 2005; Mueller & Fusenig, 2004; Wright et al., 2005). However, it is not well understood how protein expression in tissues reflect measurable levels in the serum or plasma that would allow the monitoring of the pathophysiological status of respective tissue (Anderson, 2010; Barelli, Crettaz, Thadikkaran, Rubin, & Tissot, 2007; Farrah et al., 2011; Hanash et al., 2008; Issaq, Xiao, & Veenstra, 2007). This may partially stem from the trend that the comprehensive analysis of tissue relevant proteins in less invasive clinical matrices such as the plasma or serum has been a daunting task for MS based methods despite all their latest technological advancements (Anderson, 2010; Farrah et al., 2011; Hanash et al., 2008). For example, currently available serum and plasma proteomics methods rely on the prior removal of high abundant proteins (i.e. albumin, IgGs, etc.) so that the lower abundant proteins, where potential biomarkers can be revealed, could be more easily analyzed. Several studies, however, have shown that their removal also resulted in the co-removal of a significant percentage of these lower abundant proteins due to their propensity to bind with the higher abundant proteins (S. D. Garbis et al., 2011; Granger, Siddiqui, Copeland, & Remick, 2005; Gundry, White, Nogee, Tchernyshyov, & Van Eyk, 2009; Zolotarjova et al., 2005). Additionally, these studies correctly purport than no MS based method to date has managed to fully remove albumin and other high abundant proteins despite claims made on the contrary. It is estimated that the 20 most abundant proteins in serum and plasma constitute over 99% of the total protein mass found in these matrices. In fact, the difference in endogenous concentration levels of proteins found in serum or plasma span from the mg/mL level (i.e. Albumin, IgG's) down to the low ng/mL level (i.e. Cyclin F, Interleukin 7) (Anderson, 2010; Farrah et al., 2011). This represents a 12-order of magnitude concentration range whose lower limit exceeds the detection capability of the fluorescence based ELISA technique, the most sensitive bioassay technique to date (Rissin et al., 2010). At the same token, the detection of endogenously occurring cleavage products (serum degradome) originating from both high and low abundance proteins may confer greater insight on serum biochemistry and cancer biology (van Winden et al., 2010). This is considered a very important incentive for the whole proteome wide analysis of the serum or plasma matrix in the prospecting of mechanism based biomarker panels.

In an effort to overcome these challenges, an approach coined multidimensional protein identification technology (MudPIT) has been developed (Fournier et al., 2007; S. D. Garbis et al., 2011; Hanash et al., 2008). This approach is principally based on combining two or more different types of liquid chromatographic chemistries so as to increase the separation efficiency as a result. This effect on the separation power is referred to as "orthogonal chromatography" and constitutes a very unique and powerful tool towards the more effective analysis of complex biological matrices (cell cultures, tissues, serum and plasma). Building on this theme, a three-dimensional (3-D) MudPIT variant was developed and applied to the analysis of clinical sera derived from patients with (BPH). The tissues from these BPH patients were analyzed and reported with the iTRAQ 2DLC-MS discussed in the previous section and was considered requisite for this proof-of-principle study so as to explore the possibility of finding tissue specific proteins in their respective serum (Garbis et al, 2011).

The analytical features of the 3-D MudPIT approach included (Figure 3): (1) high pressure size-exclusion chromatography (SEC) for the pre-fractionation of serum proteins followed by their dialysis exchange and solution phase trypsin proteolysis, (2) The tryptic peptides were then subjected to offline zwitterion-ion hydrophilic interaction chromatography (ZIC-HILIC) fractionation, and (3) their online analysis with reversed-phase nano ultra-performance chromatography (RP nUPLC) hyphenated to nano-electrospray ionization - tandem mass spectrometry.This orthogonal chromatographic strategy used imparts a more effective parsing, purification and enrichment of the tryptic peptides when combined with the prior SEC protein pre-fractionation stage. This has the effect on increasing their individual mass density of the tryptic peptides (higher peptide signal intensity per

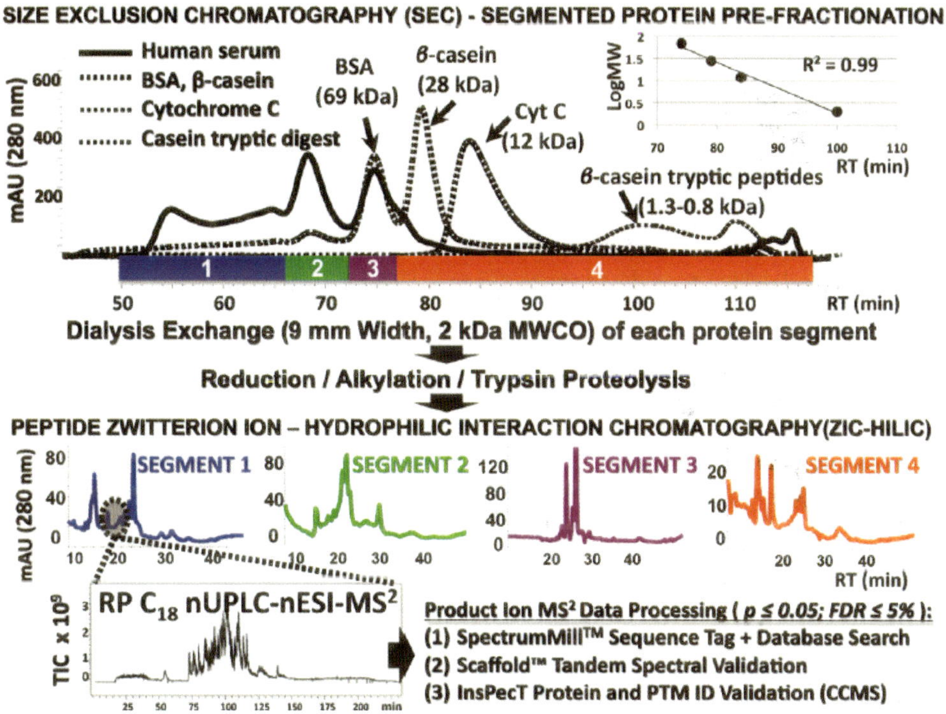

Fig. 3. **Top HPLC trace:** A representative size exclusion chromatography (SEC) trace of a pooled serum sample. Calibrant SEC traces are also shown along with their log MW vs. RT (min) linear response curve. **Middle HPLC traces:** Post-SEC sample treatment and ZIC HILIC tryptic peptide traces in concordance to SEC protein segment. The ZIC-HILIC peptide fractionation was performed in a peak-dependant manner. **Bottom HPLC trace:** Each lyophilized peptide fraction was reconstituted in MP and individually analyzed with RP C_{18} nUPLC-nESI-MS^2 analysis. The resulting product ion MS^2 peptide spectra were processed with Scaffold™ validation, SpectrumMill™ and InsPecT software programs (Garbis et al, 2011)

chromatographic retention time window) while at the same time reducing their co-elution (improved separation efficiency). It is precisely these chromatographic characteristics that allowed the enhancement of the nano-electrospray ionization of the eluting peptides followed by their tandem mass spectrometry. The end result from this process was the generation of more information rich tandem mass spectra at improved S/N ratios, which constitutes the ultimate objective for any effective MS based method.

Consequently, the collective analytical attributes of this milestone 3-D MudPIT analysis study of BPH sera resulted in the identification of proteins differing by approximately 12-orders concentration range in terms of their native abundance levels in the naturally occurring serum matrix (as measured with bioassay technique such as ELISA). In addition to this extensive dynamic range coverage, the study identified 1955 proteins with a wide spectrum of biological and physico-chemical properties. A key component however to this proteome including the detection of secreted, tissue-specific proteins also found to be differentially expressed in the respective BPH tissue reported (S. D. Garbis et al., 2008). This constitutes a hallmark feature in the effective discovery of serum protein markers that reflect the pathophysiology of a specific organ tissue of interest. An additional performance characteristic of the 3-D study method is its accuracy and sensitivity in identifying close to 400 phosphoproteins of potential importance to cancer biology. The identification of the phosphorylated variant to a potential protein marker imparts an additional molecular feature in the more precise capturing of unique chemical signatures of disease. This is based on the notion that a phosphorylated motif may signify the induction or silencing of a potential physiologic protein target already discussed. The versatility and adaptability of the method's constituent techniques permit the incorporation of label-based or label-free strategies to impart a quantitative feature for the in-depth proteome analysis of any given biological specimen derived from tissue, blood plasma or serum, and cell culture.

The tissue-surrogate serum proteins detected in this study and other MudPIT studies allow for the un-biased and in-depth discovery of useful biomarkers without recourse to the targeted antibody capture approach, as is common the case. In contrast, the Medical Therapy of Prostatic Symptoms (MTOPS) clinical trial, attempted to characterize potential biomarkers that could stratify the BPH patients according to their response to medical therapy, by using the *a priori* use of the ELISA assay (Mullins et al., 2008). However, such an *a priori* approach bypassed the possibility in observing unexpected low-abundant tissue specific and secreted proteins that might play a significant role on the differential diagnosis between BPH and PCa. Conclusively, the MudPIT approach is definitely a forward trend in the establishment of novel proteins marker that can be validated with more targeted approaches such as those based on Immuno-MRM techniques discussed below.

5. Future trends

5.1 Immuno-SRM (SISCAPA)

The comprehensive qualitative protein identification capability of the MudPIT approaches, can be extended to include relative quantitative features made possible with the use of multiplex stable isotope labelling strategies at the protein or peptide level. As already discussed, the quantitative capability will further minimize analytical systematic error and to better stratify patients in accordance to prostate pathophysiology analogous to that of the

BPH/PCa prostate tissue study reported by the authors. Such an approach can serve as part of a more systematic serum biomarker discovery study that can eventually lead to their validation over a very large number of specimens from healthy and diseased patient cohorts, typically exceeding 1000 for each group. So far, however, and despite the advancements made in analytical technologies, the discovery and validation of robust protein biomarkers with good specificity and sensitivity has been very disappointing. This low return on investment is due to several factors. One of them is due to the lack of functional or mechanistic utility of the candidate biomarkers. This lack of mechanistic relevance also applies to proteins that exhibit a significant differential expression between the healthy and disease samples. Another factor is associated with the large biological heterogeneity of the specimens tested. Unless the clinical samples have well defined inclusion and inclusion criteria along with effective sample procurement and handling protocols at statistically significant numbers to address a hypothesis at hand (i.e., power analysis), the analytical output will lack accuracy and precision to be of any value to the clinician (Adewale et al., 2008; Anderson, 2010; Barelli et al., 2007; Farrah et al., 2011). Another impediment is the lack of lower-cost and high-throughput validation protocols to compensate for the large number of samples that need to be analyzed. This is further compounded by the lack of antibodies for the vast majority of candidate proteins needed for the development of an ELISA kit, which is the only suitable bioassay for protein measurements in serum or plasma. Yet another limitation relates to the unreliability of a significant number of commercially available ELISA kits due to their lack of sufficient antibody validation in terms of their selectivity, cross-reactivity, linear dynamic range and sensitivity(Bordeaux et al., 2010; Stoevesandt & Taussig, 2007). An additional factor to the high failure rate of the effectiveness of the ELISA assay is that its development is principally based on recombinant protein standards that do not capture the level of complexity of the protein as it exists its *in vivo* modification status within the context of its biological matrix and also the level of protein purification is not high enough to compare to the behavior observed for the respective recombinant, highly purified, protein. Moreover, the ELISA assay is not conducive to multiplexing approaches that could have reduced some of the biological variation already discussed. This is where targeted tandem mass spectrometry methods can overcome these limitations (Gerber, Rush, Stemman, Kirschner, & Gygi, 2003; Jaffe et al., 2008). Examples of these methods include accurate inclusion mass spectrometry (AIMS) and quantitative selection reaction monitoring (Q-SRM). These more targeted MS methods specifically account for the amino-acid composition of surrogate tryptic peptides to which the selective monitoring of their precursor mass (i.e., with quadrupole mass filter), its fragmentation (i.e., CID, HCD, ETD), and subsequent product ions take place. This Selective towards one specific peptide MS precursor - product ion Reaction Monitoring (hence the term SRM) allows for its more full-time measurement and henceforth its enhanced detection in complex mixtures. The SRM detection is therefore based on the molecular signature (i.e. the unique amino acid composition of a peptide) traceable to an information rich, distinctively annotatable (i.e., *de novo* peptide sequencing), tandem (MS-MS) spectrum. Also, the intensity of the tandem spectrum traceable to one specific peptide depends on the relative or absolute concentration level of this peptide (Q-SRM). Such a level of selectivity and specificity is well beyond what can be attained with antibody capture technologies (i.e., ELISA assay)(Rissin et al., 2010). In addition, the detection of a biochemical assay is based on an absorption reading to a specific wavelength that is highly subject to background signal interference due to cross-reactivity or non-specific binding effects. Another innate advantage to the SRM technique is their very large linear dynamic range that exceed 4-orders of magnitude thanks to the latest developments to MS analyzer and detector technology (Cox & Mann, 2011; Nilsson et al., 2010; Zhang et al., 2011). When one accounts

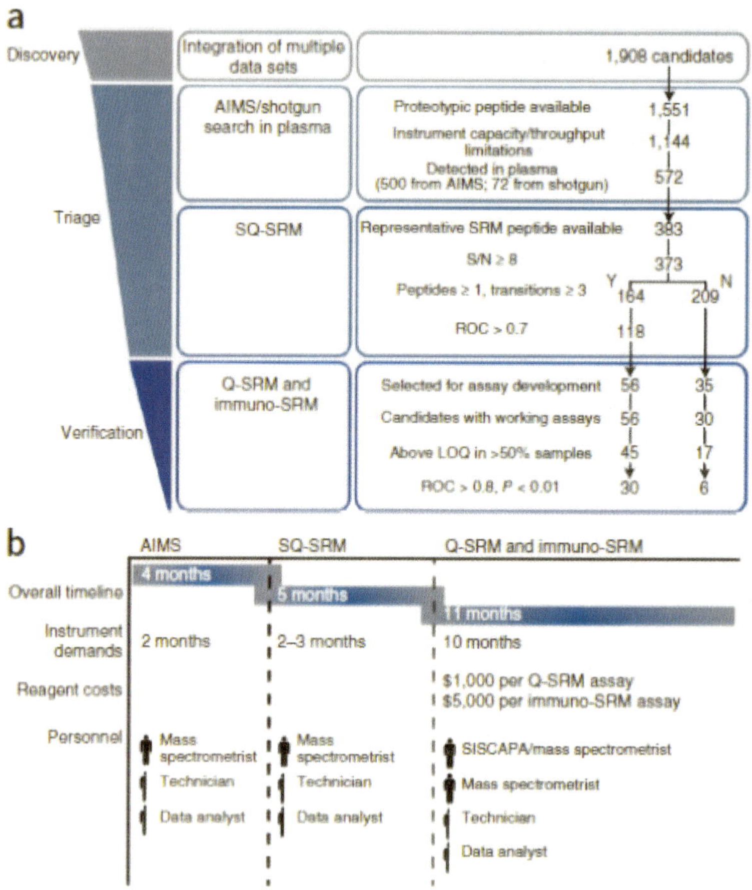

Fig. 4. Multistage, targeted proteomic pipeline for triage and verification of biomarker candidates. (a) Overview of the workflow used to triage and verify candidate biomarkers, showing the flux of candidates at each stage of the pipeline. (b) Required resources forimplementing the proteomic pipeline. The overall timeline includes time for data collection and analysis. For Q-SRM and immuno-SRM measurements, the overall timeline includes synthetic peptide quality control, development of SRM methods, acquisition of response curves and data analysis (but not the time required to generate antibodies, which can be interspersed with other activities). Instrument demands are summarized independently to provide an estimate of the required laboratory resources to carry out the study. Additional reagent costs (e.g., peptide standards and antibodies) are required for Q-SRM and immuno-SRM assays. Finally, the required personnel used in each phase of the study are denoted as full-time equivalents (Whiteaker, J.R., et al., *Nat. Biotech.* 2011).

for both the enhanced measurement selectivity and dynamic range characteristics, the SRM technique can attain > 1-2 orders of magnitude greater sensitivity compared to the fluorescence ELISA assay. These SRM advantages can be extended when combined with various targeted protein or tryptic peptide isolation techniques such as biological antibody capture (i.e., monoclonal or polyclonal based Immuno-SRM) or chemical affinity capture (i.e. chemical ligands, peptide aptamers, etc.). In the case of the Immuno-SRM variant, it can be tailored to accommodate polyclonal antibodies for the immunoaffinity capture and enrichment of proteotypic peptides mixed with their stable isotope analogs as internal standards upstream to the SRM-MS detection phase. In this scenario, the proteins found in biological extracts are tryptic digested, the resulting tryptic peptides are then immunoaffinity isolated with the polyclonal antibodies, mixed with the specific stable isotope analogues and then analyzed with SRM-MS techniques. The stable isotope peptide analogues are used as internal standards to allow for absolute or relative quantification. This particular work-flow is referred to as Stable Isotope Standards and Capture by Anti-Peptide Antibodies (SISCAPA)(Anderson, Jackson, et al.,2009; Whiteaker et al., 2011; Whiteaker, Zhao, Anderson, & Paulovich, 2010). The principles of the SISCAPA – SRM MS work-flow allows for the simultaneous capturing and analysis of over 50 tryptic peptides, uniquely traceable to over 10 proteins (Kuzyk et al., 2009). With proper experimental design and the employment of effectively trained analysts, the SISCAPA has great potential in the high-throughput with high-confidence (> 90%) analysis of thousands of clinical serum or plasma specimens for the reliable verification and validation of protein biomarker panels as unique signatures of disease prediction, diagnosis, or treatment prognosis (Figure 6). The high analysis capacity afforded by the SISCAPA - SRM MS workflow can permit the implementation of double blind, randomized and placebo controlled clinical designs (i.e., to also include a statistically significant number of healthy volunteer with diseased patient cohorts) for the more robust and comprehensive validation of such biomarker panels. Another potential advancement achievable with the SISCAPA - SRM MS workflow can be for to supersede the other currently available protein verification assays such as the Western blot, qRT-PCR, protein chip arrays, etc. This is based on the notion that workflows such as that of the SISCAPA - SRM MS can match the selectivity, specificity and sensitivity achievable by the high-precision discovery MS methods such as those based on the 3-D MudPIT and iTRAQ 2DLC-MS techniques already discussed. This especially becomes true when the same tryptic peptides including those that have undergone *in vivo* modification constitute the analytes to be measured.

5.2 Microfluidics and Lab-on-a-chip

A crucial requirement in the ability to study the content of a biomedical specimen such as clinical tissue biopsies, cell cultures or blood plasma/serum for the presence of potentially significant biomarkers is analytical sensitivity. This especially becomes prudent when the staring amount of a given clinical specimen is small. Additionally, sensitivity becomes absolutely essential given that the concentration of clinically relevant proteins and their surrogate biomolecules is exceedingly small at the progression or initiation stages of carcinogenesis already discussed. When combined with selectivity, that is an affinity to preferentially analyze one specific biomolecular entity, the availability of high sensitivity allows the targeted analysis of a naturally low abundant disease marker in complex matrices such as those typically encountered in clinical specimens. It is these requirements that drive the advancements made in microfluidic lab-on-chip (lab chip) devices (Astorga-Wells,Vollmer, Bergman, & Jornvall, 2005; Culbertson, 2006; Gottschlich, Culbertson, McKnight, Jacobson, & Ramsey, 2000; Koster & Verpoorte, 2007; Lion et al., 2003). The ever more effective bioanalyte detection is driven by the ability to integrate their extraction from complex multi-cellular matrices at decreased dilutional effects, followed by their ultra high-resolution separation, enrichment and purification upstream to the MS detection process. The lab chip devices actualize such a principle. One of several optimal characteristics of a lab chip device includes the high surface-to-volume (S/V) ratios of its microfluidic channels for analyte capture and chromatographic separation. Maintaining optimum S/V ratios is conducive toward fast and effective interaction between the solution phase bioanalyte with the stationary phase binding site. As a result, the bioanalyte to be measured exhibits

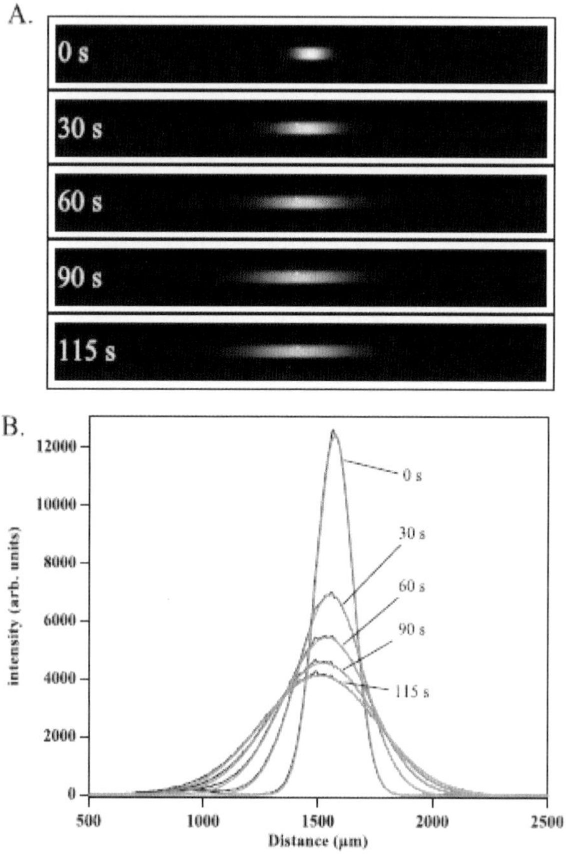

Fig. 5. Illustration of the lateral-diffusion effect of a specific amount for a given analyte species under a constant chromatographic medium. The analyte amount gets distributed over a wider distribution due to its diffusion in a time dependent manner therefore reducing its mass density at the apex. The decrease of the diffusional path of the analyte results to the increase of its mass density at the apex and consequently its improved detection at this point (Culbertson et al., 2002).

decreased lateral diffusion thus increasing its mass density leading to improved MS-based measurement sensitivity (Figure 7)(Culbertson, Jacobson, & Michael Ramsey, 2002). Other physico-chemical parameters that also play a role in achieving ideal diffusional kinetic profiles for a given chromatographic process, include the geometry of the chambers, their material properties (i.e., porous vs. non-porous), the actual chemistry (i.e. ion-exchange, hydrophilic/hydrophobic interaction, etc.) and configuration (packed vs. open tubular) of the interactive binding sites, the chemical composition of the solution phase (i.e., affecting viscosity, ion charge and mobility, etc.)(Culbertson et al., 2005; Koster & Verpoorte, 2007). Concordantly, the lab chip devices can fully exploit the very high-speed (> 40 kHz) with high-resolution (>30,000 m/Δm) signal acquisition features of the current MS platforms retrofitted with on-line or off-line ionization interfaces, such as the ESI or MALDI type, respectively.

These design features were incorporated in the development and application of a lab chip device based on a TiO_2–ZrO_2 monolithic chemical affinity chromatography format for the more selective and sensitive analysis of phosphopeptides at higher loading capacities relative to other more mainstream approaches such as those based on micropipette tips (Tsougeni et al., 2011). This monolithic column was configured on 2 mm PMMA plates, and consisted of 32 parallel microchannels with common input and output ports (Figure 8). The isolated, purified and enriched phosphopeptides were deposited onto a MALDI target and then off-line analyzed with a MALDI-MS system. The phosphopeptide binding specificity of the bidentate TiO_2–ZrO_2 chemistry at acidic pH environments, the larger number of theoretical plates (or, the density of these binding sites per unit area), and the high S/V ratio of microporous monolithic configuration all corroborated towards achieving this goal.

Conceptually, multiple chromatographic modalities can be integrated in a single lab chip format thanks to the latest developments of piezo-electric actuators, cantilevers, micro-pumps and valves, micro- and nano- mixing chambers, electroosmotically induced hydraulic pumping and other lab chip components (Figure 9). As such, these components operate under very small flow-rates (1-10 nL/min) conducive toward the optimum operation of nano-chromatographic dimensions (i.e. inner diameters < 20 μm) that also incorporate the attributes just discussed (Culbertson, Ramsey, & Ramsey, 2000; Hoeman, Lange, Roman, Higgins, & Culbertson, 2009; Jahnisch, Hessel, Lowe, & Baerns, 2004; McKnight, Culbertson, Jacobson, & Ramsey, 2001).

Another fundamental component to an integrated lab chip design is the on-line ionization source interface. In particular, the nano-electrospray ionization (nESI) source is the most suitable interface for lab chip designs when MS-based platforms are used as the detection system. Contributing factors for the ideality of the nESI source include their intrinsic non-destructive operation leading to the efficient ionization of a broad range of biomolecules including sugars, amino acids, fatty acids, nucleic acids, peptides and proteins. Therefore, the chemical integrity of these biomolecules remains intact thanks to this "soft" ionization imparted by the nESI interface (Wilm, 2011). Another contributing factor is that the nESI efficiency can be enhanced at the low nL/mL flow rate regime, provided of course that the correct geometry is utilized (Figure 10). In fact, at these flow rates, the nESI interface is less prone to the suppression effects observed when reagents essential to the operation of capillary electrophoresis and electrochromatography.

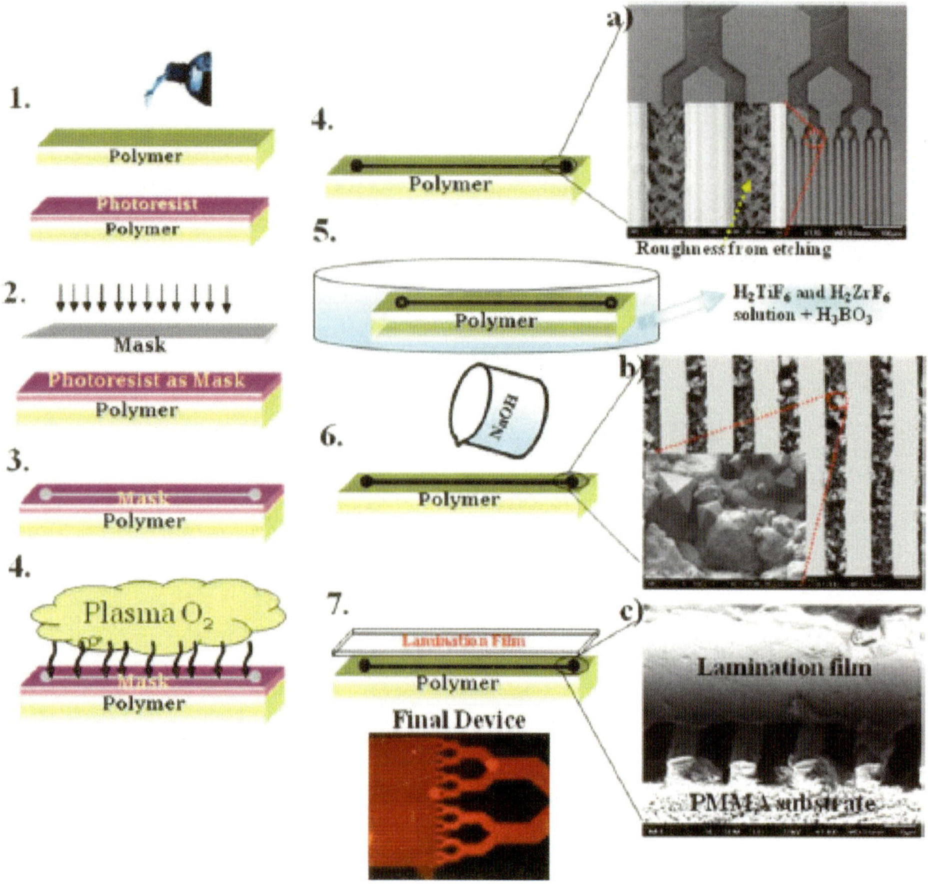

Fig. 6. Schematic representation of the fabrication process with direct lithography and plasma etching followed by liquid deposition of the TiO_2–ZrO_2 stationary phase: (1) spin coating of a thin inorganic (ORMOCER) photoresist as an etching mask on PMMA sheets, (2) lithography on photoresist polymer, using mask exposure, (3) photoresist development, (4) deep plasma etching of polymeric substrate, (5) liquid deposition of the thin TiO2–ZrO2 film and baking at 95°C, (6) rinsing with 0.1 M NaOH and DI water and baking at 95°C, and (7) sealing with lamination films. The relative thickness in the figure does not correspond to the real thickness. SEM image insets: (a) a PMMA micro-column consisting of 32 parallel microchannels after etching (a zoomed image showing the roughness at the microchannel bottom is also shown), (b) a PMMA micro-column after liquid phase deposition of TiO_2–ZrO_2 (a zoomed image of the crystallites is also shown), and (c) a cross-section of the column, after bonding with the lamination film (for details see also ESI†) (Tsougeni et al., 2011).

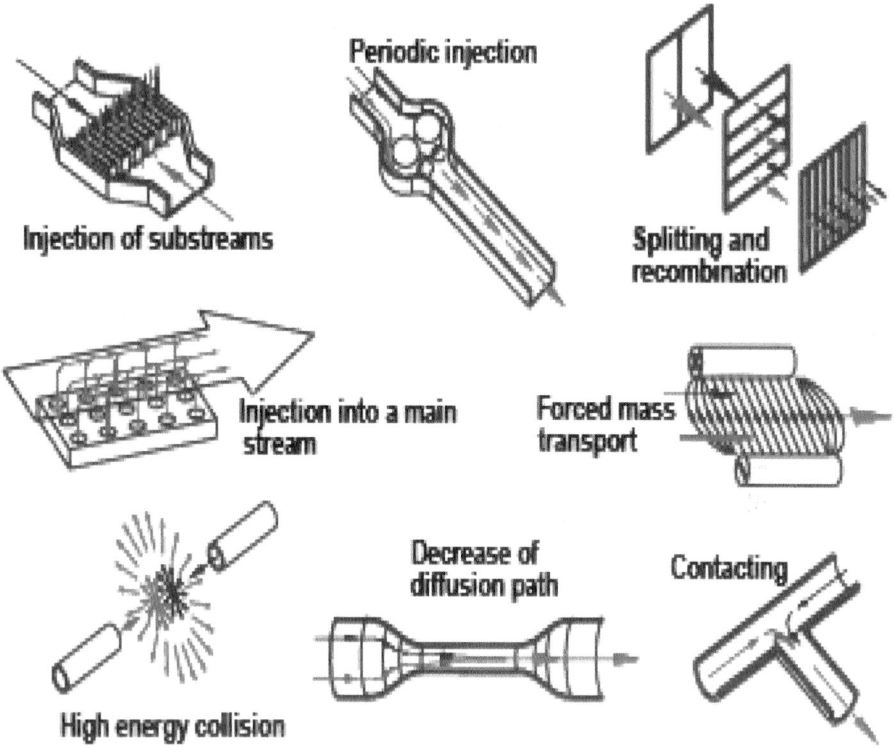

Fig. 7. Illustrative representations of various mixing chambers with different operational modes that are applicable to lab chip devices. These designs allow for the efficient mixing of reagents at nano-flow rates and assist the integration of various modes of chromatographic technique (i.e. multidimensional MudPIT) (Jahnisch et al., 2004).

Such integrated lab chip designs will allow for the effective miniaturization and automation of multi-dimensional MudPIT approaches illustrated in the previous section. Theoretically, such a lab chip reconfiguration of the more traditional lab bench analytical methodology can increase the bioanalyte sensitivity by more than several orders of magnitude. Consequently, full proteomes can be fully characterized by vastly smaller biological starting amounts (i.e. fg levels vs. μg levels). At this level of analytical sensitivity techniques such as laser capture microdissection and cell sorting can effectively be incorporated to research protocols. Also biomolecules constituting exosome entities found in plasma occurring at very low levels can also be detected. It is hypothesized that exosome biology may help explain how a particular organ secrete or shed proteins and other biomolecules such as DNA and mRNA into the systemic circulation. The exosome composition may be highly depended on the disease state of the organ (i.e. initiation stage carcinogenesis). Therefore exosomes may play a crucial role in using plasma as a biopsy source to interrogate the tissue pathophysiology status.

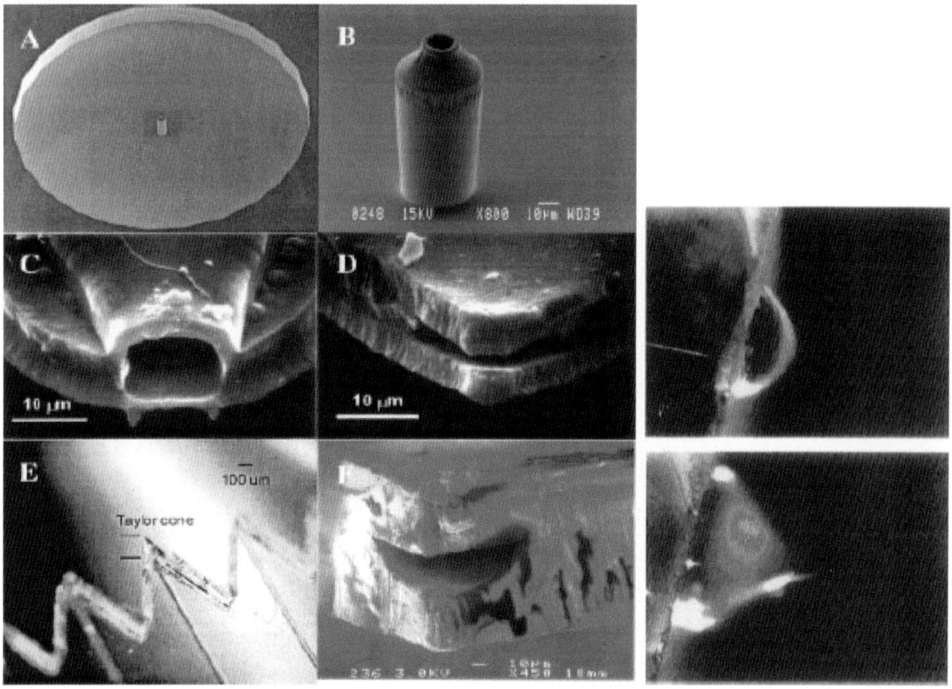

Fig. 8. Schematic nESI designs that allow its operation at the low nL/mL flow regime. Geometries, dimensions, along with their material compositions all play a pivotal role in the optimal nESI process (Lion et al., 2003).

6. Conclusion

The molecular characterization, dissection and appreciation of carcinogenesis is, undoubtedly, much more complex than we ever envisaged. The disease of cancer *per se* remains complicated, unpredictable and multifaceted - either by the impact and influence of genes, the environment, behaviour, proteins or all combined (epigenetics). In this chapter we have discussed the solid tumour of prostate cancer, a disease which falls in to two classes - indolent or aggressive. Pathologically, via immunohistology the disease 'looks' very different but at early and intermediate stages, clinically, we find it difficult to differentiate benign from malignant. We struggle to decide which glands can be left and monitored versus which that need resection and immediate therapy. The influence of 'omics and especially proteomics now has the power to categorize prostate cancer - not just the disease itself but possibly those men who may be prone to developing prostate cancer, especially the aggressive form and identify those men who need immediate intervention (Larkin et al., 2011). The next decade will see huge strides in stratifying 'normo' physiology and disease and we have presented a wealth of information here which helps to explain how the state-of-the-art methodologies and excellent clinical and patient stratification we currently have will enable this.

7. References

Ablin, R. J., Kynaston, H. G., Mason, M. D., & Jiang, W. G. (2011). Prostate transglutaminase (TGase-4) antagonizes the anti-tumour action of MDA-7/IL-24 in prostate cancer. *Journal of Translational Medicine, 9*.

Adewale, A. J., Liu, Q., Dinu, I., Lampe, P. D., Mitchell, B. L., & Yasui, Y. (2008). A cautionary note on the evaluation of biomarkers of subtypes of a single disease. *American Journal of Epidemiology, 168*(6), 559-562.

Albini, A., Ferrari, N., Tosetti, F., Fassina, G., Benelli, R., Vene, R., et al. (2007). Inflammatory angiogenesis as a target for cancer therapy and prevention. *Clinical & Experimental Metastasis, 24*(4), 230-231.

Albini, A., & Sporn, M. B. (2007). The tumour microenvironment as a target for chemoprevention. *Nature Reviews Cancer, 7*(2), 139-147.

Albini, A., Tosetti, F., Benelli, R., & Noonan, D. M. (2005). Tumor inflammatory angiogenesis and its chemoprevention. *Cancer Research, 65*(23), 10637-10641.

Alderton, G. (2007). Tumour microenvironment - Remodelling resistance. *Nature Reviews Cancer, 7*(1), 7-7.

Anderson, N. L. (2010). The clinical plasma proteome: a survey of clinical assays for proteins in plasma and serum. *Clinical Chemistry, 56*(2), 177-185.

Anderson, N. L., Anderson, N. G., Pearson, T. W., Borchers, C. H., Paulovich, A. G., Patterson, S. D., et al. (2009). A human proteome detection and quantitation project. *Molecular & Cellular Proteomics, 8*(5), 883-886.

Anderson, N. L., Jackson, A., Smith, D., Hardie, D., Borchers, C., & Pearson, T. W. (2009). SISCAPA peptide enrichment on magnetic beads using an in-line bead trap device. *Molecular & Cellular Proteomics, 8*(5), 995-1005.

Antoniades, C., Shirodaria, C., Leeson, P., Baarholm, O. A., Van-Assche, T., Cunnington, C., et al. (2009). MTHFR 677 C > T Polymorphism Reveals Functional Importance for 5-Methyltetrahydrofolate, Not Homocysteine, in Regulation of Vascular Redox State and Endothelial Function in Human Atherosclerosis. *Circulation, 119*(18), 2507-U2147.

Astorga-Wells, J., Vollmer, S., Bergman, T., & Jornvall, H. (2005). Microfluidic systems and proteomics: applications of the electrocapture technology to protein and peptide analysis. *Anal Biochem, 345*(1), 10-17.

Balk, S. P., Ko, Y. J., & Bubley, G. J. (2003). Biology of prostate-specific antigen. *Journal of Clinical Oncology, 21*(2), 383-391.

Barelli, S., Crettaz, D., Thadikkaran, L., Rubin, O., & Tissot, J. D. (2007). Plasma/serum proteomics: pre-analytical issues. *Expert Rev Proteomics, 4*(3), 363-370.

Bordeaux, J., Welsh, A., Agarwal, S., Killiam, E., Baquero, M., Hanna, J., et al. (2010). Antibody validation. *Biotechniques, 48*(3), 197-209.

Buchen, L. (2011). Missing the Mark. *Nature, 471*(7339), 428-432.

Cheung-Flynn, J., Prapapanich, V., Cox, M. B., Riggs, D. L., Suarez-Quian, C., & Smith, D. F. (2005). Physiological role for the cochaperone FKBP52 in androgen receptor signaling. *Molecular Endocrinology, 19*(6), 1654-1666.

Cox, J., & Mann, M. (2011). Quantitative, High-Resolution Proteomics for Data-Driven Systems Biology. *Annual Review of Biochemistry, Vol 80, 80*, 273-299.

Cravatt, B. F., Simon, G. M., & Yates, J. R. (2007). The biological impact of mass-spectrometry-based proteomics. *Nature, 450*(7172), 991-1000.

Culbertson, C. T. (2006). Single cell analysis on microfluidic devices. *Methods Mol Biol, 339*, 203-216.

Culbertson, C. T., Jacobson, S. C., & Michael Ramsey, J. (2002). Diffusion coefficient measurements in microfluidic devices. *Talanta, 56*(2), 365-373.

Culbertson, C. T., Ramsey, R. S., & Ramsey, J. M. (2000). Electroosmotically induced hydraulic pumping on microchips: differential ion transport. *Analytical Chemistry, 72*(10), 2285-2291.

Culbertson, C. T., Tugnawat, Y., Meyer, A. R., Roman, G. T., Ramsey, J. M., & Gonda, S. R. (2005). Microchip separations in reduced-gravity and hypergravity environments. *Analytical Chemistry, 77*(24), 7933-7940.

Dabbous, M. K., Jefferson, M. M., Haney, L., & Thomas, E. L. (2011). Biomarkers of metastatic potential in cultured adenocarcinoma clones. *Clinical & Experimental Metastasis, 28*(2), 101-111.

Das, S. K., Eder, S., Schauer, S., Diwoky, C., Temmel, H., Guertl, B., et al. (2011). Adipose Triglyceride Lipase Contributes to Cancer-Associated Cachexia. *Science, 333*(6039), 233-238.

De Leon, J. T., Iwai, A., Feau, C., Garcia, Y., Balsiger, H. A., Storer, C. L., et al. (2011). Targeting the regulation of androgen receptor signaling by the heat shock protein 90 cochaperone FKBP52 in prostate cancer cells. *Proceedings of the National Academy of Sciences of the United States of America, 108*(29), 11878-11883.

De Marzo, A. M., DeWeese, T. L., Platz, E. A., Meeker, A. K., Nakayama, M., Epstein, J. I., et al. (2004). Pathological and molecular mechanisms of prostate carcinogenesis: Implications for diagnosis, detection, prevention, and treatment. *Journal of Cellular Biochemistry, 91*(3), 459-477.

De Nunzio, C., Freedland, S. J., Miano, R., Trucchi, A., Cantiani, A., Carluccini, A., et al. (2011). Metabolic Syndrome Is Associated With High Grade Gleason Score When Prostate Cancer Is Diagnosed on Biopsy. *Prostate, 71*(14), 1492-1498.

DeMarzo, A. M., Nelson, W. G., Isaacs, W. B., & Epstein, J. I. (2003). Pathological and molecular aspects of prostate cancer. *Lancet, 361*(9361), 955-964.

DeSouza, L., Diehl, G., Rodrigues, M. J., Guo, J. Z., Romaschin, A. D., Colgan, T. J., et al. (2005). Search for cancer markers from endometrial tissues using differentially labeled tags iTRAQ and cICAT with multidimensional liquid chromatography and tandem mass spectrometry. *Journal of Proteome Research, 4*(2), 377-386.

Di Cristofano, C., Leopizzi, M., Miraglia, A., Sardella, B., Moretti, V., Ferrara, A., et al. (2010). Phosphorylated ezrin is located in the nucleus of the osteosarcoma cell. *Modern Pathology, 23*(7), 1012-1020.

Diamandis, E. P. (2004). Mass Spectrometry as a diagnostic and a cancer biomarker discovery tool - Opportunities and potential limitations. *Molecular & Cellular Proteomics, 3*(4), 367-378.

Dong, Y., Zhang, H. T., Hawthorn, L., Ganther, H. E., & Ip, C. (2003). Delineation of the molecular basis for selenium-induced growth arrest in human prostate cancer cells by oligonucleotide array. *Cancer Research, 63*(1), 52-59.

Everley, P. A., Krijgsveld, J., Zetter, B. R., & Gygi, S. P. (2004). Quantitative cancer proteomics: Stable isotope labeling with amino acids in cell culture (SILAC) as a tool for prostate cancer research. *Molecular & Cellular Proteomics, 3*(7), 729-735.

Farrah, T., Deutsch, E. W., Omenn, G. S., Campbell, D. S., Sun, Z., Bletz, J. A., et al. (2011). A high-confidence human plasma proteome reference set with estimated concentrations in PeptideAtlas. *Molecular & Cellular Proteomics, 10*(9), M110 006353.

Fournier, M. L., Gilmore, J. M., Martin-Brown, S. A., & Washburn, M. P. (2007). Multidimensional separations-based shotgun proteomics. *Chemical Reviews, 107*(8), 3654-3686.

Garbis, S., Lubec, G., & Fountoulakis, M. (2005). Limitations of current proteomics technologies. *Journal of Chromatography A, 1077*(1), 1-18.

Garbis, S. D., Melse-Boonstra, A., West, C. E., & van Breemen, R. B. (2001). Determination of folates in human plasma using hydrophilic interaction chromatography-tandem mass spectrometry. *Analytical Chemistry, 73*(22), 5358-5364.

Garbis, S. D., Roumeliotis, T. I., Tyritzis, S. I., Zorpas, K. M., Pavlakis, K., & Constantinides, C. A. (2011). A Novel Multidimensional Protein Identification Technology Approach Combining, Protein Size Exclusion Prefractionation, Peptide Zwitterion-Ion Hydrophilic Interaction Chromatography, and Nano-Ultraperformance RP Chromatography/nESI-MS(2) for the in-Depth Analysis of the Serum Proteome and Phosphoproteome: Application to Clinical Sera Derived from Humans with Benign Prostate Hyperplasia. *Analytical Chemistry, 83*(3), 708-718.

Garbis, S. D., Tyritzis, S. I., Roumeliotis, T., Zerefos, P., Giannopoulou, E. G., Vlahou, A., et al. (2008). Search for potential markers for prostate cancer diagnosis, prognosis and treatment in clinical tissue specimens using amine-specific isobaric tagging (iTRAQ) with two-dimensional liquid chromatography and tandem mass spectrometry. *Journal of Proteome Research, 7*(8), 3146-3158.

Garcia-Ramirez, M., Canals, F., Hernandez, C., Colome, N., Ferrer, C., Carrasco, E., et al. (2007). Proteomic analysis of human vitreous fluid by fluorescence-based difference gel electrophoresis (DIGE): a new strategy for identifying potential candidates in the pathogenesis of proliferative diabetic retinopathy. *Diabetologia, 50*(6), 1294-1303.

Gerber, S. A., Rush, J., Stemman, O., Kirschner, M. W., & Gygi, S. P. (2003). Absolute quantification of proteins and phosphoproteins from cell lysates by tandem MS. *Proc Natl Acad Sci U S A, 100*(12), 6940-6945.

Glen, A., Gan, C. S., Hamdy, F. C., Eaton, C. L., Cross, S. S., Catto, J. W. F., et al. (2008). iTRAQ - Facilitated proteomic analysis of human prostate cancer cells identifies proteins associated with progression. *Journal of Proteome Research, 7*(3), 897-907.

Goldstraw, M. A., Fitzpatrick, J. M., & Kirby, R. S. (2007). What is the role of inflammation in the pathogenesis of prostate cancer? *Bju International, 99*(5), 966-968.

Gonzalez-Moreno, O., Boque, N., Redrado, M., Milagro, F., Campion, J., Endermann, T., et al. (2011). Selenoprotein-P is Down-Regulated in Prostate Cancer, Which Results in Lack of Protection Against Oxidative Damage. *Prostate, 71*(8), 824-834.

Gottschlich, N., Culbertson, C. T., McKnight, T. E., Jacobson, S. C., & Ramsey, J. M. (2000). Integrated microchip-device for the digestion, separation and postcolumn labeling of proteins and peptides. *J Chromatogr B Biomed Sci Appl, 745*(1), 243-249.

Granger, J., Siddiqui, J., Copeland, S., & Remick, D. (2005). Albumin depletion of human plasma also removes low abundance proteins including the cytokines. *Proteomics, 5*(18), 4713-4718.

Grisendi, S., Mecucci, C., Falini, B., & Pandolfi, P. P. (2006). Nucleophosmin and cancer. *Nature Reviews Cancer, 6*(7), 493-505.

Gundry, R. L., White, M. Y., Nogee, J., Tchernyshyov, I., & Van Eyk, J. E. (2009). Assessment of albumin removal from an immunoaffinity spin column: critical implications for proteomic examination of the albuminome and albumin-depleted samples. *Proteomics, 9*(7), 2021-2028.

Hale, L. P., Price, D. T., Sanchez, L. M., Demark-Wahnefried, W., & Madden, J. F. (2001). Zinc alpha-2-glycoprotein is expressed by malignant prostatic epithelium and may serve as a potential serum marker for prostate cancer. *Clinical Cancer Research, 7*(4), 846-853.

Hammarsten, J., & Hogstedt, B. (2002). Calculated fast-growing benign prostatic hyperplasia - A risk factor for developing clinical prostate cancer. *Scandinavian Journal of Urology and Nephrology, 36*(5), 330-338.

Hanahan, D., & Weinberg, R. A. (2011). Hallmarks of Cancer: The Next Generation. *Cell, 144*(5), 646-674.

Hanash, S. M., Pitteri, S. J., & Faca, V. M. (2008). Mining the plasma proteome for cancer biomarkers. *Nature, 452*(7187), 571-579.

Hilario, M., & Kalousis, A. (2008). Approaches to dimensionality reduction in proteomic biomarker studies. *Briefings in Bioinformatics, 9*(2), 102-118.

Hildenbrand, Z. L., Molugu, S. K., Herrera, N., Ramirez, C., Xiao, C., & Bernal, R. A. (2011). Hsp90 can Accommodate the Simultaneous Binding of the FKBP52 and HOP Proteins. *Oncotarget, 2*(1-2), 43-58.

Hoeman, K. W., Lange, J. J., Roman, G. T., Higgins, D. A., & Culbertson, C. T. (2009). Electrokinetic trapping using titania nanoporous membranes fabricated using sol-gel chemistry on microfluidic devices. *Electrophoresis, 30*(18), 3160-3167.

Hood, B. L., Darfler, M. M., Guiel, T. G., Furusato, B., Lucas, D. A., Ringeisen, B. R., et al. (2005). Proteomic analysis of formalin-fixed prostate cancer tissue. *Molecular & Cellular Proteomics, 4*(11), 1741-1753.

Issaq, H. J., Xiao, Z., & Veenstra, T. D. (2007). Serum and plasma proteomics. *Chemical Reviews, 107*(8), 3601-3620.

Jaffe, J. D., Keshishian, H., Chang, B., Addona, T. A., Gillette, M. A., & Carr, S. A. (2008). Accurate inclusion mass screening: a bridge from unbiased discovery to targeted assay development for biomarker verification. *Molecular & Cellular Proteomics, 7*(10), 1952-1962.

Jahnisch, K., Hessel, V., Lowe, H., & Baerns, M. (2004). Chemistry in microstructured reactors. *Angew Chem Int Ed Engl, 43*(4), 406-446.

Jemal, A., Siegel, R., Xu, J. Q., & Ward, E. (2010). Cancer Statistics, 2010. *Ca-a Cancer Journal for Clinicians, 60*(5), 277-300.

Jeronimo, C., Henrique, R., Oliveira, J., Lobo, F., Pais, I., Teixeira, M. R., et al. (2004). Aberrant cellular retinol binding protein 1 (CRBP1) gene expression and promoter methylation in prostate cancer. *Journal of Clinical Pathology, 57*(8), 872-876.

Jiang, W. G., & Ablin, R. J. (2011). Prostate transglutaminase: a unique transglutaminase and its role in prostate cancer. *Biomarkers in Medicine, 5*(3), 285-291.

Joyce, J. A. (2005). Therapeutic targeting of the tumor microenvironment. *Cancer Cell, 7*(6), 513-520.

Khanna, C., Wan, X. L., Bose, S., Cassaday, R., Olomu, O., Mendoza, A., et al. (2004). The membrane-cytoskeleton linker ezrin is necessary for osteosarcoma metastasis. *Nature Medicine, 10*(2), 182-186.

Kim, C. J., Sakamoto, K., Tambe, Y., & Inoue, H. (2011). Opposite regulation of epithelial-to-mesenchymal transition and cell invasiveness by periostin between prostate and bladder cancer cells. *International Journal of Oncology, 38*(6), 1759-1766.

Kim, J., Sun, P. Y., Lam, Y. W., Troncoso, P., Sabichi, A. L., Babaian, R. J., et al. (2005). Changes in serum proteomic patterns by presurgical alpha-tocopherol and L-selenomethionine supplementation in prostate cancer. *Cancer Epidemiology Biomarkers & Prevention, 14*(7), 1697-1702.

Kocher, T., & Superti-Furga, G. (2007). Mass spectrometry-based functional proteomics: from molecular machines to protein networks. *Nature Methods, 4*(10), 807-815.

Koster, S., & Verpoorte, E. (2007). A decade of microfluidic analysis coupled with electrospray mass spectrometry: An overview. *Lab on a Chip, 7*(11), 1394-1412.

Krust, B., El Khoury, D., Nondier, I., Soundaramourty, C., & Hovanessian, A. G. (2011). Targeting surface nucleolin with multivalent HB-19 and related Nucant pseudopeptides results in distinct inhibitory mechanisms depending on the malignant tumor cell type. *Bmc Cancer, 11.*

Kuemmerle, N. B., Rysman, E., Lombardo, P. S., Flanagan, A. J., Lipe, B. C., Wells, W. A., et al. (2011). Lipoprotein Lipase Links Dietary Fat to Solid Tumor Cell Proliferation. *Molecular Cancer Therapeutics, 10*(3), 427-436.

Kuzyk, M. A., Smith, D., Yang, J., Cross, T. J., Jackson, A. M., Hardie, D. B., et al. (2009). Multiple reaction monitoring-based, multiplexed, absolute quantitation of 45 proteins in human plasma. *Molecular & Cellular Proteomics, 8*(8), 1860-1877.

Larkin, S. E., Holmes, S., Cree, I. A., Walker, T., Basketter, V., Bickers, B., et al. (2011). Identification of markers of prostate cancer progression using candidate gene expression. *Br J Cancer*. Br J Cancer. 2012 Jan 3;106(1):157-65

Lin, B. Y., White, J. T., Lu, W., Xie, T., Utleg, A. G., Yan, X. W., et al. (2005). Evidence for the presence of disease-perturbed networks in prostate cancer cells by genomic and proteomic analyses: A systems approach to disease. *Cancer Research, 65*(8), 3081-3091.

Lion, N., Rohner, T. C., Dayon, L., Arnaud, I. L., Damoc, E., Youhnovski, N., et al. (2003). Microfluidic systems in proteomics. *Electrophoresis, 24*(21), 3533-3562.

Liu, T., Belov, M. E., Jaitly, N., Qian, W. J., & Smith, R. D. (2007). Accurate mass measurements in proteomics. *Chemical Reviews, 107*(8), 3621-3653.

Lubec, G., & Afjehi-Sadat, L. (2007). Limitations and pitfalls in protein identification by mass spectrometry. *Chemical Reviews, 107*(8), 3568-3584.

Mann, M., & Kelleher, N. L. (2008). Precision proteomics: The case for high resolution and high mass accuracy. *Proceedings of the National Academy of Sciences of the United States of America, 105*(47), 18132-18138.

Martin, D. B., Gifford, D. R., Wright, M. E., Keller, A., Yi, E., Goodlett, D. R., et al. (2004). Quantitative proteomic analysis of proteins released by neoplastic prostate epithelium. *Cancer Research, 64*(1), 347-355.

McKeen, H. D., Brennan, D. J., Hegarty, S., Lanigan, F., Jirstrom, K., Byrne, C., et al. (2011). The emerging role of FK506-binding proteins as cancer biomarkers: a focus on FKBPL. *Biochemical Society Transactions, 39*, 663-668.

McKnight, T. E., Culbertson, C. T., Jacobson, S. C., & Ramsey, J. M. (2001). Electroosmotically induced hydraulic pumping with integrated electrodes on microfluidic devices. *Analytical Chemistry, 73*(16), 4045-4049.

Meehan, K. L., & Sadar, M. D. (2004). Quantitative profiling of LNCaP prostate cancer cells using isotope-coded affinity tags and mass spectrometry. *Proteomics, 4*(4), 1116-1134.

Melse-Boonstra, A., Verhoef, P., West, C. E., van Rhijn, J. A., van Breemen, R. B., Lasaroms, J. J. P., et al. (2006). A dual-isotope-labeling method of studying the bioavailability of hexaglutamyl folic acid relative to that of monoglutamyl folic acid in humans by using multiple orally administered low doses. *American Journal of Clinical Nutrition, 84*(5), 1128-1133.

Menendez, J. A., & Lupu, R. (2007). Fatty acid synthase and the lipogenic phenotype in cancer pathogenesis. *Nature Reviews Cancer, 7*(10), 763-777.

Milad, M., Sullivan, W., Diehl, E., Altmann, M., Nordeen, S., Edwards, D. P., et al. (1995). Interaction of the Progesterone-Receptor with Binding-Proteins for Fk506 and Cyclosporine-A. *Molecular Endocrinology, 9*(7), 838-847.

Miyoshi, Y., Ishiguro, H., Uemura, H., Fujinami, K., Miyamoto, H., Miyoshi, Y., et al. (2003). Expression of AR associated protein 55 (ARA55) and androgen receptor in prostate cancer. *Prostate, 56*(4), 280-286.

Moretti, R. M., Mai, S., Marelli, M. M., Rizzi, F., Bettuzzi, S., & Limonta, P. (2011). Molecular mechanisms of the antimetastatic activity of nuclear clusterin in prostate cancer cells. *International Journal of Oncology, 39*(1), 225-234.

Mueller, M. M., & Fusenig, N. E. (2004). Friends or foes - Bipolar effects of the tumour stroma in cancer. *Nature Reviews Cancer, 4*(11), 839-849.

Mullins, C., Lucia, M. S., Hayward, S. W., Lee, J. Y., Levitt, J. M., Lin, V. K., et al. (2008). A comprehensive approach toward novel serum biomarkers for benign prostatic hyperplasia: the MPSA Consortium. *J Urol, 179*(4), 1243-1256.

Nelson, W. G., DeMarzo, A. M., DeWeese, T. L., & Isaacs, W. B. (2005). The molecular pathogenesis of human prostate cancer. *Hormonal Carcinogenesis Iv*, 34-44.

Nilsson, T., Mann, M., Aebersold, R., Yates, J. R., Bairoch, A., & Bergeron, J. J. M. (2010). Mass spectrometry in high-throughput proteomics: ready for the big time. *Nature Methods, 7*(9), 681-685.

Oh, K. S., Khan, S. G., Jaspers, N. G. J., Raams, A., Ueda, T., Lehmann, A., et al. (2006). Phenotypic heterogeneity in the XPB DNA helicase gene (ERCC3): Xeroderma pigmentosum without and with Cockayne syndrome. *Human Mutation, 27*(11), 1092-1103.

Okuda, M., Horn, H. F., Tarapore, P., Tokuyama, Y., Smulian, A. G., Chan, P. K., et al. (2000). Nucleophosmin/B23 is a target of CDK2/Cyclin E in centrosome duplication. *Cell, 103*(1), 127-140.

Ong, S. E., & Mann, M. (2005). Mass spectrometry-based proteomics turns quantitative. *Nature Chemical Biology, 1*(5), 252-262.

Papayannopoulos, I. A. (1995). The Interpretation of Collision-Induced Dissociation Tandem Mass-Spectra of Peptides. *Mass Spectrometry Reviews, 14*(1), 49-73.

Pfeffer, U., Tosetti, F., Ferrari, N., Vene, R., Benelli, R., Morini, M., et al. (2002). Angioprevention: Anti-angiogenesis as a critical target for cancer chemopreventive agents. *Cancer Epidemiology Biomarkers & Prevention, 11*(10), 1235S-1235S.

Pichler, P., Kocher, T., Holzmann, J., Mohring, T., Ammerer, G., & Mechtler, K. (2011). Improved Precision of iTRAQ and TMT Quantification by an Axial Extraction Field in an Orbitrap HCD Cell. *Analytical Chemistry, 83*(4), 1469-1474.

Planche, A., Bacac, M., Provero, P., Fusco, C., Delorenzi, M., Stehle, J. C., et al. (2011). Identification of Prognostic Molecular Features in the Reactive Stroma of Human Breast and Prostate Cancer. *Plos One, 6*(5).

Rahbar, A., Rivers, R., Boja, E., Kinsinger, C., Mesri, M., Hiltke, T., et al. (2011). Realizing individualized medicine: the road to translating proteomics from the laboratory to the clinic. *Personalized Medicine, 8*(1), 45-57.

Rissin, D. M., Kan, C. W., Campbell, T. G., Howes, S. C., Fournier, D. R., Song, L., et al. (2010). Single-molecule enzyme-linked immunosorbent assay detects serum proteins at subfemtomolar concentrations. *Nat Biotechnol, 28*(6), 595-599.

Rowland, J. G., Simon, J. W., Slabas, A. R., Robson, C. N., & Leung, H. Y. (2004). Quantitative proteomic analysis of androgen & anti-androgen responses in the LNCaP prostate cancer cell line. *British Journal of Cancer, 91*, S38-S38.

Rubakhin, S. S., Romanova, E. V., Nemes, P., & Sweedler, J. V. (2011). Profiling metabolites and peptides in single cells. *Nature Methods, 8*(4), S20-S29.

Sawyers, C. L. (2008). The cancer biomarker problem. *Nature, 452*(7187), 548-552.

Seymour, S. L., Shilov, I. V., Patel, A. A., Loboda, A., Tang, W. H., Keating, S. P., et al. (2006). The application of the paragon algorithm to the study of protein modifications. *Molecular & Cellular Proteomics, 5*(10), S294-S294.

Shilov, I. V., Seymour, S. L., Patel, A. A., Loboda, A., Tang, W. H., Keating, S. P., et al. (2007). The paragon algorithm, a next generation search engine that uses sequence temperature values and feature probabilities to identify peptides from tandem mass spectra. *Molecular & Cellular Proteomics, 6*(9), 1638-1655.

Stoevesandt, O., & Taussig, M. J. (2007). Affinity reagent resources for human proteome detection: initiatives and perspectives. *Proteomics, 7*(16), 2738-2750.

Sun, C. Y., Song, C., Ma, Z. C., Xu, K., Zhang, Y., Jin, H., et al. (2011). Periostin identified as a potential biomarker of prostate cancer by iTRAQ-proteomics analysis of prostate biopsy. *Proteome Science, 9*.

Sun, C. Y., Zhao, X. J., Xu, K., Gong, J., Liu, W. W., Ding, W. H., et al. (2011). Periostin: a promising target of therapeutical intervention for prostate cancer. *Journal of Translational Medicine, 9*.

Sytkowski, A. J., Gao, C., Feldman, L., & Chen, C. (2005). Human selenium binding protein-1 (hSP56) inhibits anchorage-independent growth of PC-3 human prostate cancer cells and is down-regulated in primary human prostate tumor. *Journal of Clinical Oncology, 23*(16), 852S-852S.

Thompson, I. M., Ankerst, D. P., Chi, C., Lucia, M. S., Goodman, P. J., Crowley, J. J., et al. (2005). Operating characteristics of prostate-specific antigen in men with an initial PSA level of 3.0 ng/mL or lower. *Jama-Journal of the American Medical Association, 294*(1), 66-70.

Toki, K., Enokida, H., Kawakami, K., Chiyomaru, T., Tatarano, S., Yoshino, H., et al. (2010). CpG hypermethylation of cellular retinol-binding protein 1 contributes to cell proliferation and migration in bladder cancer. *International Journal of Oncology, 37*(6), 1379-1388.

Tsavachidou, D., McDonnell, T. J., Wen, S. J., Wang, X. M., Vakar-Lopez, F., Pisters, L. L., et al. (2009). Selenium and Vitamin E: Cell Type- and Intervention-Specific Tissue Effects in Prostate Cancer. *Journal of the National Cancer Institute, 101*(5), 306-320.

Tsougeni, K., Zerefos, P., Tserepi, A., Vlahou, A., Garbis, S. D., & Gogolides, E. (2011). TiO(2)-ZrO(2) affinity chromatography polymeric microchip for phosphopeptide enrichment and separation. *Lab on a Chip, 11*(18), 3113-3120.

Turteltaub, K. W., Davis, M. A., Burns-Naas, L. A., Lawton, M. P., Clark, A. M., & Reynolds, J. A. (2011). Identification and Elucidation of the Biology of Adverse Events: The Challenges of Safety Assessment and Translational Medicine. *Clinical Cancer Research, 17*(21), 6641-6645.

van Bentem, S. D., Mentzen, W. I., de la Fuente, A., & Hirt, H. (2008). Towards functional phosphoproteomics by mapping differential phosphorylation events in signaling networks. *Proteomics, 8*(21), 4453-4465.

van Winden, A. W., van den Broek, I., Gast, M. C., Engwegen, J. Y., Sparidans, R. W., van Dulken, E. J., et al. (2010). Serum degradome markers for the detection of breast cancer. *Journal of Proteome Research, 9*(8), 3781-3788.

Walsh, P. C. (2010). Chemoprevention of Prostate Cancer. *New England Journal of Medicine, 362*(13), 1237-1238.

Walther, T. C., & Mann, M. (2010). Mass spectrometry-based proteomics in cell biology. *Journal of Cell Biology, 190*(4), 491-500.

Weng, W. H., Ahlen, J., Astrom, K., Lui, W. O., & Larsson, C. (2005). Prognostic impact of immunohistochemical expression of ezrin in highly malignant soft tissue sarcomas. *Clinical Cancer Research, 11*(17), 6198-6204.

Whiteaker, J. R., Lin, C., Kennedy, J., Hou, L., Trute, M., Sokal, I., et al. (2011). A targeted proteomics-based pipeline for verification of biomarkers in plasma. *Nat Biotechnol, 29*(7), 625-634.

Whiteaker, J. R., Zhao, L., Anderson, L., & Paulovich, A. G. (2010). An automated and multiplexed method for high throughput peptide immunoaffinity enrichment and multiple reaction monitoring mass spectrometry-based quantification of protein biomarkers. *Molecular & Cellular Proteomics, 9*(1), 184-196.

Wilm, M. (2011). Principles of electrospray ionization. *Molecular & Cellular Proteomics, 10*(7), M111 009407.

Wright, M. E., Eng, J., Sherman, J., Hockenbery, D. M., Nelson, P. S., Galitski, T., et al. (2004). Identification of androgen-coregulated protein networks from the microsomes of human prostate cancer cells. *Genome Biology, 5*(1).

Wright, M. E., Han, D. K., & Aebersold, R. (2005). Mass spectrometry-based expression profiling of clinical prostate cancer. *Molecular & Cellular Proteomics, 4*(4), 545-554.

Wu, W. W., Wang, G. H., Baek, S. J., & Shen, R. F. (2006). Comparative study of three proteomic quantitative methods, DIGE, cICAT, and iTRAQ, using 2D gel- or LC-MALDI TOF/TOF. *Journal of Proteome Research, 5*(3), 651-658.

Yang, C. M., Yen, Y. T., Huang, C. S., & Hu, M. L. (2011). Growth inhibitory efficacy of lycopene and beta-carotene against androgen-independent prostate tumor cells xenografted in nude mice. *Molecular Nutrition & Food Research, 55*(4), 606-612.

Yang, M. H., & Sytkowski, A. J. (1998). Differential expression and androgen regulation of the human selenium-binding protein gene hSP56 in prostate cancer cells. *Cancer Research, 58*(14), 3150-3153.

Yetley, E. A., Pfeiffer, C. M., Phinney, K. W., Fazili, Z., Lacher, D. A., Bailey, R. L., et al. (2011). Biomarkers of folate status in NHANES: a roundtable summary. *American Journal of Clinical Nutrition, 94*(1), 303S-312S.

Yu, Y. P., & Luo, J. H. (2006). Myopodin-mediated suppression of prostate cancer cell migration involves interaction with zyxin. *Cancer Research, 66*(15), 7414-7419.

Zeliadt, S. B., & Ramsey, S. D. (2010). Cost-effectiveness of prostate cancer chemoprevention among high-risk men. *Expert Review of Pharmacoeconomics & Outcomes Research, 10*(5), 505-508.

Zhang, H., Liu, Q., Zimmerman, L. J., Ham, A. J., Slebos, R. J., Rahman, J., et al. (2011). Methods for peptide and protein quantitation by liquid chromatography-multiple reaction monitoring mass spectrometry. *Molecular & Cellular Proteomics, 10*(6), M110 006593.

Zolotarjova, N., Martosella, J., Nicol, G., Bailey, J., Boyes, B. E., & Barrett, W. C. (2005). Differences among techniques for high-abundant protein depletion. *Proteomics, 5*(13), 3304-3313.

16

Using miRNA as Biomarkers to Evaluate the Alcohol-Induced Oxidative Stress

Yueming Tang[1,*], Christopher B. Forsyth[1,4] and Ali Keshavarzian[1,2,3]
[1]*Division of Digestive Disease and Nutrition, Department of Internal Medicine,*
[2]*Department of Pharmacology,*
[3]*Department of Molecular Biophysics and Physiology,*
[4]*Department of Biochemistry,*
Rush University Medical Center, Chicago IL,
USA

1. Introduction

Oxidative stress is responsible for a variety of degenerative processes in many human diseases, as either cause or effect. At present, some biomarkers of oxidative stress have been used to determine an individual's oxidative status in relation to disease conditions. However, their accuracy, sensitivity, or specificity needs to be improved. The development of novel biomarkers for oxidative stress is urgent.

Micro RNAs (miRNAs) are highly conserved regulatory molecules expressed in eukaryotic cells. They are short non-coding RNAs that regulate gene expression by binding to target mRNAs, which leads to reduced protein synthesis and sometimes decreased steady-state mRNA levels. Although hundreds of miRNAs have been identified, much less is known about their biological function. There are evidences that miRNAs affect pathways fundamental to metabolic control in higher organisms such as adipocyte and skeletal muscle differentiation. Also, some miRNAs are implicated in lipid, amino acid, and glucose homeostasis. Thus, miRNA abnormalities may contribute to common metabolic and systemic diseases where oxidative stress plays a key role in their pathogenesis. Indeed, there are evidences indicated that miRNAs are able to modulate the cellular response to oxidative stress both *in vitro* and *in vivo*. Therefore, miRNA may be novel biomarkers for oxidative stress.

We hypothesize that miRNAs may be biomarkers for oxidative stress because: (1) since miRNA are post-transcriptional gene regulators, they may be able to function as 'quick responders' to oxidative stress. For example, upon exposure to stress, miRNA may rapidly localize to P-bodies or stress granules to regulate key genes involved in the oxidative stress response. After the stress is mitigated, miRNA inhibition may be promptly abated, allowing

* Correponding Author

commencement of translation and expeditive restoration of cells back to their normal state; (2) since miRNAs regulate numerous targets, they have the capacity to powerfully and efficiently coordinate a stress response involving numerous genes; (3) owing to their small size and high stability, miRNAs may be less susceptible to certain types of stress, like genotoxic insults. Hence, their ability to modulate stress response would be less likely to be compromised under oxidative-stress. Given the recent development in the field of miRNA research, we predict that miRNA will be promised biomarkers for oxidative stress.

To test our hypothesis, we chose to study Alcoholic Liver Disease (ALD) as an oxidative stress model because: (1) it has high morbidity and mortality with no satisfactory therapy; (2) we showed that oxidative damage is the major mechanism for ALD; (3) we have established and validate that ALD model in rats is a good model for studies of oxidative stress. Our studies demonstrated that: (1). Nitric oxide-induced oxidative stress is required for alcohol-induced gut leakiness and liver damage in this model; (2) The miRNA expression profile was identified by miRNA microarray analysis. The miRNAs signatures were validated by TaqMan real time PCR assay. Our research results demonstrated that the differentially expressed miRNAs are the sensitive and specific biomarkers for alcohol-induced oxidative stress. (3) We showed that oats supplementation, a diet with strong anti-oxidative effect that is widely used in diets to prevent many diseases associated with oxidative damage, prevents ALD in rats by preventing alcohol-induced oxidative tissue damage.

Numerous markers of oxidative stress and antioxidant status have been evaluated, but there has been little systematic effort to validate sensitive and specific biomarkers for oxidative damage in animal models. The application of miRNA as new biomarkers will lead to: a) identification susceptible individuals who are at risk for oxidative stress and would thus benefit from interventions that provide antioxidants; b) novel strategies to prevent and treat oxidative injury.

2. Biomarkers for oxidative stress in human disease

Oxidative/nitrosative stress, such as alcohol-induced increase of reactive oxygen/nitrogen species (ROS/NOS), is now recognized to be a common cause or a prominent feature of many acute and chronic inflammatory diseases(Dalle-Donne et al., 2006). However, up to date, there are not ideal biomarkers and/or methods available to assess oxidative stress status in human diseases. Thus, we are exploring and searching for new biomarkers of oxidative stress, such as miRNA, to objectively measure and evaluate the role of miRNA in the alcohol-induced oxidative stress.

Biomarkers may provide information on three progressive levels of disease outcome(Dalle-Donne et al., 2006): (*a*) as measurable endpoints of damage of biomolecules such as lipids and proteins; (*b*) as functional markers of, for example, cognitive function; and (*c*) as endpoints related to specific disease. In many cases, oxidative stress is an early and common pathphysiological process. Thus, it is very important to find a series of biomarkers to early detect the alcohol-induced oxidative stress. Studying the association between a biomarker and alcohol-induced oxidative stress could benefit for early detection and, therefore, prevention of diseases associated with oxidative stress.

The most intuitive goals for a biomarker are to help diagnose symptomatic and presymptomatic disease and to provide surrogate endpoints to demonstrate clinical efficacy of new treatments(Ogino and Wang, 2007). The usefulness of the ideal biomarker of oxidative damage lies in its ability to provide early indication of disease and/or its progression (Fig. 1).

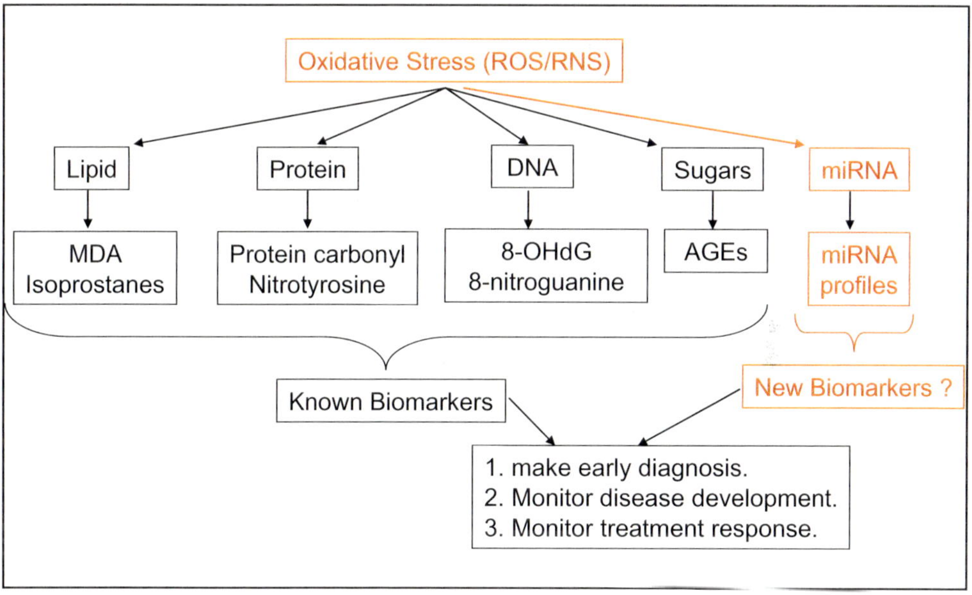

Fig. 1. Biomarkers for oxidative stress

When investigating the status of alcohol-induced oxidative stress, it is unclear what the most appropriate biomarker is and how to measure them. At present, the biomarkers of oxidative stress/damage and the methods used to measure them are different among different study groups. Thus, it is difficult to compare the study findings in different groups to determine which one is the best biomarker to evaluate an individual's oxidative status in relation to alcohol consumption.

In addition, the validity of many biomarkers remains to be established. The biomarkers that have been developed and currently been used to evaluate the oxidative stress have several shortcomings(Dalle-Donne et al., 2006), such as: (*a*) the limited specificity of the assay itself for the product of oxidative/nitrosative damage being measured; (*b*) the fact that the analyte being measured is not a specific product of a specific ROS/RNS; (*c*) the lack of sufficient sensitivity to detect concentrations of the product being measured in healthy individuals, thus not allowing the definition of a reference interval; (*d*) concentrations of the product being measured being influenced by external factors such as the lipid content of the diet; or (*e*) the assay being too invasive for in vivo investigations in humans.

So far, several oxidative stress biomarkers have been used in clinics to assess patient's reaction to oxidative stress, their accuracy, sensitivity, or specificity need to be improved

(Dalle-Donne et al., 2006; Ogino and Wang, 2007). The identification of novel biomarkers is urgently needed. miRNA may hold great promise as a biomarker for oxidative stress.

3. miRNA may be biomarkers for oxidative stress

miRNAs are highly conserved regulatory molecules expressed in eukaryotic cells. They are short noncoding RNAs that regulate gene expression by binding to target mRNAs, which leads to reduced protein synthesis and sometimes decreased steady-state mRNA levels(Ambros, 2004; Carthew, 2006; Carthew and Sontheimer, 2009; Li and Carthew, 2005). Although hundreds of miRNAs have been identified, much less is known about their biological function. There is evidence that miRNAs affect pathways fundamental to metabolic control in higher organisms such as adipocyte and skeletal muscle differentiation. Also, some miRNAs are implicated in lipid, amino acid, and glucose homeostasis. Thus miRNA abnormalities may contribute to common metabolic diseases and there may be novel therapeutic opportunities based on miRNA targeting. Indeed, the expression of certain genes can depend more on levels of regulatory miRNAs than on levels of mRNAs. miRNAs act through a mechanism similar to that of short interfering RNAs (siRNA). The expression of miRNA target genes can be fine-tuned in animals by altering the concentrations or identities of miRNAs within cells.

There are many evidences indicated that miRNAs are able to modulate the cellular response to oxidative stress both in vitro and in vivo(Babar et al., 2008). We hypothesize that miRNAs may be biomarkers for oxidative stress due to following several reasons. First, since miRNA are post-transcriptional gene regulators, they may be able to function as 'quick responders' to oxidative stress. For example, upon exposure to stress, miRNA may rapidly localize to P-bodies or stress granules to regulate key genes involved in the oxidative stress response. After the stress is mitigated, miRNA inhibition may be promptly abated, allowing commencement of translation and expeditive restoration of cells back to their normal state. Second, since miRNA regulate numerous targets, they have the capacity to powerfully and efficiently coordinate a stress response involving numerous genes. Third, owing to their small size and high stability, miRNA may be less susceptible to certain types of stress, such as genotoxic insults. Hence, their ability to modulate stress response would be less likely to be compromised under high-stress condition. Given the recent development in the field of miRNA research, we predict that miRNA will be promised biomarkers for oxidative stress.

4. Animal model of Alcoholic Liver Disease (ALD) is a good model for studying the alcohol-induced oxidative damage

ALD is one of the most common and serious complications of heavy drinking. It is a major health problem in the US, consuming 15% of total health care dollars, and associated with 20% mortality(Maher, 2002). However, the mechanisms linking Ethanol (EtOH) consumption to ALD are not completely understood.

Our in vitro, in vivo animal, and ex-vivo human studies provided compelling evidence for the central involvement of iNOS activation in EtOH-induced gut leakiness. Indeed, several of our studies (Banan et al., 2000a; Banan et al., 2000b; Banan et al., 2007; Keshavarzian et al., 2001; Keshavarzian and Fields, 2000; Keshavarzian and Fields, 2003; Keshavarzian et al., 1999; Tang et al., 2009a; Tang et al., 2009c) have shown that iNOS activation is required for EtOH-induced gut leakiness. We reported that: **1)** EtOH increases iNOS activity and NO levels in intestinal monolayers and increases monolayer permeability. A specific iNOS inhibitor (L-NIL) prevented EtOH-induced monolayer leakiness; **2)** EtOH no longer can cause leakiness in monolayers incapable of upregulating iNOS (i.e., transfected with dominant negative iNOS antisense); **3)** iNOS is increased in intestinal mucosa of alcoholics with ALD and in alcohol-treated rats with gut leakiness and endotoxemia; **4)** Daily gavage of the specific iNOS inhibitor L-NIL prevented iNOS upregulation and oxidative stress in the intestinal mucosa of alcohol-fed rats and also prevented alcohol-induced gut leakiness; **5)** Daily gavage of Lactobacillus GG or supplementation of the diet with oats prevented nitration of intestinal mucosal proteins, oxidative stress, and gut leakiness in alcohol-fed rats; **6)** A daily, alcohol-containing (Nanji) diet for 4 weeks caused gut leakiness in wild type mice but NOT in iNOS knockout mice. The unanswered question is whether miRNAs are the biomarkers for EtOH-induced oxidative injury in blood, intestinal epithelium, or liver.

5. Oats supplementation is an antioxidant

Oats, like many other plant materials, contain numerous constituents vitamins, minerals, essential fatty acids, β-glucan (fermentable fibers), and phytochemicals, including several phenolic compounds. These constituents have been found to possess many types of bioactivity, including antioxidant, antiproliferaton, anti-inflammatory, and detoxification effects, which may contribute to the promotion of good health (Chen et al., 2007).

We hypothesized that oats supplementation protects through its effects on oxidative pathways. We had two primary rationales for our hypothesis. First, it has been generally accepted that oats are of benefit to human health and normal gut growth and function not only because of their nutrient and fiber values, but also, because of their antioxidant and anti-inflammatory activities. Second, several studies have demonstrated the importance of oxidative stress and upregulated iNOS in alcohol-induced tissue injury and organ dysfunction. More specifically, several reports demonstrated the pivotal role of the upregulation of iNOS and oxidative stress in alcohol-induced gut leakiness. For example, our in vitro studies showed that preventing the upregulation of iNOS that is induced by alcohol, using both iNOS inhibitors and dominant negative mutant for iNOS, prevented alcohol-induced disruption of the barrier integrity of intestinal cell monolayers.

Furthermore, we recently showed that inhibition of iNOS by L-NIL reduces EtOH-induced NO overproduction, oxidative tissue injury and gut leakiness in alcohol-treated rats. Our current study, which uses immunohistochemical staining, provides direct evidence that EtOH induces iNOS activation in colonic epithelium and that oats prevent this effect and prevent alcohol-induced intestinal mucosal oxidative stress.

We confirmed our in vitro findings in an animal model of alcoholic steatohepatitis (ASH). We showed that chronic, daily alcohol administration to rats caused gut leakiness. More importantly, we showed that EtOH-induced gut leakiness in rats was associated with endotoxemia and alcoholic steatohepatitis. Furthermore, we showed that oats supplementation prevents loss of intestinal barrier integrity, endotoxemia and steatohepatitis(Keshavarzian et al., 2001; Tang et al., 2009a). However, the mechanism for the protective effects of oats is unclear.

6. Opportunity and potential impact

Numerous markers of oxidative stress and antioxidant status have been evaluated, but there has been little systematic effort to validate sensitive and specific biomarkers for oxidative damage in animal models.

Development of miRNA as a new biomarker for alcohol-induced oxidative stress is limited by the lack of easy access to the tissues from patient populations. Therefore, the majority of discovery work will need to be carried out in the animal model of ALD. The advantage provided by animal models is the ability to control and define disease stages. We have to correlate these model diseases to the clinical status of actual patient populations. The process of biomarker discovery in animal models will be validated by clinical studies. As the technology develops to allow higher throughput screening of miRNA, these candidate biomarkers can be more easily tested and applied to larger patient populations.

The *long term goal* of our laboratory is to design an effective therapeutic intervention to prevent and treat oxidant-induced disorders. Increasing our understanding of the mechanism of oxidant-induced gut leakiness should lead to identification of optimal targets for development of new preventive and therapeutic strategies for alcohol-induced, endotoxin mediated, tissue damage such as ALD. Our studies should thus lead to development of: **a)** miRNA as biomarkers for identifying susceptible individuals who are at risk for endotoxemia & ALD and would thus benefit from interventions that prevent gut leak; **b)** novel strategies to prevent ALD by preventing gut leakiness and endotoxemia in alcoholics; **c)** novel therapies to treat advanced alcoholic and non-alcoholic liver disease, because gut leakiness can perpetuate the hepatic necroinflammatory cascade (via feedback loops) and thereby contribute to the progression of liver injury. Since our model involves oxidative stress and iNOS, the results could have relevance to other pathological conditions where gut leakiness and oxidative stress play key roles like non-alcoholic liver disease, inflammatory bowel disease & food allergy to name a few.

7. Results

7.1 Relative miRNA expression in rat intestine of ALD model

Fluorescence signals of the hybridized miRXploreTM Microarrays were detected using a laser scanner from Agilent (Agilent Technologies). In figure 2 a representative false-color image of the microarray experiment is shown as an example; Red color indicates that the Hy5 signal intensity is higher than the Hy3 signal intensity. Therefore, the corresponding gene is overexpressed in the Hy5-labeled sample. Green spots, however, indicate that the fluorescence intensity in the control sample is stronger than in the experimental sample. Yellow spots indicate that the signal intensities are equal for both samples. The signal intensities of each spot/miRNA that passed the quality filtering are shown in a double-logarithmic scale (Fig.3), represented by a dot. X-axis: Hy3 signal intensity, y-axis: Hy5 signal intensity. Dashed diagonal lines define the areas of x-fold differential signal intensities. Approximately 30 miRNAs including miR-212, miR-7, miR-145, and miR-146a are expressed primarily in digestive tract tissues.

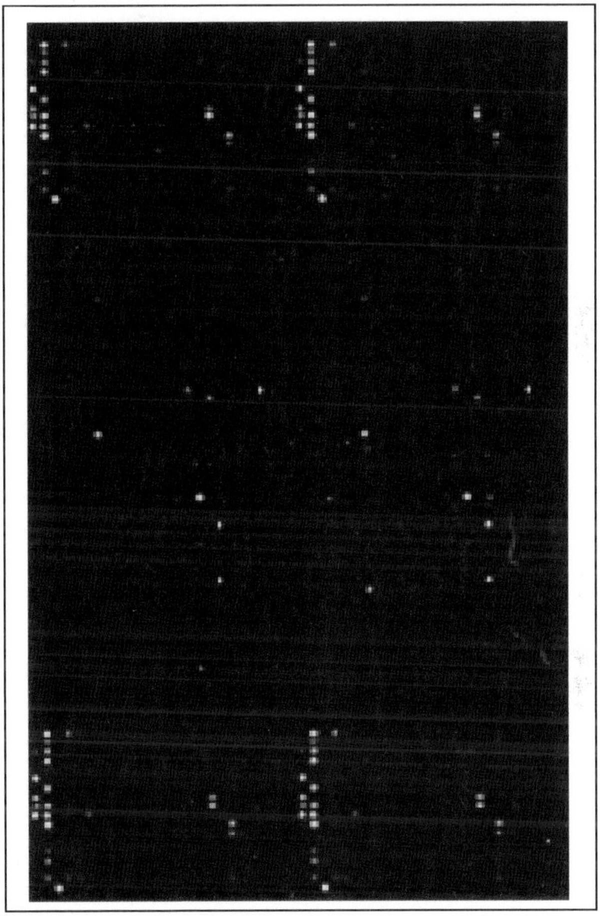

Fig. 2. Hy5/Hy3 false-color image after scanning of microarray

The successful development of effective antioxidant therapies remains a key goal, the attainment of which is required to elucidate the role played by accumulation of oxidized molecules in clinical picture of disease associated with oxidative stress. The use of miRNA as a biomarker provides a logical scientific basis for major intervention trials of antioxidants; such trials could in turn eventually validate or disprove the biomarker concept.

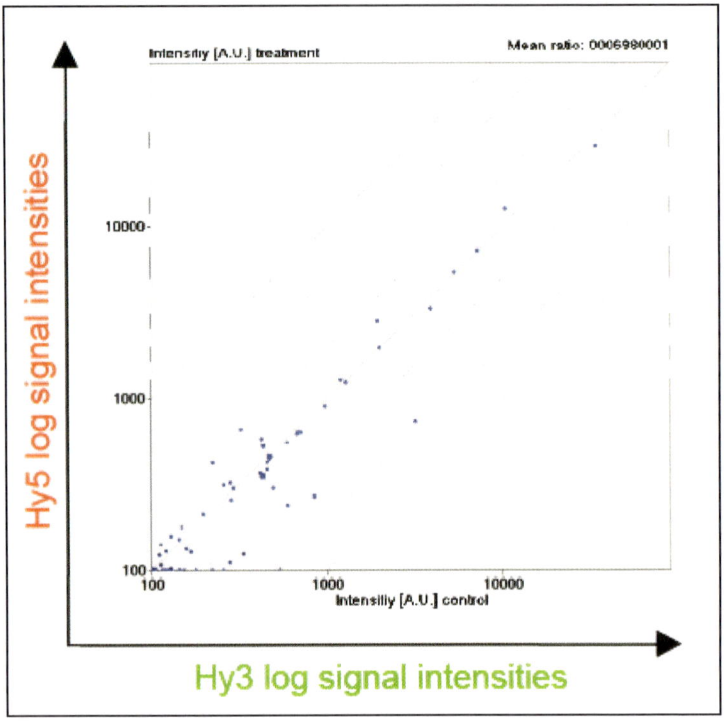

Fig. 3. Duble-log scatter plot

7.2 miR-212 expression in animal model of ALD

To translate our in vitro observation to an in vivo model to establish the key role of miRNA-212 in EtOH-induced gut leakiness, we turned to use an animal model of alcohol-induced gut leakiness. This model has been established and validated in our previous studies. Recently, to determine whether gut leakiness and endotoxemia are one of the key co-factors for development of alcoholic steatohepatitis (ASH), we studied time courses for development of gut hyperpermeability, endotoxemia, and liver injury and showed that gut leakiness and endotoxemia occurred several weeks prior to development of ASH. These data support the notion that gut leakiness causes endotoxemia, which leads to alcoholic steatohepatitis and serious ALD.

In this animal model, rats were given daily EtOH (6 g/kg, by gastric gavage) for 10 weeks. The miRNAs expression levels in the intestine mucosa were assayed by miRNA microarray analysis (Miltenyi Biotec, Auburn CA). The data show that miR-212 expression in EtOH treated group was up regulated by 1.5 fold compared with control group (**Fig.4**).

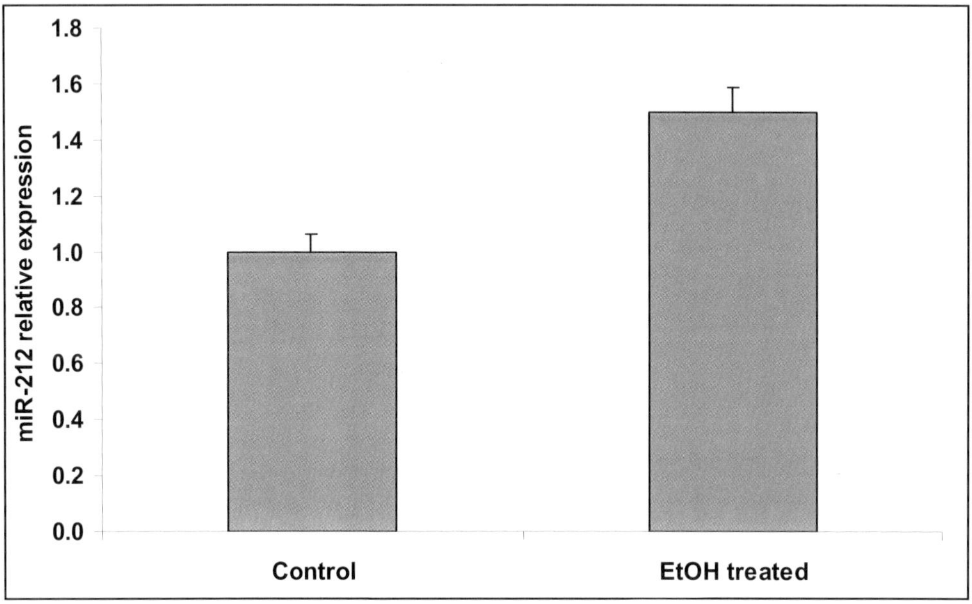

Fig. 4. miR-212 expression levels in intestinal mucosa were increased in rats of ALD model. The rats were fed with EtOH (6 g/kg, by gastric gavage) for 10 weeks. The miR-212 expression levels were assayed by miRNA microarray analysis

8. Our recent publications related to the role of miRNA in the alcohol-induced oxidative stress (Keshavarzian et al., 2009; Tang et al., 2008; Tang et al., 2009a; Tang et al., 2009c)

8.1 Effect of alcohol on miR-212 expression in intestinal epithelial cells and its potential role in alcoholic liver disease (Tang et al., 2008)

Alcoholic liver disease (ALD) is commonly associated with intestinal barrier dysfunction. Alcohol-induced dysregulation of tight junction proteins such as zonula occluden 1 (ZO-1) in intestinal epithelial cells, plays an important role in regulation of intestinal permeability. MicroRNAs (miRNAs) are recently discovered small noncoding RNAs that can regulate gene expression by targeting mRNAs and triggering either translational repression or RNA degradation. ZO-1 is predicted to be a target gene of one such miRNA, miR-212. We previously showed that miR-212 levels in colon biopsy samples in ALD patients were higher than in healthy controls; while ZO-1 protein levels were lower. Here, we studied the mechanisms for the involvement of miR-212 in alcohol-induced gut leakiness. We showed that miR-212 is highly expressed in intestinal tissues using a TaqMan microRNA real time PCR assay. Alcohol-induced miR-212 over-expression is accompanied by reductions in ZO-1 protein expression, disruption of tight junction protein (ZO-1), and increased permeability of Caco-2 cell monolayers. Alcohol-induced miR-212 over-expression correlated with alcohol-induced disruption of monolayer integrity. To demonstrate that miR-212 acts directly at the ZO-1 3'UTR, we inserted the miR-212 target site of ZO-1 3'UTR into luciferase reporter construct and transfected it into Caco-2 cells. The expression of luciferase was significantly decreased when cotransfected with miR-212. This suppression was relieved by a single base mutantion in the UTR binding site. To see if miR-212 regulates ZO-1 levels, we did both overexpression studies using miR-212 precursors and inhibition studies using miR-212-specific antisense oligonucleotide inhibitors (anti-miR-212). miR-212 over-expression significantly inhibited ZO-1 protein expression. Knocking down of miR-212 expression in Caco-2 cells using anti-miR-212 inhibited alcohol-induced hyperpermeability by 50% ($p<0.05$). Our studies suggest a novel mechanism for alcohol-induced gut leakiness. Alcohol induces miR-212 over-expression which disrupts intestinal barrier integrity by inhibiting ZO-1 translation. This cascade could lead to dysfunction of tight junction and increase intestinal permeability. This mechanism provides a potential therapeutic target for preventing the leaky gut in patients with ALD.

8.2 Oxidative stress is required for alcohol-induced gut leakiness and liver damage (ALD model)(Keshavarzian et al., 2009)

Thus ALD model is excellent model for studying the biomarkers of oxdative stress. Time courses for development of gut hyperpermeability, nitric oxide production, oxidative injury to the gut, endotoxemia, and liver injury were assessed in these ALD medol. Liver fat and serum transaminase increased after 2 weeks, but evidence of liver cell injury and inflammation occurred after 8 weeks. Gut leakiness, intestinal oxidative injury, and endotoxemia occurred in weeks 2-4 and progressed thereafter. Our data support the hypothesis that oxidative stress is a key co-factor (trigger) for ALD.

8.3 Nitric oxide mediated oxidative injury is required for ALD (Tang et al., 2009c)

We hypothesized that iNOS inhibitors (L-NAME, L-NIL) in vivo will inhibit the above cascade and liver injury in an animal model of alcoholic steatohepatitis (ASH). Male Sprague-Dawley rats were gavaged daily with alcohol (6 g/kg/day) or dextrose for 10 weeks ± L-NAME, L-NIL or vehicle. Systemic and intestinal NO levels were measured by nitrites and nitrates in urine and tissue samples, oxidative damage to the intestinal mucosa by protein carbonyl and nitrotyrosine, intestinal permeability by urinary sugar tests, and liver injury by histological inflammation scores, liver fat, and myeloperoxidase activity. The results showed that alcohol caused tissue oxidation, gut leakiness, endotoxemia and ASH. L-NIL and L-NAME, but not the D-enantiomers, attenuated all steps in the alcohol-induced cascade including NO overproduction, oxidative tissue damage, gut leakiness, endotoxemia, hepatic inflammation and liver injury. *Conclusions:* The mechanism we reported for alcohol-induced intestinal barrier disruption in vitro – NO overproduction, oxidative tissue damage, leaky gut, endotoxemia and liver injury – appears to be relevant in vivo in an animal model of alcohol-induced liver injury. That iNOS inhibitors attenuated all steps of this cascade suggests that prevention of this cascade in alcoholics will protect the liver against the injurious effects of chronic alcohol and that iNOS may be a useful target for prevention of ALD.

8.4 Oats supplementation prevents alcohol-induced oxidative tissue damage in rats (Tang et al., 2009b)

We previously reported that oats supplementation prevents gut leakiness and alcoholic steatohepatitis in our rat model of ALD. Since oxidative stress is implicated in the pathogenesis of both alcohol-induced gut leakiness and ASH, and since oats have anti-oxidant properties, we tested the hypothesis that oats protect by preventing alcohol-induced oxidative damage to the intestine. Oxidative stress and injury were assessed by measuring colonic mucosal iNOS (by immunohistochemistry), nitric oxide, (colorimetric assay) and protein carbonylation and nitrotyrosination (immunoblotting). Colonic barrier integrity was determined by assessing the integrity of the actin cytoskeleton (immunohistochemistry) and the integrity of tight junctions (electron microscopy). Oats supplementation prevented alcohol-induced upregulation of iNOS, nitric oxide overproduction in the colonic mucosa, and increases in protein carbonyl and nitrotyrosine levels. This protection was associated with prevention of EtOH-induced disorganization of the actin cytoskeleton and disruption of tight junctions. We conclude that oats supplementation attenuates EtOH-induced disruption of intestinal barrier integrity, at least in part, by inhibiting EtOH-induced increases in oxidative stress and oxidative tissue damage. This inhibition prevents alcohol-induced disruption of the cytoskeleton and tight junctions. This study suggests that oats may be a useful therapeutic agent - a nutriceutical - for the prevention of alcohol-induced oxidative stress and organ dysfunction.

9. Conclusion

Our research results demonstrated that the differentially expressed miRNAs are the sensitive and specific biomarkers for alcohol-induced oxidative stress. MiRNAs are potential biomarkers to accurately measure the degree of oxidative stress, early detect the indication of disease, and evaluate the effectiveness of antioxidant therapy (fig.5). The validation of miRNAs as biomarkers for alcohol-induced oxidative stress requires further studying. The key steps for validation of miRNA as suitable biomarkers for alcohol-induced oxidative stress are summarized in Fig.6. The application of miRNA as new biomarkers will lead to: a) identification susceptible individuals who are at risk for oxidative stress and would thus benefit from interventions that provide antioxidants; b) novel strategies to prevent and treat oxidative injury.

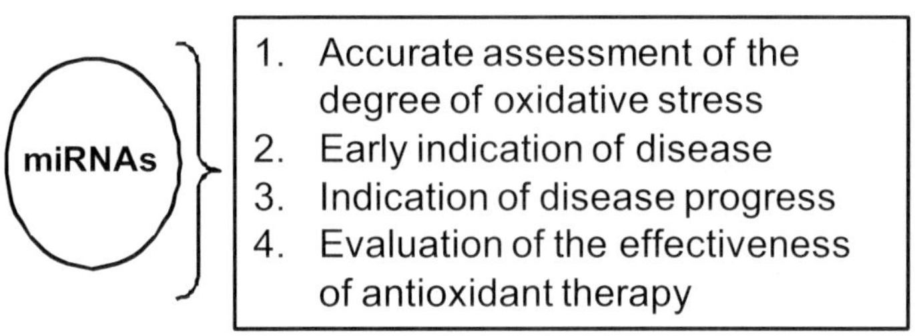

Fig. 5. Potential uses of miRNA as biomarkers for oxidative stress

1. Selection of miRNAs as biomarkers for oxidative stress
2. Measuring miRNAs (microarray and real time PCR)
3. Verification of miRNAs as biomarkers in suitable animal model (ALD)
4. Test the sensitivity, simplicity, and specificity of miRNAs for oxidative stress-induced injury
5. Validation of miRNAs as biomarkers for oxidative stress using antioxidants (oats)

Fig. 6. Key steps for validation of miRNAs as suitable biomarkers of oxidative stress

10. Future direction

In last two decades, there has been great progress in development of biomarkers of oxidative stress that may eventually be useful in disease prevention. The challenges for future miRNA studies are (1) to validate available biomarkers for oxidative stress in animal and human studies based on their specificity, stability for storage, reproducibility, causal relation with disease, and response to antioxidant intervention; (2) to examine the basal lebels of oxidative damage in healthy subjects; and (3) to assess the long-term effect of antioxidants, such as oats, on oxidative damage by well-designed, randomized, controlled trials in human and as well as to examine the consistency of the findings among various studies. The identification of miRNAs as biomarkers of oxidative damage, if validated, may open the way for the development of early detection and prevention strategies for oxidative stress-associated human diseases.

11. Acknowledgement

This work was supported by National Institute of Health grants AA18729 (Y.T.), AA019405 (A.K.) and AA020216 (A.K.), and in part by mentoring program of Department of Internal Medicine of Rush University Medical Center (Y.T.).

12. References

Ambros V (2004) The functions of animal microRNAs. Nature 431(7006):350-5.

Babar IA, Slack FJ, Weidhaas JB (2008) miRNA modulation of the cellular stress response. Future Oncol 4(2):289-98.

Banan A, Choudhary S, Zhang Y, Fields JZ, Keshavarzian A (2000a) Oxidant-induced intestinal barrier disruption and its prevention by growth factors in a human colonic cell line: role of the microtubule cytoskeleton. Free Radic Biol Med 28(5):727-38.

Banan A, Fields JZ, Decker H, Zhang Y, Keshavarzian A (2000b) Nitric oxide and its metabolites mediate ethanol-induced microtubule disruption and intestinal barrier dysfunction. J Pharmacol Exp Ther 294(3):997-1008.

Banan A, Keshavarzian A, Zhang L, Shaikh M, Forsyth CB, Tang Y, Fields JZ (2007) NF-kappaB activation as a key mechanism in ethanol-induced disruption of the F-actin cytoskeleton and monolayer barrier integrity in intestinal epithelium. Alcohol 41(6):447-460.

Carthew RW (2006) Gene regulation by microRNAs. Curr Opin Genet Dev 16(2):203-8.

Carthew RW, Sontheimer EJ (2009) Origins and Mechanisms of miRNAs and siRNAs. Cell 136(4):642-55.

Chen CY, Milbury PE, Collins FW, Blumberg JB (2007) Avenanthramides are bioavailable and have antioxidant activity in humans after acute consumption of an enriched mixture from oats. J Nutr 137(6):1375-82.

Dalle-Donne I, Rossi R, Colombo R, Giustarini D, Milzani A (2006) Biomarkers of oxidative damage in human disease. Clin Chem 52(4):601-23.

Keshavarzian A, Choudhary S, Holmes EW, Yong S, Banan A, Jakate S, Fields JZ (2001) Preventing gut leakiness by oats supplementation ameliorates alcohol-induced liver damage in rats. J Pharmacol Exp Ther 299(2):442-8.

Keshavarzian A, Farhadi A, Forsyth CB, Rangan J, Jakate S, Shaikh M, Banan A, Fields JZ (2009) Evidence that chronic alcohol exposure promotes intestinal oxidative stress, intestinal hyperpermeability and endotoxemia prior to development of alcoholic steatohepatitis in rats. J Hepatol 50(3):538-47.

Keshavarzian A, Fields J (2000) Alcohol: "ice-breaker" yes, "gut barrier-breaker," maybe. Am J Gastroenterol 95(5):1124-5.

Keshavarzian A, Fields J (2003) Alcoholic liver disease: is it an "extraintestinal" complication of alcohol-induced intestinal injury? J Lab Clin Med 142(5):285-7.

Keshavarzian A, Holmes EW, Patel M, Iber F, Fields JZ, Pethkar S (1999) Leaky gut in alcoholic cirrhosis: a possible mechanism for alcohol-induced liver damage. Am J Gastroenterol 94(1):200-7.

Li X, Carthew RW (2005) A microRNA mediates EGF receptor signaling and promotes photoreceptor differentiation in the Drosophila eye. Cell 123(7):1267-77.

Maher JJ (2002) Alcoholic steatosis and steatohepatitis. Semin Gastrointest Dis 13(1):31-9.

Ogino K, Wang DH (2007) Biomarkers of oxidative/nitrosative stress: an approach to disease prevention. Acta Med Okayama 61(4):181-9.

Tang Y, Banan A, Forsyth CB, Fields JZ, Lau CK, Zhang LJ, Keshavarzian A (2008) Effect of alcohol on miR-212 expression in intestinal epithelial cells and its potential role in alcoholic liver disease. Alcohol Clin Exp Res 32(2):355-64.

Tang Y, Forsyth CB, Banan A, Fields JZ, Keshavarzian A (2009a) Oats supplementation prevents alcohol-induced gut leakiness in rats by preventing alcohol-induced oxidative tissue damage. J Pharmacol Exp Ther.

Tang Y, Forsyth CB, Banan A, Fields JZ, Keshavarzian A (2009b) Oats supplementation prevents alcohol-induced gut leakiness in rats by preventing alcohol-induced oxidative tissue damage. J Pharmacol Exp Ther 329(3):952-8.

Tang Y, Forsyth CB, Farhadi A, Rangan J, Jakate S, Shaikh M, Banan A, Fields JZ, Keshavarzian A (2009c) Nitric Oxide-Mediated Intestinal Injury Is Required for Alcohol-Induced Gut Leakiness and Liver Damage. Alcohol Clin Exp Res.

17

Serum Peptidomics

Kaihua Wei[1], Qingwei Ma[2], Yunbo Sun[1], Xiaoming Zhou[1], Weirong Guo[2] and Jian Yuan[1]
[1]State Key Lab of Proteomics, Beijing Proteome Research Center,
[2]Bioyong (Beijing) Technologies Limited, Beijing, China

1. Introduction

1.1 Concept

1.1.1 Proteomics

The performer of life functions is the dynamically-changing protein, rather than the relatively-static gene. Accordingly, the study of protein is of practical significance in the explication of vital phenomena, especially in the revelation of onset, deterioration and outcome of human diseases, which is also a driving force for the emergence of proteomics. Wilkins and Williams (Wasinger VC. et al, 1995) initiated the study of proteomics by putting forward the concept of proteomics for the first time. The proteome is the set of expressed proteins in a given type of cells, tissues or an organism at a given time under defined conditions. Proteomics is the large-scale study of proteomes, to discover composition and expression of proteins in organism, to understand interactions between proteins and explore functions of proteins and laws of vital activities of cells. It covers expression proteomics, functional proteomics and cell-localization proteomics etc. The proteomics technologies has provided a new tool for studying the biomarkers, pathogeny mechanism, diagnostic methods of diseases.

1.1.2 Serum proteomics

When proteomics comes to the clinical applications, it mainly refers to serum proteomics. The features of serum proteome research: firstly, it is easily to access samples, which means that it is able to meet the research requirements and easy to standardize; secondly, the dynamic variation in serum proteins is capable to reflect the pathological changing state of human organs; this is of far-reaching importance for disease diagnosis and curative effect monitoring. Human Proteome Organization (HUPO) brought the human plasma/serum proteome plan under the first-phase of the human proteome plans, which is showing the significance of studying serum proteomics for healthy and sick states of human.

Taking all proteins expressed in the serum of selected target clusters as the object, the serum proteomics, based on the normal protein expression profiles, aims to look for the differential proteins and define disease-associated proteins, the structures and functions of which will further be studied. In the hope of presenting a new approach for studying the pathological and physiological mechanisms of severe diseases, specific protein markers are expected to be found for early diagnosis and drug targets. Compared with the tissue proteins and cell proteins, serum proteins are unique in many aspects such as the largest number (tens of thousands of varieties), extremely great difference in contents of proteins (with a difference of more than 10^8-10^{12}), extremely instable variety and content of low-abundance proteins. The main components of serum proteins are albumin and immunoglobulin, which share the features like high abundance, large molecular weight and easy-to-detect. Besides, non-protein substances like lipids and salts also exist in the serum. All other components will interfere with the study of small-molecular-weight proteins in the serum. Usually, all the important information come from the low-abundance proteins and small-molecular-weight proteins with great varieties and different properties, on the other hand, the features of these proteins make them difficult to be separated and identified.

1.1.3 Serum peptidomics

With the deepening of biological study of proteins, a kind of non-protein intermediate that composes of amino acid is discovered and described as polypeptide. According to biochemists, peptides are short polymers of amino acids linked by amino bonds (also called peptide bonds). Polypeptide is a kind of peptides with more than 10 amino acids (if fewer than 10, they are called oligo-peptides). In our study here, proteins with the molecular weight less than 10KDa fall into the category of the polypeptides. Besides molecular weights, the polypeptides are also different from proteins in functions: firstly, the polypeptide are information messenger, which can arouse various physiological activities and regulate biochemical response; secondly, polypeptide have high bioactivity; thirdly, as smaller molecule, the structure of polypeptide is easier to rebuild and simpler for artificial synthesis and chemosynthesis; fourthly, fragments of polypeptide can be used for further research of protein features and changing and synthesizing proteins as basic materials. The polypeptide is a sort of biologically active substance related to cell functions of organisms. Tens of thousands of polypeptides have been found existing in organisms and can be synthesized in all cells. Moreover, nearly all cells are regulated by polypeptides, which play a role in hormone, nerves, cell growth and reproduction, etc. Presently, in company with the instant development of proteomics and mass-spectrometric technology, more and more researchers are turning their eyes to polypeptide, which thereby bring about the proteomics-based peptidomics.

The main clinical application of peptidomics is the serum peptidomics. The serum peptidome, generally referring to serum peptidome profiling, is to detect the accurate mass value of polypeptide in serum by mass spectrometry and process mass spectrum with the bioinformatics method to build a polypeptide profiling. In the profiling, the peptidome identified by an accurate mass value can be further analyzed into amino acid sequence through tandem mass spectrometer, thereby used to identify the precursor proteins and their biogenetic derivation. Through contrasting differences in the serum peptidome profiling of the patients and the healthy controls, proteins or polypeptides specifically expressed in disease state and the biomarkers associated with diseases can be discovered to perform the studies of proteins related to early diagnosis, classification and subtype, onset mechanism of diseases. The serum polypeptide profiling is reputed to be a "brand-new health fingerprinting library" technology (Tarnaris A et al, 2006) and has become a research hotspot of proteomics.

1.2 History of serum peptidomics platform

Such are three major technical approaches for proteomics study as two-dimensional gel electrophoresis (2-DE), mass spectrometry (MS) and bioinformatics. Similar to the proteomics technology, serum peptidomics technology also involves in technical advancement and upgrade in sample preparation, detection and result analysis, which jointly constitute a platform in serum peptidomics research. Most of studies rely on matrix-assisted laser desorption/ionization time of flight mass spectrometry (MALDI-TOF-MS). The working principle of MALDI-TOF-MS is: the pulse laser is utilized to force the matrix to absorb energy from laser so that the solid-phase polypeptide samples are ionized; the ionized peptides are put into the TOF mass analyzer and separated due to difference in the mass-to-charge ratio (m/z); the peptide mass fingerprint (PMF), peptide sequence tag (PST) or the amino acid sequences can be obtained through measuring peptide ions; qualitative identification or quantitative analysis of peptides can be accomplished through searching in the proteome database with corresponding software. On this basis, three serum peptidomics research platforms have been developed successfully.

1.2.1 The 1st generation of serum peptidomics platform: SELDI

Different from MALDI-TOF-MS, the surface enhanced laser desorption/ionization(SELDI) time of flight mass spectrometry platform combines the protein chip with multiple high technologies (highly integrated, ultra-micro, computerized, automat-zed) based on the chromatogram principle, thereby to strengthen the affinity and capture ability of the chip so that proteins are selectively absorbed by the chemically-modified solid surface. The proteins captured by the chip surface are ionized in the ion source and their weight is detected by referring to the different flight time in the flight tube. In this platform, protein chip is the core of the whole system.

Distinguished by chemical modification, the protein chip is divided into hydrophobic surface (H4), normal phase (NP), weak cation exchange (WCX), strong anion exchange (SAX) and immobilized metal affinity capture (IMAC) which are aim to fit for different detecting requirement. Different chemisorption media allows an extremely large amount of proteins to be reduced to a relatively low level, those remained proteins can be absorbed by the surface of chip. They are characterized by: (1) can be directly used for crude biological samples, such as serum, urine, body fluid and cell lysis solution, etc. (2) low dosage of sample is required, generally is 0.5-15μl or 2000 cells; (3) high throughput with automatic operation; (4) rapid discovery for multiple biomarkers and some low-abundance, small-molecular-weight proteins; (5)high sensitivity lower the limitation of detection (LOD) to 1fmol (10^{-15}mol); (6) special identification ability for hydrophobic protein, especially for membrane proteins; (7) a high-efficiency and cost-effective system integrates all the protein separation, purification, identification, detection and data analysis process.

The processing and analysis system produces the results in forms like scanning profiling, bar graph and electrophoresis patterns (simulation gel image) and analyses the difference among two or more groups of results to find out the special mass spectra of identification information. The procedure includes: (1) database building; (2) internal and external information calibration; (3) data processing and analysis.

The data processing of serum protein profiles commonly includes peak detection, data grouping, marker selection, marker evaluation and composite mode building. In information analysis and processing, two algorithms will be used: (1) non-monitoring algorithm, like self-organizing cluster analysis; (2) monitoring algorithm, like artificial neural network (ANN). These two, especially the latter one, are more and more found in studies regarding tumor diagnosis with satisfying results.

SELDI, however, has some disadvantages: it is incapable of identifying differential proteins screened online; in the profiling, the peak height and protein concentration not always have a linear relationship; in the detection process, many factors are involved but the control method hasn't been standardized yet, which leads to poor reproduction quality of characteristic peaks of the same disease among different researchers.

1.2.2 The 2nd generation of serum peptidomics research technology system: ClinProt

To overcome the defects of SELDI, the ClinProt platform with functional magnetic beads, AnchorChip technology, MALDI-TOF-MS and ClinProTools has been developed. This platform has magnetic bead separating system, MS detecting system, analysis software and optional body fluid sample automatic processing system. The basic procedure is as follows: first of all, samples like serum, plasma, urine and cerebrospinal fluid, etc. from patients or the healthy controls have their high-abundance proteins and other impurities like salts to be eliminated and have the low-abundance proteins to be enriched with the magnetic bead. After separation and purification, samples are mixed with matrixes and directly drip on the AnchorChip target plate, and then protein mass spectrogram can be obtained through time-of-flight-MS (TOF-MS). The analysis software is employed to compare the differential expressed proteins of the patients or the healthy controls to get the specific mass spectra of the both for predicting the category of unknown samples (sick or healthy). Therefore, the core of this platform is the magnetic bead system and the software system.

Magnetic reagents include magnetic beads based Weak Cation Exchange (MB-WCX), Immobilized Metal Ion Affinity Chromatography Cu (MB-IMAC Cu) and Reverse Phase C18 (MB-RPC18), etc. The principle of magnetic beads is that the target proteins firstly combine with the magnetic microsphere surface ligand reversibility; secondly they will move in an outer magnetic field with a set direction by utilizing the magnetism of the magnetic beads to rapidly separate from surrounding medium. Compared with conventional technologies, the features of magnetic beads are: with large total surface area of magnetic beads, the specific basic groups on the surface can sufficiently combine with the low-abundance proteins in the serum to enhance the varieties of proteins, thereby to ensure the favorable specificity of the system; with simple and rapid operation, preliminary treatment can be finished through the simple blending, washing and elution process, which is suitable for clinical examination; the magnetic bead system has very high repetitiveness due to its large surface area; the liquid automatic processing system is a high throughput platform, it is capable to handle as many as 30,000 samples per day.

ClinProTools is a bioinformatics software boasting of all functions of biomarker detection and evaluation and capable of performing pre-processing of data, obtaining powerful, intuitive and visualized data from massive sample groups, carrying out peak statistics and pattern recognition, cluster analysis and independent test of data sensitivity, cross validation of specificity and meeting the classification demand of unknown samples.

Compared with SELDI, the magnetic bead particles have a larger total surface area due to their shapes and have stronger combining capacity, higher sensitivity and accuracy, so they perfectly cater for the research requirement of serum small-molecular proteins. Furthermore, biomarkers combined with the magnetic beads can be eluted, so this technology is suitable for MS and satisfy the requirement of sequential analysis in the further study. ClinProt system is able to perform the sequence identification task for the differentially expressed polypeptides/proteins to clearly distinct whether they are known or not.

1.2.3 The 3rd generation of serum peptidomics research platform: ClinTOF

Considering features of the serum polypeptide profiling and defects of the ClinProt system, it is fair to say that ClinTOF is the representative of the latest platform up to now.

On one hand, ClinTOF is capable of detecting the biomarker pattern or biomarker profiling indicating specific diseases in the biological liquid; on the other hand, this technology can identify the candidate for a single biomarker. ClinTOF composes of three parts, including magnetic beads, time-of-flight mass spectrometer (TOF MS) and analysis software BioExploer ™.

1. Magnetic Beads

The magnetic beads includes hydrophobic magnetic beads, metal affinity magnetic beads, ion exchange magnetic beads, glycoprotein magnetic beads and immunoaffinity magnetic beads. Further, SPE-C magnetic beads, the reagent dedicated for the serum polypeptide fingerprint diagnosis is available. Presently, magnetic beads have been found in biomedicine fields like immuno-magnetic separation (IMS), cell and cell organelle separation, microorganism detection and nucleic acid hybridization. The whole system is used in the clinical research of serum peptidomics.

2. TOF MS

Time-of-flight mass spectrometer (TOF MS) is used to obtain mass ratio and content of proteins captured by magnetic beads. ClinTOF, the clinical mass spectrometer, has adopted the cutting-edge 60Hz pulsed nitrogen laser which allows the data generated at the fastest speed compared with its counterparts. The zoom optics technology is employed with the laser speckle ranging from 50μm to 200 μm (adjustable), also the greatest adjustable range among like products, so that the size of laser speckles can meet the demands of different samples. The unique gap design in ion source has been utilized, keeping ion sources from contaminations and greatly reducing maintenance frequency. The laser system has been added with the laser energy leveling function, presenting more stable light intensity of the laser and more accurate data. The unique touch screen design has integrated MALDI-TOF control system and the PC system, making operations more simple and handy.

3. Analysis Software BioExploer™

BioExploer™ software is used both in processing genetic data and also protein data. BioExploer™ has combined visualized analysis and multiple mathematical algorithms to build pattern recognition models for MS data classification and forecast, and hunt the disease markers from data. It can perform data visualization, data reduction and data mining over various types of MS data and build category prediction models. This software features: data of multiple forms can be analyzed with this software even if they have converted their formats; signal spectrogram can be visualized through the virtual gel graph and stack diagram; wavelet transform is used to deal with the mass spectrogram, including baseline elimination, spectrogram smoothing, peak selection and normalization; random statistical analysis can be made on one and more groups of spectrogram protein peaks; compatibility analysis is designed for the pairing data; the building and verification of the pattern recognition models involve in optimistic algorithms including genetic algorithm, radial basis neural network and the support vector machine and allow users to select the modeling space; output of data analysis reports and backup and storage at any moment.

The BioExploer™ control and analysis system adopts the display forms of scanning profiling (Fig.1) and electrophoresis patterns (simulation gel graph) (Fig.2). Statistical analysis graphs include the 3D sample distribution diagram (Fig.3), typical value-variogram (Fig.4) and 3D stack diagram (Fig.5). The user may switch the three graphs by clicking the three buttons at the lower left corner.

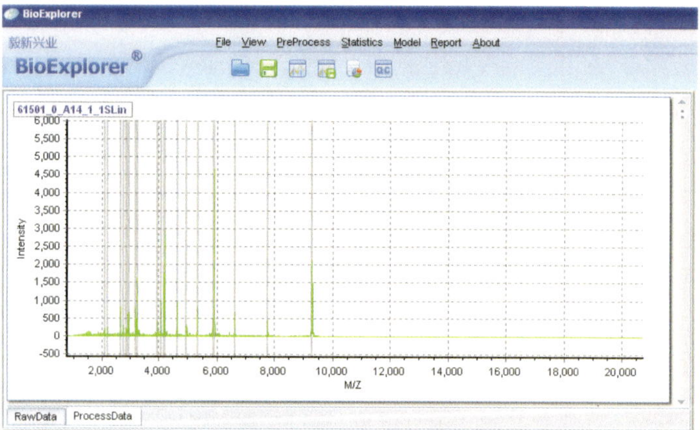

Fig. 1. ClinTOF System Scanning Profiling

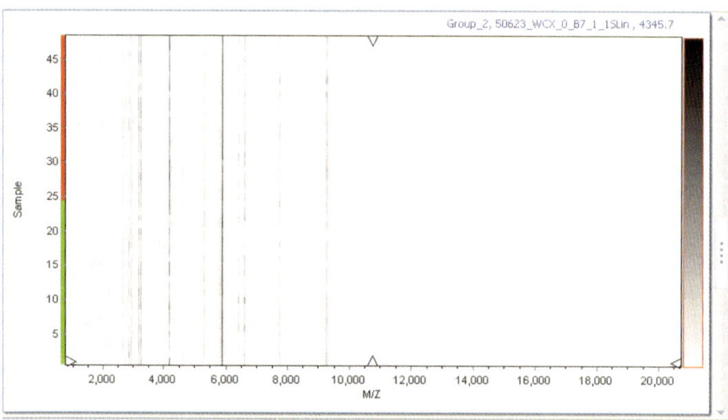

Fig. 2. Electrophoresis Graph of the ClinTOF System

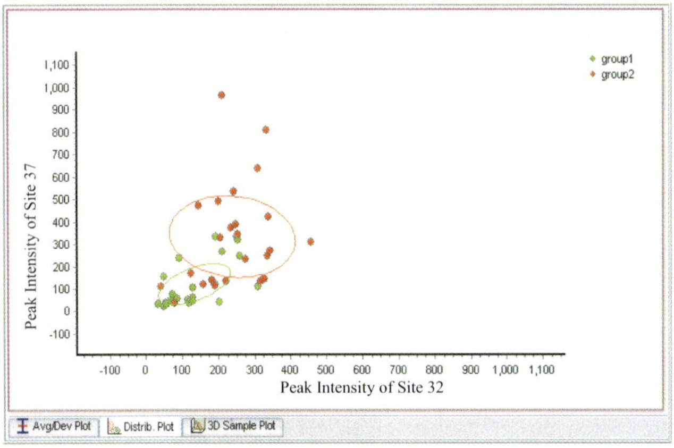

Fig. 3. ClinTOF System 3D Sample Distribution Diagram

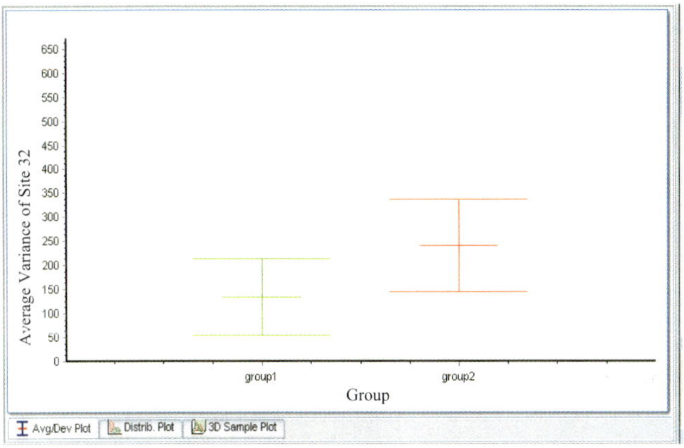

Fig. 4. ClinTOF System Typical Value Variogram

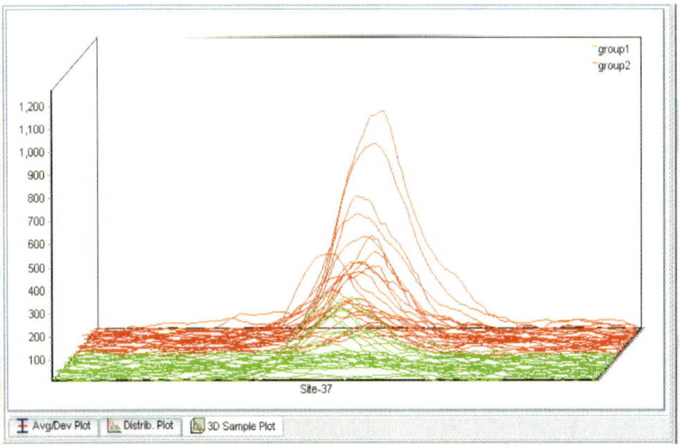

Fig. 5. ClinTOF System 3D Stack Diagram

4. Applications of ClinTOF Platform

ClinTOF can be used in disease peptidomics, early tumor diagnosis and curative effect evaluation, mental disease diagnosis, biomarker discovery, microorganism identification, single nucleotide polymorphism (SNP) detection and medicine quality control. This system as a breakthrough can detect more than 200 polypeptides at the same time by utilizing magnetic bead reagent, mass spectrometry and pattern analysis. BIOYONG is the only manufacturer in China for ClinTOF system development and certification and has obtained many patents. For the moment, this technology has been widely used in the clinical based researches, granted a solid scientific foundation for future promotion.

Besides the intrinsically strength of MALDI-TOF, the ClinTOF system has improved its stability and repeatability for clinical analysis. So far, it has detected more than 10,000 clinical samples and established detection models for colon and rectal cancers, lung cancer, hepatic carcinoma and brain glioma. Its accuracy for the early detection of cancers is above 85% and its specificity and sensitivity exceed 80%. MS models for some tumors based on the Clin TOF system have been built and many patents have gained authorization.

The ClinTOF system has been widely applied in studies on the early diagnosis of ovarian cancer, prostatic cancer, breast cancer, brain glioma, head and neck squamous cell carcinomas (HNSCC) and carcinoma of urinary bladder and disease diagnosis models have been built. For the colon and rectal cancers, the model is shown in Table 1. In the model built in the experiment, 70 of the normal cases and 60 of colon and rectal cancer cases are used; 31 of the normal cases and 35 of colon and rectal cancer cases are used; the sensitivity of the model is 84.17% and the specificity, 95.95%. For the model verified by blind samples, the normal/colon and rectal cancer cases is (31/35) and the sensitivity and specificity of the model both exceed 80%, with the accuracy reaching 84.85%. For the hepatic carcinoma, the diagnosis model is shown in Table 2. According to the established standard operating

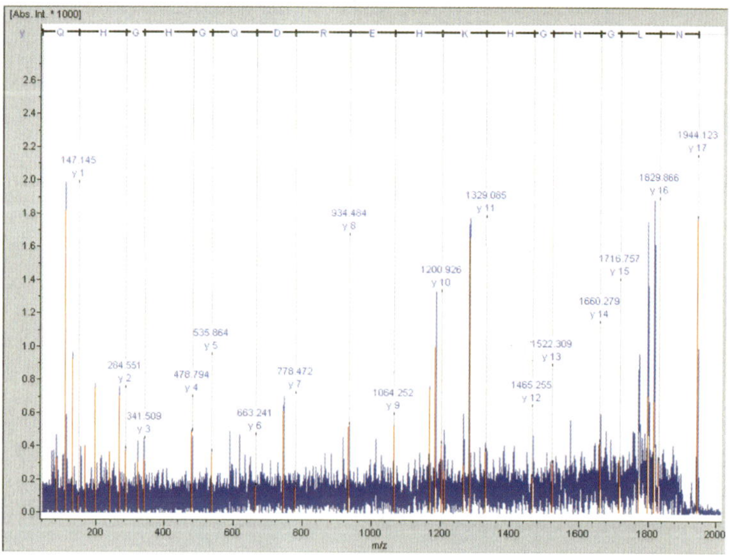

Fig. 6. Hepato Carcinoma Diagnosis Model of the ClinTOF System

procedure (SOP), BIOYONG has studied the polypeptide profiling of the 200 hepatic carcinoma cases and 200 normal serum cases. 28 differential polypeptides (P<0.0001) were obtained, with the molecular weight of 900 ~5000Da (Fig.6). Among them, 9 were down regulated (2.5~8 times) and 19 up-regulated (2.5~20 times). For the model built with SNN, the recognition rate is 100% and predictive ability, 98.39%. 100 samples were used for double-blind determination, with the correctness rate exceeding 90%.

	Training Set	Testing Set
Sensitivity	84.17%	77.4%(24/31)
Specificity	95.95%	91.4%(32/35)
Positive Predictive Value (PPV)	---	88.89%(24/27)
Negative Predictive Value (NPV)	---	82.1%(32/39)
Accuracy	---	84.85(56/66)

Table 1. Colon and Rectal Cancer Diagnosis Model of the ClinTOF System

Performance	Bruker microflex	Bioyong ClinTOF	CipherGen PBSII/C	CipherGen PCS4000
Laser light source	nitrogen 337nm 1-20Hz adjustable	nitrogen 337nm 1-60Hz adjustable	nitrogen 337nm 10Hz	
Ion source technology	Delayed extraction technology			
Ion source pattern	Positive and negative ion sources			
Vacuum system capacity	10^{-6}pa		10^{-7}pa	10^{-4}pa
Detection system	Micro-channel plate detector		Electron multiplier	
	Shielding the "gate" function of noise peaks			
Mass range	>600KDa	>500KDa	>500KDa	>380KDa
Sensitivity	<1fmol		<10fmol	
Resolution	>3500FWHM	>2500FWHM	>700FWHM	>1000FWHM
Accuracy (inner calibration)	≤50ppm	≤50ppm	≤100ppm	
Accuracy (outer calibration)	≤150ppm	≤100ppm	≤2500ppm	≤250ppm
Other features	Patented AnchorChip MALDI sample target	Zoom optics technology, with the laser speckle ranging 50um to 200um adjustable	Coaxial laser technology	
	WishperMode technology reduces lab sound pollution	Unique remote ion source design of big gap, keeping ion source from contamination		
Applications	Proteomics, SNP, biomarker analysis	Proteomics, SNP, biomarker analysis, tissue imaging, microorganism, organ-small molecules, clinical examination in hospitals		

Table 2. Serum Peptidomics Research Technical Systems

1.2.4 Comparison of serum peptidomics research platform

The three systems, namely, SELDI system, ClinProt system and ClinTOF system, of the serum peptidomics research platform are compared in Table 2.

1.3 Main application areas of serum peptidomics

For the moment, the serum peptidomics is clinically used in complex diseases involved in polygene and featuring multi-cause heterogeneity, like cancer (including colon and rectal cancer, lung cancer, hepatic carcinoma, esophagus cancer, stomach cancer, cervical carcinoma and nasopharyngeal carcinoma), nerve degenerative diseases (including Alzheimer disease, Parkinson's disease, Huntington's Disease), autoimmune diseases (rheumatoid arthritis, system lupus erythematosus syndromes), cardio-cerebrovascular disease and palsy, to discover protein/polypeptide profiling and biomarker profiling as well as the single biomarker in the serum of sufferers of these diseases, making breakthroughs and providing a new tool for the researches of disease pathogeny, drug target, diagnosis and treatment.

2. Research method of serum peptidomics

The research of serum peptidomics involves in sample detection and data analysis. Fig.7 is the work flow of serum peptidomics. As shown in Fig.7, blood samples from the

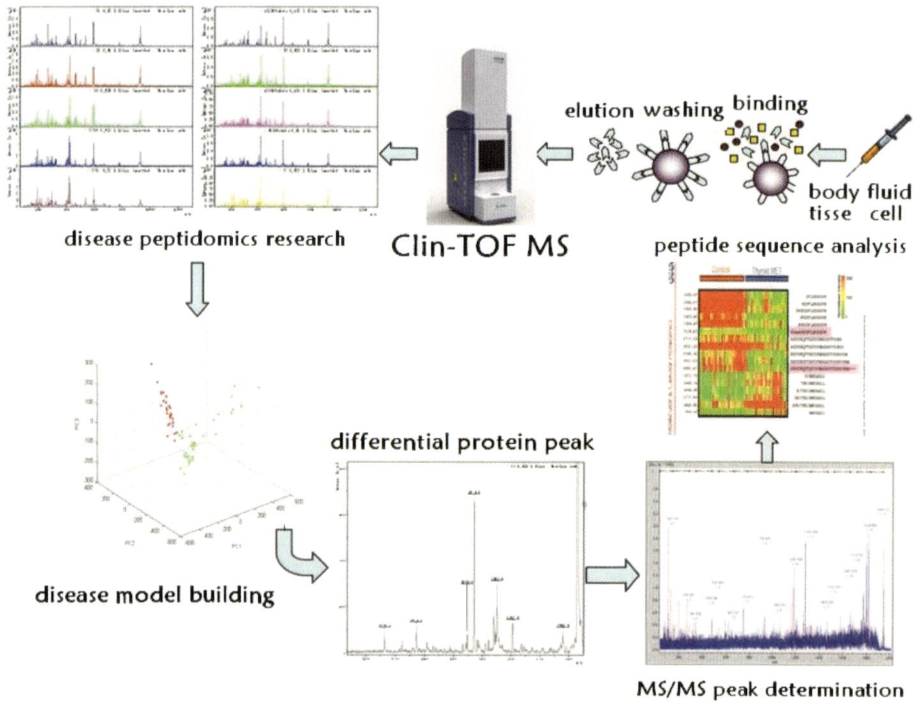

Fig. 7. Technical Process for Serum Peptidomics

pathological group and the healthy control group are collected and then the serum is separated from the blood. The serum is mixed with magnetic beads to extract serum polypeptides for detection with the mass spectrometry. The spectra obtained can produce characteristic spectrum peaks. The meaningful characteristic spectrum peaks are screened out with the statistical method. A prediction model is built with the pattern recognition method and validated with test data. After continuous optimization, a disease diagnosis model and a group of characteristic spectrum peaks can be obtained.

Briefly, the research includes magnetic beads, detection instrument, analysis software, polypeptide identification and clinical model.

2.1 Polypeptide extraction

The separation and purification methods adopted in the serum peptidomics research depend on the nature of the extracted substance. The commonly used methods for polypeptide extraction and separation include: salting removal method, ultra-filtration process, gel filtration, isoelectric point precipitation method, ion-exchange chromatography, affinity chromatography, adsorption chromatography, countercurrent distribution and enzymolysis method. These methods often work together to separate and purify specific substances.

2.1.1 High Pressure Liquid Chromatography (HPLC)

HPLC is a favorable method for peptides separation, because the HPLC can complete the separation in a short time under suitable chromatographic conditions, and more importantly, HPLC is capable of producing polypeptide of bioactivity at the preparative scale. Many scholars therefore have done substantive work in looking for the best conditions for separating and preparing polypeptide substances. How to maintain the activity of polypeptide, how to select stationary phase material and eluent type, how to make analytic determination are all contents of the present study. Common methods include: reversed phase high pressure liquid chromatography (RP-HPLC), hydrophobic interaction chromatography (HIC), Size-Exclusion chromatography (SEC), Ion-Exchange chromatography (IEC), Chromatography of Membrane Protein (CMP), High-Performance Displacement Chromatography (HPDC) and Perfusion Chromatography (PC).

2.1.2 Affinity Chromatography

Affinity Chromatography (AC) is the method of separating substances based on the specific affinity between ligand connecting to the stationary phase matrix and the ligand having interaction with the specificity. Since 1968 when Cuatrecasas put forward the concept of affinity chromatography, in searching for the specific affinity interaction substances many combinations have been found, like antigen-antibody, enzyme-substrate, agglutinin-polyose, oligonucleotides and their complementary strands. For the separation of polypeptide substances, currently the monoclonal antibody or biological simulation ligand can be used for affinity to such substances. These ligands can be natural or artificially synthesized according to their structure. Immobilized Metal Affinity Chromatography (IMAC) is an affinity method developed in recent years. Some metal ions are chelated on the stationary phase substrate, like Cu^{2+}, Ni^{2+} and Fe^{3+}. The magnetic beads can be chelated through the coordination bond to connect polypeptides that contain Lys, Met, Asp, Arg, Tyr, Glu and His on the side chain. In particular, structures with the peptide sequences containing His-X-X-X-His are easiest combined to the metal ion affinity column, featuring good purification effect.

2.1.3 Capillary Electrophoresis

Capillary electrophoresis (CE) was invented by Hjerten at the 1960s on the basis of the conventional electrophoretic technology and improves the electrophoresis efficiency by dozens of times by replacing the large electrophoresis tanks with the capillaries. This technology developed rapidly from 1980 and became a good tool for separation and determining the nature of polypeptides and protein substances by bio-chemical analysts and biochemical scholars. By application principles, CE can be divided into: Capillary Zone Electrophoresis (CZE), Capillary Isoelectric Focusing (CIEF), Capillary Gel Electrophoresis (CGE) and Micellar Electrokinetic Electrophoresis Chromatography(MECC).

2.1.4 Solid phase protein chip technology

The solid phase protein chip technology usually refers to the sample separation part of the SELDI system. The SELDI can not only use the enzyme, antibody, receptor and DNA as the sorting basis of chips, but also take chemical mediators of different natures as the protein sorting basis according to the different chemical natures of proteins, thereby to reduce the requirement on the sample purification and enlarge the sorting range of samples. SELDI chips can be divided into the chemical surface chips and biological surface chips according to the detection purpose. The former include hydrophobic surface (H4), normal phase (NP), weak cation exchange (WCX), strong anion exchange (SAX) and immobilized metal affinity capture (IMAC) and the latter include antibody-antigen surface chips, receptor-ligand surface chips, enzyme-substrate surface chips and DNA-protein surface chips, specifically for detecting the corresponding polypeptide molecules.

2.1.5 Liquid phase protein chip technology – Magnetic bead

The magnetic bead is a new multifunctional reagent developed in recent years and widely used in biomedicine. Owing to diversified surfaces of macromolecular coat, magnetic beads can be coupled with various biologically active substances (like antibody, antigen, receptor, enzyme and nucleic acid), which can be fixed to the magnetic beads to further identify corresponding antigen or antibody, ligand, substrate, nucleic acid in the reaction medium, thereby to realize separation or detection. The results show magnetic beads have functions of both the carrier and separation performer. They can simplify complicated operations by utilizing the physical, chemical and biomedicine principles, thereby to greatly shorten the period of conventional test. Different from protein chips, magnetic beads are composed of many magnetic spherical granules, which provide them with greater surface area and enable them to combine more specific proteins and to have higher sensitivity and accuracy.

To be detailed, the disease associated differential protein liquid chip SPE-C magnetic beads; hydrophobic MB-HI C 1 (suitable for purification and enrichment of proteins more-than-20kDa), MB-HI C 3 (suitable for purification and enrichment of 8-20kDa proteins), MB-HI C 8 (suitable for purification and enrichment of 1-10 kDa proteins/polypeptide), MB-HI C 18 (suitable for purification and enrichment of less-than-4kDa polypeptide); metal affinity magnetic beads include MB-IMAC-Fe (for capture and enrichment of phosphorylation proteins) and MB-IMAC-Cu (for the capture and enrichment of specific affinity proteins/polypeptides); ion exchange magnetic beads include MB-WCX (purification and enrichment of acid proteins with the cation-exchange chromatography technology) and MB-WAX (purification and enrichment of basic proteins with the anion-exchange chromatography technology); glycoprotein magnetic beads include ConA and ConB (for purification and enrichment of glycoprotein); the immune fishing liquid chips include immune affinity magnetic bead ProteinG (the ProteinG on the magnetic bead can combine with any one antibody, for screening specific antigens).

2.1.6 Systematic applications of polypeptide separation engineering

Polypeptide separation technologies mentioned above are combined to use in practice. Different separation tools will be used according to the nature of polypeptide. In particular in the post genome era, researches on the proteome are deepened and people are making continuous progress in tools for separating polypeptides and proteins. They have comprehensively utilized natures of proteins and polypeptides and adopted both the routine protein and polypeptide extraction methods aforementioned and also the high efficiency liquid chromatography, capillary electrophoresis and 2-d electrophoresis, to get as many polypeptides as possible.

2.2 Sample detection

2.2.1 Detection of N-terminal sequence with Edman degradation method

The Edman degradation method used for sequencing can obtain a precise peptide sequence, therefore making it a major method for protein identification. Yet its sequencing speed is slow and expansive. With technical breakthroughs in microsequencing and speed, Edman degradation method will exert a major role in proteome researches. The C-terminal Maxam-Gilbert method, similar to Edman, has been studied for years and produced automated analyzers, but its reaction efficiency is low and usually requires more samples.

2.2.2 Amino acid composition analysis

Amino acid composition analysis is frequently used for protein identification owing to its low cost. Different from the peptide mass or sequence tags, amino acid composition analysis identifies proteins by utilizing the specific amino acid component of different proteins. This method can be used for identifying 2-DE separated proteins. The radio-labeled amino acid is used to determine amino acid components of proteins, or the proteins are converted to the PVDF membrane and after the automatic derivation of amino acid, undergo chromatographic separation to obtain data. Then, inquiries are made to the database to rank proteins in the database by the amount of difference of two components, as a result, the top ranking proteins having greater reliability. Yet this method has some defects: slow speed and require a great amount of proteins or peptides; restricted in the ultramicro analysis;the possible amino acid variation due to the incomplete acidic hydrolysis or partial degradation.

2.2.3 Mass Spectrometry

Mass Spectrometry (MS): MS is an analytical technique that measures the mass-to-charge ratio (or mass) of charged particles, molecules or molecular fragments. MS provides information of molecular weight, molecular formula, isotopic element composition of molecules and molecular structure of samples analyzed. It has been widely applied in protein and polypeptide analysis. In particular, it is suitable for the analysis and identification of polypeptide substances in the online analysis after separation and purification due to its hypersensitivity and rapidity. Commonly, MS includes electrospray MS (in the spray process, the continuous ionization method makes the polypeptide samples ionized), fast atom bombardment MS (FAB MS) and isotopic element MS. Among them, the Continuous-Flow Fast Atom Bombardment, cf-FAB) and the Electrospray Ionization (ESI) have just been developed in recent years.

Continuous-Flow Fast Atom Bombardment(cf-FAB): a kind of weak ionization technology, it is capable of ionizing peptides or small-molecular-weight proteins into the form of MH+ or (M-H). It is mostly applied in the separation and detection of peptides and has moderate resolution, with the accuracy greater than +0.2amu and flow rate of 0.5-1.5μl ·Ml-1. In the determination, the mobile phase shall be added with 0.5%-10% substrate like glycerol and high organic solvents, so that samples can be sensitized at the detection probe. The cf-FAB is usually used together with HPLC and CEZ, to realize the purpose of isolation analysis. The cf-FAB analysis methods have been built for many polypeptides and well applied.

Electrospray Ionization (ESI): able to generate multivalent ionized proteins or polypeptides, allowing analyzing of proteins with the molecular weight reaching 100kD; its resolution is 1500-2000 amu and accuracy about 0.01 %. ESI is more suitable for the online analysis of proteins with large molecular weight and requires gasification or organic solvents for the sample sensitization. It has been a success to combine ESI and HPLC for separation and analysis of GH and hemoglobin. ESI can also be used together with CEZ.

MALDI-TOF MS: in this method, the ionization of polypeptide samples is realized with the substrate absorbing the laser energy. It is a tool for accurately determining the molecular mass in the current protein identification and particularly suitable for the determination of the molecular weight of mixed proteins and polypeptides, featuring high sensitivity and resolution. For the moment, it is a necessary tool for the proteomics research. Working with the coupling technique of the liquid chromatography, this method can identify polypeptides at a high efficiency. Especially, when MS technologies of different principles are coupled, they can not only obtain the molecular weight of polypeptides, but also determine the sequential structure. This technology will exert a decisive effect in the future proteomics study.

2.2.4 Nuclear Magnetic Resonance

Nuclear Magnetic Resonance (NMR): NMR profiling has purely digital signals, excessive overlapping range (due to the large molecular weight) and weak signals, so it is seldom used in analysis of proteins and polypeptides. In company with the application of 2D, 3D and 4D NMR and the progress of molecular biology and computer processing technology, NMR has gradually become a main approach for analysis of proteins and polypeptides. NMR can be used for determining amino acid sequence and the content of components in mixtures. Yet some problems need solving if this method is used for protein analysis, for instance, how to give proteins with large molecular weight a specific shape to facilitate quantitative and qualitative analysis and how to reduce the data processing time, which are being studied by many scholars. Despite of its infrequent use in the protein analysis, NMR is extremely useful in analyzing small peptides with the molecules having less than 30 amino acids, in which case, it can overcome the foregoing defects and realize rapid and accurate analysis.

2.2.5 Others

Besides the foregoing methods, amino acid composition analysis, amino acid sequence analysis, Field Desorption Mass Spectrometer (FDMS), IR, UV spectra, circular dichroism spectrum, bioassay technique, tagging method and immunologic method have also been used for the result identification, analysis and detection of polypeptides.

2.3 Analysis method

Regarding research on serum peptidomics, the analysis of data collected shall have: high-efficient analysis technical platform, computer and network have become a necessary tool of biological research; high throughput technical platform, mainly targeting at how to use the information technology to analyze the giant data; data mining technical platform, which shall be able to mine knowledge from the massive data saved in database or other information banks for the analysis; data visualization technical platform, in describing the systematic relations, the functions of nucleic acid, protein, cell, organ and tissue shall be considered, that is to say, a systematic method shall be used to learn about vital activities.

Currently, databases used for proteomics research include SWISS-PROT, BLOCKS, SMART, PROSITE, WORLD-2D-PAGE, EMBL, GenBank, DDBJ, ProClass, PR INTS, MASCOT, PROTO-MAP, DOMO, PDB and NCBI. Among them, SWISS-PROT is a real protein sequence database and also the largest and most diversified proteome database in the world. EMBL is to collect protein sequences that have been translated from nucleic acid automatically and not yet entered the SWISS-PROT. NCBI contains protein sequences translated from DNA in the GenBank and from the PDB, SWISS-PROT and PIR databases.

Presently, many tools and methods used for MS data process and analysis of serum peptidomics have been developed, mainly including:

2.3.1 Bioconductor

Bioconductor is an open source and open development software project, with the broad goals of providing widespread access to a broad range of powerful statistical and graphical methods for the analysis of genomic data, facilitating the inclusion of biological metadata and driving comprehensive analysis and application of data. Its application function is to provide users with the integrated packages. It has also provided many packages of MS data processing and analysis for users. Bioconductor is based on the R language, so it requires that users must be familiar with the R-language working environment and have some knowledge of programming, that is to say, it will be difficult for the general clinical and lab workers.

2.3.2 MATLAB

MATLAB is a piece of commercial software integrating statistical analysis and engineering computation. Taking MATLAB as the development platform, it will be possible to realize the pretreatment, display and statistical analysis of MS data. In the research of serum peptidome profiling of prostatic cancer, breast cancer and bladder cancer, this tool together with the GENESPRING of Agilent has achieved good results in data analysis (Villanueva et al, 2005).

2.3.3 TOF-MS Based Software

1. Spectrogram Pretreatment

Due to many influencing factors in the MS experiment, the original spectrogram produced by MS must be pretreated to eliminate disturbance. Pretreatment of the MS data includes baseline elimination, filtration and noise elimination, standardization, peak detection and peak quantification. The comparison of commonly-used pretreatment methods and tools are shown in Table 3 (Cruz-Marcelo et al, 2008).

Algorithm and Tool	Main Functions	Relevant Information
ProteinChip Software 3.1 and Biomarker Wizard	Commercial software of Ciphergen Biosystems, designed for analyzing SELDI-TOF MS data	http://www.vermillion.com/
PROcess	An R-language based package of BioConductor, designed for pretreatment of SELDI-TOF MS	http://www.bioconductor.org/packages/bioc/1.8/html/PROcess.html
Cromwell	MatLab script to realize MS data pretreatment	http://bioinformatics.mdanderson.org/cromwell.html
SpecAlign	MS data pretreatment and peak alignment	http://physchem.ox.ac.uk/~jwong/specalign/index.htm
MassSpecWavelet	An R-language based package of BioConductor, using continuous wavelet transform for peak detection	http://www.bioconductor.org/packages/2.0/bioc/html/MassSpecWavelet.html

Table 3. Commonly-used MS Pretreatment Algorithms and Tools

2. Peak Alignment

The spectrograms after pretreatment shall undergo peak alignment. Many spectrograms are combined into a matrix file similar to the gene expression profile, namely the serum peptidome profiling. In the profiling, the line represents the peak of some specific charge-mass ratio (m/z), namely, the relative content of specific proteins or polypeptides, and the column represents samples. This is the foundation for follow-up bioinformatics analysis and its data quality directly influences the analysis results.

3. Bioinformatics Analysis

Usually, the first step is to make cluster analysis, mainly including shortest distance method, longest distance method, median method, centroid method, average linkage and Ward's minimum-variance method. Also, the data classification is carried out. The commonly-used methods include support vector machine (SVM), decision tree, neural networks and k nearest neighbor (kNN).

The research process based on serum peptidomics classification is first to divide the mass spectrometric data after pretreatment into a group of modeling data and the other group of validation data. The modeling data fall into the training set and testing set. Then, analysis will be performed over the training set with t-test, Pearson correlation analysis and genetic algorithm, to find peaks of higher specificity to build a sorter. Then, the testing set makes tests, which shall be repeated and optimized. Finally, the validating data are used for validating to get a stable model.

4. TOF-MS System Based Softwares

Softwares based on the TOF-MS system mainly includes: (1) for the SELDI system, the ProteinChip Software 3.1 and Biomarker Wizard taking the decision tree as the core; (2) for the ClinProt system, the ClinProTools software taking cluster analysis as the core; (3) for the ClinTOF system, the BioExploer™ software taking specific vector machine (SVM), decision, tree, neural networks and k nearest neighbor (kNN) as the core.

Other bioinformatics tools for MS correlation analysis include: MapQuant, MASPECTRAS, SpecArray, msInspect and MZMine. These tools or softwares haven't realized seamless connection with serum peptidomics data, so they fail to perfectly accomplish the data management and analysis based on MS serum peptidome profiling.

3. Disease serum peptidomics research progress

Nowadays in clinical detection, the serum biochemical indicators fail to accomplish the task of diagnosing complex diseases. For instance, there are only one or two serological diagnosis indicators available for specific cancers; even worse, these indicators cannot diagnose diseases independently and sometimes confuse the cancer with benign tumors or inflammation. For example, the prostate specific antigen (PSA) is a major diagnosis indicator for prostatic cancer, but not a biomarker for the prostatic cancer specificity, for the reason that 15%~25% prostatic cancer patients see their serum PSA falling into the normal range. Besides, PSA may also rise due to the benign hyperplasia of prostate, urinary infection, acute prostatitis, retention of urine and the per rectum operations. Accordingly, serum peptidomics analysis, as a new clinical diagnosis method, has made great progress in early diagnosis of complex diseases like tumor, neurological degenerative diseases and autoimmune disease.

3.1 Tumor

3.1.1 Ovarian cancer

Ovarian cancer is the most maligne tumor among all malignant tumors of the reproductive system, with the pathogenic factors unclear yet but possibly relating to the reproductive and hereditary factors. Most ovarian cancer cases are detected in the late stage and seldom cured. For the moment, the universally-ratified specificity biomarker CA125 for ovarian cancer diagnosis, as the single biomarker, sees the positive predicted value less than 10%. Therefore it is urgent to develop an approach for the early-stage clinical diagnosis so as to enhance the survival rate. The serum based peptidomics has seen great progress in researches of ovarian cancer diagnosis.

Pleasantly, based on findings of the SELDI system, the US Vermilion Company and Quest Diagnostics worked together to develop the OVA1, which can determine the onset of ovarian cancer by detecting the cavum pelvis enclosed mass and decide whether operations are needed, what operations are needed and who shall perform the operations if applicable. OVA1 ovarian cancer qualitative serum test forms a single digital grading system by combining the five immunoassay combinations. The test has shown that female older than 18, requiring operations of ovarian enclosed mass and not examined by the oncologist can undergo examination with OVA1. This immune test has determined five tried and true biomarkers, namely, thyroxin, apolipoprotein A-1, β2-microglobulin, transferin and cancer antigen 125. One algorithm is decided to determine the probability of tumor onset of female cavum pelvis enclosed mass. Quest Diagnostics exclusively provides OVA1 to the US clinical lab for three years. Food and Drug Administration (FDA) has approved OVA1 to be used for the high-sensitivity testing of ovarian cancer, with effect better than biopsy or operation examination, even if the radiation test results cannot show whether malignant tumors exist. Vermilion is devoted to discovering, developing and commercializing new-style high-value diagnostic tests, to help doctors diagnose, cure and perfect prognoses of the patient. Vermilion provides approaches for diagnosis of tumor, blood and heart disease and for ensuring women health (OVA1, Fremont, CA: Vermillion, Inc; 2009).

Petricoin et al., with the fund from the clinical proteome plan of the US FDA/NIH, has successfully applied the serum polypeptide profiling technology to make diagnosis of early-stage ovarian cancer. The ovarian cancer serum proteomics findings with the hydrophobic chips were reported: they discover that the content of five types of proteins in the serum of ovarian cancer patients and the healthy people is changing at the same time, which is of far reaching importance to the diagnosis of ovarian cancer. This proteome worked as the specificity biomarker for diagnosing ovarian cancer and double-blind researches were done to the serum of the healthy people, ovarian cancer patients and ovarian benign pathological changes, with results showing that the sensitivity of this method is 100%, specificity 95% and positive predicted value 94%; by contrast, the positive predicted value of CA125 was only 35% (Petricoin et al, 2002).

Katherine et al. utilized the protein fingerprint technology to load 184 serum samples on the strong anion exchange (SAX) chips. The 184 cases included 109 ovarian cancer cases, 19 benign ovarian tumor cases and 56 healthy people. The univariate and multivariate statistics method has been applied for analysis. From the protein fragments from the 140 serum samples, 3 groups of protein markers of diagnosis significance were obtained: the first group included 5 candidate protein markers, with the ovarian cancer sensitivity of 95.7%, specificity of 82.6% and accuracy of 89.2%; the other two groups of protein markers included 5 and 4 candidate protein markers respectively, with the sensitivity of 81.7% and 72.8%, specificity 94.9% and of 94.9% and accuracy of 88.2% and 83.9% respectively. After screening out 3 groups of protein markers, the rest 44 unknown serum samples were used for blind validation, showing that when the three groups were employed together, 41 serum cases were diagnosed correctly, to be detailed, 21 ovarian cancers were correctly diagnosed, 11 ovarian cancers of the progressive stage were correctly diagnosed and 10 of the 11 ovarian cancers of the early stage were confirmed; 6 low-malignancy potential tumors were diagnosed, 5 of the 6 benign tumors were excluded the possibility of ovarian cancer, 1 of the 10 serum cases of healthy people had a wrong diagnosis. In this sense, Katherine et al. believed that they had found ovarian cancer protein marker groups of diagnosis significance and can effectively distinguish healthy people from the benign/malignant ovarian tumors.

Ye et al. utilized the protein chip technology to analyze the serum of 80 ovarian cancer patients and 91 healthy people, discovering the differential protein peak at the position with the molecular mass of 11700 Da, which was obviously higher than the density peak value of the control group. Then, the affinity chromatography method was used for purification of it and the protein sequence was then determined with the fluid chromatography and mass spectrometer. A polypeptide chain was synthesized. Finally, it was identified that this polypeptide fragment was haptoglobin chain and corresponding antibody was derived. Combined with CA125, this method saw the ovarian tumor diagnosis sensitivity of 95.7%, specificity 82.6%, enhanced the early diagnosis rate of ovarian cancers and lowered false positive of CA125. Currently, relevant technologies started being applied in screening ovarian cancers.

In addition, theses published on Lancet indicated the MS technology was used to analyze the composition pattern of serum peptidome and based on the pattern, found out differential points for detection of ovarian cancer clinically. Results showed that 50 ovarian cancer patients were all detected, with 18 patients suffering stage-I ovarian cancer; 63 of 66 gynecologic benign tumors were diagnosed correctly. In detection of ovarian cancer, the sensitivity, specificity and positive predicted value of this method were 100%, 95% and 94% respectively, much better than the conventional CA125 detection. In particular, it was successful in diagnosing the early-stage ovarian cancer (stage I), indicating that this technology may be used for the early-stage or early warning detection of ovarian cancer hopefully. Thereafter, a series of theses on the serum peptide profiling technology for disease diagnosis were published in the world. For instance, in 2004, Soltys et al. with the Stanford University published results of using serum peptidome profiling to diagnose squamous carcinoma on Clinical Cancer Research; in 2005, Kaz'ufumiHonda et al. with the Japanese National Cancer Center published thesis on utilizing low-resolution MS and high-resolution MS to diagnose pancreatic cancer on Cancer Research. At the beginning of 2006, Villanueva et al. with the US Sloan-Kettering Cancer Center published an article on using serum peptide profiling technology to diagnose bladder cancer, breast cancer and prostatic cancer; at the end of 2006, Nature published remarks on this article, signaling its support for this technical development and application. Lately, Lancet published an article on using the serum peptide profiling technology to diagnose tuberculosis, which produced sensitivity and specificity greater than 950k.

3.1.2 Breast cancer

We employed the ClinTOF system in the research of breast cancer, with the experimental design as shown in Fig.8. The serum polypeptides were extracted with magnetic beads and then the polypeptide profiling was obtained with MS detection, to build a disease model. Significant difference was found with the software analysis and the reliability of the model was validated with a certain number of blind samples. At the same time, the reliability of the difference was confirmed. Multiple tandem mass spectrometry were used to identify differential polypeptides. FlexAnalysss2.4, BioExplorer, SIMCAP+ and ClinProTools2.0 were used to analyze results, as shown in Fig.9, finding out 4 differential peaks; identification and functional forecast were performed on differential polypeptides.

Most of the polypeptide sequences identified lacked of only one or several amino acids. After comparing them with results and discussions in literatures, it was concluded that under different disease response conditions, the activity of external peptidase would undergo changes, thereby to obtain a series of polypeptides by cutting different protein loca. These polypeptides might share the same modif.

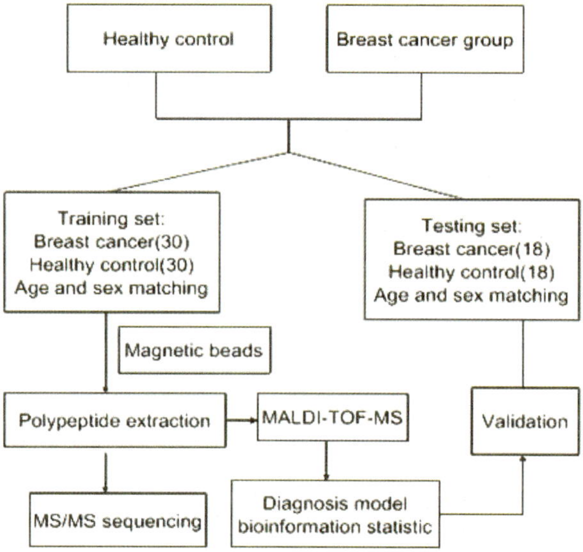

Fig. 8. Experimental Design of ClinTOF System for Breast Cancer Research

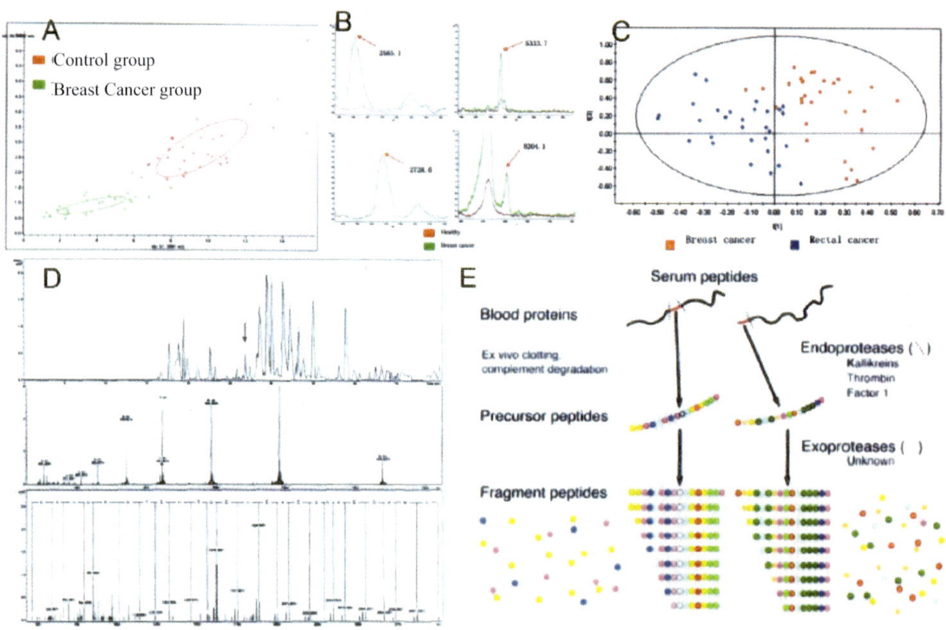

A: sample distribution diagram; B: average profiling of significantly differential peaks; C: distribution of samples obtained by SIMCAP+; D: results of MS identificdatin of differential polypeptides; E: description of mechanism according to distribution of identified polypeptides

Fig. 9. Findings of Using the ClinTOF System to Breast Cancer Research

Some researchers have also shown that protein MS peaks obtained by the SELDI system can effectively screen and distinguish the breast cancer and non-breast cancer patients. Van Winden et al. adopted the SELDI technology to determine the density difference between the breast cancer group and the control group, making new progress compared with the previous breast cancer marker protein reseraches (van Winden et al, 2009). Gast et al. utilized the SELDI technology to detect the protein profiling in tissues and serum to diagnose breast cancer, showing that 3 peaks are significantly correlated to breast cancer. 27 tissues were detected to have differential peaks. These protein fragments presented potential pathological and physiological mechanisms related to breast cancer, which is helpful for raising the diagnosis rate of the breast cancer (Gast et al., 2009). Taku et al employed the SELDIS technology to detect 65 breast cancer patients as a group, concluding that the overexpression of a non-identified protein and the underexpression of the other are related to the lymphatic metastasis of breast cancer (Taku et al., 2006).

3.1.3 Nasopharyngeal carcinoma

In the early stage, if nasopharyngeal carcinoma fails to show some disease features due to disturbance of some factors, the test method is so insensitive that the patient cannot get timely and correct diagnosis, it will delay the treatment and cause unfavorable prognosis. In the research on nasopharyngeal carcinoma serum peptidome, some progress has been made.

We employed the ClinTOF system to research the marker of early-stage nasopharyngeal carcinoma. The magnetic bead system was SPE-C. By comparing 40 nasopharyngeal carcinoma cases and 61 healthy people, 65 significantly differential peaks were observed in the mass range of 1,000Da-10,000Da. The peak with the most obvious difference of expression has the mass-to-charge ratio of 1262.67 and is identified with the LTQ -Orbitrap to be the fragment of fibrinopeptide A. Fibrinogen is a kind of glycoprotein rich in blood and a symmetrical dimer composed of 6 polypeptide chains; it plays a major role in blood coagulation and hemostasis. So far, more than 300 fibrinogen natural mutants have been discovered, among which, about 55% are subclinical, 25% have hemorrhagic tendency and 20% have thrombophilia. Among these mutants, the most common expression is that one amino acid is replaced by another. At the molecular biology level, expressions are point mutation, deletion, insertion and nonsense mutation. Moreover, the polymorphism of the fibrinogen results in the overexpression, which raises the fibrinogen level of plasma and closely relates to diseases.

Researchers have also indicated that this system has a higher repeatability than the IMAC Cu^{2+} chips (Ciphergen Company) and is capable of finding more differential peaks in proteins with the molecular weight ranging 2,000Da -5,000Da.

Wei et al., using the SELDI system, screened out the mass-to-charge ratios of four proteins, to be detailed, 4 097Da, 4 180 Da, 5 912Da and 8 295Da, which make a marker combination to build a classification tree model for diagnosis of nasopharyngeal carcinoma. In diagnosing nasopharyngeal carcinoma, the sensitivity and specificity of this model were 94.5 % and 96.7% respectively and for the blind screening group, the two figures were 92% and 92.9% respectively. Using the protein MS peaks with the mass-to-charge ratio of 4 581Da and 7802Da to predict the stage I and stage II nasopharyngeal carcinoma, the accuracy proved to be 80% and for the stage III and stage IV, this figure was 86% (Wei et al, 2008).

Guo et al. applied the SELDI system and the artificial neural network technology to analyze serum of 58 type-A (cranial nerve type: featured by basicranial destruction and cranial nerve violation, no lymphonodi cervicales metastasis) and type-D (lymphonodi cervicales metastasis type: widespread metastasis of one- or two-sided lymphonodi cervicales, no cranial nerve violation or basicranial bone destruction) nasopharyngeal carcinoma patients and obtained 11 potential biomarkers, with the mass-to-charge ratio of 4 053, 5 885, 4 072, 5 798, 4 209, 8 689, 2 382, 9 357, 2 221, 4 230Da and 5 901Da respectively. The MS peaks of these proteins saw accuracy for distinguishing type A and type D reach 90% (Guo et al, 2005).

Cho et al. employed IMAC3-Cu protein chips to detect the serum of the healthy people, modified nasopharyngeal carcinoma patients after treatment and the relapse nasopharyngeal carcinoma patients before and after chemotherapy, discovering 13 meaningful protein MS peaks. Protein MS peaks with the mass-to-charge ratio of 2950Da and 6 701Da were selected to build a classification tree model for predicting chemotherapy response, with the sensitivity and specificity of 80% and 87% respectively. In detection and analysis of serum protein profiling of the healthy people and the relapse nasopharyngeal carcinoma patients, it is newly discovered that the MS peaks with the mass-to-charge ratio of 3803Da and 3953Da were found in the serum of both patients taking the initial diagnosis and treatment, and the modified nasopharyngeal carcinoma patients after treatment. In addition, the protein MS peaks with the mass-to-charge ratio of 3953Da and 7765Da were identified to be the inter-alpha trypsin inhibitor heavy chain H4 precursor (ITIH4) fragments and platelet factor 4 (PF4) with the method of MS/MS sequence and immune affinity capture test, thus presuming that they are related to the onset, development, metastasis and relapse of nasopharyngeal carcinoma (Cho et al., 2004).

Huang et al. adopted the CM 10 chip and SELDI technology to detect squamous epithelial cells of the nasopharyngeal carcinoma patients and made contrast with serum of the healthy people. 94 protein MS peaks were detected, among which, 26 were obviously different from the serum of healthy people ($P<0.05$, Mean>SD), 5 of overexpression and 21 underexpression. Three protein MS peaks with the mass-to-charge ratio of 3159 83, 5 187 65 and 1 3738.6Da were selected to build a diagnosis model. Verified by the blind method, this diagnosis model has accuracy of 90.63%, sensitivity 95.00%, specificity 83.33%, positive predicted value 90.48% and negative predicted value 90.90%, indicating that this model has a higher diagnosis value for NPC (Huang et al, 2008).

Doustjalali adopted the ClinProt system and the MASCOT database retrieval, discovering that in the serum of nasopharyngeal carcinoma patients, the content of CPL showed overexpression compared with the control group; further, after the ELISA method validation, it was discovered that in the nasopharyngeal carcinoma tissues, CPL showed overexpression. After 6 months' treatment, the CPL content in tissues reduced. CPL is a kind of copper-bearing glycoprotein and considered to be a key molecule for activating angiogenesis factor, which can promote growth of tumors, as shown by studies. This research monitored the changes of ceruloplasmin in company with the ease of the disease with the proteome technology, which would play a role in diagnosis, curative effect observation and prognoses evaluation, observation and monitoring of nasopharyngeal carcinoma (Doustjalali et al., 2006).

Liao et al. adopted 2-DE /MALDI-TOF-MS technology to screen tumor specific antigens of nasopharyngeal carcinoma. High-abundance protein elimination and desalting pretreatment were performed over serum of the nasopharyngeal carcinoma metastasis group, nasopharyngeal carcinoma non-metastasis group and the control group. Then, analysis was made to the 3 groups of serum profiling, obtained 29 differential protein spots and identified 23 proteins. Through comparison of the cancer profiling and the profiling of the control group, it is discovered that the transferrin, zinc finger protein 544, thyroid hormone binding protein, NM 23H 1 protein and FAD synthetase showed underexpression in nasopharyngeal carcinoma patients. Yet lipoxygenase (LOX), serum amyloid protein A1, cytochrome P450, sICAM1, cathepsin G and histone lysine specific demethylase 1 showed overexpression in the two groups of nasopharyngeal carcinoma patients; the LOX, sICAM1, cathepsin G and histone lysine specific demethylase 1 showed higher expression in the nasopharyngeal carcinoma metastasis group than in the non-metastasis group, while the heat shock protein 70 was only expressed in the nasopharyngeal carcinoma metastasis group. In addition, by combining the immune histochemical technique and ELISA method, it is concluded that HSP70, sICAM1 and serum amyloid protein A (SAA) were potential serological markers for mediating nasopharyngeal carcinoma metastasis and also exerted an important role in clinical detection and control of nasopharyngeal carcinoma (Liao et al, 2008).

3.1.4 Cervical carcinoma

The serum peptidomics technology has been used in the research of endometrial carcinoma and is of guidance significance for the early diagnosis and clinical grading of diseases.

Our researches using the ClinTOF system have indicated that in the cervical carcinoma group and the control group, the protein peak intensify difference of only 21 proteins had statistical significance ($P<0.05$). M1450.35Da, M1778.7Da, M1896.65Da and M5520.42Da were taken as the classified variables to build a classification predictive model, to make classification diagnosis over the cervical carcinoma group and the control group, with the identification rate and predictive ability of 90.45% and 81.75% respectively. By contrasting the proteome of different pathological differentiation degrees, it is discovered that the protein peak intensity difference of 2 proteins had statistical significance ($P<0.05$). M5904.14Da and M5264.26Da were taken as the classified variables to build a classification model, to make classification diagnosis on different differentiation degrees, with the identification rate and predictive ability of 81.48% and 78.89% respectively.

Yoshizaki et al. adopted the SELDI system to analyze the protein profiling of 19 endometrial carcinoma cases and 20 normal tunica intima tissues, discovering two differential proteins, namely EC1 and EC2. The former had overexpression in the endometrial carcinoma tissues and the latter on the contrary. These differential proteins may be used for diagnosing endometrial carcinoma hopefully (Yoshizaki et al., 2005).

3.1.5 Leukemia

The treatment of acute leukemia (AL) depends on minimal residual disease (MRD) diagnosis and detection. However there has been no serum biomarker that can be used by the clinicians for diagnosing AL and evaluating MRD. Yang et al. analyzed serum of AL patients, discovering two peptides (m/z of 1778 and 1865) reduced with the rise in the modification degree and that 1865 was related to AL types. After further FT-ICR-MS detection, the two peptides are the C3F fragment. The linear regression analysis has indicated that the combined use of the peptides could distinguish PML / RARα positive molecules from M3. Findings show that the two C3F fragments are significantly correlated with the MRD level and can be used for evaluating clinical MRD (Liang et al., 2010).

3.1.6 Brain glioma

Our forward-looking researches on brain spongiocytoma diagnosis have indicated: using the SPE-C magnetic bead separation and liquid automatic processing robot operations of the ClinTOF system, after MS, 74 differential peaks occurred in the serum of 84 patients and 72 healthy people. 55 samples were taken randomly to build the MS model of patients and healthy people, with the diagnosis specificity for the healthy people reaching as high as 96.4% (Fig.10).

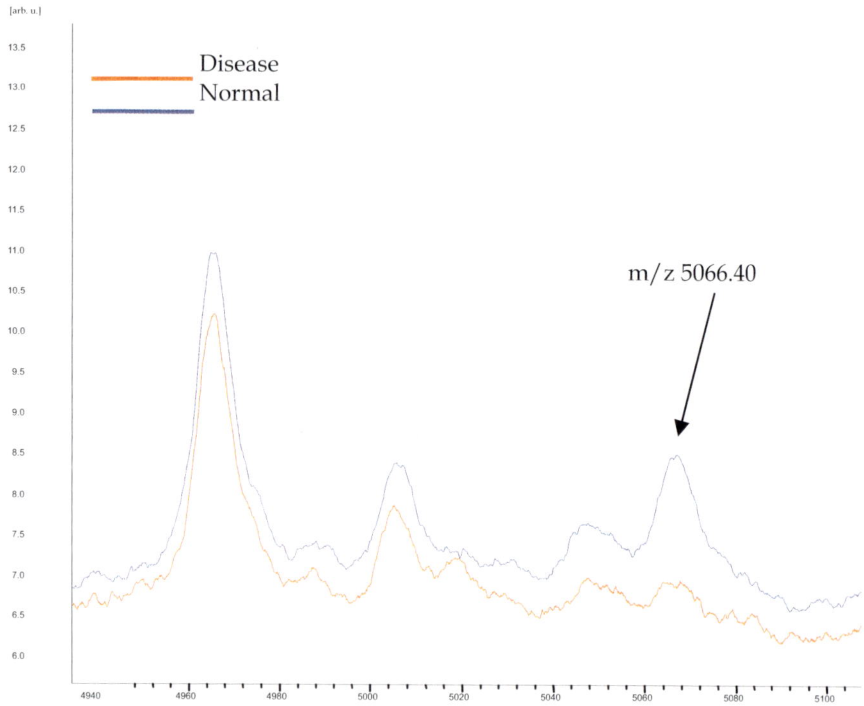

Fig. 10. Differential Polypeptide Peaks of Brain Glioma

3.2 Nerve and mental diseases

Alzheimer disease (AD) is a degenerative disease with unclear causes and mainly disturbing cerebral cortex neurons. Zhang et al. discovered that in the serum of AD patients, the haptoglobin and complement factor H were overexpressed. Haptoglobin is a kind of acute phase reactive protein and an antioxidant, featuring multiple biological activities and is considered to have participated in the inflammation process together with lymphocyte, neutrophilic granulocyte and monocyte and played a vital role in regulating host defense. Complement factor H is an important complement modulation substance and can also work as a significant effector molecule of congenital immunity. It is capable of distinguishing self and non-self and the activated and non-activated cell surfaces. In the research, the overexpression of two proteins indicates the inflammatory reaction, oxidation stress and immunologic mechanism are participating in the onset process of AD (Zhang et al., 2004). Hye et al. made case-control study to the plasma of 50 AD patients and the control group, discovering many disease pathology related proteins, including complement factor H (CFH) precursor and α22 macroglobulin and pointing out that the expression of CFH is related to the cognitive dysfunction of AD patients. α22 macroglobulin (A2M) is a pan-protease inhibitor. In case of brain damages, the immunological activity of A2M of the neuron and colloid cells will rise, especially at the levels of senile plaques, nerve fiber matting and auantic neuron neurite (Hye et al., 2006).

We utilized the SPE-C magnetic beads and ClinTOF system to compare 85 two-way patients having no medicine and 100 healthy people, discovering 5 significantly differential peaks in the mass range of 800Da-12,000Da among the mental disease patients and the healthy people. The serum polypeptide MS standard model profiling has a predictive sensitivity of 100% for the healthy people and for the mental disease patients, 87%.

3.3 Healthy people screening

To study relevancy between some disease and polypeptide, we introduced serum polypeptide profiling into health screening. The ClinTOF system was used to study 1980 healthy people related polypeptide profiling researches, covering the age of 18-75, large sample statistics of both sexes, with the experimental design work shown in Fig.11 With

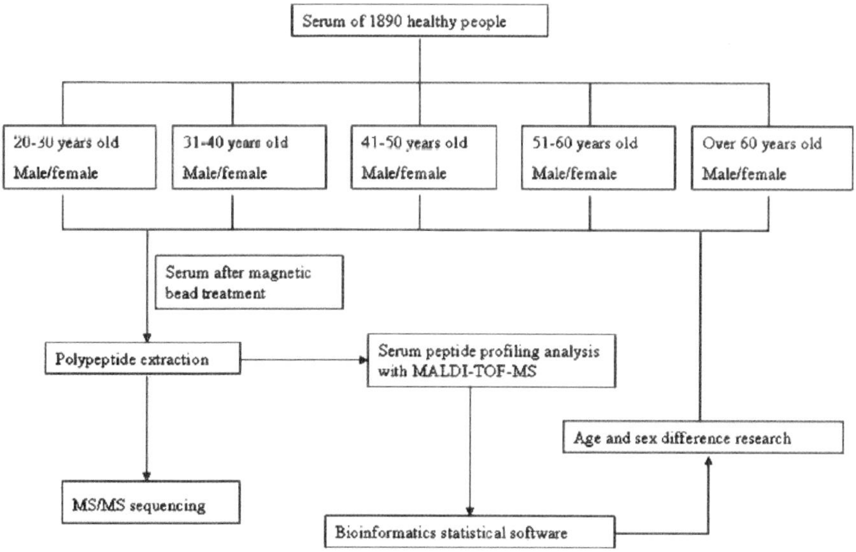

Fig. 11. Experimental Design of Healthy People Screening with the ClinTOF System

the SPE-C magnetic bead, MS profiling (Fig.12) for age 5 ranges was built and 10 peaks with the most significantly mass-to-charge ratio were identified. The online search of database with Mascot indicated that most polypeptide protein precursors were isogenous with the human prokinin precursors. After the analysis of serum peptidome profiling and bioinformatics data mining of 1890 healthy people, for the healthy people, the profiling has no obvious difference regardless of age and sex, but for people younger than 30, the sex difference factor shall be considered, that is, the elder the person is, the more different the serum peptidome profiling will be. Therefore, in researching the disease peptidome profiling, the age and sex matching factors shall be considered. It has also discovered that 50 polypeptides have a higher frequency of occurrence (more than 30%) in the serum of healthy people, indicating that these polypeptides can work as reference for health controls.

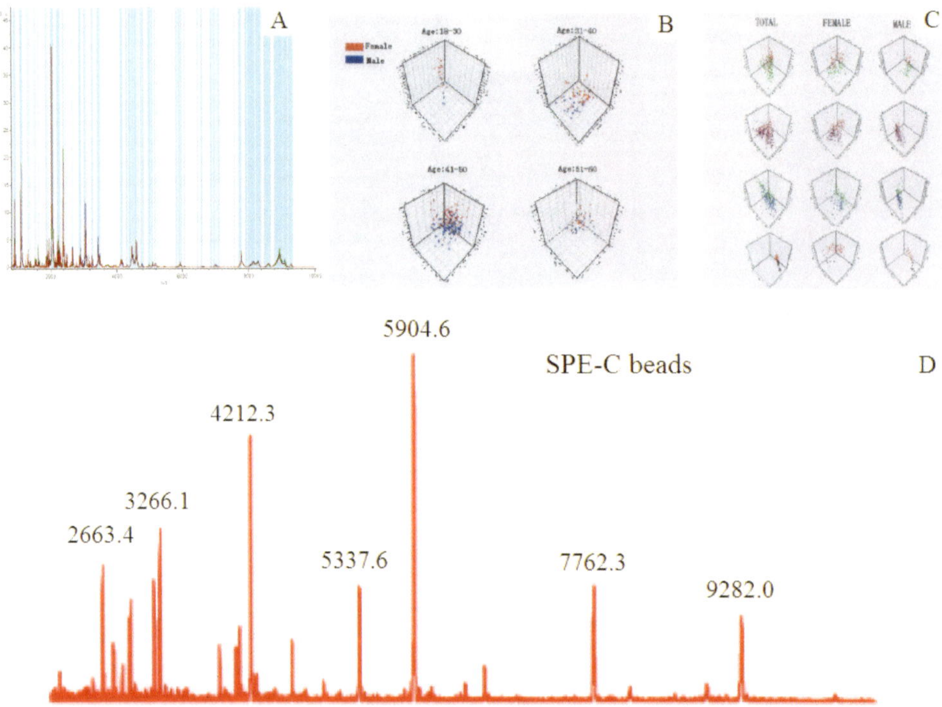

A: average profiling of 1890 healthy people; B and C: results from PCA analysis by age and sex; D: some peaks of highly-frequent occurrence detected by MS after the treatment by SPE-C magnetic beads

Fig. 12. Results of Healthy People Screening with the ClinTOF System

3.4 Fetal congenital aplasia

We have used the ClinTOF system to study fetal congenital aplasia, with the research protocol shown in Fig.13. This thinking has generalized the sample collection strategies and the result expectations sufficiently indicating the diversification and universality of serum peptide method, and can be used for most research areas. Secretion leukoprotease inhibitory factor (SLPI) is an endogenic immunity related protein, capable of specifically inhibiting elastolytic enzyme, cathepsin G, trypsin and fibrinolysin and boasts of antiphlogistic response and antibiosis/antiviral activity. The detection of the content of SLPI protein in serum may have great clinical significance for diagnosis. Differential polypeptides were obtained (Fig.14) and their functions were explained (Table 4).

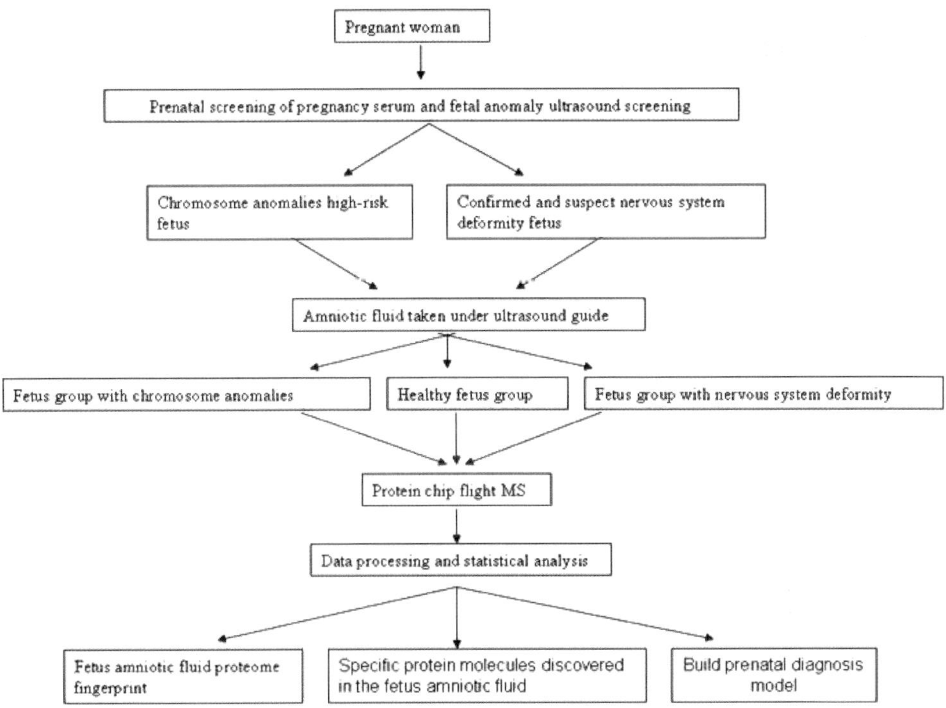

Fig. 13. Research Protocol for **Fetal Congenital Aplasia** with ClinTOF System

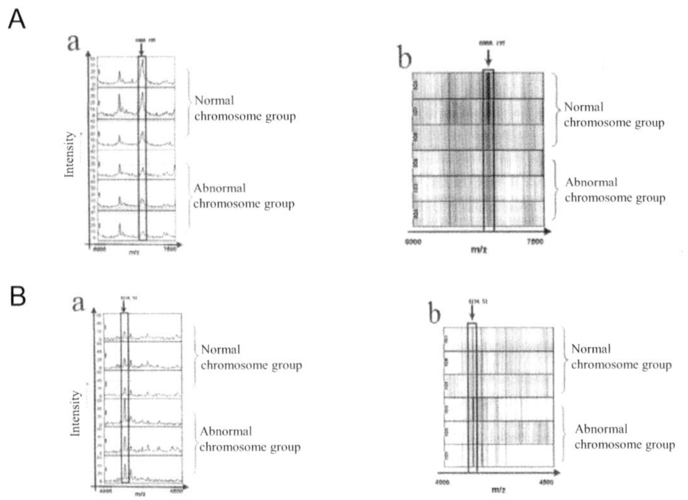

A and B: gel image of differential polypeptides

Fig. 14. Findings of Rsearching **Fetal Congenital Aplasia** with the ClinTOF System

biomarkers (Mw)	Meaningful matching information in Swiss-Prot database: Protein Name	Mw	pI	comments
3107.1	GLCM1_HUMAN(Q8IVK1) Putative glycosylation-dependent cell adhesion molecule 1.	3109	8.23	ALTERNATIVE PRODUCTS
4967.526	HMHB1_HUMAN (O97980) histocompatibility protein HB-1	4965	4.95	Precursor of the histocomplatibility Minor antigen HB-1
5589.2	CO031_HUMAN (Q13653) Putative uncharacterized protein C15orf31.	5583	7.59	Expressed at higher level in total thymocytes than in mature T or NK cells, especially in CD8+ cells.
11717.0	LV201_HUMAN (P01704) Ig lambda chain V-II region TOG	11713	8.66	MISCELLANEOUS: This is a Bence-Jones protein. SIMILARITY: Contains 1 Ig-like (immunoglobulin-like) domain.
	HV308_HUMAN (P01769)	11706	9.80	MISCELLANEOUS: This chain was isolated from a Waldenstrom's macroglobulin. SIMILARITY: Contains 1 Ig-like (immunoglobulin-like) domain.
	SLPI_HUMAN (P03973) Antileukoproteinase	11726	9.10	Acid-stable proteinase inhibitor with strong affinities for trypsin, chymotrypsin, elastase, and cathepsin G May prevent elastase-mediated damage to oral and possibly other mucosal tissues.

Table 4. Retrieval Results from Swiss-Prot Protein Database

Besides diseases studied by the ClinTOF system above, for the moment, we have finished the detection of near 10000 samples. Diseases are not only restricted to tumors, but covering almost all clinical aspects, as shown in Table 5.

Disease	Case Load	Source
Lung cancer, lung squamous carcinoma, adenocarcinoma of lung	1678	PLA 301 Hospital, Guangzhou People's Hospital, Xian Jiaotong University, Hebei Medical University Fourth Hospital
Stomach cancer	117	Fudan University, Shanghai Ruijin Hospital
Esophagus cancer	48	West China University of Medical Science, CICAMS
Nasopharyngeal carcinoma	238	Sun Yat-Sen University Cancer Center
Breast cancer	156	Beijing Cancer Hospital, Xinjiang Medical University
Pancreatic cancer	120	Guangzhou People's Hospital
Endometrial carcinoma Endometrial carcinoma	283	Beijing Obstetrics and Gynecology Hospital, Capital Medical University
Leukemia	103	Shanghai Fifth Hospital
Intestinal cancer	185	Shanghai Jiaotong University, Capital Medical University
Rheumatosis, lupus erythematosus	75	Shenzhen People's Hospital
Cirrhosis, hepatic carcinoma, hepatitis B	303	PLA 301 Hospital, Tianjin Third Hospital
Cognitive dysfunction	230	Zhongnan Hospital of Wuhan University, Shanghai Jiaotong University
Endometriosis uterine	137	Beijing People's Hospital
Diabetes	188	Shanghai Changzheng Hospital
Test-tube baby tracking	102	Beijing University Third Hospital
Mental disease	1220	Chongqing Medical University
Healthy people	2473	Capital Medical University
Athletes	1995	PLA 301 Hospital

Table 5. Diseases and Case Load Applied by the ClinTOF System (alterable)

4. Prospect

Clinically, the high incidence and mortality rate of complex diseases like tumors cry for the new early-diagnosis patterns and effective early-diagnosis markers. In the mining of the mass spectrometric data, the cluster analysis and classification analysis have been used, but many problems still need further studies. In particular, the pretreatment of MS profiling, there is no standard method available. These issues are critical for putting serum peptidome into clinical detection. Secondly, along with the instant development and application of mass spectrometer and serum peptidome technology, a lot of serum polypeptide profiling data have been produced. It has become an international competition focus in the post-genome era how to develop an effective bioinformatics instrument to determine proteins related to some vital phenomena (like growth, upgrowth, tumor onset) from the substantive data including peptide mass and intensity and their functions. It is believed that with the progressive development and application of serum peptidomics technology and the ClinTOF system, better clinical models will appear and more early-stage tumor biomarkers will be discovered and identified. Also, great breakthroughs will be made in the pathogeny, diagnosis and treatment of complex diseases, to cultivate new hope for research, diagnosis and treatment of many diseases.

5. References

[1] Andrew Tarnaris, Laurence D Watkins and Neil D Kitchen. Biomarkers in chronic adult hydroce-phalus. Cerebrospinal Fluid Research, 2006,3:11.

[2] Brichory F, Beer D, Le Naour F, et al. Proteomics- based identification of protein gene product as a tumor antigen that induces a humoral immune response in lung cancer. *Cancer Res*, 2001, 61(21) : 7908- 7912.

[3] Cho WC, Yip TT, Yi PC, et al. Identification of serum amyloid a protein as a potentially useful biomarker to monitor relapse of nasopharyng eal cancer by serum proteomic profiling. *Clin Cancer Res*, 2004, 10: 43-52.

[4] Cruz-Marcelo A, Guerra R, Vannucci M, et al. Comparison of algorithms for pre-processing of SELDI-TOF mass spectrometry data. *Bioinformatics*, 2008, 24:2129-2136.

[5] Cubizolles M, Laurendeau I, Bedossa P. Identification of a new marker of hepatocellular carcinoma by serum protein profiling of patients with chronic liver diseases. *Hepatology*, 2005; 41: 40-47.

[6] Doustjalali SR, Yuso f R, Gov indasamy GK, et al. Patients with nasopharyngea carcinoma demonstrate enhanced serum and tissue cerulo plasm in expression. *J Med Invest*, 2006, 53: 20-28.

[7] Gast M C, van Du lken E J, van Loenen TK, et al. Detection of breast cancer by surface enhanced laser desorption/ionization time of flight mass spectrometry tissue and serum protein profiling. *Int J BioMarkers*, 2009, 24 (3): 130 -141.

[8] Guo X, Cao SM, Y u JK, et al. Distinct seruma proteomic patterns between ascending and descending types of locoregionally advanced nasopharyng eal carcinoma assessed by surface enhanced laser desorption ionization and analyses. *Chin Med J*, 2005, 118(22): 1912-1917.

[9] Huang Y J, Xuan C, Zhang BB, e t al. SELDI-TOF-MS profiling of serum for detection of nasopharyngea carcinoma.*Cancer*, 2008 , 112(3): 544-551.

[10] Hye A , Lynham S, Thambisetty M , et al. Proteome based plasma biomarkers for Alzheimer 's disease. *Brain* , 2006,129 (Pt11): 3042-3050.

[11] Liao QL, Zhao L, Chen X, et al. Serum proteome analysis for profiling protein markers associated with carcinogenesis and lymph nodemetastasis in nasopharyngea l carcinoma. *Clinical and Experimental Metastasis*, 2008, 25(4): 465-476.

[12] Paradis V, Degos F, Dargère D, Pham N, Belghiti J, Degott C, Janeau JL, Bezeaud A, Delforge D, Poon TC, Yip TT, Chan AT, Yip C, Yip V, Mok TS, Lee CC, Leung TW, Ho SK, Johnson PJ. Comprehensive proteomic profiling identifies serum proteomic signatures for detection of hepatocellular carcinoma and its subtypes. *Clin Chem,* 2003, 49: 752-760.

[13] Petricoin EF, Ardekani AM, Hitt BA, Levine PJ, Fusaro VA, Steinberg SM, Mills GB, Simone C, Fishman DA, Kohn EC et al: Use of proteomic patterns in serum to identify ovarian cancer. *Lancet,* 2002, 359(9306):572-577.

[14] Taku N, Sharon KH , Steve RM, et al. Proteomic profiling of primary breast cancer predicts axillary lymph node metastasis. *Cancer Res,* 2 0 0 6, 6 6 (2 4) : 1 1 82 5 - 1 1 8 3 0.

[15] van Winden AW, Gast MC, Beijnen JH, Rutgers EJ, Grobbee DE, Peeters PH, van Gils CH. Validation of previously identified serum biomarkers for breast cancer with SELDI-TOF MS: a case control study. *BMC Med Genomics,*2009,2:4.

[16] Villanueva J, Philip J, Chaparro CA, Li Y, Toledo-Crow R, DeNoyer L, Fleisher M, Robbins RJ, Tempst P. Correcting common errors in identifying cancer-specific serum peptide signatures. *J Proteome Res,*2005, 4(4):1060-1072.

[17] Wasinger VC, Cordwell S J, Cerpa PA, et al. Progress with gene product mapping of the Mollicutes: Mycoplasma genitalium. Electrophoresis, 1995, 16 (7): 1090-1094.

[18] Wei YS, Zheng YH, Zhang ZH, et al. Identification of serum biomarkers for nasopharyngea carcinoma by proteomic analysis. *Cancer,* 2008, 12 (3): 544-551.

[19] Yoshizaki T, Enomoto T, Nakashima R, e t al. Altered protein expression in endometrial carcinogenesis. *Cancer Lett,* 2005, 226 (2):1012 - 1061.

[20] Zhang R, Barker L, Pinchev D, et al. Mining biomarkers in human sera using proteomic tools. *Proteomics,* 2004, 4(1): 244-256.

[21] Johnson, KL, Mason, CJ, Muddiman, DC, etal. Analysis of the low molecular weight fraetion of serum by LC-Dual ESI-FT-ICR mass speetrometry:spectrometry: Precision of time, mass, and ion abundance. Anal Chem, 2004, 76:5097-5103.

[22] Soltys SG, Le QT, Shi G, etal. The Use of plasma Surface-Enhanced Laser Desorption/ionization Time-of-Flight Mass Spectrometry proteome patterns for detection of head and neck squamous cell cancers, Clinical Cancer Research, 2004, 10:4806-812.

[23] Honda K, Hayashida Y, Umaki T, et al.Possible detection of pancreatic cancer by plasma protein profiling. Cancer Res, 2005, 65 : 10613-10622.

[24] Villanueva J, Shaffer DR, Philip J, et al. Differential exoprotease activity confer tumor-specific serum Peptidome Patterns. J Clin Invest, 2006, 116:271-284.

[25] Novak K. Biomarkers:Taking out the Trash. Nature, 2006, 6:92.

[26] Cheng AJ, Chen LC, Chien KY, et al. Oral Cancer Plasma Tumor Marker identified with Bead-Based Affinity Fractionated Proteomic Technology. Clin Chem, 2005, 51:2236-2244.

[27] YIP T TC, Chan J WM, Cho W CS, et al. Protein chip array profiling analysis in patients with severe acute respiratory syndrome identified serum amyloid: a protein as a a biomarker potentially useful in monitoring the extent of pneumonia. Clin Chem, 2005, 51(l):47-55.

[28] Semmes OJ, Feng Z, Adam BL, et al. Evaluation of serum protein profiling by surface-enhanced laser desorption/ionization time-of-flight mass spectrometry for the detection of Prostate cancer: assessment of platform reproducibility. Clin Chem,, 2005, 51:102-12.

[29] Dekker LJ, Boogerd W, Stockhammer G, Et al. MALDI-TOF mass spectrometry analysis of cerebrospinal fluid tryptic peptide profiles to diagnose leptomeningeal metastases in patients with breast cancerMol Cell Proteomics, 2005, 4:1341-1349.

[30] Villanueva J, Martorella AJ, Lawlor K, et al. Serum peptidome patterns that distinguish metastatic thyroid carcinoma from cancer-free controls are unbiased by gender and age. Mol Cell Proteomic, 2006, 5(10):1840-1852.

[31] Dobrin N, Urban A.K, Erie E.N., et al. Population Proteomics. Mol Cell Proteomics 2006, 5(10):1811-1818

[32] Agranoff D, Delmiro FR, Papadopoulos MC, et al.. Identification of diagnostic markers for tuberculosis by proteomic fingerprinting of serum. Lancet, 2006,368(9540):1012-1021

[33] Emanuel FP, Claudio B, Robyn P, et al. The blood peptidome: a higher dimension of information content for cancer biomarker discoverNat Rev Cancer,2006,6(12):961-967

Permissions

The contributors of this book come from diverse backgrounds, making this book a truly international effort. This book will bring forth new frontiers with its revolutionizing research information and detailed analysis of the nascent developments around the world.

We would like to thank Tapan Kumar Khan, PhD, for lending his expertise to make the book truly unique. He has played a crucial role in the development of this book. Without his invaluable contribution this book wouldn't have been possible. He has made vital efforts to compile up to date information on the varied aspects of this subject to make this book a valuable addition to the collection of many professionals and students.

This book was conceptualized with the vision of imparting up-to-date information and advanced data in this field. To ensure the same, a matchless editorial board was set up. Every individual on the board went through rigorous rounds of assessment to prove their worth. After which they invested a large part of their time researching and compiling the most relevant data for our readers. Conferences and sessions were held from time to time between the editorial board and the contributing authors to present the data in the most comprehensible form. The editorial team has worked tirelessly to provide valuable and valid information to help people across the globe.

Every chapter published in this book has been scrutinized by our experts. Their significance has been extensively debated. The topics covered herein carry significant findings which will fuel the growth of the discipline. They may even be implemented as practical applications or may be referred to as a beginning point for another development. Chapters in this book were first published by InTech; hereby published with permission under the Creative Commons Attribution License or equivalent.

The editorial board has been involved in producing this book since its inception. They have spent rigorous hours researching and exploring the diverse topics which have resulted in the successful publishing of this book. They have passed on their knowledge of decades through this book. To expedite this challenging task, the publisher supported the team at every step. A small team of assistant editors was also appointed to further simplify the editing procedure and attain best results for the readers.

Our editorial team has been hand-picked from every corner of the world. Their multi-ethnicity adds dynamic inputs to the discussions which result in innovative outcomes. These outcomes are then further discussed with the researchers and contributors who give their valuable feedback and opinion regarding the same. The feedback is then collaborated with the researches and they are edited in a comprehensive manner to aid the understanding of the subject.

Apart from the editorial board, the designing team has also invested a significant amount of their time in understanding the subject and creating the most relevant covers. They scrutinized every image to scout for the most suitable representation of the subject and create an appropriate cover for the book.

The publishing team has been involved in this book since its early stages. They were actively engaged in every process, be it collecting the data, connecting with the contributors or procuring relevant information. The team has been an ardent support to the editorial, designing and production team. Their endless efforts to recruit the best for this project, has resulted in the accomplishment of this book. They are a veteran in the field of academics and their pool of knowledge is as vast as their experience in printing. Their expertise and guidance has proved useful at every step. Their uncompromising quality standards have made this book an exceptional effort. Their encouragement from time to time has been an inspiration for everyone.

The publisher and the editorial board hope that this book will prove to be a valuable piece of knowledge for researchers, students, practitioners and scholars across the globe.

List of Contributors

Vanessa Deschoolmeester, Filip Lardon, Patrick Pauwels and Marc Peeters
Center for Oncological Research (CORE) Antwerp, Laboratory of Cancer Research and Clinical Oncology, University of Antwerp, Belgium

Muhammad Imran Aslam, Maleene Patel and Baljit Singh
Department of Cancer Studies and Molecular Medicine, University of Leicester, Robert Kilpatrick Clinical Sciences Building, Leicester Royal Infirmary, United Kingdom
Department of Colorectal Surgery, University Hospitals of Leicester NHS Trust, Leicester General Hospital, Gwendolen Road, Leicester, United Kingdom

James Howard Pringle
Department of Cancer Studies and Molecular Medicine, University of Leicester, Robert Kilpatrick Clinical Sciences Building, Leicester Royal Infirmary, United Kingdom

John Stuart Jameson
Department of Colorectal Surgery, University Hospitals of Leicester NHS Trust, Leicester General Hospital, Gwendolen Road, Leicester, United Kingdom

Teresa de Souza Fernandez and André Mencalha
National Cancer Institute (INCA), Bone Marrow Transplantation Center (CEMO) Laboratory Division, Rio de Janeiro, RJ, Brazil

Cecília de Souza Fernandez
Mathematics and Statistics Institute, Federal Fluminense University (UFF), Niteroi, RJ, Brazil

Tsutomu Fukuwatari and Katsumi Shibata
The University of Shiga Prefecture, Japan

Björn Gerdle and Britt Larsson
Rehabilitation Medicine, Faculty of Health Sciences, Linköping University, Linköping, and Pain and Rehabilitation Centre, University Hospital, Linköping, Sweden

Lydia Finney
Advanced Photon Source, Argonne National Laboratory, USA

R. Lozano, R. Marin, A. Pascual, MJ. Santacruz, A. Lozano and F. Sebastian
Pharmacy and Psychiatry Services, Hospital Real Ntra. Sra. De Gracia, Zaragoza, Spain

Carina Ladeira and Susana Viegas
Escola Superior de Tecnologia da Saúde de Lisboa, Instituto Politécnico de Lisboa, Portugal
Centro de Investigação e Estudos em Saúde Pública, Universidade Nova de Lisboa, Portugal

Elisabete Carolino and Miguel Brito
Escola Superior de Tecnologia da Saúde de Lisboa, Instituto Politécnico de Lisboa, Portugal

Manuel Carmo Gomes
Faculdade de Ciências, Universidade de Lisboa, Portugal

Brian T. Luke and Jack R. Collins
SAIC-Frederick, NCI at Frederick, Frederick, USA

Egle Machtejeviene
Lithuanian University of Health Sciences, Lithuania

Egidijus Machtejevas
Merck KGaA, Germany

Shusaku Nomura
Nagaoka University of Technology, Japan

Ning Ma
Faculty of Health Science, Suzuka University of Medical Science, Suzuka, Mie, Japan

Shosuke Kawanishi, Shiho Ohnishi and Raynoo Thanan
Faculty of Pharmaceutical Sciences, Suzuka University of Medical Science, Suzuka, Mie, Japan

Yusuke Hiraku and Mariko Murata
Department of Environmental and Molecular Medicine, Mie University Graduate School of Medicine, Tsu, Mie, Japan

Zinaida Sergueeva, Heather Collins, Sally Dow, Mollie McWhorter and Mark L. Parrish
Covance Genomics Laboratory, Seattle, Washington, USA

Flemming Lund, György Sölétormos and Merete Frejstrup Pedersen
Department of Clinical Biochemistry, Hillerød Hospital, University of Copenhagen, Denmark

Per Hyltoft Petersen
Department of Clinical Biochemistry, Hillerød Hospital, University of Copenhagen, Denmark
Norwegian Quality Improvement of Primary Care Laboratories (NOKLUS), Section for General Practice, University of Bergen, Bergen, Norway

Spiros D. Garbis
Cancer Sciences, Faculty of Medicine, University of Southampton, Southampton, UK
Biomedical Research Foundation, Academy of Athens, Athens, Greece

Paul A. Townsend
Cancer Sciences, Faculty of Medicine, University of Southampton, Southampton, UK

Yueming Tang
Division of Digestive Disease and Nutrition, Department of Internal Medicine, USA

Ali Keshavarzian
Division of Digestive Disease and Nutrition, Department of Internal Medicine, USA

Department of Pharmacology, USA
Department of Molecular Biophysics and Physiology, USA

Christopher B. Forsyth
Division of Digestive Disease and Nutrition, Department of Internal Medicine, USA
Department of Biochemistry, Rush University Medical Center, Chicago IL, USA

Kaihua Wei, Yunbo Sun, Xiaoming Zhou and Jian Yuan
State Key Lab of Proteomics, Beijing Proteome Research Center, China

Qingwei Ma and Weirong Guo
Bioyong (Beijing) Technologies Limited, Beijing, China